# Blood Conservation with Aprotinin

# Blood
# Conservation
# with Aprotinin

### Roque Pifarré, MD
Professor and Chairman
Department of Thoracic
  and Cardiovascular Surgery
Loyola University of Chicago
  Stritch School of Medicine
Maywood, Illinois

HANLEY & BELFUS, INC./Philadelphia

Publisher:                 HANLEY & BELFUS, INC.
                           210 South 13th Street
                           Philadelphia, PA 19107
                           (215) 546-7293
                           FAX (215) 790-9330

**Library of Congress Cataloging-in-Publication Data**

Blood conservation with aprotinin / [edited by] Roque Pifarré.
    p.      cm.
Includes bibliographical references and index.
ISBN 1-56053-151-7
    1. Cardiopulmonary bypass–Complications.   2. Aprotinin–Therapeutic use.   3. Hemostasis.
4. Blood–Coagulation.
    I. Pifarré, Roque.
    [DNLM: 1. Cardiopulmonary Bypass.   2. Hemostasis. 3. Blood Coagulation.   4. Aprotinin–
    therapeutic use.  WG 168 B654 1995]
RD598.B58 1995
617.4 ' 1201–dc20
DNLM/DLC
for Library of Congress                                                          95-6759
                                                                                 CIP

**Blood Conservation with Aprotinin**                         ISBN 1-56053-151-7

Last digit is printed number: 9 8 7 6 5 4 3 2 1

# Dedication

To my wife Teresa

# Contents

# Contributors

**Theodore A. Alston, M.D., Ph.D.**
Assistant Professor, Harvard Medical School; Massachusetts General Hospital, Boston, Massachusetts

**Rodger L. Bick, M.D.**
Clinical Professor, Departments of Medicine and Pathology, University of Texas Southwestern Medical Center; Medical Director of Hematology and Oncology, Presbyterian Comprehensive Cancer Center, Dallas, Texas

**Benjamin Peter Bidstrup, FRACS, FRCSEd**
Senior Lecturer in Surgery, North Queensland Clinical School, University of Queensland, Townsville, Queensland, Australia

**Bradford P. Blakeman, M.D.**
Associate Professor, Department of Thoracic and Cardiovascular Surgery, Loyola University of Chicago Stritch School of Medicine, Maywood, Illinois

**Günther Blümel, M.D.**
Professor of Surgery, Institute for Experimental Surgery, Technical University of Munich, Munich, Germany

**Jodi Cava, C.C.P.**
Department of Thoracic and Cardiovascular Surgery, Loyola University of Chicago Stritch School of Medicine, Maywood, Illinois

**Manuel Concha, M.D., Ph.D.**
Titular Professor of Surgery, Department of Cardiovascular Surgery, Cordoba Faculty of Medicine, Cordoba, Spain

**Jack G. Copeland, M.D.**
Michael Drummond Distinguished Professor of Cardiothoracic Surgery, University of Arizona College of Medicine, Tucson, Arizona

**Michael Nicholas D'Ambra, M.D.**
Assistant Professor, Department of Anesthesiology, Harvard Medical School; Associate Anesthetist, Massachusetts General Hospital, Boston, Massachusetts.

**Wulf Dietrich, M.D.**
Staff Anesthesiologist, Department of Anesthesiology, German Heart Center, Munich, Germany

**L. Henry Edmunds, Jr., M.D.**
Julian Johnson Professor of Cardiothoracic Surgery, Chief, Division of Cardiothoracic Surgery, University of Pennsylvania School of Medicine, Philadelphia, Pennsylvania

**Berit Edsberg, M.D.**
Manager, Novo Nordisk A/S, Medical Department, Bagsvverd, Denmark

**León Eijsman, M.D., Ph.D.**
Professor of Cardiopulmonary Surgery, Academic Medical Center; OLVG-Hospital; Free University; University of Amsterdam, Amsterdam, The Netherlands

**Jawed Fareed, Ph.D.**
Professor of Pathology and Pharmacology, and Director, Hemostasis and Thrombosis Research Laboratories, Loyola University of Chicago Stritch School of Medicine, Maywood, Illinois

**Jordi Fontcuberta, M.D.**
Chief, Hemostasis and Thrombosis Unit, Department of Hematology, Hospital Sant Pau, Barcelona, Spain

**John L. Francis, Ph.D., M.R.C.Path.**
Director, Hemostasis and Thrombosis Research; Professor of Chemistry, Walt Disney Memorial Cancer Institute at Florida Hospital, University of Central Florida, Altamonte Springs, Florida

**Michael J. Gallimore, Ph.D.**
Director, Institute for Diagnostic Research, Walmer, Deal, Kent, England; Department of Thoracic and Cardiovascular Surgery, University of Tübingen, Tübingen, Germany

**David Green, M.D., Ph.D.**
Professor, Department of Medicine, Northwestern University Medical School, Chicago, Illinois

**Sylvia Haas, M.D.**
Professor of Medicine, Institute for Experimental Surgery, Technical University of Munich, Munich, Germany

**Wolfgang Heller, Ph.D.**
Professor Doctor, Department of Thoracic and Cardiovascular Surgery, University of Tübingen, Tübingen, Germany

**H. Coenraad Hemker, M.D., Ph.D.**
Professor of Biochemistry, Cardiovascular Research Institute, University of Limburg, Maastricht, The Netherlands

**Debra A. Hoppensteadt, M.S., M.T.(A.S.C.P.)**
Technical Specialist, Department of Pathology, Loyola University of Chicago Stritch School of Medicine, Maywood, Illinois

**Philip Hornick, B.Sc.(Hons), M.B., B.Chir, FRCS**
British Heart Foundation Research Fellow in Cardiothoracic Surgery, Department of Cardiothoracic Surgery, Royal Postgraduate Medical School, Hammersmith Hospital, London, United Kingdom

**Maher Istanbouli, C.C.P.**
Director, School of Perfusion, Department of Thoracic and Cardiovascular Surgery, Loyola University of Chicago Stritch School of Medicine, Maywood, Illinois

**Marc Janssens, M.D., D.Sc.**
Assistant Professor, Department of Anesthesiology and Intensive Care Medicine, University Hospital of Liège, Liège, Belgium

**Walter Jeske, B.S.**
Department of Pharmacology, Loyola University of Chicago Stritch School of Medicine, Maywood, Illinois

**James K. Kirklin, M.D.**
Professor of Surgery, University of Alabama at Birmingham, Birmingham, Alabama

**Michael J. Koza, B.S., M.T.(A.S.C.P.)**
Research Associate, Department of Thoracic and Cardiovascular Surgery, Loyola University of Chicago Stritch School of Medicine, Maywood, Illinois

**Maurice Lamy, M.D.**
Professor, Department of Anesthesiology and Intensive Care Medicine, University Hospital of Liège, Liège, Belgium

**Ulana Leskiw, M.D.**
Fellow in Cardiothoracic and Vascular Anesthesia, Department of Anesthesia, Emory University Hospital, Atlanta, Georgia

**Jerrold H. Levy, M.D.**
Associate Professor of Anesthesiology, Division of Cardiothoracic Anesthesia and Critical Care, Emory University School of Medicine, Atlanta, Georgia

**David C. McGiffin, M.D.**
Associate Professor of Surgery, University of Alabama at Birmingham, Birmingham, Alabama

**José Mateo, M.D.**
Staff Physician, Hemostasis and Thrombosis Unit, Department of Hematology, Hospital Sant Pau, Barcelona, Spain

**Harry L. Messmore, Jr., M.D.**
Professor of Medicine, Departments of Medicine and Pathology, Loyola University of Chicago Stritch School of Medicine, Maywood, Illinois

**Alvaro Montoya, M.D.**
Professor, Department of Thoracic and Cardiovascular Surgery, Loyola University of Chicago Stritch School of Medicine, Maywood, Illinois

**Hansjörg Mössinger, M.D.**
Institute for Anesthesiology, German Heart Center, Munich, Germany

**Ignacio Muñoz, M.D.**
Cordoba University Medical Center, Reina Sofia Hospital, Cordoba, Spain

**John Michael Murkin, M.D., F.R.C.P.C**
Professor, Department of Anaesthesia, University Hospital, University of Western Ontario, London, Ontario, Canada

**Gregory A. Nuttall, M.D.**
Instructor in Anesthesiology, Mayo Medical School; Department of Anesthesiology, Mayo Clinic, Rochester, Minnesota

**William C. Oliver, Jr., M.D.**
Assistant Professor of Anesthesiology, Mayo Medical School; Department of Anesthesiology, Mayo Clinic, Rochester, Minnesota

**Roque Pifarré, M.D.**
Professor and Chairman, Department of Thoracic and Cardiovascular Surgery, Loyola University of Chicago Stritch School of Medicine, Maywood, Illinois

**Hanno Riess, M.D.**
Professor, Department of Internal Medicine, University Hospital Rudolf Virchow, Berlin, Germany

**Miquel L.L. Rutllant, M.D., Ph.D.**
Professor of Medicine, Department of Hematology, Hospital Sant Pau, University of Barcelona, Barcelona, Spain

**Friedrich Schumann, Dr. rer. nat.**
International Clinical Project Manager, Bayer AG, HealthCare, Pharma, Wuppertal, Germany

**Jamal Sinno, C.C.P.**
Assistant Director, School of Perfusion, Department of Thoracic and Cardiovascular Surgery, Loyola University of Chicago Stritch School of Medicine, Maywood, Illinois

**Joan Carles Souto, M.D.**
Staff Physician, Hemostasis and Thrombosis Unit, Department of Hematology, Hospital Sant Pau, Barcelona, Spain

**Henry J. Sullivan, M.D.**
Professor and Vice Chairman, Department of Thoracic and Cardiovascular Surgery, Loyola University of Chicago Stritch School of Medicine, Maywood, Illinois

**Kenneth M. Taylor, M.D., FRCS**
British Heart Foundation Professor of Cardiac Surgery, Department of Cardiothoracic Surgery, Royal Postgraduate Medical School, Hammersmith Hospital, London, United Kingdom

**Jeanine M. Walenga, Ph.D.**
Associate Professor, Department of Thoracic and Cardiovascular Surgery and Pathology, and Co-Director, Hemostasis and Thrombosis Research Laboratories, Loyola University of Chicago Stritch School of Medicine, Maywood, Illinois

**Ch.R.H. Wildevuur, M.D., Ph.D.**
Professor, Department of Cardiopulmonary Surgery, Cardiopulmonary Surgical Center of Amsterdam, Groningen, The Netherlands

**Hans Peter Wendel, M.Sc.**
Dipl.-Biologist, Department of Thoracic and Cardiovascular Surgery, University of Tübingen, Tübingen, Germany

**Isabel Zuazu-Jausoro, M.D.**
Professor of Medicine, Department of Hematology, University of Murcia, Murcia, Spain

# Foreword

This volume is of interest not only because it provides extensive pharmacologic and clinical information about the role of aprotinin in reducing bleeding during cardiopulmonary bypass surgery, but also because it illustrates how a drug develops from concept to clinical utility. A polypeptide serine protease inhibitor derived from bovine lung, aprotinin has a variety of inhibitory actions on proteolytic enzymes such as trypsin, plasmin, and kallikrein. These enzymes are widely distributed and catalyze many biologic reactions. In patients whose blood has been altered by extracorporeal circulation assist devices, defects in platelet function and fibrinolysis lead to perioperative bleeding. It was postulated that aprotinin might beneficially reduce these defects, resulting in less bleeding.

The "Hammersmith" high-dose regimen now approved in the United States was first employed by Royston and colleagues in London. Studies of this dose regimen as well as a "half Hammersmith" regimen were begun in the U.S., and the interest in the drug was quite apparent to those of us at FDA involved in the investigations. The possibility, noted in selected patients, that no blood or little blood might be needed during cardiopulmonary bypass surgery caused a large number of requests for what is known as compassionate use. These individual studies as well as the formal investigations contributed to an increased appreciation of the risks of using the drug, such as thrombosis due to inadequate heparinization and renal toxicity.

Null trials, such as those in cardiac valve replacement and liver transplantation, made it clear that benefits were not everywhere established. Nevertheless, in properly selected patients undergoing cardiopulmonary bypass the benefits of the drug were clearly greater than the risks, although even in those cases the drug had to be used with knowledge and caution.

Approval by the FDA in December, 1993 has not been the end of the process. We have evaluated the "half Hammersmith" as an alternative dose regimen, and we continue to monitor toxicity and add safety information to the labeling where appropriate. In time to come, other agents may prove more effective and/or safer. Aprotinin, then, is a beginning, showing us what can be done to reduce or eliminate the need for transfusion in this setting, and this volume codifies information about this important drug.

Stephen Fredd, M.D.
Director
Division of Gastrointestinal and Coagulation Drug Products
Office of Drug Evaluation I

# Preface

The majority of cardiac operations are performed under cardiopulmonary bypass using heparin as an anticoagulant. The large surface area of extracorporeal perfusion systems provides a massive thrombotic stimulus. Heparin acts near the end of the coagulation cascade by inhibiting activated factor X and accelerating antithrombin III, inhibiting thrombin; therefore, heparin does not inhibit the early reactions.

Cardiopulmonary bypass activates the contact system of plasma proteins, the platelets, and the fibrinolytic system. The consequences of these early reactions are potential bleeding, thrombotic complications, and inflammatory reactions associated with cardiopulmonary bypass. Contact activation generates factor XII to produce kallikrein, plasmin, and complement activation that is not inhibited by heparin during cardiopulmonary bypass. The conversion of fibrinogen and fibrin to their respective degradation products is mediated by plasmin. The circulation of these degradation products is increased during cardiopulmonary bypass, as well as in the period after cardiopulmonary bypass. The elevated levels of fibrin degradation products are associated with increased postoperative bleeding. These degradation products can impair platelet aggregation. Plasmin impairs the function of glycoprotein receptors on platelet membranes. In order to diagnose and manage the perioperative coagulation problems we need to continue research on the role of von Willebrand factor (vWF) and the glycoprotein 1b (GP1b) in platelet adhesion, platelet aggregation and the release of granules, the generation of thrombin on the platelet membrane, and the action of thrombin in the clearing of fibrinogen to fibrin and stimulating the release of tissue plasminogen activator (TPA) and the generation of plasmin.

The use of antifibrinolytic drugs can prevent this plasmin-mediated conversion of fibrinogen and fibrin to their degradation products. The perioperative use of the protease inhibitor aprotinin may produce hemostatic results because adhesive receptors of the platelets (GP1b) are preserved.

Blood conservation in cardiovascular surgery has to start with meticulous surgical technique. Surgical hemostasis is the first step to minimize blood loss. Blood salvage is the next step: the blood that is shed is processed and reinfused to the patient. Complementing this approach, an attempt can be made to prevent blood loss by reducing the propensity for perioperative bleeding. This has been accomplished with the serine protease inhibitor aprotinin. It has been shown to be highly effective in reducing blood loss and blood requirements.

The purpose of this book is to familiarize the cardiovascular surgeon with the blood reactions and hemostatic defects associated with cardiopulmonary bypass and to provide a state-of-the-art review of the role of aprotinin in correcting these defects. The complexity of anticoagulation, hemostasis, and blood conservation during cardiopulmonary bypass are discussed by experts in this field.

Monitoring of anticoagulation during cardiopulmonary bypass, especially when aprotinin is being used, is most important in order to avoid potential thrombotic complications. The need to maintain adequate anticoagulation, especially in prolonged reoperations, cannot be overemphasized.

Aprotinin is a useful and powerful drug. For the first time we can modify the tendency to increased bleeding during and after cardiac operations. Its mode of action is not totally defined. We would like to emphasize the need for further studies to clarify its effects on the blood coagulation mechanism, the ideal dosage, and the indications for its use.

I would like to express my gratitude and appreciation to the authors for their efforts and cooperation. There is no doubt in my mind that their expertise, expressed in these chapters, will contribute significantly to the noble task of blood conservation.

Roque Pifarré, M.D.

# Rodger L. Bick, MD

# 1

# Physiology and Pathophysiology of Hemostasis during Cardiac Surgery

The property of the circulation by which blood retains its fluidity within the vasculature and by which the system prevents excessive blood loss upon injury is hemostasis. Three anatomic compartments—**tissues** (vasculature), **blood cells** (platelets), and **plasma** (proteins)— are involved in a series of delicately orchestrated biochemical interplays which, under normal conditions, modulate responses in a fashion compatible with maintaining the finely tuned equilibrium of hemostasis.

## Physiology of Hemostasis

The three specific hemostatic compartments are: (1) the **platelets**, which must be normal in both number and function; (2) the **plasma proteins**, which include procoagulants, anticoagulants, and fibrinolytic proteins; and (3) the **vasculature**, which remains the last frontier and most poorly understood for disorders of hemostasis. During injury, the vessel wall constricts and generates compounds which activate platelets and plasma proteins. Platelets adhere and cohere at the site of injury, initiating a complex process that promotes further platelet aggregation, vascular constriction, and activation of coagulation components resulting in fibrin formation. Many chemical signals designed to initiate or terminate various events serve as a system of checks and balances. Disturbances (inherited or acquired) are reflected in appropriate responses, predisposing to either thrombosis or hemorrhage, and sometimes both.

To appreciate the complexity of the inter- and intracompartmental interactions, we will discuss the normal hemostatic aspects of the vasculature, platelets, and plasma proteins separately. The reader is encouraged, however, to maintain a perspective of integrated function, as this is the basis for efficient diagnosis of hemostatic dysfunction and the mainstay for the development of targeted pharmacologic (therapeutic) agents.

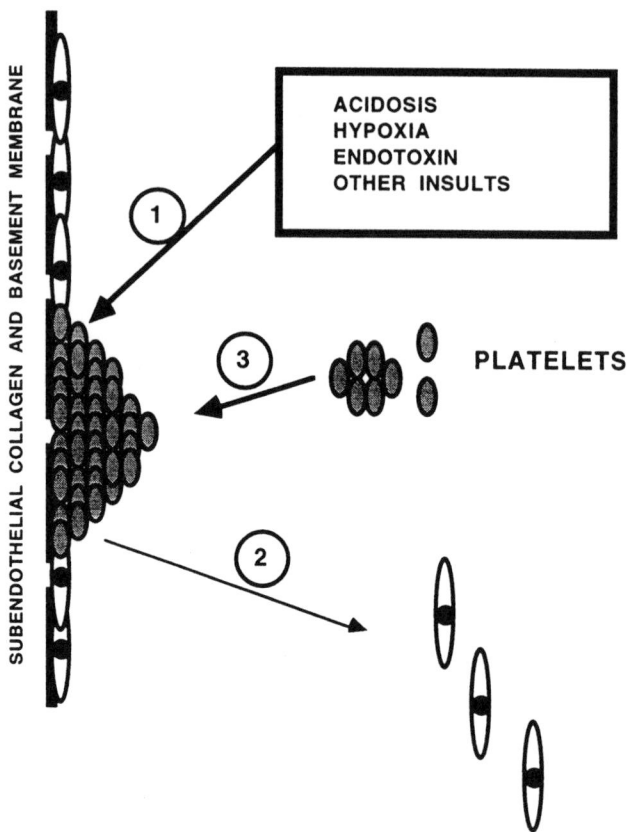

**FIGURE 1.** Steps in endothelial sloughing and "activation." **1.** Endothelial sloughing is induced by a variety of triggers, including acidosis, hypoxia, and endotoxins. **2.** Subendothelial collagen and basement membrane are exposed. **3.** Platelets fill the gap in endothelium, forming a primary hemostatic plug to stop the escape of blood from the vessel.

## Vascular Function

Normal vascular morphology is comprised of three discrete layers: the intima, media, and adventitia. The intima consists of a monolayer of nonthrombogenic endothelial cells and an internal elastic membrane. The media consists of smooth muscle cells; the size of the media varies depending on the type (arterial/venous) and size of the vasculature. The adventitia comprises an external elastic lamina or membrane and supportive connective tissue.

Figure 1 illustrates the first event occurring when endothelial sloughing occurs (induced by a variety of insults, or triggers, including acidosis, hypoxia, endotoxin, circulating antigen–antibody complexes) with the subsequent exposure of subendothelial collagen and basement membrane. Platelets are immediately recruited to fill this endothelial gap,[1-4] with the goal of forming a primary hemostatic plug to stop blood from leaving the vascular compartment. Subsequent reparative events include smooth muscle or other cells from the media migrating through the internal elastic membrane and differentiating into new nonthrombogenic endothelial cells. If this bleed is a one-time event, the reparative process is completed. It should be noted, however, that forming the primary hemostatic plug may constitute an overwhelming event, leading to a large platelet/fibrin thrombus and impedance of blood flow with resultant end-organ damage via ischemia. This event is particularly alarming when the process evolves repeatedly in the same area over a protracted period. As smooth muscle or other cells differentiate and migrate into the intima, compounds are released, attracting macrophages which, in turn, ingest cholesterol and other materials—the fundamental construct of an atherosclerotic plaque.[5-8]

Potential events consequent to vascular injury are summarized in Figure 2. **Permeability, fragility**, and **vasoconstriction** are properties of the vasculature. Increased permeability results in blood leaving the vessel and manifests as petechiae and purpura or, sometimes, large ecchymoses. Increased fragility results in rupture of the vasculature with ensuing petechiae, purpura (especially in the integument and mucous membranes), and large ecchymoses with potential serious deep-tissue hemorrhage. Vasoconstriction is under local, neural, and humoral control. Most important is humoral control, effected primarily by compounds released from platelets including epinephrine, norepinephrine, ADP kinins, and thromboxanes. Fibrin(ogen) degradation products (FDPs) also modulate vasoconstriction.[9,10]

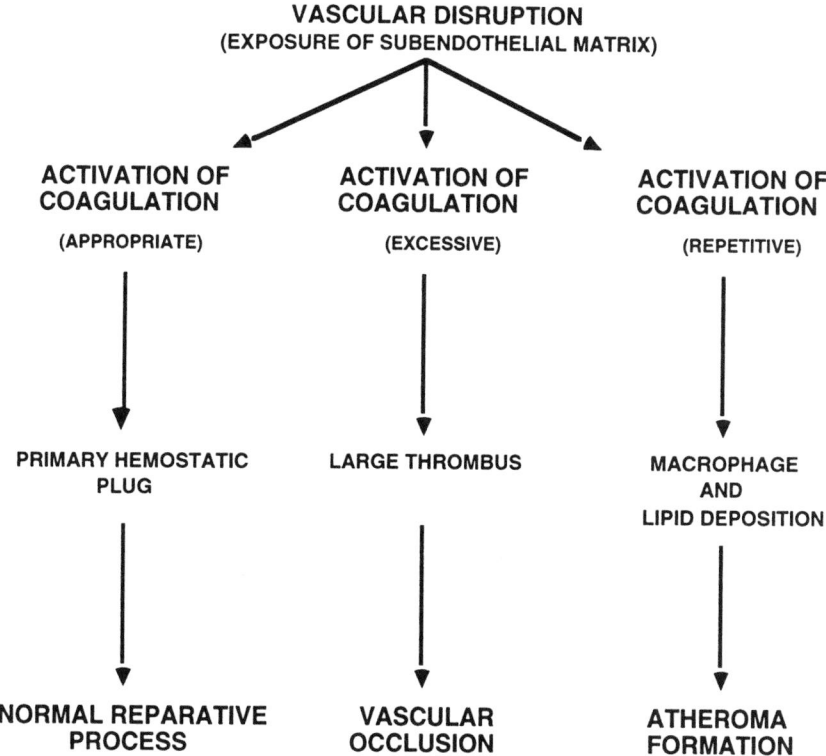

**FIGURE 2.** Potential consequences of vascular injury. The response depends on the nature of activation of coagulation—appropriate excessive, or repetitive—leading to a normal reparative process, vascular occlusion, or atheroma formation, respectively.

Endothelial cells are contractile, responding when stimulated by histamine, serotonin, kinins, or thromboxanes. The endothelial cell has been identified as a primary site for the biosynthesis of critical hemostatic proteins, specifically von Willebrand factor, plasminogen activator, thrombomodulin inhibitor of active protein C, and prostaglandins.[11-15] Platelet attraction and subsequent activation happen when subendothelial basement membrane or collagen is exposed. Also, this can directly activate factor XII to factor XIIa as well as factor XI to factor XIa.[16,17] Clearly, any of these processes, if left unmodulated, can give rise to a generalized activation of the coagulation system.[18-22]

## Platelet Function

Morphologically, the platelet can be envisioned as comprising three primary zones: (1) peripheral zone, (2) sol-gel zone, and (3) organelle zone.[9] The **peripheral zone** comprises an extramembranous glycocalyx inside of which is a plasma membrane, similar to other triamellar cellular plasma membranes. Under this membrane is an open canalicular system. The **sol-gel zone** is composed of microtubules and microfilaments, and a dense tubular system which contains primarily adenine nucleotides and calcium ions. Also, in the sol-gel zone is the contractile protein, thrombosthenin, which is similar to actomyosin. The **organelle zone** is composed of dense bodies, alpha granules, mitochondria, and the usual array of organelles found in other cellular systems, including lysosomes and endoplasmic reticula. Alpha granules contain and release fibrinogen and lysosomal enzymes, whereas dense bodies contain and release adenine nucleotides, serotonin, catecholamines, and platelet factor 4.[23-25]

An adequate number of platelets must be present for normal platelet function, in vivo and in vitro, usually approximately $100,000/mm^3$. With a platelet count of $<100,000/mm^3$, abnormal laboratory tests results will be noted, e.g., prolonged template bleeding times and abnormal platelet aggregation profiles. For normal function, platelets require (1) adequate energy metabolism; (2) an adequate number of (and contents of) storage granules capable of releasing their contents when appropriate stimuli are presented; (3) cationic proteins such as thrombosthenin; (4) membrane receptors responsive to appropriate stimuli; (5) divalent cations, the most important of which is calcium; and, of course, (6) adequate physical conditions, such as pH and temperature.

Table 1 lists the common platelet proteins. Some are not platelet-specific, and the list includes many plasma proteins that are found in or on the surface of platelets, including clotting factors II, V, VII, VIII, IX, X, XI, XII, and XIII.[26] Sometimes, these proteins are found in a slightly different molecular form in platelets when compared to the molecular species found in plasma (e.g., factor XIII). Platelet-specific

**TABLE 1.**   A Partial List of Key Platelet Proteins

| Nonspecific (plasma) proteins | Specific platelet proteins |
|---|---|
| Fibrinogen | Thrombosthenin |
| Factors II, V, VII, VIII, IX, X, XII, XIII | Platelet glycoproteins |
| Albumin | Platelet factors 2 and 4 |
| Plasminogen | Platelet antiplasmin |
| Complement components | Cathepsin A |
| | Beta thromboglobulin |

**TABLE 2.**   Specific Platelet Factors and Their Function

| Platelet Factor | Function |
| --- | --- |
| 1 | Coagulation factor V |
| 2 | Thromboplastic material |
| 3 | Platelet thromboplastin |
| 4 | Antiheparin factor |
| 5 | Fibrinogen coagulant factor |
| 6 | Antifibrinolytic factor |
| 7 | Platelet cothromboplastin |

proteins are also present, including thrombosthenin, platelet factor 4, beta thromboglobulin, and cathepsin A.

Table 2 lists the seven platelet-specific factors that have been identified and characterized. The essential two of these are platelet factor 3 (platelet thromboplastin/phospholipid) and platelet factor 4 (antiheparin factor), which has become an important molecular marker of platelet reactivity.[27-29]

Compounds released from platelets include the biogenic amines serotonin, catecholamines, and histamine; the adenine nucleotides cyclic AMP, ADP, and ATP; various enzyme activities including acid hydrolases; specific ions including calcium, magnesium, and potassium; and platelet factors, including platelet factor 4, beta thromboglobulin, and platelet factor 3. Also, other proteins including fibrinogen, other clotting factors, and albumin are released from platelets during activation.

### Platelet Activation and Adhesion

Multiple stimuli induce platelet activation.[30,31] Potent inducers of a platelet release reaction, besides subendothelial collagen and basement membrane, are thrombin, soluble fibrin monomer, some FDPs (especially fragment X), endotoxin, circulating antigen–antibody complexes, gammaglobulin-coated surfaces, various viruses, ADP, catecholamines, and free fatty acids.[32-35] Many proteolytic enzymes including trypsin, snake venoms, papain, and elastase are used in vitro to induce platelet release. Other in vitro release reaction techniques include the use of centrifugation, cold fracture, latex particles, carbon particles, kaolin, and celite.

Figure 3 shows a moderately activated (and accidentally fractured) platelet. With activation, platelets contract and form pseudopods. During contraction, the numerous intraplatelet compounds and granules are concentrated at the center of the platelet, where organelle membranes disrupt and their contents are released and subsequently transported outside the platelet via the open canalicular system. These compounds then interact with neighboring platelet membrane receptors or adjacent endothelium, causing further platelet activation and thereby amplifying the process. Pseudopod formation enhances platelet–surface interactions (adhesion) and platelet–platelet interaction (cohesion).

Figure 4 is a scanning electron micrograph of venous endothelium which has been rendered hypoxic. Endothelial cells are missing in several areas. Note that these gaps are filled by activated platelets (contracted and with marked pseudopod formation).

Platelet function is summarized in Figure 5. The process of **platelet adhesion** refers to a platelet adhering to something other than another platelet, e.g., an artificial surface or collagen basement membrane exposed upon injury. This adhesion results in an initial release reaction, generating ADP. This is a reversible process and

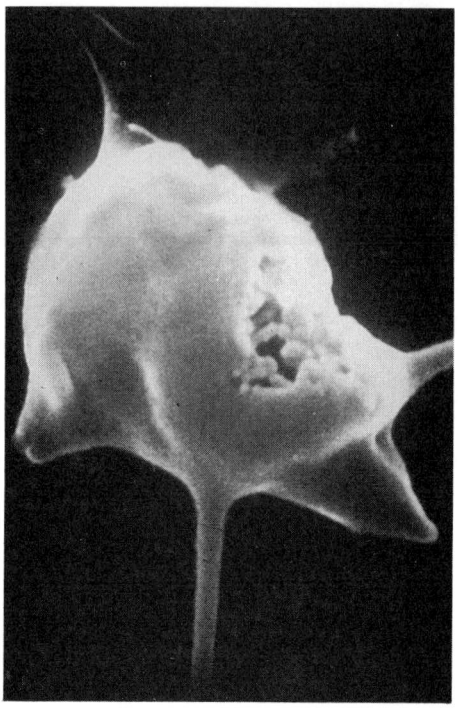

**FIGURE 3.** Scanning electron micrograph of a moderately activated platelet. The platelet has been accidentally fractured during preparation.

accounts for the primary wave on an aggregation pattern (primary reversible aggregation). As the concentration of ADP increases, platelet cohesion happens, which is platelets sticking to each other. As the process continues, released compounds (including serotonin) not only activate adjacent platelets but also induce vascular constriction. In this advanced phase of activation, there follows an irreversible conformational change in the platelet membrane, making available platelet factor 3 (platelet membrane phospholipid). This material serves as a primary "surface" mediating the formation of complexes in the coagulation protein sequence.

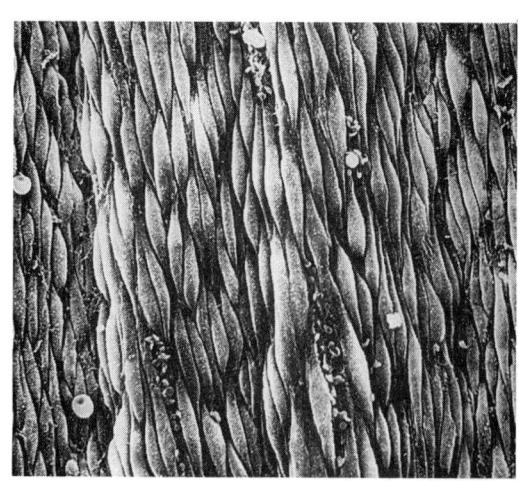

**FIGURE 4.** Scanning electron micrograph of hypoxic venous endothelium. Endothelial cells are missing in several areas, and these are filled with activated platelets showing marked pseudopod formation.

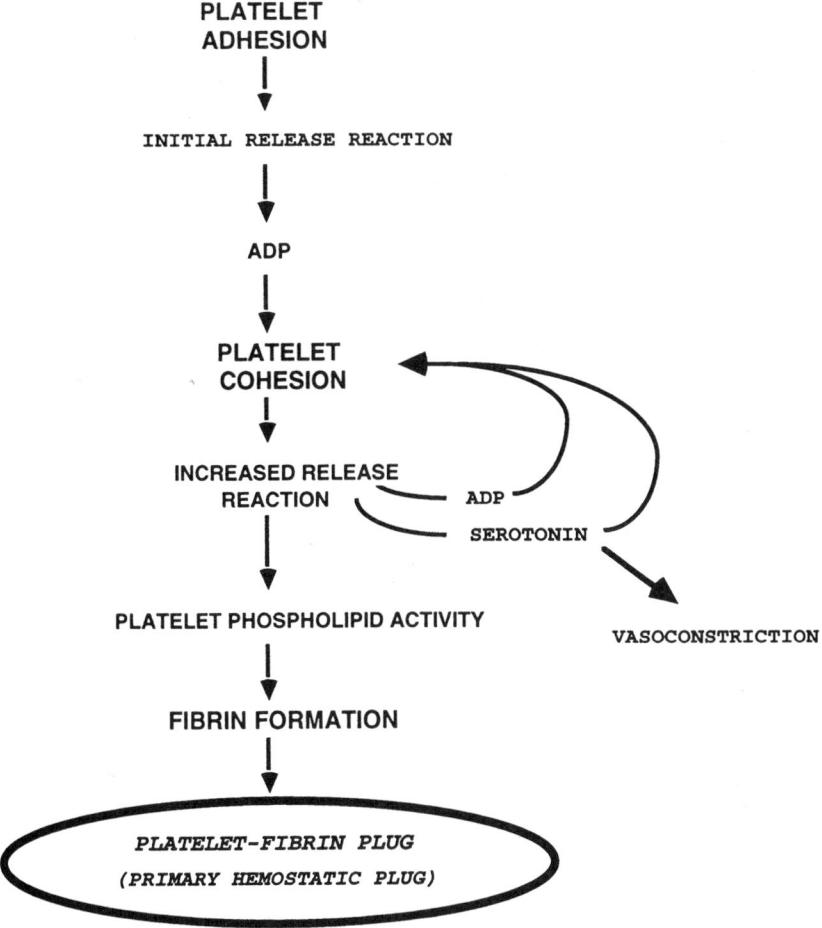

**FIGURE 5.** Platelet function. When a platelet adheres to the collagen basement membrane or an artificial surface (not another platelet, which is termed cohesion), the platelet generates an initial release reaction, producing ADP which, in turn, induces platelet–platelet cohesion. As cohesion continues, compounds are released that activate adjacent platelets and induce vasoconstriction. The platelet membrane then releases or presents platelet membrane phospholipid (platelet factor 3), which mediates the formation of complexes and platelet/fibrin thrombus.

This irreversible process accounts for the secondary wave seen in a platelet aggregation pattern. In vivo, the result is the eventual formation of a platelet/fibrin thrombus, or primary hemostatic plug, the function and integrity of which is facilitated by vasoconstriction.

### Intraplatelet Biochemical Activity

Intraplatelet functional biochemical sequences are outlined in Figure 6. The key modulator of intraplatelet function is **cAMP**.[36,37] The role of this compound is to combine with a cAMP-dependent protein to generate kinase activity, the role of which is to phosphorylate a receptor protein which then binds (sequesters) calcium

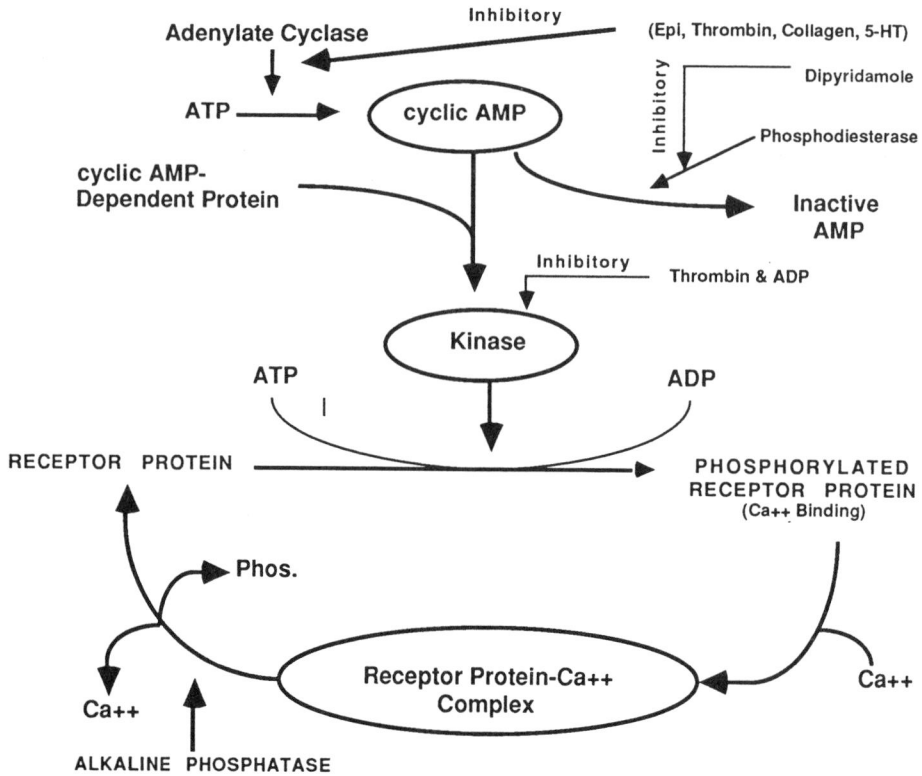

**FIGURE 6.** Abbreviated sequence of biochemical events modulating intraplatelet function. cAMP combines with cAMP-dependent protein to generate kinase, which phosphorylates a receptor protein. This receptor protein then binds calcium ions, making the platelet hypoaggregable and hypoadhesible. Various factors, such as epinephrine, serotonin (5-HT), phosphodiesterase, and alkaline phosphatase, help regulate this sequence by inhibiting compounds at different sites in this sequence, with their effects balancing one another.

ions, rendering the platelet hypoaggregable and hypoadhesible. Epinephrine, thrombin, collagen, and serotonin inhibit the enzyme adenylate cyclase, which is responsible for the conversion of ATP to cAMP. This inhibition results in a decrease in kinase concentration, a decrease in phosphorylated receptor protein, and an increase in ionized (free) calcium which renders the platelet hyperaggregable.

Balancing this biochemical sequence is the enzyme **phosphodiesterase,**[38,39] responsible for destroying cAMP. Agents such as dipyridamole, caffeine, and papaverine inhibit this enzyme, resulting in decreased free calcium and making the platelet hypofunctional. Yet another mechanism for regulating the availability of ionized calcium may relate to the activity of membrane-bound alkaline phosphatase, which is responsible for dephosphorylation of the receptor protein–$Ca^{2+}$-complex.

The role of prostaglandins and derivatives in platelet function are summarized in Figure 7. Platelet and endothelial cell membrane phospholipids are converted into arachidonic acid by the enzyme phospholipase $A_2$,[40] which is activated by both thrombin and collagen. Arachidonic acid is converted into prostaglandin intermediates, prostaglandin $G_2$ ($PGG_2$) and prostaglandin $H_2$ ($PGH_2$), by the enzyme cyclo-oxygenase. In the platelet membrane, thromboxane synthetase converts $PGH_2$

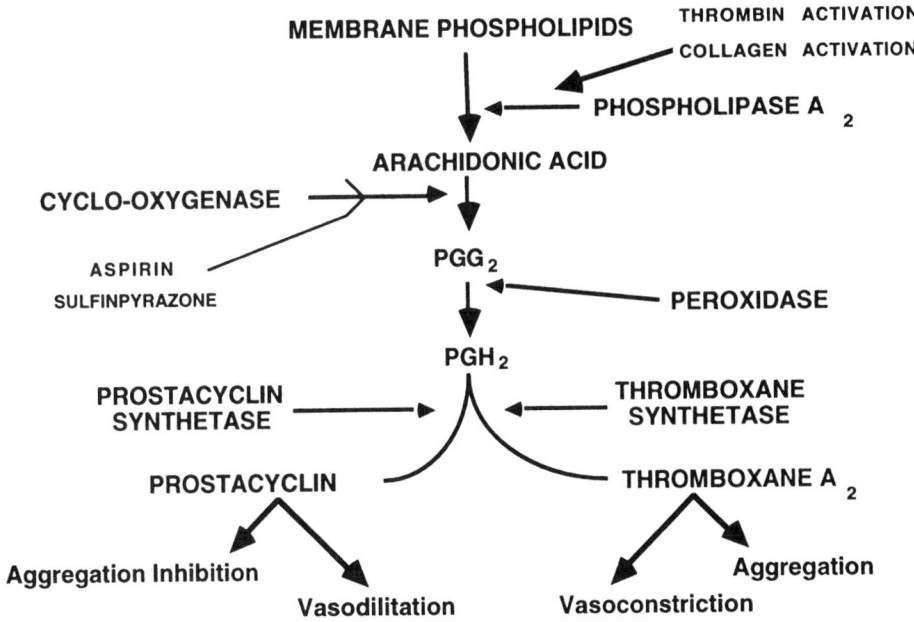

**FIGURE 7.** The role of prostaglandins and their derivatives in platelet function.

into thromboxane $A_2$, a potent inhibitor of adenylate cyclase and, therefore, one of the most potent aggregating agents. Thromboxane $A_2$ also has very potent vasoconstricting activity. In the endothelial cell and in some subendothelial muscle cells, prostacyclin synthetase converts $PGH_2$ into prostacyclin, which is a potent stimulator of adenylate cyclase and, therefore, a very potent aggregation inhibitor and a potent vasodilator.[41,42]

This scheme represents an exquisitely balanced biological system whereby platelets are synthesizing and releasing into the adjacent milieu a compound (thromboxane $A_2$) that promotes platelet function, and the adjacent endothelium is synthesizing and releasing prostacyclin which inhibits platelet function. Therefore, the predisposition to bleeding or thrombosis may depend on the relative equilibrium between these two compounds.

Cyclo-oxygenase is inhibited by aspirin and sulfinpyrazone, two popular antiplatelet agents.[43] Evidence suggests that these two antiplatelet agents function selectively because their activity is directed primarily toward platelets. Also, in their presence, endothelium continues to synthesize prostaglandins, but platelets do not. The precise mechanisms for this selectivity have not yet been elucidated.

### Platelet Membrane Glycoproteins

Platelet interactions with the vasculature (adhesion) with other platelets (cohesion) and with plasma proteins occur at the platelet membrane surface, mediated by various platelet membrane glycoproteins (PMGPs).[44] The major PMGPs and their functions, where known, are summarized in Table 3. PMGP Ia is complexed to PMGP IIa and functions to adhere platelets to subendothelial collagen, independent of von Willebrand factor.[45,46] PMGP Ib has been associated with multiple functions. It has a molecular weight of about 170,000 and is composed of an alpha and beta

**TABLE 3.** Platelet Membrane Glycoproteins

| Glycoprotein | Function | Characteristic |
|---|---|---|
| Ia | von Willebrand-independent receptor for subendothelium | — |
| Ib | von Willebrand receptor; quinidine-antibody receptor | Missing in Bernard-Soulier |
| Ic, IIa | No defined function | — |
| IIb, IIIa | von Willebrand and fibrinogen receptor Platelet-antigen-1 antibody receptor | Missing in Glanzmann's |
| V | Thrombin receptor | Missing in Bernard-Soulier |
| IX | — | Missing in Bernard-Soulier |
| G | Thrombin- and collagen-induced aggregation | — |

subunit, one of which fixes it to the platelet membrane. PMGP Ib exists in complex with PMGP IX and V.[47] PMGP Ib and IX are absent from platelets in Bernard-Soulier syndrome.[48] PMGP Ib serves as a receptor for von Willebrand factor, the first step in platelet adhesion to subendothelial surfaces.[46,49] Also, PMGP Ib is the receptor for quinine and quinidine drug-dependent antibody, which is present in quinine and quinidine-induced thrombocytopenia.[50] PMGP Ib is also a part of the thrombin receptor complex of platelets, and although its role is unclearly defined, PMGP V is of vital importance in this mechanism of platelet activation.[51] PMGP IIb/IIIa complex is found in platelet alpha granules, as well as on the membrane.[52] PMGP IIb has a molecular weight of about 125,000, and PMGP IIIa, about 93,000. Both appear to be subunits of a single glycoprotein, heavily dependent upon calcium for binding of the complex.[53] PMGP IIb/IIIa is absent or markedly reduced in Glanzmann's thrombasthenia, is the binding site for fibrinogen, and serves as the apparent binding site for platelet antigen 1 antibody.[54,55] The binding of fibrinogen to PMGP IIb/IIIa is needed for optimal ADP-induced platelet aggregation. Glycoprotein G, also called thrombospondin, has a molecular weight of about 180,000 and is partly responsible for thrombin- and collagen-induced aggregation.[56,57] PMGPs Ic and IIa have been identified but are thus far without known functions in hemostasis.

## Plasma Protein Function

Plasma protein function in hemostasis comprises multiple interactive systems: (1) coagulation, (2) fibrino(geno)lysis, (3) kinin generation, (4) complement activation, and (5) inhibitors for these systems. Although normally not considered an integral part of "hemostasis" pathophysiologically, kinin generation and complement activation assume considerable importance, especially in syndromes of disseminated intravascular coagulation (DIC).[58]

### Coagulation Protein System

The coagulation proteins are listed in Table 4. The Roman numeral system is most widely used and is preferred. The chromosomal location for genetic information for synthesis of almost all the coagulation factors is known[59] and is summarized in

**TABLE 4.**  Coagulation Factors

| Factor | Synonym |
|---|---|
| I | Fibrinogen |
| II | Prothrombin |
| V | Accelerator globulin |
| VII | Prothrombin conversion accelerator |
| VIII:C | Antihemophilic factor |
| IX | Christmas factor |
| X | Stuart-Prower factor |
| XI | Thromboplastin antecedent |
| XII | Hageman (contact) factor |
| XIII | Profibrinoligase |
| Fletcher factor | Prekallikrein |
| Fitzgerald factor | HMW kininogen |
| Protein C | Xa inhibitor |

Table 5. The formation of a fibrin clot is best thought of as consisting of four key reactions involving the generation of several proteolytic enzymes (serine proteases): (1) formation of factor IXa, (2) formation of factor Xa, (3) formation of thrombin, and (4) formation of fibrin.

**Formation of Factor IXa:** The "contract activation" phase of coagulation begins with the generation of active Hageman factor (factor XIIa). "Surfaces" (phospholipids, subendothelial collagen) and kallikrein can convert factor XII to factor XIIa which, in turn, converts factor XI into factor XIa.[60,61] This reaction happens quickly in the presence of high-molecular-weight kininogen (a significantly prolonged activated

**TABLE 5.**  Chromosomal Locations for Coagulation and Fibrinolytic Factor Information

| Factor | Inheritance | Chromosome | Region |
|---|---|---|---|
| I | AD | 4 | q26–31 |
| II | AD | 11 | p11–q12 |
| V | AR | 1 | q21–25 |
| VII | AR | 13 | q34 |
| VIII:C | SLR | X | q28 |
| vWF | AD | 12 | p12–13 |
| IX | SLR | X | q27 |
| X | AR | 13 | q34 |
| XI | AR | 4 | q35 |
| XII | AR | 5 | q33 |
| XIII | AD | 6 | p24–25 |
| Antithrombin | AD | 1 | p23 |
| Protein C | AD | 2 | q13–14 |
| Protein S | AD | 3 | p21 |
| Plasminogen | AD | 6 | q26–27 |
| TPA | AD | 8 | p12 |
| TPA-I-1 | AD | 7 | q21–22 |
| TPA-I-2 | AD | 18 | q21–22 |
| Antiplasmin | AR | 18 | ? |
| Prekallikrein | AR | ? | ? |
| HMW kininogen | AR | ? | ? |
| Heparin cofactor II | AD | 22 | ? |

*Usual mode of inheritance: AD = autosomal dominant; AR = autosomal recessive; SLR = sex-linked recessive.

partial thromboplastin time is noted in its absence).[62] The role of factor XIa is to convert inactive factor IX (in the presence of calcium ions) to the active form, factor IXa, which is the enzyme responsible for the second key reaction, the generation of factor Xa. Factor XIIa itself converts prekallikrein into kallikrein, which further enhances the generation of factor XIIa.[63]

**Formation of Factor Xa:** The second key reaction involves two major pathways: intrinsic and extrinsic. **Intrinsic** formation of factor Xa involves a five component system: substrate (factor X), enzyme (factor IXa), determiner or cofactor (factor VIII:C), surface (platelet factor 3), and calcium ions.[64] The complex formed is mediated by calcium ions. The enzyme factor IXa cleaves a peptide from the substrate (factor X) with resultant exposure of an active serine site. Factor Xa is the product of this reaction. Factor VIII:C is modified and rendered dysfunctional in the process.

The **extrinsic** pathway of factor Xa formation involves the participation of thromboplastin (tissue factor), factor VII, and calcium ions. Tissue factor is a membrane-bound protein (lipoprotein) existing in a protected state within the plasma membrane of endothelial cells. Upon injury, it is released into the circulation, where it forms a complex with coagulation factor VII in the presence of calcium ions. The activity of the complex seems to depend largely on the concentration of tissue factor. However, the enzymatic activity responsible for the proteolytic activation of factor Xa resides in the factor VII molecule.[65,66] Aprotinin, the primary topic of this book, has been shown to inhibit the factor VIIa–tissue factor complex.[67]

Factor VII exists in plasma as a single-chain glycoprotein with close structural homology to prothrombin, factor IX, and factor X. Contrary to its analogs, however, factor VII is not a zymogen in the true sense, because it has proteolytic activity, although to a limited extent. In the presence of thrombin or factor Xa and lipids and calcium ions, this activity may be increased as much as 400-fold and is accompanied by the formation of a two polypeptide chain molecule. Upon further incubation, the two-chain form of factor VII becomes inactive, and the rate of inactivation is dependent on the concentration of factor Xa. It has been proposed that in the activation of factor X by factor VII, the continuing generation of factor Xa results in a "pulse of factor X-converting activity that can quickly disappear."[65,66]

**Formation of Thrombin:** The third key reaction is the formation of thrombin. Similar to the generation of factor Xa (intrinsic), a five component system is involved: substrate (prothrombin), enzyme (factor Xa), determiner/cofactor (factor V), platelet factor 3, and calcium ions.[68] These components form a complex on the phospholipid surface, and a product, thrombin (factor IIa), the new enzyme, is generated. Factor V, like factor VIII:C in the previous reaction, is modified and loses biological activity. The role of the determiner/cofactor in both reactions is to ensure that the correct enzyme and substrate enter into complex formation. The enzymes thrombin, factor Xa, factor IXa, factor VIIa, and others (such as protein C and protein S) are synthesized in liver parenchymal cells in precursor forms by a vitamin-K-dependent process, which involves the post-ribosomal attachment of calcium-binding prosthetic groups to the N-terminal region of each of these proteins. The process involves the introduction of an extra carboxyl group on the side chain (gamma position) of several glutamic acid residues, forming gamma-carboxyglutamic acid.[69] In the absence of vitamin K (e.g., in a patient on vitamin K antagonist therapy[70]), although a protein is synthesized, it is dysfunctional. These abnormal vitamin-K-dependent factors are called PIVKAs, or proteins induced by vitamin K absence/antagonists.[71]

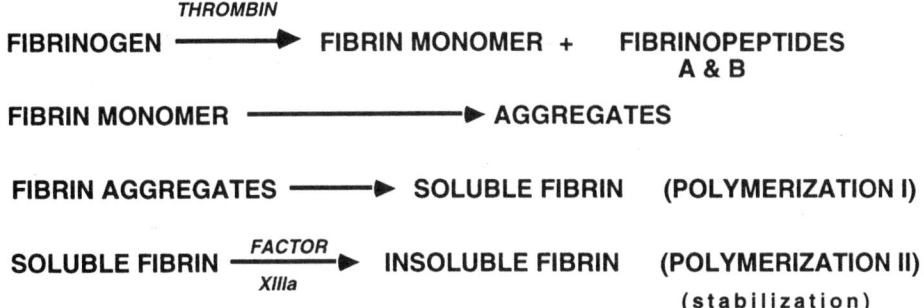

**FIGURE 8.** Conversion of fibrinogen to fibrin. From fibrinogen, thrombin removes fibrino-peptides A and B, yielding fibrin monomer. This fibrin monomer then polymerizes into aggregates, which are subsequently stabilized by noncovalent bonds into "soluble fibrin" (soluble in dispersing agents). Factor XIIIa then acts on soluble fibrin to render it more elastic and less amenable to lysis, yielding an "insoluble fibrin."

**Formation of Fibrin:** The fourth key reaction is the formation of fibrin.[72] Figure 8 summarizes the sequence in the conversion of fibrinogen to fibrin. Thrombin specifically removes fibrinopeptides A and B from fibrinogen, a dimeric structure composed of six covalently linked polypeptide chains (two A alpha, two B beta, and two gamma chains), leaving fibrin monomer.[73,74] Fibrin monomer (fibrinogen minus peptides A and B) polymerizes by aggregating end to end and side to side; these aggregates are stabilized by noncovalent bonds. This fibrin is called "soluble fibrin" since it dissolves in 5 M urea or 1% monochloroacetic acid. This is polymerization I. Thrombin, in its multiple roles as a pivotal enzyme in hemostasis,[72] also activates factor XIII to factor XIIIa. This enzyme, functioning as a transpeptidase in the presence of calcium ions, introduces isopeptide bonds between the epsilon amino groups of certain lysine residues and the gamma carboxyamide groups of certain glutamines in neighboring gamma and alpha chains of the fibrin polymer. This renders the fibrin more elastic and less amenable to lysis.[75,76] This is called polymerization II, yielding "insoluble fibrin." Figure 9 illustrates schematically a nascent, stabilized fibrin matrix. Figure 10 summarizes the pathways of activation for the four key reactions in coagulation.

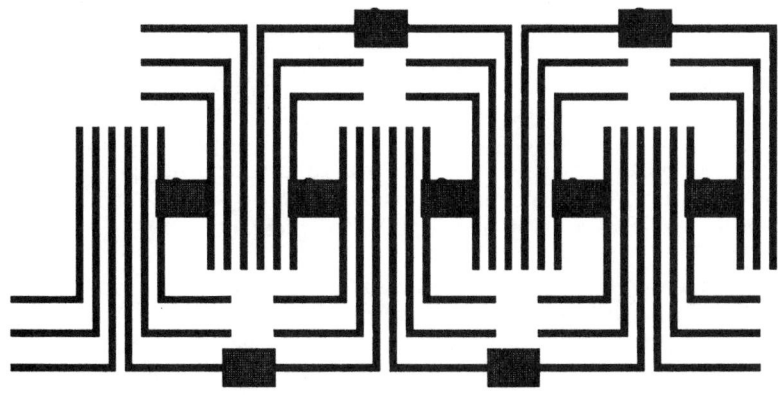

**FIGURE 9.** A stabilized fibrin matrix.

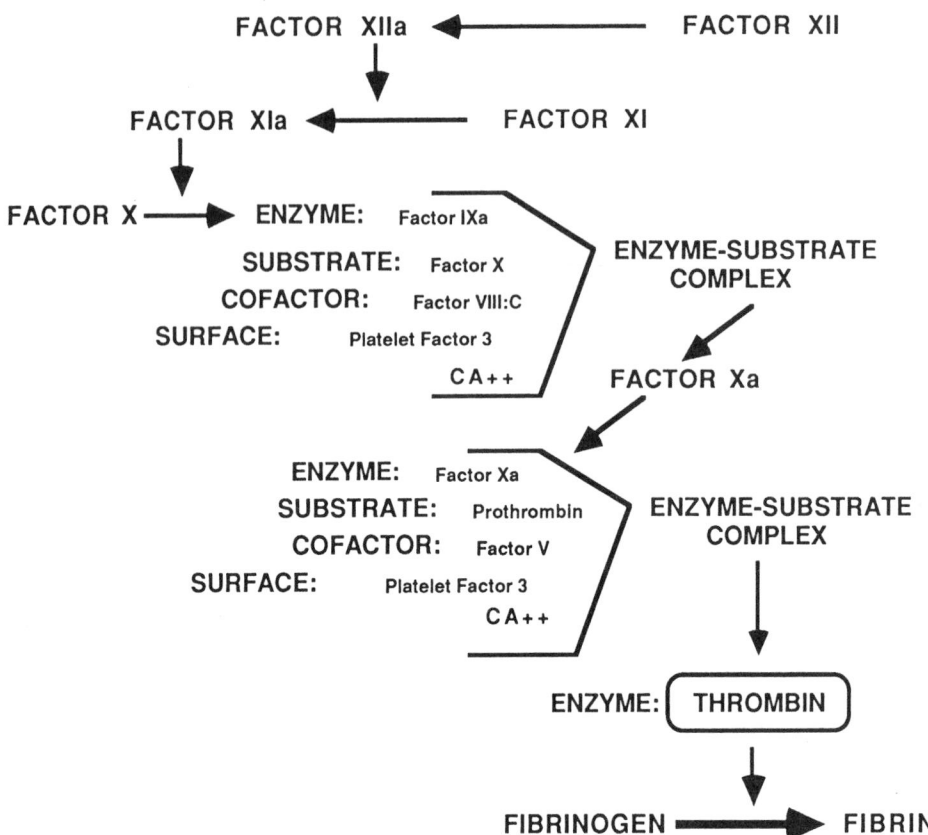

**FIGURE 10.** Summary of the activation pathways in coagulation.

## The Fibrinolytic System

With fibrin deposition considered as a fundamental mechanism of injured tissue repair, fibrinolysis may be viewed as its physiologic antithesis—the destruction of a fibrin clot.[77,78] Hemorrhage or thrombosis thus may depend upon a delicate balance between the procoagulant system and the fibrinolytic system. Figure 11 summarizes the biology of the fibrinolytic system. It consists of a proenzyme, plasminogen, which is converted via many pathways into the active enzyme, **plasmin**.[79] Unlike the enzyme thrombin, which has a relatively narrow substrate specificity, the serine protease plasmin has a much broader spectrum of activity with a number of substrates. Indeed, it hydrolyzes both fibrinogen and fibrin into degradation products (FDPs) and degrades factors V, VIII, IX, and XI, ACTH, growth hormone, insulin, components of the complement system, and many other proteins.[80–92]

There are two recognized and well-characterized physiologic activation pathways of the fibrinolytic system. A primary one involves endothelial cell-derived plasminogen activator (TPA) which converts plasminogen to plasmin directly.[83] A second pathway, probably of less physiologic significance, involves factor XIIa (generated by many triggers) which converts a proactivator (prekallikrein) into an activator (kallikrein) which, in turn, converts plasminogen into plasmin.[84–86]

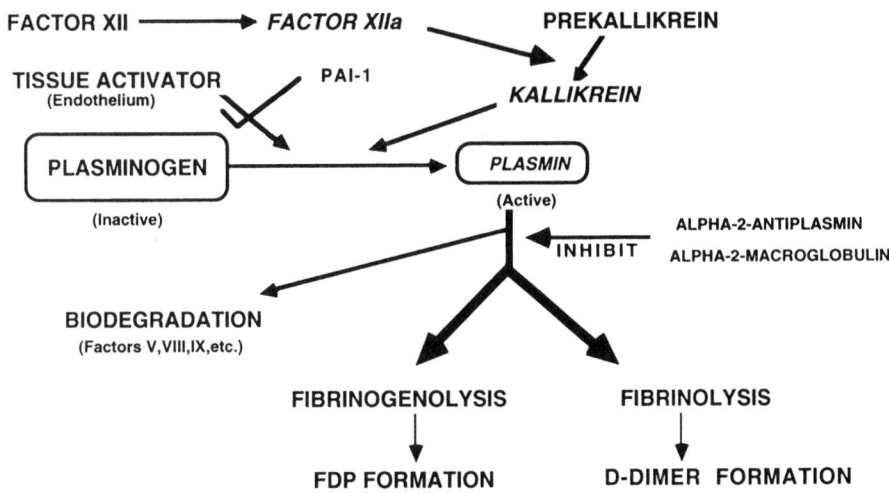

**FIGURE 11.** Biology of the fibrinolytic system. The key compound, plasminogen, is converted primarily by endothelium-derived tissue plasminogen activator (TPA) to the active enzyme, plasmin, which hydrolyzes fibrinogen and fibrin into FDPs and degrades other compounds. PAI-1 (plasminogen inhibitor-1) serves to inhibit TPA and fibrinolysis.

The fibrinolytic system is modulated by many inhibitors. **Alpha-2 antiplasmin** is an extraordinarily rapid inhibitor of plasmin activity.[77,87] Although present in very low concentration in plasma, alpha-2 antiplasmin, with its extraordinary affinity for plasmin (resulting in an irreversible covalent complex), is the primary candidate for the major regulator of fibrinolysis in vivo. There are two known inhibitors of TPA[88,89]: plasminogen inhibitors 1 and 2 (PAI-1 and PAI-2). PAI-1 is the primary modulator. A number of cells produce this protein, including platelets, supporting the hypothesis that at sites of injury, platelet aggregation facilitates the survival of the fibrin and thus the integrity of the hemostatic plug.[90] Aprotinin is a potent exogenous (pharmacologic) inhibitor of plasmin.[91]

In contrast to thrombin which cleaves fibrinopeptides A and B from the amino terminus of fibrinogen, creating fibrin monomer, plasmin begins to degrade fibrin(ogen) at the carboxy terminus of the A-alpha chain and continues to further hydrolyze the matrix in various other loci, yielding soluble degradation products. Figure 12 depicts the characterized FDPs. The presence of FDPs in the circulation may seriously compromise hemostasis by interfering with fibrin monomer polymerization and platelet function.[90,92,93]

### Complement Activation

Although complement activation is generally not considered an integral part of the hemostatic system, its role in the pathophysiology of thrombohemorrhagic disorders is of considerable importance. The complement system is a multimolecular self-assembling system constituting the primary humoral mediators of inflammation and tissue damage.[94,95] It involves a series of sequential reactions similar to those of the coagulation system and is depicted in Figure 13. There is a primary "classical" activation pathway that involves the activation of C1 by antigen–antibody complexes and an "alternate" (properdin) activation pathway that involves the direct activation

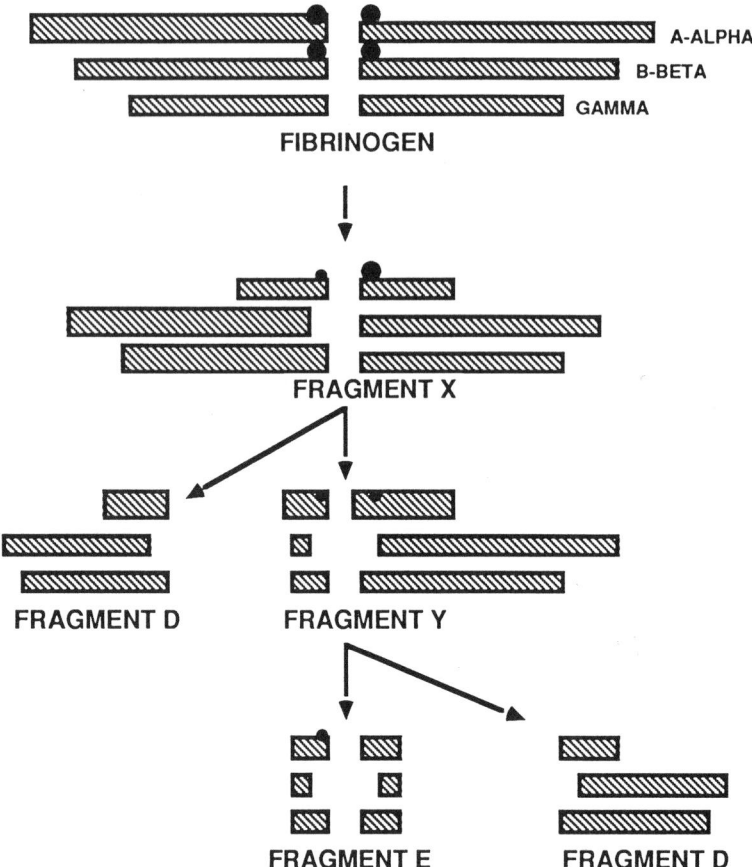

**FIGURE 12.** The fibrin(ogen) degradation products (FDPs) are listed in decreasing order of molecular size: fibrogen has an MW of ~340,000; fragment X; ~265,000; fragment Y, ~155,000; fragment D, ~95,000; and fragment E, ~50,000.

of C3. The activation of C1–C4 is called the **activation phase**, and the activation of C5–C9 is called the **attack phase**, leading to cell lysis or the destruction of pathogens by phagocytes (opsonization). This includes osmotic lysis of red cells and platelets, releasing procoagulant material in the form of membrane lipoprotein, as well as ADP, both serving to accelerate the coagulation process.[96-98] It is of interest to note that while difficult to assess its pathophysiologic relevance, plasmin generated either by TPA or via the Hageman factor pathway can directly activate C1 or C3 independently of antigen–antibody complexes. Aprotinin is capable of the inhibition of kallikrein–C1-inhibitor complexes and C1–C1-inhibitor complexes.[99] In many instances of pronounced activation of the fibrinolytic system, one might envision significant plasmin-induced activation of the complement system, leading to serious clinical consequences.[58]

### Kinin Generation

The importance of kinin generation during thrombohemorrhagic disorders has been appreciated only recently. Kinins increase vascular permeability and induce

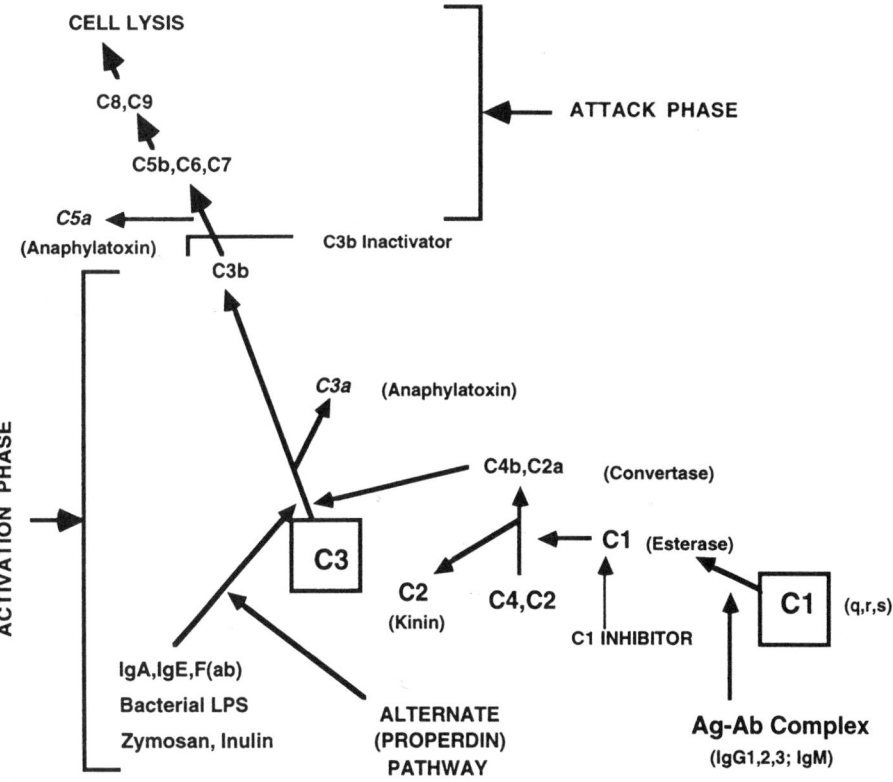

**FIGURE 13.** Sequence of reactions in complement activation. The "classic" activation pathway involves activation of C1 by antigen–antibody (Ag-Ab) complexes, such as immunoglobulin G1 (IgG1), whereas the alternate pathway involves direct activation of C3 by immunoglobulins or bacterial cell-wall lipopolysaccharide (LPS). Activation of C1–C4 constitutes the "activation phase," and activation of C5–C9 is the "attack phase," leading to cell lysis or opsonization of pathogens.

vascular dilation leading to hypotension, shock, and potential end-organ damage—common occurrences in syndromes of disseminated intravascular coagulation.[58,100-102] Like complement activation, generation of kinins centers around Hageman factor (factor XII) activation. As noted earlier, factor XIIa, in addition to activating factor XI to factor XIa, converts prekallikrein (Fletcher factor) into kallikrein, which converts kininogens into kinins. Also, factor XIIa is further digested into factor XIIa fragments by plasmin; these fragments, while void of procoagulant activity, can further activate prekallikrein to kallikrein with ensuing generation of kinins. Aprotinin is a potent inhibitor of kallikrein.[103]

Figure 14 illustrates the important interrelationships between the coagulation system, the fibrinolytic system, the complement system, and the kinin system. Factor XII is converted to active factor XIIa by various compounds ("surfaces") including collagen and phospholipids; factor XIIa converts prekallikrein to kallikrein which converts plasminogen to plasmin. Plasmin activates C1 and/or C3 of the complement system. Also, plasmin-induced factor XIIa fragments convert prekallikrein to kallikrein which, in addition to generating more plasmin, converts kininogen to kinin. These activation pathways, although difficult to assess quantitatively, have

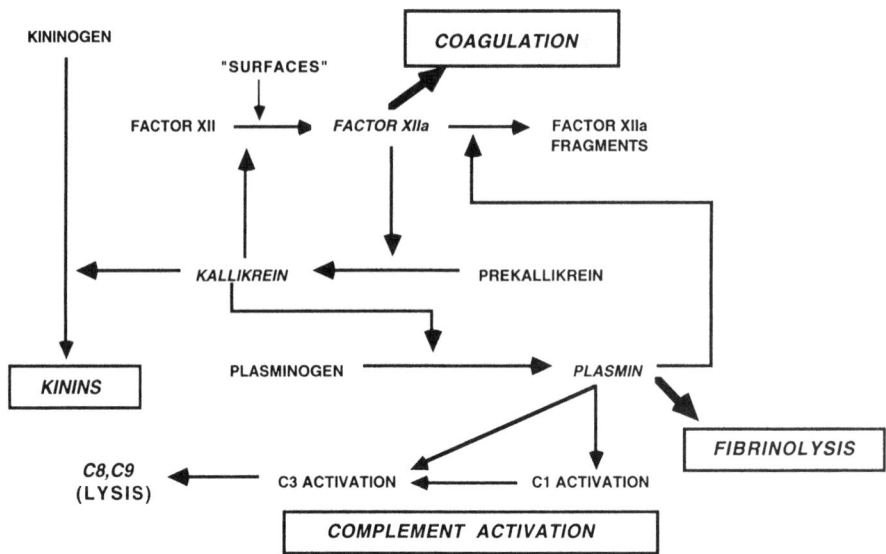

**FIGURE 14.** Interaction of coagulation, fibrinolysis, complement, and kinin systems.

been shown in a multitude of clinical observations to likely play important roles in the pathophysiology of DIC, often leading to catastrophic clinical consequences.[58]

### Inhibitor Systems

Like other biologic processes, the blood coagulation system is governed by many inhibitory mechanisms designed to limit the extent of the various biochemical reactions and possible dissemination of the coagulation process. To this extent, the regulation of coagulation is effected by a number of negative feedback loops, the involvement of specific inhibitors, and the compartmentalization of function, all of which serve to restrict clotting to a localized process.

Table 6 summarizes the inhibitory systems in hemostasis.[104,105] Many of these machanisms assume major importance in pathophysiology. First, there is the inactivation of factors V and VIII:C by the activated protein C and protein S system.[106] This mechanism involves the interaction of the enzyme thrombin with an endothelial cell component, thrombomodulin, resulting in an in situ complex (a proenzyme) to protein Ca (an enzyme). Protein Ca, in turn and in the presence of another protein (protein S), inactivates (by proteolysis) factors V and VIII:C, essentially

**TABLE 6.** Inhibitory Systems in Hemostasis

1. Inactivation of factors V and VIII by thrombin and activated protein C and protein S system
2. Inhibition of thrombin, factor Xa, IXa, XIa, XIIa, and kallikrein by antithrombin III
3. Inhibition of prothrombin activation and fibrin formation by prothrombin fragments
4. Inhibition of thrombin or factor Xa formation by suboptimal "complex" components
5. Inhibition of thrombin activity by absorbing to fibrin
6. Inhibition of fibrin monomer polymerization and platelet function by products of fibrino(geno)lysis (FDP)

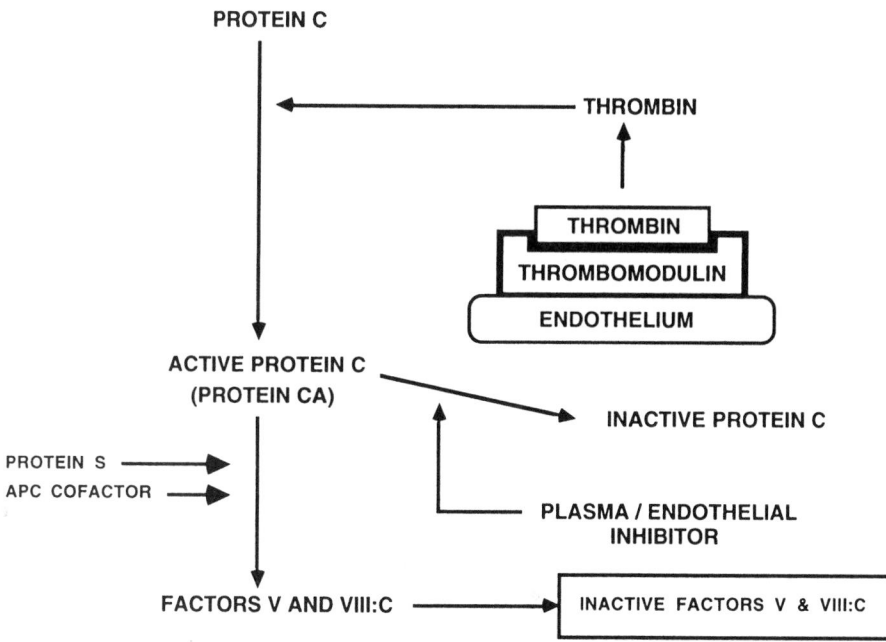

**FIGURE 15.**   Regulation of the blood coagulation system. Thrombin and an endothelial cell component, thrombomodulin, interact to form a complex that converts protein C (proenzyme) to protein Ca (active enzyme). Protein Ca, in the presence of protein S and an activated protein C (APC) cofactor, inactivates factors V and VIII:C, thereby halting fibrin deposition.

halting further fibrin deposition (Fig. 15). Recently, Dahlback and associates have identified an activated protein C cofactor, the absence of which leads to familial thrombosis.[107] In concert with procoagulant inhibitor activity is the observation that protein Ca enhances fibrinolysis, perhaps by depressing the activity of naturally occurring fibrinolytic inhibitors and/or by enhancing the activity of plasminogen activators. Also, aprotinin is a potent inhibitor of activated protein C.[108] The inhibitory activity of active protein C is itself modulated by another endothelial cell-derived inhibitor.

Another mechanism playing a primary role in modulating hemostasis is the inhibition of the serine proteases thrombin, factor Xa, factor IXa, factor XIIa, and kallikrein by antithrombin. The inhibitory activity of antithrombin is markedly enhanced by heparin.[109-113] Figure 16 depicts a model illustrating the interaction of antithrombin with serine proteases. Arginine-rich centers in antithrombin react irreversibly with the serine center of serine proteases. In the figure, thrombin serves as an example. Heparin, when used in therapy, reacts with lysine sites in antithrombin, making the arginine-rich center more available and thereby enhancing antithrombin inhibitory activity. This ternary complex then dissociates to yield an inactive thrombin–antithrombin complex and free heparin. The complex is then cleared from the circulation. The elucidation of this mechanism has served as a fundamental premise rationalizing heparin/miniheparin therapy.

Whereas the vast majority of evidence shows that these two systems (protein C and antithrombin) likely are the most important modulators of coagulation, the contribution by other mechanisms listed in Table 6 is probably not trivial. For

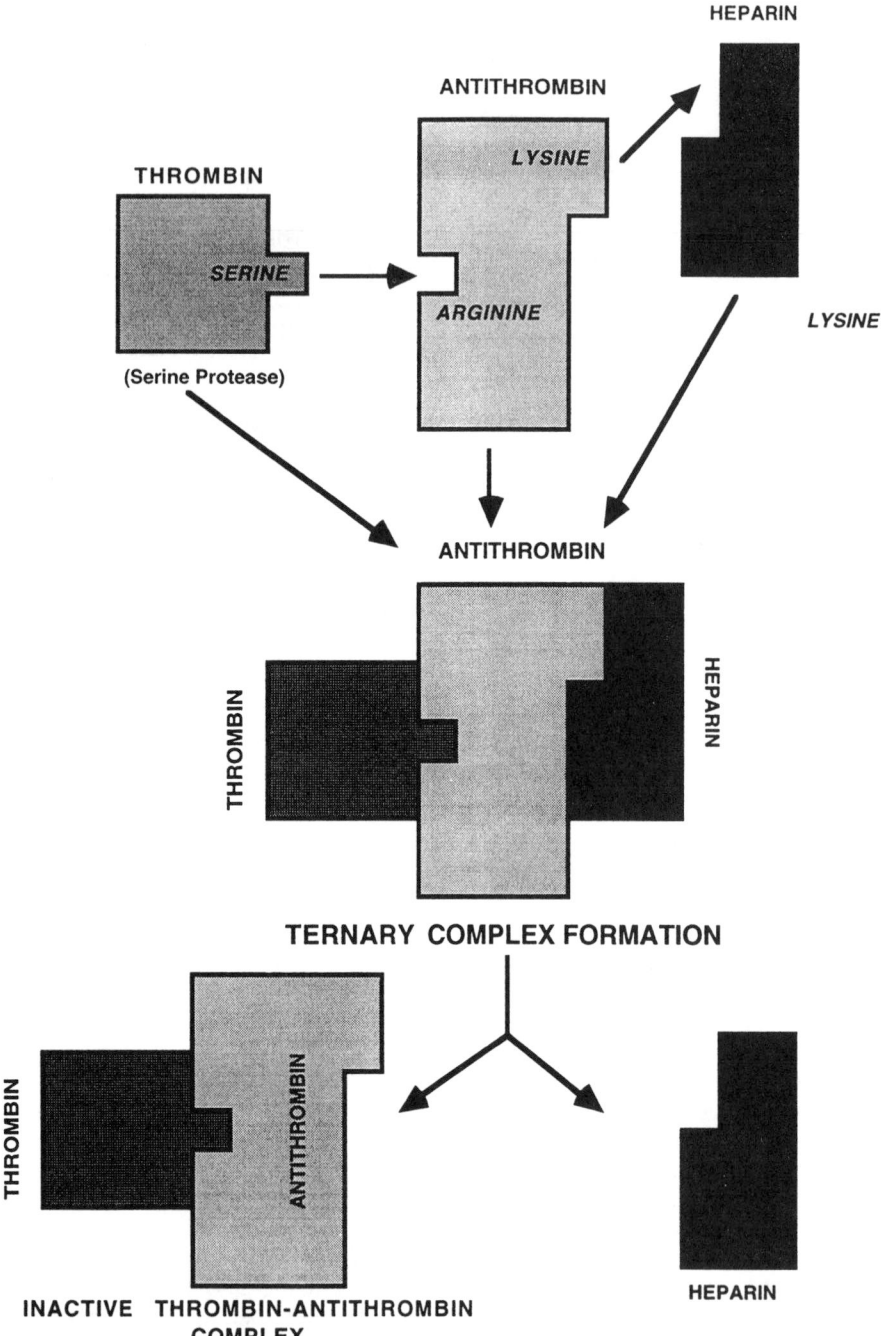

**FIGURE 16.** Inhibition of serine proteases (thrombin; factors Xa, IXa, and XIIa; and kallikrein) by antithrombin. Heparin, by making the arginine-rich centers in antithrombin more available to bind with the serine proteases, thereby enhances antithrombin's inhibitory activity. The ternary complex then dissociates, yielding an inactive thrombin–antithrombin complex, which is cleared from the circulation, and free heparin.

instance, prothrombin fragments produced when thrombin is generated are known to interfere with further prothrombin conversion and with fibrin polymerization. As fibrin is formed, it absorbs thrombin, thus decreasing thrombin availability. Also, inhibition of fibrin monomer polymerization and platelet function by FDPs may occur. If FDPs complex with fibrin monomer, it becomes "solubilized" and unavailable for polymerization. Late degradation products, especially fragments D and E, have a high affinity for platelet membranes and render platelets markedly dysfunctional. Sometimes, this activity can lead to significant clinical hemorrhage.[114]

### Other Interactive Components

Evidence is mounting that many other interactive components, including the vascular proteoglycans, fibronectin, complement derivatives, neutrophils/monocytes, and other thus-far-uncharacterized agents, may play important roles in modulating hemostasis.

**Fibronectin** is a high-molecular-weight glycoprotein that is soluble in plasma.[115] An insoluble form is found in connective tissue and basement membranes.[116] It binds to collagen, fibrin, fibrinogen, and intact cells, especially fibroblasts.[116–118] It is synthesized by vascular endothelium and is also found in the alpha granules of platelets.[29] It is cleaved by thrombin and trypsin, coprecipitates with fibrin, and is covalently cross-linked to fibrin by factor XIIIa.[119–121] Fibronectin is needed to support cell growth, enhances cellular migration into a fibrin clot, and provides an extracellular matrix which eventually replaces a fibrin clot. As clot formation occurs, approximately 50% of plasma fibronectin is lost.[120] This loss is because of cross-linking of fibronectin to the alpha chain of fibrin (by factor XIIIa), thus accounting for approximately 5% of the total protein of a fibrin clot. Fibronectin is necessary for cryoprecipitation of fibrinogen/fibrin complexes and accounts for the laboratory "cryoprecipitation" seen in DIC. Fibronectin is commonly decreased not only in DIC but also in postoperative states, in patients sustaining major trauma (especially burns), and in patients with solid tumor metastases.[121]

Other activities associated with fibronectin relate to the potentiation of plasminogen activators, thus mediating clot lysis and matrix turnover; the mediation of activation of platelets by damaged tissue; opsonization of bacteria by neutrophils; attachment of bacteria to damaged tissues; and inhibition of the endothelial uptake of low density lipoprotein. The fibronectin associated with alpha granules of platelets is released during collagen- or thrombin-induced platelet aggregation; following release, it binds to the platelet surface, further enhancing collagen-platelet adhesion and further stimulating collagen-induced platelet aggregation and release. The interaction with collagen[119] and probably other vascular proteoglycans (heparan sulfate, hyaluronic acid, and chondroitin sulfate) is mediated by cross-linking by factor XIIIa. Heparin may accelerate the binding of fibronectin to both fibrinogen and collagen; however, the binding of heparin to fibronectin does not appear to change the "anticoagulant" nature of the bound haparin.[121]

**Vascular proteoglycans** are a heterogeneous group of high-molecular-weight protein polysaccharides consisting of carbohydrate polymers (glycosaminoglycans) covalently linked to a protein core.[122] The common vascular proteoglycans are hyaluronic acid, chondroitin-4-sulfate, chondroitin-6-sulfate, dermatan sulfate, keratin sulfate, heparin sulfate, heparan sulfate, and heparin.[123] Heparan sulfate is a low-sulfated, D-glucuronic, acid-rich polysaccharide, whereas heparin is a highly sulfated, L-iduronic, acid-rich polysaccharide. The amount of each particular type of proteoglycan differs in various regions of the vasculature. Most are concentrated in the intimal layer. The concentrations of dermatan and heparan sulfate correlate closely with antithrombotic activity. Selected proteoglycans inhibit collagen- and thrombin-induced platelet aggregation, accelerate antithrombin inhibitory activity, and induce the release of platelet factor 4. Their concentrations change with the development of atherosclerotic plaques. Physiologically, vascular proteoglycans support vascular integrity, maintain the viscoelastic properties of vessels, regulate permeability of macromolecules, and regulate arterial lipid deposition. All these properties encompass modulating functions in the interaction of blood proteins with the vascular wall.

Several **complement derivatives**, especially C3a and C5a, may play key roles in hemostasis. These components not only regulate vascular tone but also may induce a neutrophil/monocyte release of enzymes like elastases and collagenases, important in the degradation of fibrinogen, fibrin, and FDPs. Also, complement derivatives modulate release of granulocyte/monocyte procoagulant activity, may modulate platelet reactivity, and influence the neutrophil/monocyte interaction with fibronectin.[124] Granulocytes and monocytes contain procoagulant activity which may be released under pathological conditions, such as in acute leukemia.[125,126]

## Concluding Remarks

The consequences of acute insults to the hemostatic system, whether congenital or acquired, often present a considerable challenge in diagnosis and therapy. Logical and effective management depends upon (1) the proper identification of the hemostatic compartments involved; (2) an appreciation for the complex, delicately modulated interplays of various enzyme/inhibitor systems; and (3) knowledge of the mechanism by which various apparently unrelated disease processes precipitate sometimes catastrophic events (thrombosis, embolism, hemorrhage). The section on plasma proteins pays particular attention to biocybernetic principles (positive/negative feedback loops) and to the interrelationship of enzyme systems involved in coagulation, fibrinolysis, kinin generation, and complement activation, as these systems are often disrupted during cardiac surgery. A working knowledge of basic mechanisms provides not only advantages in diagnostic and therapeutic mangement, but also serves as a firm foundation for the development of novel diagnostic and therapeutic modalities, particularly as relate to prevention, diagnosis, and management of hemorrhage associated with cardiac surgery.

## Pathophysiology of Hemostasis during Cardiac Surgery

Cardiopulmonary bypass (CPB) surgery has become conventional in clinical medicine, and the severe defects in hemostasis that can occur with CPB may dramatically compromise morbidity or mortality of patients.

### Prevention of Cardiac Surgical Bleeding

Hemorrhage associated with cardiac surgery may be devastating and life-threatening; over-cautiousness regarding prevention, differential diagnosis, and rapid effective therapy is essential. Awareness must be given to preventing surgical hemorrhage by uncovering hereditary, acquired, or drug-induced bleeding tendencies before CPB. A preexisting bleeding diathesis, although mild, when coupled with the changes of hemostasis induced by cardiac surgery may lead to calamitous results.[127] Recently, there has been great interest in aprotinin as an agent to decrease blood loss during cardiac surgery.[128-132]

## Laboratory Screening

Any preoperative laboratory and hemostasis screen should generally be simple and incur a minimum of expense to the patient while providing adequate information; however, presurgical or precardiac bypass hemostasis screens are often insufficient.[133-135] As with an adequate history and physical examination, one must be knowledgeable in screening for defects in hemostasis when a surgical procedure is planned. When preexisting hemostatic defects are combined with the defects in hemostasis created by CPB, the resultant hemorrhage is often catastrophic but often can be averted by wise screening of the patient. The usually ordered SMA-12/60 biochemical screening survey, electrolytes, and complete blood and platelet count will detect the common acquired disorders often associated with a bleeding tendency, such as chronic liver disease, renal disease, and instances of "hypersplenism" or bone marrow failure. Most commonly, a presurgical screen consists only of a prothrombin time (PT), activated partial thromboplastin time (aPTT) and platelet count. Although these simple tests will detect most coagulation protein problems and thrombocytopenia, they provide absolutely no information about vascular or platelet function and ignore the possibility of pathologic fibrinolysis.

Most nontechnical hemorrhage associated with cardiac surgery is caused by platelet function defects and, less commonly, coagulation protein or vascular defects; it is important to realize platelet defects are a more common cause of surgical bleeding than are coagulation protein problems! Therefore, one simple procedure is added to the routine preoperative surgical screen—the standardized template bleeding time, as described by Mielke and coworkers.[136] It is done on all patients before a cardiac surgical procedure and provides a reasonable screen for adequate vascular function and platelet function.[137] The template bleeding time should not be done until adequate platelet numbers ($>100,000/mm^3$) are documented by count or smear evaluation. For CPB patients, a thrombin time is added to the preoperative screen.[138,139] In addition, the resultant clot should be observed for 5 minutes after the test is done. A normal thrombin time assures the absence of significant hypofibrinogenemia, dysfibrinogenemia, fibrinolysis, or FDP elevation. The use of these tests in the presurgical screen adds only minimal cost and laboratory time while providing valuable information not given by a simple PT, aPTT, or platelet count. If hypothermic perfusion is to be done, cryoglobulins and cold agglutinins should also be assessed before bypass.[140-145] The preoperative surgical and bypass hemostasis screen is summarized in Table 7.[136,146-149]

**TABLE 7.** Presurgical Hemostasis Screen (Minimal Requirements)

| | |
|---|---|
| Complete blood and platelet count (CBC) | Thrombin time (CPB surgery) |
| Prothrombin time | (observe clot for 5 min) |
| Partial thromboplastin time (PTT) | Cryoglobulins and cold agglutinins |
| Template bleeding time (duplicate) | (hypothermic CPB) |

## Hemostasis in Cardiac Surgery

Hemorrhage during or after bypass is of more than fleeting significance, as it may lead to substantial morbidity and mortality from an elective procedure, places formidable demands on blood bank facilities, and can lead to prolonged, costly hospitalization.[139,150-153] The actual incidence of life-threatening hemorrhage associated with CPB varies from 5–25%.[139,150-156]

Formerly, the pathophysiology of altered hemostasis created by CPB was poorly understood. Various investigators attributed the hemorrhagic syndrome of CPB surgery to an assorted spectrum of defects; each investigator, moreover, prioritized diverse degrees of importance on each defect, depending on which particular hemostatic parameters were monitored. In the past, the abnormalities most often cited to account for CPB hemorrhage included (1) inadequate heparin neutralization, (2) protamine excess, (3) heparin rebound, (4) thrombocytopenia, (5) hypofibrinogenemia, (6) primary fibrinolysis, (7) DIC, (8) isolated coagulation factor deficiencies, (9) transfusion reactions, and (10) hypocalcemia. The suggestion that all these defects may contribute to CPB hemorrhage clearly shows that despite the finding of multiple defects in hemostasis, the basic pathophysiology of altered hemostasis during CPB is bewildering to many. It is equally clear that basic mechanisms of altered hemostasis associated with CPB must be completely understood and appreciated before a useful approach to rapid diagnosis and effective therapy can be rationally designed.

### *Thrombocytopenia*

Early studies of hemostasis during CPB noted significant thrombocytopenia, about 50,000/ml, in patients undergoing bypass surgery; many authors thought this low count responsible for bypass hemorrhage. Kevy et al. noted that thrombocytopenia was related to time on bypass, being more pronounced with perfusions lasting > 60 minutes.[157] A relationship between thrombocytopenia and time on bypass was also reported by Signori and colleagues[158] and later studies.[159,160] Porter and Silver[159] observed that in most patients undergoing CPB, the platelet count fell to one-third of the preoperative levels and that thrombocytopenia did not abate until several days after CPB. Earlier studies by Wright and coworkers[161] and von Kaulla and Swan[162] also recognized thrombocytopenia in association with CPB, but these investigators decided that thrombocytopenia bore little, if any, relationship to actual bypass hemorrhage. Other studies finding thrombocytopenia during CPB concluded that this represented thrombocytopenia of DIC.[163-166] Bick[135,139,151,167-170] and others[171-173] have failed to find significant thrombocytopenia during CPB. This wide variability in experience probably represents different surgical and pumping techniques, such as flow rates, normothermic or hypothermic perfusion, oxygenation system used, time on bypass, and priming solution.

Figure 17 shows changes in platelet number during CPB for membrane-oxygenation-pumped patients versus bubble-oxygenation patients.[135,151,174] In our experience, the type of oxygenation mechanism used plays little role, if any, in causing clinically significant thrombocytopenia.[135,151,174] Thrombocytopenia occurs slightly more frequently with bubble oxygenators than with membrane oxygenators, but this does not often reach clinical significance. The most commonly cited mechanisms for the development of CPB thrombocytopenia are (1) hemodilution, (2) formation of intravascular platelet thrombi, (3) platelet utilization in the pump

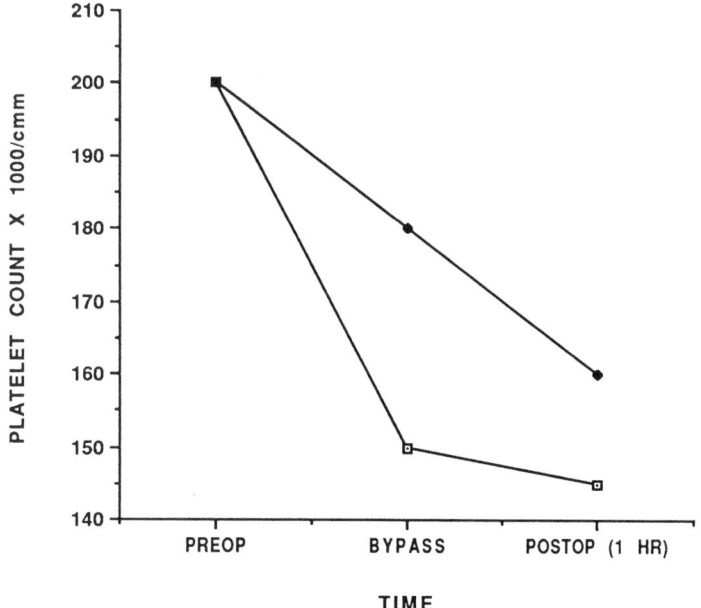

**FIGURE 17.**   Platelet counts during CPB, comparing membrane (*solid circles*) versus bubble oxygenation (*open boxes*) in 300 consecutive patients.

or oxygenation system, and (4) peripheral utilization because of DIC. We have failed to find a correlation between CPB hematocrit and platelet count, suggesting that hemodilution is not a major factor.[134,170,175] Indeed, the role, if any, of these mechanisms in producing CPB thrombocytopenia is unclear.

### Platelet Function Defects

In contrast to the prolific investigations of platelet number during CPB, platelet function has received little attention during this procedure. Early investigators suspected that abnormalities of platelet function might happen, as faulty clot retraction was noted.[158] These results were of unclear significance, however, because other changes known to affect clot retraction, such as hypofibrinogenemia and thrombocytopenia, were also present. Another early study assessed platelet function in patients before CPB but not during or after bypass; in this study, abnormal preoperative platelet adhesion in glass bead columns was associated with increased postoperative bleeding.[176] Salzman[177] studied platelet adhesion before, during, and after bypass and noted decreased adhesion to glass bead columns in patients during bypass. However, the significance of this defect was difficult to evaluate, because all patients had marked thrombocytopenia, which is known to alter adhesion studies,[178-180] and in addition, adhesion studies are now generally thought to be without any particular clinical significance.[137,181,182] Further information from this study was that heparin, in doses used during CPB, did not alter platelet adhesion. This study concluded that a circulating anticoagulant might be responsible for the platelet function defect noted, as plasma from CPB patients altered adhesion when added to normal platelets. This circulating anticoagulant probably represented FDPs.[139] Salzman's study also noted that perfusion temperature and the type of priming solution did not correlate with the development of abnormal platelet function.

Platelet adhesion studies have also been performed in patients undergoing CPB without significant thrombocytopenia.[167,169,170,175] In these studies, platelet function, as measured by adhesion, decreased profoundly in all patients at the initiation of bypass; most patients showed adhesion which decreased to 17% of preoperative levels. In one study, little correlation was noted between hematocrit, fibrinogen level, or FDP titer and abnormal adhesion.[169] Also, poor correlation was noted between chest tube blood loss and abnormal platelet function, as assessed by adhesion. Again, recent studies have questioned the clinical importance of platelet adhesion by the glass bead column technique.[137,181,182] However, this degree of abnormal platelet function would surely be expected to compromise hemostasis severely. The platelet function defect is slightly more severe and tends to correct more slowly when a membrane oxygenator is used as compared to a bubble oxygenator. Platelet function as assessed by template bleeding times or by platelet aggregation or lumi-aggregation is abnormal in patients with platelet function defects,[137,180] von Willebrand's syndrome (ristocetin aggregation only),[179] and myeloproliferative disorders.[183]

Many factors, some possibly altered by CPB, may affect platelet function, including (1) pH, (2) absolute platelet count, (3) hematocrit, (4) drugs, (5) presence of FDPs, (6) type of pump prime, and (7) type of oxygenation system used.[139,184-190] Although most studies do not clearly define the reasons for abnormal platelet function during CPB, they do suggest that several of these mechanisms are probably not involved. The finding of platelet counts $> 100,000/mm^3$ and hematocrits $> 30\%$ in most patients with marked platelet dysfunction 1 hour after CPB suggests that the absolute platelet count and hematocrit do not account for altered platelet function. Also, most patients have a normal or near-normal pH 1 hour after bypass surgery, so a change in pH is unlikely to account for abnormal platelet function during bypass surgery. Heparin, at levels higher than those attained in patients undergoing CPB, has been shown to not alter platelet function.[150,177,180] Circulating FDPs are known to interfere with platelet function, and these are present in about 85% of patients undergoing CPB.[139,185,189] However, there is poor correlation between levels of circulating FDP and abnormal platelet function during bypass surgery.[169,175] In addition, defective platelet functions happens in 100% of patients undergoing CPB, and thus circulating FDP cannot account for many cases.[134,139,151,169,175]

Other possible mechanisms of altered platelet function during CPB include platelet membrane damage by shearing force or contact with foreign material, resulting in a partial release of platelet contents, platelet membrane coating with nonspecific proteins or protein degradation products, or incomplete release reaction or nonspecific platelet damage induced by flow rates. More recent studies have shown selective platelet degranulation to occur during bypass surgery.[191] However, no studies reported yet allow conclusions to be drawn regarding the contribution of any of these mechanisms to altered platelet function during CPB. In one preliminary study of 29 patients, only 20% developed aggregation abnormalities during CPB; however, after heparin reversal with protamine sulfate, 90% of patients developed aggregation abnormalities. These authors attributed this finding to a protamine/platelet interaction and not to bypass itself.[192] We have evaluated platelets by lumi-aggregation in patients undergoing CPB surgery, and in all patients platelet aggregation and platelet release were markedly altered.[150,151,193] Typical mid-byass and post-bypass lumi-aggregation patterns seen in these patients are depicted in Figures 18A and B. In all patients assessed, the aggregation and release reaction defect happened within 10–15 minutes of starting bypass. Also, we noted that in all

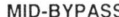

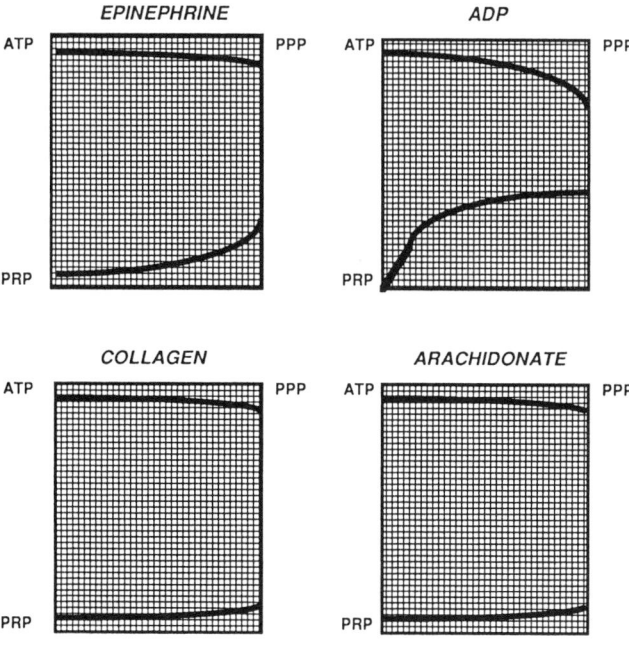

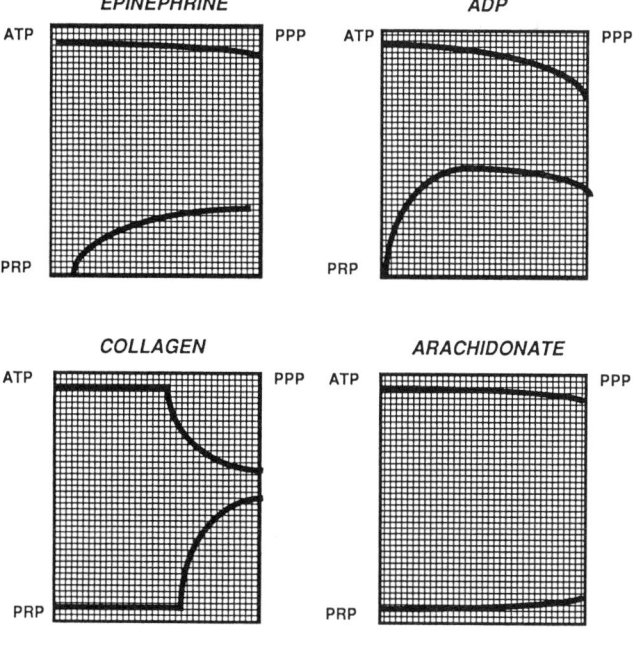

**FIGURE 18.** Platelet lumi-aggregation patterns in CPB as assessed at mid-bypass and post-bypass. PRP = platelet-rich plasma; PPP = platelet-poor plasma; ATP = ATP release.

patients, platelet factor 4 levels rose rapidly with the initiation of bypass. The aggregation defects appear to be similar with both membrane and bubble oxygenators, although the type of priming solution, albumin versus hydroxyethyl starch, does seem to change the type of defects seen.[193]

Despite the mechanism(s) involved, studies to date clearly disclose a significant platelet function defect that is induced in all patients undergoing CPB surgery. The magnitude of this defect certainly would be expected to have potential serious consequences for hemostasis during and after bypass. In addition, patients who have ingested drugs known to interfere with platelet function would be expected to have more blood loss than those not ingesting such agents, with these drugs compounding the defects already induced by CPB and potentiating the chance for hemorrhage; one small study has supplied evidence for this conclusion.[188] Although diagnosis and management of hemorrhage associated with CPB will be discussed later, it should be pointed out that this platelet function defect is of major importance in post-CPB hemorrhage. The use of platelet concentrates in the face of a normal platelet count usually promptly corrects or significantly reduces most episodes of CPB or post-CPB hemorrhage. DDAVP (desmopressin acetate) was initially thought to decrease bleeding after open-heart surgery, thus leading many surgeons to begin the empirical, and sometimes irrational, use of DDAVP during and after open-heart surgery. However, more recent blinded randomized trials have failed to show any significant differences in post-CPB blood loss between DDAVP and placebo.[194-196] Also, DDAVP releases tissue (endothelial) plasminogen activator, potentially activating the fibrinolytic system and enhancing or inducing hemorrhage; so, many using this agent recommend the concomitant use of aminocaproic acid to abort any possible hemorrhage.[197-200] Because of current evidence, there appears to be little, if any, rationale for the empiric use of DDAVP during CPB; those using this agent should be aware of the potential for enhancing hemorrhage and for increasing risk of coronary artery and cerebrovascular thrombosis.

### Isolated Coagulation Factor Defects

Many studies have examined and reported coagulation factor deficiencies during CPB. A wide variety of findings have been observed and, like the finding of thrombocytopenia, may only reflect differences in surgical or pumping techniques, such as flow rate or priming solution. Most studies have noted significant hypofibrinogenemia that does not seem to be correlated with perfusion time.[154,159-161, 169,170] We[169,170,185] and others[154,160] have found fibrinogen levels to be closely correlated with CPB fibrinolysis; however, other investigators report little correlation.[157,201] Figure 19 depicts correlations noted between fibrinogen, plasminogen, circulating plasmin, and FDP during CPB.[134,151,174] Some studies have concluded that hypofibrinogenemia happens primarily because of DIC during pump surgery[163,165,166]; however, others found no hypofibrinogenemia during CPB.[202,203]

It seems reasonable to conclude from the studies reported that hypofibrinogenemia secondary to hyperfibrinolysis may be a frequent event during CPB. Fibrinolysis occurs in about 85% of patients undergoing bypass surgery. Most studies have also noted other coagulation deficiencies in association with CPB, most commonly factor II, factor V, and factor VIII:C.[154,157,160,161,163,166] It has been noted that some patients undergoing CPB for valvular heart disease have low factor VIII:von Willebrand factor high-molecular-weight monomers; also, these monomers may increase during the CPB procedure.[195] Some conclude that these

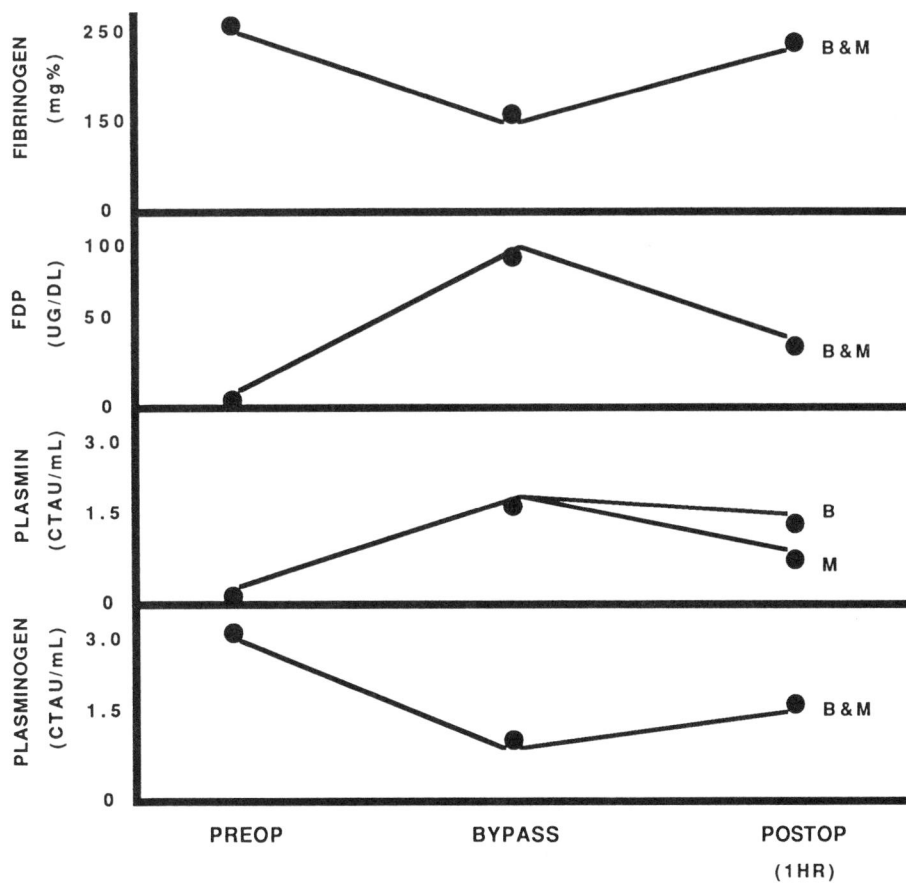

**FIGURE 19.** Fibrinolytic activity during CPB, comparing membrane (*M*) versus bubble (*B*) oxygenation techniques.

changes are secondary to DIC,[163,173] whereas others describe these decreases to a primary fibrinolytic syndrome and plasmin-induced degradation of coagulation proteins.[134,139,154,169,170,185] Still others find no signficant decrease in most coagulation factors during bypass surgery,[157,202,203] and two authors have reported increased factor VIII:C levels during perfusion.[202,204]

### Disseminated Intravascular Coagulation

The question of DIC developing during bypass surgery has caused much confusion regarding altered hemostasis both during and after bypass. Many early studies of hemostasis during CPB concluded that DIC occurred.[163,165,166,205,206] However, many such studies monitored only isolated coagulation factors; the measured decreases were empirically ascribed to presumed DIC, as no other clear explanation was evident. Specifically, the findings of isolated fribinogen, factor VIII:C,[161,165] or prothrombin complex factor deficiencies[172] were often assumed, usually erroneously, to be secondary to DIC without proper confirmatory laboratory testing. Also, two recent reports have concluded that DIC accounts for altered hemostasis during CPB.[173,207] In these reports of nine patients, it was concluded that DIC was present after several parameters of hemostasis worsened following heparin reversal with protamine. Specifically, FDP elevation, hypofibrinogenemia, and hypoplasminogenemia appeared to accentuate following the infusion of protamine. However, our experience[134,135,139,150,169,170] and that of others[154,158,159,162,203,208] have been the opposite: hypofibrinogenemia, hypoplasminogenemia, and FDP elevation are usually noted to correct rapidly and uniformly after the administration of protamine sulfate.

These findings would suggest that DIC is not generally associated with CPB surgery. DIC during cardiac surgery also seems unlikely in view of massive heparinization and the absence of significant or uniform thrombocytopenia reported in many studies in which hemostasis appears to be markedly abnormal. Another finding which would surely suggest that DIC is not present during CPB is the presence of normal or near-normal antithrombin III levels during CPB[134,150,154,175]; evidence suggests that decreased antithrombin III levels are a good indicator of the development of acute or chronic DIC.[209-212]

Only one study has shown decreased antithrombin III during CPB[173]; however, in the nine patients described, all had low levels of antithrombin III before bypass was started. Also, the method used was quite old and possibly influenced by the presence of FDP or heparin, making interpretation of these results unclear. Another consideration negating the probability that DIC happens during cardiopulmonary bypass is that if DIC were present in patients undergoing CPB, the infusion of intravenous protamine sulfate would be expected to cause a massive precipitation of soluble fibrin monomer, with resultant extensive micro- or macrovascular occlusion. In this author's experience, only two out of several thousand patients have had true DIC in association with CPB.[134,139,151] Both patients developed DIC before CPB, one from cardiac arrest and the other from septicemia. In these two instances, bypass surgery was finished without incidence; however, when protamine sulfate was infused, massive vascular occlusion including carotid and renal artery thrombosis occurred.

To summarize, although most early and several recent studies have detected primary fibrinolysis in association with CPB, few have concluded that DIC might occur. These conclusions probably emanate from the marked superficial similarities between primary fibrinolysis and DIC and the usual secondary fibrinolytic response and from the difficulty in making a clear-cut differential diagnosis between these two states without sophisticated and complete coagulation studies.

### Primary Fibrinolysis

Fibrinolytic activity is generally decreased or inhibited during and following most general surgical procedures.[213-216] However, most studies using a variety of laboratory modalities have found increased fibrinolysis during and after CPB surgery.[134,139,151,154,169-171,185-187,193,201,208,217] Many earlier studies of hemostasis during CPB assessed fibrinolysis with the euglobulin lysis time, and the finding of fibrinolysis was of unclear significance for a long time.[218,219] More recent studies of CPB hemostasis,[134,150,151,159,169,170,175] which have used more specific methods for assessing fibrinolysis (primarily synthetic substrate assays[211,220-224]), have confirmed earlier reports of a primary fibrino(geno)lytic syndrome in most patients undergoing CPB surgery. Figure 19 depicts changes in the fibrinolytic system in patients undergoing CPB. Because of early reports detecting primary fibrinolysis during CPB, the empirical use of antifibrinolytics, usually epsilon-aminocaproic acid, has become commonplace. Despite the attendant hazards of this agent, which include hypokalemia, hypotension, ventricular arrhythmias, local or disseminated thromboses, and DIC syndromes,[225,226] many cardiovascular surgeons have often used this drug. Controlled studies with and without antifibrinolytics have failed to show any clear-cut differences in CPB hemorrhage,[154,160,201,227,228] and Gomes and McGoon[208] and Tsuji et al.[203] have shown a definite increase in post-CPB hemorrhage with the empirical use of antifibrinolytics. In fact, the need to use aminocaproic acid to control CPB hemorrhage is extremely rare[134,135,139,151]; this agent should only be used when clear laboratory evidence of primary fibrinolysis is noted in the severely hemorrhaging CPB patient who does not respond to adequate platelet transfusions.

Several investigators finding primary fibrinolysis during CPB have concluded this to be inconsequential as a cause of post-perfusion hemorrhage,[158,160] whereas others have thought that this syndrome is triggered only by specific events, such as pyrogenicity of equipment, the use of dextran 40, or induction of anesthesia.[162,229,230] Because primary fibrinolysis happens in most patients subjected to CPB surgery, it seems likelier that activation of the fibrinolytic system may be happening in the oxygenation mechanism or, alternatively, that pump-induced accelerated flow rates may activate the plasminogen-plasmin system or may alter endothelial plasminogen activator/inhibitor activity. There is marked activation of factor XII in patients undergoing CPB surgery, with about 70% of factor XII being converted to factor XIIa.[231] This is another potential activation pathway for the initiation of a primary fibrinolytic syndrome. However, the pathogenesis of fibrinolytic activation during CPB is unclear. Although many investigators have noted enhanced fibrinolysis during CPB, few studies have found only elevated fibrinolytic activator activity with no systemically circulating plasmin.[157,201,205] Also, a few studies have failed to find any evidence of primary fibrinolysis in association with CPB.[160,161,205,227]

### Other Defects in Cardiac Surgery

Heparin "rebound" has received significant attention as a potential cause of CPB hemorrhage,[230,232-235] usually in earlier studies. With today's generally accepted doses of both heparin and protamine, both heparin rebound and inadequate heparinization are rarely, if ever, seen.[134,139,151,164,170,173,175] Neither heparin rebound nor inadequate heparin neutralization has ever been documented as an actual cause of CPB hemorrhage.[134,135,151,164,165] Similarly, protamine excess has occasionally been incriminated as a cause of CPB hemorrhage, but several studies have failed to note this phenomenon in a single patient undergoing CPB.[139,156,169,170,171,233,236] Also, although protamine sulfate is a well-known in vitro anticoagulant, it is unlikely that this agent is the cause of clinical hemorrhage.[237]

Several authors have reported that both coagulation defects and significant CPB hemorrhage may be associated with hypothermic perfusion[160,162,227,230]; our experience in comparing normothermic to hypothermic perfusions has led to the same conclusion.[217] Gomes and McGoon[208] and Porter and Silver[159] found no increased incidence of CPB hemorrhage resulting from hypothermic perfusion. Many patients undergoing coronary artery bypass grafting for coronary occlusive disease have been on warfarin-type drugs. Verska and associates[227] have noted that although the prothrombin time returns to normal before CPB, patients previously receiving warfarin therapy show more hemorrhage than those not earlier on these agents. This observation applies to general surgery patients as well. One study[149] noted that increased hemorrhage was associated with a repeat bypass procedure; others, however, noted no increased hemorrhage in association with a second procedure.[166,208] Also, patients undergoing CPB for correction of cyanotic heart disease appear to have more severe derangements in hemostasis during perfusion and a propensity to hemorrhage than those operated on for noncyanotic heart disease.[158,208] Advancing age does not appear to be associated with increased risk of hemorrhage with CPB.[238,239]

### Summary of CPB Hemostasis

Many conclusions regarding altered hemostasis and resultant hemorrhage during CPB surgery are of questionable significance. For example, it appears that over-heparinization, heparin rebound, inadequate protamine neutralization, and protamine excess, although receiving at least theoretical attention as potential causes of CPB hemorrhage, have not been documented as causes of bleeding associated with bypass surgery. Similarly, thrombocytopenia, almost surely a potential source of hemorrhage, is an inconsistent finding during bypass surgery. The finding of isolated coagulation defects during CPB has added little except confusion to an understanding of altered hemostasis during bypass surgery; probably, these findings simply represent isolated measurements of the results of fibrinolysis and systemically circulating plasmin.

Although DIC has been thought by some to happen during CPB, most carefully done studies have not documented this. The significant doses of heparin used during CPB, the absence of consistent thrombocytopenia, and the general correction of hypofibrinogenemia, hypoplasminogenemia, and elevated FDPs after heparin neutralization all suggest that the presence of DIC during cardiac surgery is a very rare event. DIC may be associated with cardiac surgery when another triggering event is provided, such as sepsis, shock, massive transfusions, or a frank hemolytic transfusion reaction.

Predisposing factors which are associated with enhanced CPB hemorrhage are (1) long perfusion times, (2) prior ingestion of warfarin-type drugs, (3) cyanotic heart disease, (4) hypothermic perfusions, (5) preoperative ingestion of drugs known to interfere with platelet function, and (6) prolonged perfusion times. These predisposing risk factors are summarized in Table 8. Prevailing evidence suggests that most patients undergoing CPB bypass surgery develop a primary fibrinolytic syndrome, although the exact triggering mechanisms are unclear but may be resulting from factor XII activation. However, the resultant secondary derangements in hemostasis will certainly create a potential for CPB hemorrhage. Also, most patients undergoing CPB procedures develop severe platelet dysfunction. It is unclear if this defect results from coating of platelet surfaces by FDP, membrane damage from the oxygenation mechanism, platelet damage from fast flow rates, or other unrecognized mechanisms. Whatever the triggering mechanism(s), it is quite clear that the most important alterations in hemostasis associated with CPB surgery

**TABLE 8.**   Factors Predisposing to Hemorrhage during Cardiopulmonary Bypass

| | |
|---|---|
| Long perfusion times | Hypothermic perfusion |
| Prior use of warfarin-type agents | Preoperative ingestion of antiplatelet drugs |
| Cyanotic heart disease | Repeat bypass procedure |

**TABLE 9.** Hemorrhagic Syndromes Seen with Cardiopulmonary Bypass Surgery*

| | |
|---|---|
| Severe platelet dysfunction | Thrombocytopenia |
| CPB-induced | Hyperheparinemia or rebound (??) |
| Drug-induced | Disseminated intravascular coagulation (DIC) |
| Primary fibrinolytic syndrome | (exceedingly rare) |

*Listed in descending order of probability.

are defective platelet function and primary fibrinolysis. These two defects, alone or in combination, certainly account for most nonsurgical and nontechnical hemorrhage in patients undergoing CPB; platelet function defects account for far more hemorrhagic episodes than primary fibrinolysis.

## Diagnosis of CPB Hemorrhage

When bleeding happens during or after bypass, obviously it is extremely important to define the defect as quickly as possible; only in this manner can specific and effective therapy be delivered.[135,139,151,156,240] As earlier mentioned, many instances of CPB hemorrhage are clearly because of inadequate surgical technique, but alterations of hemostasis may also be responsible for accentuating CPB hemorrhage. This discussion is limited to nontechnical causes of CPB hemorrhage. The types of hemorrhage that happen during CPB are somewhat limited and are listed in Table 9.

The primary distinction to be made is between strictly surgical bleeding, defects in hemostasis, or a combination of the two. This distinction becomes more difficult and more important after the patient has left the operating room; during this period, a decision must be made regarding re-exploration and the adequacy of hemostasis for re-exploration. In distinguishing between surgical and nonsurgical bleeding, many physical findings are helpful: Is the bleeding localized or systemic? If the patient is already in the recovery room, the recognition of hematuria in association with petechiae and purpura and of oozing from intravenous sites in conjunction with increased chest tube blood loss and oozing from surgical sites (including the sternotomy wound and saphenous vein harvest site) means a defect in hemostasis. However, increased chest tube blood loss alone often signifies a technical bleeding problem. When the patient is in the operating room, these same findings hold true, and the surgeon will usually note bleeding or oozing throughout the surgical field in nontechnical bleeding. It is important, therefore, that communication between the surgeon and hematologist or internist occur. Clinical suggestions of a systemic, instead of local, cause of CPB hemorrhage are noted in Table 10.

When CPB hemorrhage is seen or suspected, the following laboratory tests are ordered: PT, aPTT, complete blood count and platelet count, examination of a

**TABLE 10.** Clinical Evaluation of Hemorrhage in the CPB Patient

Chest tube blood loss only?
*Or associated with:*

| | |
|---|---|
| Petechiae, purpura, or ecchymoses | Oozing from sternotomy wound |
| Hematuria | Oozing from saphenous vein |
| Oozing from intra-arterial line sites | graft site |
| Oozing from intravenous sites | Other systemic bleeding sites |
| Oozing form venipunctures | Clots forming in chest tube |

peripheral smear, FDP and D-dimer level, heparin assay by synthetic substrate, thrombin or reptilase time, and plasminogen/plasmin levels by synthetic substrate methods.[136,150,151,156] Evaluation of the heparin level will provide rapid information regarding the status of heparin and its potential effects on other tests of hemostasis. The resultant clot from the thrombin or reptilase time is always observed for 5 minutes for evidence of lysis, supplying rapid additional information regarding the presence or absence of a clinically significant primary figrino(geno)lytic syndrome. More evidence for or against primary lysis is obtained by noting the FDP and D-dimer level.[210,241-243] A peripheral blood smear and platelet count are invaluable to rapidly evaluate the potential for thrombocytopenic bleeding. Plasminogen and plasmin levels obtained by synthetic substrate technique are not time-consuming but are not used for an immediate diagnosis; however, they are invaluable in making decisions regarding antifibrinolytic therapy later.[136,150,151,156] If significant primary fibrinolysis is present, FDPs will be significantly elevated and the D-dimer level normal or near-normal, and hypoplasminogenemia and circulating plasmin will be detected. If available, fibrinopeptide A levels will not be elevated but B-beta 15–42-related peptides will be elevated. If on the other hand, excess heparin is a potential problem, this is noted by the heparin assay and, in addition, the thrombin time will be markedly prolonged. If no significant clot lysis is observed and the clot formed during measurement of the thrombin time, and significant FDP elevation is not present, primary fibrinolysis should not be dwelled upon.

All patients undergoing CPB have a platelet function defect; when bleeding occurs, this author assumes this defect is always present, and although it might not be the primary reason for hemorrhage, platelet dysfunction can be assumed to be additive to any other defect whether surgical or resulting from altered hemostasis. No tests of platelet function are routinely done, therefore, but platelets are immediately ordered for any patient who demonstrates intra-bypass or post-bypass hemorrhage.[134,135,151] The time period when hemorrhage occurs—i.e., intraoperatively, after heparin neutralization, or in the recovery room—appears to bear little relationship to the etiology of the primary hemostatic defect responsible for hemorrhage. Exceptions to this are thrombocytopenic bleeding, which usually happens after the patient is in the recovery room, and a significant drug-induced platelet function defect, which is usually manifest as significant oozing immediately after the operative procedure is started. Tests ordered for the differential diagnosis of the etiology of hemorrhage during CPB surgery are listed in Table 11.

## Management of CPB Hemorrhage

When a patient with CPB hemorrhage is first encountered, whether intraoperatively or postoperatively, it is of prime importance (1) to note the type of bleeding (systemic versus local), (2) to order a stat laboratory screen as outlined earlier, and

**TABLE 11.** Laboratory Evaluation of Bypass Hemorrhage (Ordered "Stat")

| | |
|---|---|
| Platelet count and CBC | D-Dimer assay |
| Peripheral blood smear evaluation | Heparin assay* |
| Prothrombin time (PT) | Thrombin time† |
| Partial thromboplastin time (PTT) | Plasminogen assay* |
| FDP titer | Plasmin assay* |

* Synthetic substrate assay
† Observe for clot lysis for 5 min.

(3) to administer 6–8 units of platelet concentrates as quickly as possible. Although the use of platelet concentrates is somewhat empirical at this point, it is done for several sound reasons: all patients have a significant platelet function defect which may be the primary reason for hemorrhage (and usually is if it is a nontechnical bleed) or this defect is likely to be accentuating bleeding from other causes, whether it be a surgical defect or defective hemostasis. The quick administration of platelet concentrates while awaiting the laboratory evaluation often will stop or significantly reduce most instances of nontechnical CPB hemorrhage.[134,135,151] Recently, a fibrin glue in paste or spray form has been applied with reasonable success to bleeding sites in patients undergoing CPB hemorrhage; the source for this fibrin glue may be autologous or allogeneic.[244-247]

When bleeding begins immediately upon initiation of surgery, a platelet function defect, usually drug-induced, can be assumed to be present until further laboratory investigation can be done. In this instance, the patient should be given 6–8 units of platelet concentrates as quickly as possible, and the surgical wound should be closed if feasible. If a platelet function defect is responsible for the hemorrhage (no laboratory evidence of significant fibrinolysis or hyperheparinemia), 6–8 units of platelet concentrates should be repeated the evening after surgery and for 2 postoperative mornings. Thrombocytopenic CPB hemorrhage should be controlled in the same manner, although greater numbers of platelet concentrates may be needed as dictated by the initial platelet count, the site and severity of hemorrhage, and the response to platelet transfusions. Hyperheparinemia and heparin rebound, if thought to be a real clinical problem as documented by synthetic substrate assays, are managed by delivering 25% of the originally calculated protamine sulfate dose; this is repeated every 30–60 minutes until bleeding stops. It should again be stressed that hyperheparinemia and heparin rebound are unlikely to be responsible for bleeding and should not be dwelled upon unless concrete laboratory proof of hyperheparinemia is present and evidence of primary fibrinolysis is clearly absent. This author has seen many instances of excessive heparinization resulting from mistakes in calculations and solution preparation; none of these instances was associated with significant cardiac surgical hemorrhage. Similarly, protamine excess is rarely, if ever, a clinical problem. This situation should never call for therapy and should not be dwelled upon at the risk of ignoring other potential defects in hemostasis.

Primary fibrinolysis is commonly present and may or may not be responsible for hemorrhage. This syndrome should not be treated empirically; antifibrinolytic therapy should be considered if the patient has failed to respond to platelet concentrates and there is documented laboratory evidence for this syndrome, as noted by the presence of hypoplasminogenemia, circulating plasmin, and elevated FDPs. Also, for those having appropriate testing systems available, the absence of elevated fibrinopeptide A, the absence of elevated D-dimer, and the presence of elevated B-beta 15–42 related peptides offer further evidence for primary lysis. Primary fibrino(geno)lytic bleeding is generally treated with epsilon-aminocaproic acid given as an initial dose of 5–10 g by slow intravenous push followed by 1–2 g/hr until bleeding stops or slows to a non-life-threatening level. It should be recalled that this agent may be associated with ventricular arrhythmias (tachycardia or fibrillation), hypotension, hypokalemia, localized or diffuse thrombosis, and frank DIC. It should be injected slowly, and patients should be monitored carefully for cardiac status, renal output, blood pressure, and electrolytes. A newer and more potent antifibrinolytic agent is tranexamic acid; this is usually delivered at a dose of about 3–6 g intravenously per 24 hours.[248]

## Summary

This discussion has provided a review of altered hemostasis associated with CPB surgery. The key to prevention of CPB hemorrhage is to obtain an adequate preoperative evaluation. An adequate history for bleeding tendencies and thrombotic tendencies in both the patient and family is of importance; also, a careful history regarding the use of drugs effecting hemostasis, especially drugs known to interfere with platelet function, should be obtained. A careful physical examination, searching for clues of a real or potential bleeding diathesis, may also prevent catastrophic cases of hemorrhage. An adequate presurgical screen must be done in CPB candidates. Besides the usual PT, PTT, and platelet count, a standardized template bleeding time and thrombin time should be done. The use of these simple testing modalities will guard against significant defects in vascular and platelet function. Most instances of nontechnical cardiovascular surgical hemorrhage are because of several well-defined defects in hemostasis which should be easily controlled if approached in a logical manner as a team effort among cardiac surgeons, pathologists, and hematologists. It is hoped the new promises of aprotinin will develop with time, making cardiac surgery an even safer procedure.

## References

1. Muller-Berghaus G: Pathophysiologic and biochemical events in disseminated intravascular coagulation: Dysregulation of procoagulant and anticoagulant pathways. Semin Thromb Hemost 15:58, 1989.
2. Ryan TJ: The investigation of vasculitis. In: Microvascular Injury. Philadelphia, W.B. Saunders, 1976, p 333.
3. Sheppard B, French JE: Platelet adhesion in the rabbit abdominal aorta following the removal of endothelium: A scanning and transmission electron microscopic study. Proc R Soc Lond 176:427, 1971.
4. Wessler S, Yin ET: On the mechanism of thrombosis. Prog Hematol 4:201, 1969.
5. Friedman RJ, Burns ER: Role of platelets in the proliferative response of the injured artery. Prog Hemost Thromb 4:249, 1978.
6. Harker LA, Schwartz SM, Ross R: Endothelium and arteriosclerosis. Thromb Clin Haematol 10:283, 1981.
7. Roberts WC, Ferrans VJ: The role of thrombosis in the etiology of atherosclerosis (a positive one) and in precipitating fatal ischemic heart disease (a negative one). Semin Thromb Hemost 2:123, 1976.
8. Sinzinger H: Role of platelets in atherosclerosis. Semin Thromb Hemost 12:124, 1986.
9. Bick RL, Murano G: Physiology of hemostasis. In Bick RL, Bennett JM, Brynes RK, et al (eds): Hematology: Clinical and Laboratory Practice. St. Louis, Mosby, 1993, p 1285.
10. Triplett DA: The platelet: A review. In Triplet DA (ed): Platelet Function. Chicago, ASCP Press, 1978, p 1.
11. Astrup T: Fibrinolysis: An overview. In Davidson JF, Rowan RM, Samama MM, Desnoyers PE (eds): Progress in Chemical Fibrinolysis, vol. 3. New York, Raven Press, 1978, p 1.
12. Kwaan HC: The role of fibrinolysis in disease states. Semin Thromb Hemost 10:71, 1984.
13. Mammen EF: Inhibitor abnormalities. Semin Thromb Hemost 9:42, 1983.
14. Ruggeri ZM, Zimmerman TS: Von Willebrand factor and von Willebrand disease. Blood 70:895, 1987.
15. White GC, Shoemaker CB: Factor VIII gene and hemophilia. Blood 73:1, 1989.
16. Walsh P: The effect of collagen and kaolin on the intrinsic coagulation activity of platelets: Evidence for an alternative pathway in intrinsic coagulation not requiring factor XII. Br J Haematol 22:393, 1972.
17. Wilner GD, Nossel HL, LeRoy EL: Activation of Hageman factor by collagen. J Clin Invest 47:2608, 1968.
18. Ginbrane MA: Vascular Endothelium in Hemostasis and Thrombosis. London, Churchill Livingstone, 1986, p 250.

19. Leonard EF, Turitto VT, Vroman L (eds): Blood in contact with natural and artificial surfaces. Ann NY Acad Sci 516:688, 1987.
20. Ruggeri ZM, Fulcher CA, Ware J (eds): Progress in vascular biology, hemostasis and thrombosis. Ann NY Acad Sci 614:311, 1991.
21. Stern DM, Nawroth PP (eds): Vessel wall. Semin Thromb Hemost 13:391–536, 1987.
22. Ulutin ON, et al (eds): Modulation of endothelium and control of vascular and thrombotic disorders. Semin Thromb Hemost 14(suppl):114, 1988.
23. Droller MJ: Ultrastructure of the platelet release reaction in response to various aggregating agents and their inhibitors. Lab Invest 29:595, 1973.
24. Stuart MJ: Inherited defects of platelet function. Semin Hematol 12:233, 1975.
25. White JG: Identification of platelet secretion in the electron microscope. Ser Haematol 6:429, 1973.
26. Nachman RL: Platelet proteins. Semin Hematol 5:18, 1968.
27. Day NJ, Stormorken, Holmsen H: Subcellular localization of platelet factor 3 and platelet factor 4. In: Proceedings of the 12th Congress of the International Society of Hematology, Mexico City, 1968, p 172.
28. Packham MA, Mustard JF: Platelet reactions. Semin Hematol 8:30, 1971.
29. Thomas DP, Niewiarowski S, Ream VJ: Release of adenosine nucleotides and platelet factor 4 from platelets of man and four other species. J Lab Clin Med 75:607, 1970.
30. Born GVR, Cross MJ: The aggregation of blood platelets. J Physiol 168:178, 1963.
31. Zucker MB, Peterson J: Serotonin, platelet factor 3 activity and platelet aggregating agent released by adenosine diphosphate. Blood 30:556, 1967.
32. Davis RB, Mecker WR, Bailey WL: Serotonin release after injection of *E. coli* endotoxin in the rabbit. Fed Proc 20:261, 1961.
33. Des Prez RM, Horowitz HI, Hoo EW: Effects of bacterial endotoxin on rabbit platelets: I. Platelet aggregation and release of platelet factors in vitro. J Exp Med 114:857, 1961.
34. Mueller-Eckhardt C, Luscher EF: Immune reactions of human blood platelets: I. A comparative study on the effects on platelets of heterologous antiplatelet antiserum, antigen-antibody complexes, aggregation gamma-globulin, and thrombin. Thromb Diath Haemorrh 20:155, 1968.
35. Pfueller SL, Luscher F: The effects of immune complexes on blood and their relationship to complement activation. Immunochemistry 9:1151, 1972.
36. Haslam RJ: Interactions of the pharmacological receptors of blood platelets with adenylate cyclase. Ser Haematol 6:333, 1973.
37. Salzman EW: Cyclic AMP and platelet function. N Engl J Med 286:358, 1972.
38. Cole R, Robison GA, Hartman RC: Effects of prostaglandin E and theophylline on aggregation and cyclic AMP levels of human blood platelets. Fed Proc 29:316, 1970.
39. Horlington M, Watson PA: Inhibition of 3′-5′-cyclic-AMP, phosphodiesterase by some platelet aggregation inhibitors. Biochem Pharmacol 19:955, 1970.
40. Gerrard JM, White JG: Prostaglandins and thromboxanes: "Middlemen" modulating platelet function in hemostasis and thrombosis. Prog Hemost Thromb 4:87, 1978.
41. Gryglewski RJ, Bunting S, Moncada S, et al: Arterial walls are protected against deposition of platelet thrombi by a substance (prostaglandin X) which they make from prostaglandin endoperoxides. Prostaglandins 12:685, 1976.
42. Moncada S, Gryglewski R, Bunting S, Vane JR: A lipid peroxide inhibits the enzyme in blood vessel microsomes that generate from prostaglandin endoperoxides the substance (prosta-glandin x) which prevents platelet aggregation. Prostaglandins 12:715, 1976.
43. Turpie AGG: Antiplatelet therapy. Thromb Clin Haematol 10:497, 1981.
44. Berndt MC, Caen JP: Platelet glycoproteins. Prog Hemost Thromb 7:111, 1984.
45. Davies GE, Palek J: Platelet protein organization: Analysis by treatment with membrane-permeable cross-linking reagents. Blood 59:502, 1982.
46. Lusher JM, et al (eds): Factor VIII/VWF and platelet formation and function in health and disease. Ann NY Acad Sci 509:223, 1987.
47. Berndt MC, Gregory C, Chong BH: Additional glycoprotein defects in Bernard-Soulier syndrome: Confirmation of genetic basis by parental analysis. Blood 62:800, 1983.
48. Clemetson KJ, McGregor JL, James E: Characterization of the platelet membrane glycoprotein abnormalities in Bernard-Soulier syndrome and comparison with normal by surface-labeled techniques and high-resolution two-dimensional gel electrophoresis. J Clin Invest 70:304, 1982.
49. Meyer D, Baumgartner HR: Role of von Willebrand factor in platelet adhesion to the subendothelium. Br J Haematol 54:1, 1983.

50. Kunicki TJ, Russell N, Nurden AT: Further studies of the human platelet receptor for quinine and quinidine-dependent antibodies. J Immunol 126:398, 1981.
51. Berendt MC, Phillips DR: Interaction of thrombin with platelets: Purification of the thrombin substrate. Ann NY Acad Sci 370:87, 1981.
52. Gogstad GO, Hagen J, Korsmo R: Characterization of the proteins of isolated human platelet alpha granules: Evidence for a separate alpha granule pool of the glycoproteins IIb and IIIa. Biochem Biophys Acta 670:150, 1981.
53. Fujimura K, Phillips DR: Binding of Ca$^{++}$ to glycoprotein IIb from human platelet plasma membranes. Thromb Haemost 50:251, 1983.
54. McMillan R, Mason D, Tani P: Evaluation of platelet surface antigens: Localization of the PLA-1 alloantigen. Br J Haematol 51:297, 1981.
55. White JG: Inherited disorders of the platelet membrane and secretory granules. Hum Pathol 18:123, 1987.
56. Lawler J, Hynes RO: Structural organization of the thrombospondin molecule. Semin Thromb Hemost 13:245, 1987.
57. Santoro SA: Thrombospondin and the adhesive behavior of platelets. Semin Thromb Hemost 13:290, 1987.
58. Bick RL: Disseminated intravascular coagulation: Objective criteria for diagnosis and management. Med Clin North Am 78:511, 1994.
59. McKusick VA: Mendelian Inheritance in Man: Catalogs of Autosomal Dominant, Autosomal Recessive and X-Linked Phenotypes, 9th ed. Baltimore, Johns Hopkins University Press, 1990.
60. Kaplan AP: Initiation of the intrinsic coagulation and fibrinolytic pathways of man: The role of surfaces, Hageman factor, prekallikrein, high molecular weight kininogen, and Factor XI. Prog Hemost Thromb 4:127, 1978.
61. Kaplan AJ, Meier HL, Mandle R: The Hageman factor dependent pathways of coagulation, fibrinolysis, and kinin-generation. Semin Thromb Hemost 3:1, 1976.
62. Griffin JH, Cochrane CG: Recent advances in the understanding of contact activation reactions. Semin Thromb Hemost 5:254, 1979.
63. Manuhalter CH (ed): Contact phase coagulation disorders. Semin Thromb Hemost 13:130, 1987.
64. Irwin JF, Seegers WH, Andary JTJ, et al: Blood coagulation as a cybernetic system: Control of autoprothrombin C (Xa) formation. Thromb Res 6:431, 1975.
65. Jesty J, Maynard JR, Radcliffe RD, et al: Initiation and control of the extrinsic pathway of coagulation. In Reich E, Rifkin DB, Shaw E (eds): Proteases and Biological Control. Cold Spring Harbor, NY, Cold Spring Harbor Labs, 1975, p 171.
66. Silverberg AS, Nemerson Y, Zur M: Kinetics of the activation of bovine Factor X by components of the extrinsic pathway. J Biol Chem 252:8481, 1977.
67. Chabbat J, Porte P, Tellier M, Steinbuch M: Aprotinin is a competitive inhibitor of the Factor VIIa–tissue factor complex. Thromb Res 71:205, 1993.
68. Seegers WH: Prothrombin complex. Semin Thromb Hemost 7:291, 1981.
69. Stenflo J: Vitamin K, prothrombin, and gamma-carboxy-glutamic acid. N Engl J Med 296:624, 1977.
70. Denson KWE: The levels of factor II, VII, IX, and X by antibody neutralization techniques in the plasma of patients receiving phenindione therapy. Br J Haematol 20:643, 1971.
71. Mackie MJ, Douglas AS: Drug induced disorders of coagulation. In Ratnoff OD, Forbes CD (eds): Disorders of Hemostasis. Philadelphia, W.B. Saunders, 1991, p 493.
72. Walz DA, Fenton JW, Shuman MA (eds): Bioregulatory functions of thrombin. Ann NY Acad Sci 485:1–450, 1986.
73. Fenton JW (ed): Thrombin and hemostasis. Semin Thromb Hemost 19:321–424, 1993.
74. Mosesson MW, Doolittle RF (eds): Molecular biology of fibrinogen and fibrin. Ann NY Acad Sci 408:1–672, 1983.
75. Alami SY, Hampton JW, Race GH, Speer RJ: Fibrin stabilizing factor (factor XIII). Am J Med 44:1, 1968.
76. Ratnoff OD: The molecular basis of hereditary clotting disorders. Prog Hemost Thromb 1:39, 1972.
77. Aoki N, Harpel PC: Inhibitors of the fibrinolytic enzyme system. Semin Thromb Hemost 10:24, 1984.
78. Wiman B, Hamsten A: The fibrinolytic enzyme system and its role in the etiology of thromboembolic disease. Semin Thromb Hemost 16:207, 1990.
79. Castellino FJ: Biochemistry of human plasminogen. Semin Thromb Hemost 10:18, 1984.
80. Aoki N (ed): Fibrinolysis. Semin Thromb Hemost 10:107, 1984.

81. Ratnoff OD, Naff GB: The conversion of C'1s to C'1 esterase by plasmin and trypsin. J Exp Med 125:337, 1967.
82. Robbins KM: Present status of the fibrinolytic system. In Fareed J, Messmore HL, Fenton J, Brinkhous KM (eds): Perspectives in Hemostasis. New York, Pergamon Press, 1980, p 53.
83. Bachmann F, Kruithof KO: Tissue plasminogen activator: Chemical and physiological aspects. Semin Thromb Hemost 10:6, 1984.
84. Goldsmith GN, Saito H, Ratnoff OD: The activation of plasminogen by Hageman, factor (factor XII) and Hageman factor fragments. J Clin Invest 21:54, 1978.
85. Kaplan AP, Austin F: The fibrinolytic pathway of human plasma: Isolation and characterization of the plasminogen proactivator. J Exp Med 135:1378, 1972.
86. Stump DC, Taylor FB, Neshein ME: Pathologic fibrinolysis as a cause of clinical bleeding. Semin Thromb Hemost 16:260, 1990.
87. Schreiber AD: Plasma inhibitors of the Hageman factor dependent pathways. Semin Thromb Hemost 3:43, 1976.
88. Astedt B, Lecander I, Ny T: The placental type plasminogen activator inhibitor: PAI-2. Fibrinolysis 1:203, 1987.
89. Loskutoff DJ, Sawdey M, Mimuro J: Type 1 plasminogen activator inhibitor. Prog Hemost Thromb 9:87, 1989.
90. Emeis JJ, Brommer EJP, Kluft C: Progress in fibrinolysis. In Poller L (ed): Recent Advances in Blood Coagulation. Edinburgh, Churchill Livingstone, 1985, p 11.
91. Yee JA, Yan L, Dominguez JC, et al: Plasminogen-dependent activation of latent transforming growth factor beta (TGF-beta) by growing cultures of osteoblast-like cells. J Cell Physiol 157:528, 1993.
92. Marder VJ: Molecular aspects of fibrin formation and dissolution. Semin Thromb Hemost 8:74, 1982.
93. Marder VJ, Shulman NR: High molecular weight derivatives of human fibrinogen produced by plasmin: Mechanism of their anticoagulant activity. J Biol Chem 244:2120, 1969.
94. Rosse WF: Complement. In Williams WJ, Beutler E, Erslev AJ, Rundles RW (eds): Hematology. New York, McGraw Hill, 1977, p 87.
95. Ruddy S. Gigli I, Austen KF: The complement system in man: I. Activation, control, and products of the reaction sequences. N Engl J Med 278:489, 1972.
96. Gotze O: Proteases of the properdin system. In Reich E, Rifkin DB, Shaw E (eds): Proteases and Biological Control. Cold Spring Harbor, NY, Cold Spring Harbor Symposium, 1975, p 255.
97. Muller-Eberhard HJ: Complement. Annu Rev Biochem 44:667, 1975.
98. Pillimer L, Blum L, Lepow IH: The properdin system and immunity: I. Demonstration and isolation of a new serum protein, properdin, and its role in immune phenomena. Science 120:279, 1954.
99. Wachtfogel YT, Kucich U, Hack CE, et al: Aprotinin inhibits the contact, neutrophil, and platelet activation systems during simulated extracorporeal circulation. J Thorac Cardiovasc Surg 106:1, 1993.
100. Bennett B, Ogston D: Role of complement, coagulation, fibrinolysis, and kinins in normal haemostasis and disease. In Bloom AL, Thomas DP (eds): Haemostasis and Thrombosis. London, Churchill Livingstone, 1981, p 236.
101. Ryan JW, Ryan US: Biochemical and morphological aspects of the actions and metabolism of kinins. In Pisano JJ, Austen KF (eds): Chemistry and Biology of the Kallikrein-Kinin System in Health and Disease. (DHEW publ #76-791.) Bethesda, MD, US Department of Health, Education, and Welfare, 1974, p 315.
102. Van Arman CG, Bohidar HR: role of the kallikrein kinin system in inflammation. In Pisano JJ, Austin KF (eds): Chemistry and Biology of the Kallikrein-Kinin System in Health and Disease. (DHEW publ #71-791.) Bethesda, MD, US Department of Health, Education, and Welfare, 1974, p 471.
103. Swies J, Chopicki S, Gryglewski RJ: Kinins and thrombolysis. J Physiol Pharmacol 44:171, 1993.
104. Comp PC: Hereditary disorders predisposing to thrombosis. Prog Hemost Thromb 8:71, 1986.
105. Bick RL, Pegram M: Syndromes of hypercoagulability and thrombosis. Semin Thromb Hemost 20:109, 1994.
106. Esmon CT: Protein-C. Semin Thromb Hemost 10:109–172, 1984.
107. Dahlback B, Carlsson M, Svensson PJ: Familial thrombophilia due to a previously unrecognized mechanism characterized by poor anticoagulant response to activated protein C: Prediction of a cofactor to activated protein C. Proc Nat Acad Sci USA 90:1004, 1994.
108. Taby O, Chabbat J, Steinbuch M: Inhibition of activated protein C by aprotinin and the use of the insolubilized inhibitor for its purification. Thromb Res 59:27, 1990.

109. Bick RL: Clinical relevance of antithrombin III. Semin Thromb Hemost 8:276, 1982.

110. Jaques LB, McDuffie NM: The chemical and anticoagulant nature of heparin. Semin Thromb Hemost 4:277, 1978.

111. Rosenberg RD: The effect of heparin on factor XIa and plasmin. Thromb Diath Haemorrh 33:51, 1975.

112. Rosenberg RD, Damus P: The purification and mechanism of action of human antithrombin-heparin cofactor. J Biol Chem 248:6490, 1973.

113. Seegers WH: Antithrombin III. Semin Thromb Hemost 7:263, 1981.

114. Bick RL: The clinical significance of fibrinogen degradation products. Semin Thromb Hemost 8:302, 1982.

115. Moseson MW: Cold-insoluble globulin: A circulating cell surface protein. Thromb Haemost 38:742, 1977.

116. Pearlstein E. Gold LI, Garcia-Pardo A: Fibronectin: A review of its structure and biological activity. Mol Cell Biochem 29:103, 1980.

117. Couchman JR, Austria MR, Woods A: Fibronectin-cell interactions. J Invest Dermatol 94:7, 1990.

118. Moser DF: Fibronectin. Prog Hemost Thromb 5:111, 1980.

119. Moser DF, Schad PE, Kleinman HK: Cross-linking of fibronectin to collagen by blood coagulation factor XIIIa. J Clin Invest 64:781, 1979.

120. Moseson MW, Umfleet RA; The cold-insoluble globulin of plasma. Biol Chem 254:5728, 1970.

121. Wagner DD, Hynes RO: Domain structure of fibronectin and its relationship to function. J Biol Chem 254:6746, 1979.

122. Wight TN: Vessel proteoglycans and thrombogenesis. Prog Hemost Thromb 5:1, 1980.

123. Ofusu FA, Danishefsky I, Hirsh J (eds): Heparin and related polysaccharides. Ann NY Acad Sci 556:1–501, 1989.

124. Goldstein IM, Perez HD: Biologically active peptides derived from the fifth component of complement. Prog Hemost Thromb 5:41, 1980.

125. Galloway MJ, Mackie MJ, McVerry BA: Combinations of increased thrombin, plasmin, and non-specific protease activity in patients with acute leukemia. Haemostasis 13:322, 1983.

126. Lisiewicz J: Disseminated intravascular coagulation in acute leukemia. Semin Thromb Hemost 14:339, 1988.

127. Bick RL, Murano G: Physiology of hemostasis. In Bick RL, Bennett JM, Brynes RK, et al (eds): Hematology: Clinical and Laboratory Practice. St. Louis, Mosby, 1993, p 1285.

128. Teylor KM: Effect of aprotinin on blood loss and blood use after cardiopulmonary bypass. In Pifarre R (ed): Anticoagulation, Hemostasis, and Blood Conservation in Cardiovascular Surgery. Philadelphia, Hanley & Belfus, 1993, p 129.

129. Orchard MA, Goodchield CS, Prentice CR, et al: Aprotinin reduces cardiopulmonary bypass-induced blood loss and inhibits fibrinolysis without influencing platelets. Br J Haematol 85:533, 1993.

130. Schonberger JP, Bredee JJ, van Oeveren W, et al: Preoperative therapy of low-dose aspirin in internal mammary bypass operations with and without aprotinin. J Thorac Cardiovasc Surg 106:262, 1993.

131. Hardy JF, Desroches J, Belisle S, et al: Low-dose aprotinin infusion is not clinically useful to reduce bleeding and transfusion of homologous blood products in high-risk cardiac surgical patients. Can J Anaesth 40:625, 1993.

132. Royston D: Controversies in the practical use of aprotinin. In Pifarre R (ed): Anticoagulation, Hemostasis, and Blood Conservation in Cardiovascular Surgery. Philadelphia, Hanley & Belfus, 1993, p 147.

133. Bick RL, Tse N: Hemostasis abnormalities associated with prosthetic devices and organ transplantation. Lab Med 23:462–486, 1992.

134. Bick RL: Hemostasis defects with cardiac surgery, general surgery, and prosthetic devices. In Bick RL: Disorders of Thrombosis and Hemostasis: Clinical and Laboratory Practice. Chicago, ASCP Press, 1992, p 195.

135. Bick RL: Hemostasis defects associated with cardiac surgery, prosthetic devices, extracorporeal circuits, and transplanation. In Bick RL, Bennett JM, Brynes RK, et al (eds): Hematology: Clinical and Laboratory Practice. St. Louis, Mosby, 1993, p 1501.

136. Mielke CH, Kaneshiro MM, Maher LA, et al: The standardized normal Ivy bleeding time and its prolongation by aspirin. Blood 34:204, 1969.

137. Bick RL: Platelet defects. In Bick RL: Disorders of Hemostasis and Thrombosis: Principles of Clinical Practice. New York, Thieme, 1985, p 65.

138. Bick RL, Murano G: Primary hyperfibrino(geno)lytic syndromes. In Murano G, Bick RL (eds): Basic Concepts of Hemostasis and Thrombosis. Boca Raton, FL, CRC Press, 1980, p 181.
139. Bick RL: Syndromes associated with hyperfibrino(geno)lysis. In: Disseminated Intravascular Coagulation. Boca Raton, FL, CRC Press, 1983, p 105.
140. Shahian DM, Wallach SR, Bern MM: Open heart surgery in patients with cold-reactive proteins. Surg Clin North Am 65:315, 1985.
141. Landymore R, Isom W, Barlam B: Management of patients with cold agglutinins who require open-heart surgery. Can J Surg 26:79, 1983.
142. Guena L, Kwabena KA, Addei A: Intraoperative hypothermia in a patient with cold agglutinin disease. JAMA 74:691, 1982.
143. Klein HG, Faltz LL, McIntosh CL, et al: Surgical hypothermia in a patient with a cold agglutinin. Transfusion 20:354, 1980.
144. Leach AB, Van Hasselt GL, Edwards JC: Cold agglutinins and deep hypothermia. Anaesthesia 38:140, 1983.
145. Moore RA, Geller EA, Mathews ES, et al: The effect of hypothermic cardiopulmonary bypass on patients with low-titer, non-specific cold agglutinins. Ann Thorac Surg 37:233, 1984.
146. Brecker G, Cronkite EP: Morphology and enumeration of human blood platelets. J Appl Physiol 3:365, 1950.
147. Hougie C: Fundamentals of Blood Coagulation in Clinical Medicine. New York, McGraw-Hill, 1963, p 241.
148. Proctor RR, Rapaport SI: The partial thromboplastin time with kaolin: A simple screening test for first stage plasma clotting factor deficiencies. Am J Clin Pathol 36:212, 1961.
149. Quick AJ, Stanley-Brown M, Bancroft FW: A study of the coagulation defect in hemophilia and in jaundice. Am J Med Sci 190:501, 1935.
150. Bick RL: Alterations of hemostasis associated with surgery, cardiopulmonary bypass surgery, prosthetic devices and transplantation. In Ratnoff OD, Frobes CD (eds): Disorders of Hemostasis, 2nd ed. Philadelphia, W.B. Saunders, 1991, p 382.
151. Bick RL: Physiology and pathophysiology of hemostasis during cardiac surgery. In Pifarre R (ed): Anticoagulation, Hemostasis, and Blood Conservation in Cardiovascular Surgery. Philadelphia, Hanley & Belfus, 1993, p 23.
152. Beall C, Yow EM, Blodwell RD, et al: Open heart surgery without blood transfusion. Arch Surg 94:567, 1967.
153. Cordell AR: Hematological complications of extracorporeal circulation. In Cordell AR, Ellison RG (eds): Complications of Intrathoracic Surgery. Boston, Little, Brown, 1979, p 27.
154. Mammen EF: Natural proteinase inhibitors in extracorporeal circulation. Ann NY Acad Sci 146:754, 1968.
155. Koets MH, Washington BC, Wolk LW, et al: Hemostasis changes during cardiovascular bypass surgery. Semin Thromb Hemost 11:281, 1985.
156. Bick RL: Pathophysiology of hemostasis and thrombosis. In Sodeman WA Jr, Sodeman TM (eds): Sodeman's Pathologic Physiology: Mechanisms of Disease, 7th ed. Philadelphia, W.B. Saunders, 1985, p 705.
157. Kevy SV, Glickman RM, Bernhard WF, et al: The pathogenesis and control of the hemorrhagic defect in open-heart surgery. Surg Gynecol Obstet 123:313, 1966.
158. Signori EE, Penner JA, Kahn DR: Coagulation defects and bleeding in open heart surgery. Ann Thorac Surg 8:521, 1969.
159. Porter JM, Silver D: Alterations in fibrinolysis and coagulation associated with cardiopulmonary bypass. J Thorac Cardiovasc Surg 56:869, 1968.
160. Tice DA, Worth MH: Recognition and treatment of postoperative bleeding associated with open heart surgery. Ann NY Acad Sci 146:745, 1968.
161. Wright TA, Darte J, Mustard WT: Postoperative bleeding after extracorporeal circulation. Can J Surg 2:142, 1959.
162. von Kaulla KN, Swan H: Clotting deviations in man during cardiac bypass: Fibrinolysis and circulating anticoagulants. J Thorac Surg 36:519, 1958.
163. Blomback M, Noren I, Senning A: Coagulation disturbances during extracorporeal circulation and the postoperative period. Acta Chir Scand 127:433, 1964.
164. Deiter RA, Neville WE, Piffare R, Jasuja M: Preoperative coagulation profiles and posthemo-dilution cardiopulmonary bypass hemorrhage. Am J Surg 121:689, 1971.
165. Penick GD, Averette HE, Peters RM, Brinkhous KM: The hemorrhagic syndrome complicating extracorporeal shunting of blood: An experimental study of its pathogenesis. Thromb Diath Haemorrh 2:218, 1958.

166. Trimble AS, Herst R, Grady M, Crookston J: Blood loss in open heart surgery. Arch Surg 93:323, 1966.

167. Bick RL, Arbegast NR, Holtermann N, et al: Platelet function abnormalities in cardiopulmonary bypass. Circulation 50(suppl):301, 1974.

168. Bick RL, Schmalhorst WR, Crawford L, et al: The hemorrhagic diathesis created by cardiopulmonary bypass. Am J Clin Pathol 63:588, 1975.

169. Bick RL, Arbegast NR, Crawford L, et al: Hemostatic defects induced by cardiopulmonary bypass. Vasc Surg 9:228, 1975.

170. Bick RL, Schmalhorst WR, Arbegast NR: Alterations of hemostasis associated with cardiopulmonary bypass. Am J Clin Pathol 63:588, 1975.

171. Casteneda AR: Must heparin be neutralized following open heart operations? J Thorac Cardiovasc Surg 52:716, 1966.

172. deVries SI, von Creveld S, Green P, et al: Studies on the coagulation of the blood in patients treated with extracorporeal circulation. Thromb Diath Haemorrh 5:426, 1961.

173. Muller N, Popov-Cenić S, Buttner W, et al: Studies of fibrinolytic and coagulation factors during open-heart surgery: II. Postoperative bleeding tendencies and changes in the coagulation system. Thromb Res 7:589, 1975.

174. Bick RL: Alterations of hemostasis during cardiopulmonary bypass: A comparison between membrane and bubble oxygenators. Am J Clin Pathol 73:300, 1980.

175. Bick RL, Schmalhorst SW, Arbegast NR: Alterations of hemostasis associated with cardiopulmonary bypass. Thromb Res 8:285, 1976.

176. Holswade GR, Nachman RL, Killip T: Thrombocytopathies in patients with open-heart surgery: Preoperative treatment with corticosteroids. Arch Surg 94:365, 1967.

177. Salzman WE: Blood platelets and extracorporeal circulation. Transfusion 3:274, 1963.

178. Bick RL, Adams T, Schmalhorst WR: Bleeding times, platelet adhesion, and aspirin. Am J Clin Pathol 65:69, 1976.

179. Bowie EJW, Owen CA, Thompson JH: Platelet adhesiveness in von Willebrand's disease. Am J Clin Pathol 52:69, 1969.

180. Bowie EJW, Owen CA: The value of measuring platelet adhesiveness in the diagnosis of bleeding diseases. Am J Clin Pathol 60:302, 1973.

181. Hirsh J: Laboratory diagnosis of thrombosis. In Colman RW, Hirsh J, Marder VJ, Salzman EW (eds): Hemostasis and Thrombosis: Basic Principles and Clinical Practice. Philadelphia, J.B. Lippincott, 1982, p 789.

182. Zimmerman TS, Meyer D: Factor VIII-von Willebrand factor and the molecular basis of von Willebrand's disease. In Colman RW, Hirsh J, Marder VJ, Salzman EW (eds): Hemostasis and Thrombosis: Basic Principles and Clinical Practice. Philadelphia, J.B. Lippincott, 1982, p 54.

183. Adams T, Schultz L, Goldberg L: Platelet function abnormalities in the myeloproliferative disorders. Scand J Haematol 13:215, 1975.

184. Mustard JF, Packham MA: Factors influencing platelet function: Adhesion, release, and aggregation. Pharmacol Rev 23:97, 1970.

185. Bick RL: The clinical significance of fibrinogen degradation products. Semin Thromb Hemost 8:302, 1982.

186. Sarin CL, Yalav E, Clement AJ, Braimbridge MV: Thromboembolism after Starr valve replacement. Br Heart J 33:111, 1971.

187. Hellem AJ: The advances of human blood platelets in vitro. Scand J Clin Lab Invest 51(suppl):1, 1960.

188. Bick RL, Fekete LF: Cardiopulmonary bypass hemorrhage: Aggravation by pre-op ingestion of antiplatelet agents. Vasc Surg 13:277, 1979.

189. Kowalski E, Kopeć M, Wegrzynowicz Z: Influence of fibrinogen degradation products (FDP) on platelet aggregation, adhesiveness, and viscous metamorphosis. Thromb Diath Haemorrh 10:406, 1963.

190. Kowalski E: Fibrinogen derivatives and their biologic activities. Semin Hematol 5:45, 1968.

191. Harker LA, Malpass TW, Branson HE, et al: Mechanisms of abnormal bleeding in patients undergoing cardiopulmonary bypass: Acquired transient platelet dysfunction associated with selective alpha-granule release. Blood 56:824, 1980.

192. Stass S, Bishop C, Fosberg R, et al: Platelets as affected by cardiopulmonary bypass [abstract]. Trans Am Soc Clin Pathol 35, 1976.

193. Saunders CR, Carlisle L, Bick RL: Hydroxyethyl starch versus albumin in cardiopulmonary bypass prime solutions. Ann Thorac Surg 35:532, 1983.

194. Salzman EW, Weinstein MJ, Weintraub RM, et al: Treatment with desmopressin acetate to reduce blood loss after cardiac surgery. N Engl J Med 314:1402, 1986.
195. Weinstein M, Ware JA, Troll J, Salzman EW: Changes in von Willebrand factor during cardiac surgery: Effect of desmopressin acetate. Blood 71:1648, 1988.
196. Rocha E, Llorens R, Paramo JA, et al: Does desmopressin acetate reduce blood loss after surgery in patients on cardiopulmonary bypass? Circulation 77:1319, 1988.
197. Mannucci PM: Desmopressin (DDAVP) for treatment of disorders of hemostasis. Prog Hemost Thromb 8:19, 1986.
198. Warrier I, Lusher JM: DDAVP: A useful alternative to blood components in moderate hemophilia A and von Willebrand's disease. J Pediatr 102:228, 1983.
199. Mariani G, Ciavarella N, Mazzucconi MG: Evaluation of the effectiveness of DDAVP in surgery and in bleeding episodes in hemophilia and von Willebrand's disease: A study of 43 patients. Clin Lab Haematol 6:229, 1984.
200. De La Fuente B, Kasper CK, Rickles FR: Response of patients with mild hemophilia A and von Willebrand's disease to treatment with desmopressin. Ann Intern Med 103:6, 1985.
201. Derman UM, Rand PW, Barker N: Fibrinolysis after cardiopulmonary bypass and its relationship to fibrinogen. J Thorac Cardiovasc Surg 51:223, 1966.
202. Bachmann F, McKenna R, Cole ER, Maiafi HJ: The hemostatic mechanisms after open-heart surgery: I. Studies on plasma coagulation factors and fiibrinolysis in 512 patients after extracorporeal circulation. J Thorac Cardiovasc Surg 70:76, 1975.
203. Tsuji HK, Redington JV, Kay JH, Goesswald RK: The study of fibrinolytic and coagulation factors during open heart surgery. Ann NY Acad Sci 146:763, 1968.
204. Woods JE, Kirklin JW, Owen CA, et al: The effect of bypass surgery on coagulation sensitive clotting factors. Mayo Clin Proc 42:724, 1967.
205. Gans H, Subramanian V, John S, et al: Theoretical and practical (clinical) considerations concerning proteolytic enzymes and their inhibitors, with particular reference to changes in the plasminogen-plasmin system during assisted circulation in man. Ann NY Acad Sci 146:721, 1968.
206. Palester-Chlebowzyk M, Strzyzewska E, Sitowski W, Olender K: Detection of the intravascular coagulation of blood clotting: II. Results of the paracoagulation test in patients undergoing open-heart surgery with extracorporeal circulation. Pol Med J 11:59, 1972.
207. Kladetsky RG, Popov-Cenić S, Buttner W, et al: Studies of fibrinolytic and coagulation factors during open-heart surgery with ECC. Thromb Res 7:579, 1975.
208. Gomes MM, McGoon D: Bleeding patterns after open heart surgery. J Thorac Cardiovasc Surg 60:87, 1970.
209. Bick RL: Disseminated intravascular coagulation and related syndromes. In Bick RL, Bennett JM, Brynes RK, et al (eds): Hematology: Clinical and Laboratory Practice. St. Louis, Mosby, 1993, p 1463.
210. Bick RL: Disseminated intravascular coagulation and related syndromes: A clinical review. Semin Thromb Hemost 14:299, 1988.
211. Bick RL: Clinical hemostasis practice: The major impact of laboratory automation. Semin Thromb Hemost 9:139, 1983.
212. Bick RL, Kovacs I, Fekete LF: A new two stage functional assay for antithrombin III (heparin cofactor): Clinical and laboratory evaluation. Thromb Res 8:745, 1976.
213. Lackner H, Javid JP: The clinical significance of the plasminogen level. Am J Clin Pathol 60:175, 1973.
214. Tsitouris G, Bellet S, Eilberg R, et al: Effects of major surgery on plasmin-plasminogen systems. Arch Intern Med 108:98, 1961.
215. Wuelfing D, Brandau KP: Fibrinolytic activity after surgery. Minn Med 51:1503, 1968.
216. Ygge J: Changes in blood coagulation and fibrinolysis during the postoperative period. Am J Surg 119:225, 1970.
217. Bick RL, Bishop RC, Warren M, Stemmer E: Changes in fibrinolysis and fibrinolytic enzymes during extracorporeal circulation. Trans Am Soc Hematol 109, 1971.
218. Graeff H, Beller FK: Fibrinolytic activity in whole blood, dilute blood, and euglobulin lysis time tests. In Bang N, Beller FK, Deutsch E (eds): Thrombosis and Bleeding Disorders: Theory and Methods. New York, Academic Press, 1970, p 328.
219. Menon IS: A study of the possible correlation of euglobulin lysis time and dilute blood clot lysis time in the determination of fibrinolytic activity. Lab Pract 17:334, 1968.
220. Bick RL, Bishop RC, Shanbrom ES: Fibrinolytic activity in acute myocardial infarction. Am J Clin Pathol 57:359, 1972.

221. Bishop RC, Ekert H, Gilchrist G, et al: The preparation and evaluation of a standardized fibrin plate for the assessment of fibrinolytic activity. Thromb Diath Haemorrh 23:202, 1970.
222. Fareed J: New methods in hemostatic testing. In Fareed J, Messmore H, Fenton J (eds): Perspectives in Hemostasis. New York, Pergamon Press, 1981, p 310.
223. Fareed J, Messmore HL, Bermes EW: New perspectives in coagulation testing. Clin Chem 26:1380, 1980.
224. Huseby RM, Smith RE: Synthetic oligopeptide substrates: Their diagnostic application in blood coagulation, fibrinolysis, and other pathologic states. Semin Thromb Hemost 6:173, 1980.
225. Naeye RL: Thrombotic state after a hemorrhagic diathesis: A possible complication of therapy with epsilon aminocaproic acid. Blood 19:694, 1962.
226. Ratnoff OD: Epsilon aminocaproic acid: A dangerous weapon. N Engl J Med 280:1124, 1969.
227. Verska JJ, Lonser ER, Brewer LA: Predisposing factors and management of hemorrhage following open-heart surgery. J Cardiovasc Surg (Torino) 13:361, 1972.
228. Verska J: Letter to the editor. Ann Thorac Surg 13:87, 1972.
229. Brooks DH, Bahnson HT: An outbreak of hemorrhage following cardiopulmonary bypass. J Thorac Cardiovasc Surg 63:449, 1972.
230. O'Neill JA, Ende N, Collins IS, Collins HA: A quantitative determination of perfusion fibrinolysis. Surgery 60:809, 1966.
231. Bick RL, Frazier BL, Saunders CL, Arbegast NR: Alterations of hemostasis during cardiopulmonary bypass: The potential role of factor XII activation in inducing primary fibrino(geno)lysis. Blood 64:926, 1984.
232. Akkerman JW, Runne WC, Sixma JJ, Zimmerman AE: Improved survival rates in dogs after extracorporeal circulation by improved control of heparin levels. J Thorac Cardiovasc Surg 68:59, 1974.
233. Ellison N, Betty CP, Blake DR, et al: Heparin rebound: Studies in patients and volunteers. J Thorac Cardiovasc Surg 67:723, 1974.
234. Gollub S: Heparin rebound in open-heart surgery. Surg Gynecol Obstet 124:337, 1967.
235. Jaberi M, Bell WR, Benson DW: Control of heparin therapy in open-heart surgery. J Thorac Cardiovasc Surg 67:133, 1974.
236. Ellison N, Ominsky AJ, Wollman H: Is protamine a clinically important anticoagulant? A negative answer. Anesthesiology 35:621, 1971.
237. Ollendorff P: The nature of the anticoagulant effect of heparin, protamine, Polybrene, and toluidine blue. Scand J Clin Lab Invest 14:267, 1962.
238. Tsai TP, Matloff JM, Gray RJ, et al: Cardiac surgery in the octagenerian. J Thorac Surg 91:924, 1986.
239. Horneffer PJ, Gardner TJ, Manolio TA, et al: The effects of age on outcome after coronary bypass surgery. Circulation 76:V-6, 1987.
240. Soloway HB, Cornett BM, Donahoo JV, Cox SP: Differentiation of bleeding diathesis which occurs following protamine correction of heparin anticoagulation. Am J Clin Pathol 60:188, 1973.
241. Lewis JH, Wilson HJ, Brandon JM: Counterelectrophoresis test for molecules immunologically similar to fibrinogen. Am J Clin Pathol 58:400, 1972.
242. Salzman EW: The events that lead to thrombosis. Bull NY Acad Med 48:225, 1972.
243. Bick RL, Baker WF: Diagnostic efficacy of the D-dimer assay in DIC and related disorders. Blood 68:329, 1986.
244. Rousou JA, Engelman RM, Breyer RH: Fibrin glue: An effective hemostatic agent for nonsuturable intraoperative bleeding. Ann Thorac Surg 38:409, 1984.
245. Rousou J: Randomized clinical trial of fibrin glue sealant in patients undergoing resternotomy or reoperation after cardiac operations: A multicenter study. J Thorac Surg 97:194, 1989.
246. Garcia-Rinaldi R, Simmons P, Salcedo V, Howland C: A technique for spot application of fibrin glue during open heart operations. Ann Thorac Surg 47:59, 1989.
247. Dresdale A, Bowman FO, Malm JR, et al: Hemostatic effectiveness of fibrin glue derived from single-donor fresh frozen plasma. Ann Thorac Surg 40:385, 1985.
248. Verstraete M: Clinical application of inhibitors of fibrinolysis. Drugs 29:236, 1985.

**L. Henry Edmunds, Jr., MD**

# 2

# Cardiopulmonary Bypass and Blood

Cardiopulmonary bypass (CPB) is prerequisite for open heart surgery and has the potential to sustain circulatory and respiratory function indefinitely. However, CPB makes patients sick and is associated with unique complications that increase morbidity and mortality. Blood mediates most of the trouble, because only blood touches the plastic and metal surfaces of the heart-lung machine. CPB causes massive fluid retention and intercompartmental fluid shifts,[28,104] multiple organ dysfunction,[1,3,105,106,111] showers of emboli,[82] and unique bleeding complications.[43] Blood is circulated without a pulse[44] by a mechanical pump that is independent of physiologic controls. Intravascular pressures stray outside normal ranges. Blood elements are activated; plasma proteins are diluted and denatured; contaminants and foreign materials are introduced. A host of vasoactive substances[39] that affect capillary permeability[116] and vasomotor tone are generated. Temporary dysfunction of nearly every organ ensues. A massive defense reaction—aptly termed "the whole-body inflammatory response"—is initiated.[12] Homeostasis becomes chaos.

## Heparin

CPB is not possible without heparin, but heparin is not an ideal anticoagulant. Heparin acts near the end of the coagulation cascade, not at the beginning. This is a serious deficiency because the coagulation cascade is a series of enzymatic reactions that are amplified and accelerated at each step. Consequently, a number of powerful serine proteases are produced during CPB, even though clotting does not occur. Heparin prevents clotting by activating the natural plasma protein, antithrombin III (AT-III). AT-III is a large (62,000 daltons), abundant (290 $\mu$g/ml) plasma protease inhibitor of factors IXa, Xa, and thrombin. AT-III primarily complexes with thrombin; inhibition of factor Xa is partial and even less with factor IXa. Heparin accelerates the action of AT-III approximately 1000-fold to achieve a second-order rate constant for thrombin of $3.7 \times 10^7$/M/s.[103] Thus AT-III–heparin

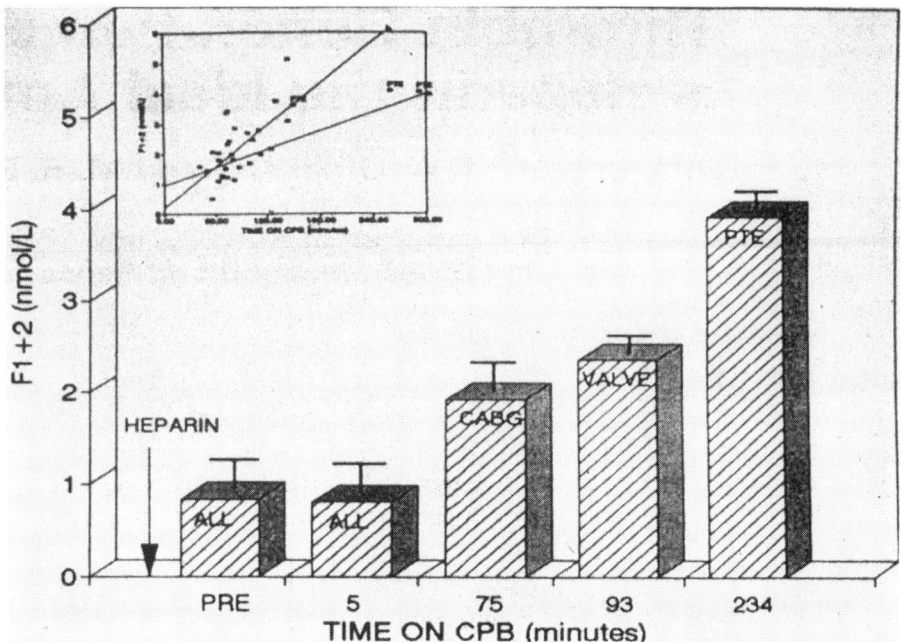

**FIGURE 1.** Plasma prothrombin fragment F1.2 concentrations (mean ± SEM) in patients before, during, and after CPB stratified for coronary artery bypass grafting (CABG), valve repair/replacement (VALVE), and pulmonary thromboendarterectomy (PTE). (From Brister SJ, Ofosu FA, Buchanan MR: Thrombin generation during cardiac surgery: Is heparin the ideal anticoagulant? Thromb Haemost 70:259–262, 1993; with permission.)

inhibits soluble thrombin very rapidly but does not become part of the complex. After the reaction, heparin is released to catalyze another coupling and the AT-III–thrombin complex is excreted through liver and kidney. AT-III–heparin does not inhibit thrombin bound to fibrin and cannot prevent thrombin activation of platelets and fibrinogen conversion within clots.[134]

Despite activated clotting times over 400 seconds, thrombin is progressively formed during CPB in every patient (Fig. 1).[16,20] CPB produces a massive thrombotic stimulus that overwhelms the ability of AT-III–heparin to prevent thrombin production and circulation. F1.2, a marker of the conversion of prothrombin to thrombin, and fibrinopeptide A, a fragment produced by conversion of fibrinogen to fibrin, increase progressively during CPB despite very rapid inhibition of thrombin and partial inhibition of factor Xa. As discussed below, thrombin is not a nice enzyme to circulate.

Hirudin is a natural protein produced by leeches and is now available in various forms from recombinant technology. Hirudin is a rapid, tight-binding thrombin inhibitor that can inhibit clot-bound thrombin. However, in extracorporeal perfusion systems, the drug is less effective than heparin in suppressing thrombin formation.[8] This is probably because hirudin has no effect on factor Xa. Low-molecular-weight heparins are less effective thrombin inhibitors and better factor Xa inhibitors than standard heparin.

Heparin has additional drawbacks. Heparin preparations vary in anticoagulant effectiveness. Heparin also increases the sensitivity of platelets to various agonists.[47]

Heparin-induced thrombocytopenia is a serious postoperative problem for some patients (2–5%),[77] and on rare occasions, heparin-induced thrombosis is a catastrophic problem.[71] Heparin also contributes to the activation of neutrophils[133]; the heparin–protamine complex is a major stimulus to complement activation.[23] Thus, heparin is not an ideal anticoagulant, but it is the only one we have.

## Initial Events in the CPB-Related Coagulation

When heparinized blood touches a nonendotheial cell surface, plasma proteins are instantaneously adsorbed onto the surface to produce a protein layer approximately 200 Angstroms thick.[4] The chemical and physical characteristics of this surface influence the amounts and distribution of surface-adsorbed proteins, but so far no physical or chemical attribute or attributes predict the molecular topography of the resulting protein mosaic.[5,122] All nonendothelial cell surfaces produce a thrombotic stimulus, but the intensity of the stimulus seems to vary between surfaces; some materials stimulate thrombosis more slowly than others.[5] Surface-bound heparin, which carries a negative charge, may be one of these "thromboresistant" surfaces, but the mechanism may be due to the pattern of surface-adsorbed proteins on top of buried heparin molecules rather than to heparin contact with flowing blood. Beyond the need for smoothness and chemical inertness, the physical and chemical characteristics of surfaces that reduce the thrombotic stimulus are not defined.

The amounts of adsorbed proteins are not proportional to bulk plasma concentrations. Fibrinogen is selectively adsorbed, but the amounts vary between synthetic materials.[122] Hydrophobic surfaces adsorb more fibrinogen than hydrophilic materials.[122] Adsorbed fibrinogen, however, rapidly undergoes conformational changes, so that antifibrinogen antibody is no longer recognized.[19] In addition, some adsorbed fibrinogen is rapidly displaced by an activated form of high-molecular-weight (HMW) kininogen.[19] Other plasma proteins are also adsorbed. Albumin, factor XII, prekallikrein, HMW kininogen, von Willebrand factor, fibronectin, thrombospondin, hemoglobin, and immunoglobulins all adsorb onto the surface in various amounts that differ between surfaces.[138] In general, amounts of specific proteins adsorbed to specific synthetic surfaces differ if the surface is exposed to plasma or to purified protein solutions. A dynamic equilibrium between circulating and adsorbed surface proteins is quickly established for each synthetic material. Over time, adsorbed proteins desorb or are degraded and replaced by new proteins.[138]

## Activation of Blood Elements

CPB activates at least five plasma protein systems and five "blood cells" during perfusion of heparinized blood. The vasoactive substances, enzymes, and microemboli produced by activation of these protein systems and cells mediate much of the morbidity associated with CPB.

**Contact System.** The contact system consists of four primary plasma proteins: factors XII and XI, prekallikrein, and HMW kininogen.[30] When blood contacts a nonendothelial-cell negatively charged surface, factor XII cleaves into XIIa and factor XIIf. Prekallikrein and HMW kininogen must be present. Surface-adsorbed proteins provide sufficient negative charges to activate factor XII. The activated forms of factor XII are serine proteases and directly initiate activation of the intrinsic coagulation pathway, complement, and neutrophils. Activation of the extrinsic coagulation pathway and monocytes is not, at present, throught to be related to activation of the contact system.[42]

In the presence of prekallikrein and HMW kininogen, factor XIIa cleaves prekallikrein to produce kallikrein.[30] Kallikrein greatly accelerates cleavage of factor XII in a feedback loop and thus amplifies activation of the contact system. Kallikrein is also involved in other important reactions initiated by activation of the contact proteins and directly activates neutrophils.

**Intrinsic Coagulation Pathway.** In the presence of HMW kininogen, factor XIIa also activates factor XI, the fourth protein of the contact system. Activation of factor XI to factor XIa initiates the intrinsic coagulation pathway that proceeds through factor IX to activate factor X. Factor Xa converts prothrombin to thrombin. Thrombin catalyzes the conversion of fibrinogen to fibrin but is also an agonist for platelets and endothelial cells.[113] The reactions outlined above that culminate in activation of factor X represent the intrinsic coagulation pathway. This pathway provides the major coagulation stimulus during all applications of extracorporeal perfusion technology.

**Extrinsic Coagulation Pathway.** Until recently, the extrinsic coagulation pathway was not thought to be important during CPB. This pathway is the major pathway that provides hemostasis in wounds. Although there is overlap of the two pathways,[42] the intrinsic pathway is not particularly involved in wound hemostasis. However, open heart operations produce a sizable wound that produces tissue factor. There is also evidence of tissue factor expression that tissue factor is present in blood aspirated from the pericardial well during CPB.[119] Tissue factor is an integral membrane glycoprotein that is present and expressed on most nonvascular cells and is induced by various agonists in endothelial cells and monocytes. Tissue factor rapidly binds to factor VII and VIIa to initiate the extrinsic pathway that proceeds to activate factor X.[42] Factor X, produced by both the intrinsic and extrinsic coagulation pathways, is the gateway protein of the common coagulation pathway.

**Complement.** The fourth plasma protein system activated during extracorporeal perfusion is the complement system.[24] Like the coagulation system, two separate pathways activate the gateway complement protein C3 to form C3a and C3b. Factor XIIa, produced by the contact system, activates C1 of the classical pathway. The alternative system, thought to be the principal complement activation pathway during CPB,[24] is activated by generation of C3b by the classical pathway or by hydrolysis of a third bond of C3.[114] Plasma factor B binds to C3b. Factor D, which circulates in its active state, cleaves bound factor B to produce C3bBb. C3bBb activates C5 to C5a and C5b. C5a directly activates neutrophils, C5b initiates formation of the membrane attack complex that is capable of producing cell lysis and death.

There is also direct evidence of complement activation by the classical pathway during CPB.[133] The classical pathway requires three complement proteins, C1, C2 and C4, which in sequential steps form C4b2a, which in turn cleaves C3 to form C3a and C3b.[114] C4b2a, with the help of C3b, also activates C5 to form C5a and C5b. The classical pathway proceeds in sequential steps, but the alternative pathway contains a feedback loop that serves to amplify complement activation.

Both the alternative and classical pathways are activated during CPB, but amplification of the alternative system predominates. C4a, a product of the classical pathway, does not increase during CPB but does increase afterwards.[67]

C3a and terminal complement proteins[25] increase progressively during CPB. Protamine also activates complement.[78,133] C3a and C5a, produced during CPB, and C4a, produced by the heparin–protamine complex, are anaphylatoxins which have vasoactive properties. C3a also impairs cardiac function.[35] C5a activates neutrophils.[25] Complement activation during CPB is associated with significant morbidity.[79]

**Fibrinolysis.** The fifth plasma protein system activated during CPB is the fibrinolytic system. During CPB, endothelial cells stimulated by thrombin[88] produce tissue plasminogen activator (tPA),[59] which cleaves plasminogen to plasmin. tPA primarily activates plasminogen adsorbed onto fibrin. Fibrinolysis, as demonstrated by detection of plasma D-dimer,[59] occurs during and after open heart surgery.

**Platelets.** Platelets do not contain a nucleus but, as cellular structures, are activated during CPB and extracorporeal perfusion. The degree of activation and the effect of a decrease in platelet numbers and function on bleeding time and wound hemostasis appear to vary between perfusion systems and patients[43,139] and are currently under active investigation.[75]

Platelets are probably activated during CPB by thrombin, but this has not been proved. Thrombin is a potent platelet agonist, stimulates a specific platelet membrane receptor,[32] and is produced during CPB. Once activated, platelets undergo shape change, aggregate, adhere to synthetic surfaces, and release granule contents and cause an increase in bleeding times.[43,139]

During CPB, platelets adhere to binding sites located on the alpha chain and C terminal domain of the gamma chain of surface-adsorbed fibrinogen.[135] The attachment of platelets to synthetic surfaces primarily involves the glycoprotein (GP) IIb/IIIa receptor complex (fibrinogen receptor)[56] and does not involve the GPIb receptor. Platelet adhesion occurs almost instantly,[109] but the density of platelet accumulation varies with the chemical and physical attributes of the surface.[89,109] Rough surfaces accumulate more platelets than smooth surfaces.[38] Platelet adhesion, platelet aggregation, and blood dilution are the major causes of thrombocytopenia during CPB.

Platelets also form aggregates which circulate and form microemboli.[42] Activated platelets with exposed GPIIb/IIIa receptor complexes bind together using bridges of fibrinogen. Platelets also express GMP-140 receptors and form aggregates with circulating monocytes and, to a lesser extent, neutrophils, but not with lymphocytes.[107]

During CPB, aggregation studies indicate decreased platelet sensitivity to various agonists, but studies utilizing whole blood flow cytometry do not suggest a decrease.[75] A small percentage of platelets, both attached and circulating, release granule contents. Alpha granules contain several coagulation proteins, including HMW kininogen, von Willebrand factor, and thrombospondin, platelet factor 4, and factors that increase capillary permeability and smooth muscle cell proliferation and attract neutrophils. Dense granules contain ADP and ATP, calcium, and serotonin. Lysosomes contain potent acid hydrolases and neutral proteases. Release of these granules[2] into the circulation contributes to the systemic inflammatory response.

Activated platelets also synthesize and release thromboxane $A_2$, a potent vasoconstrictor and powerful platelet agonist. Thromboxane $A_2$ is the product of arachidonic acid metabolism, which requires cyclooxygenase to produce prostaglandin $G_2$ and $H_2$, the precursors of thromboxane and prostacyclin. Platelets primarily produce thromboxane $A_2$, which has a critical role in platelet hemostasis and a half-life in plasma of approximately 30 seconds. Most studies show an increase in plasma thromboxane $B_2$ during CPB.[48] Aspirin, by inhibiting cyclooxygenase, inhibits thromboxane $A_2$ production for the life of the platelet.

As perfusion continues, some adherent platelets detach, leaving behind fragments of platelet membrane.[135] Platelet membrane fragments also detach and circulate.[55] Some studies indicate a decrease in mean GPIb, GPIIb/IIIa (Fig. 2), and adrenergic receptors[130,135] of circulating platelets, but recent flow cytometry studies show little change in the mean numbers of platelet membrane receptors.[75]

At the end of CPB, the platelet population is a heterogeneous mixture that probably varies between patients and perfusion systems. Hemodilution, adhesion, aggregation, release, and destruction reduce platelet number by 30–50% (43,139). Some platelets are intact and discoid; others show pseudopod formation.[139] Some larger platelets recently arrived from the bone marrow are present.[84] Partially and completely degranulated platelets are also present, as are platelet membrane

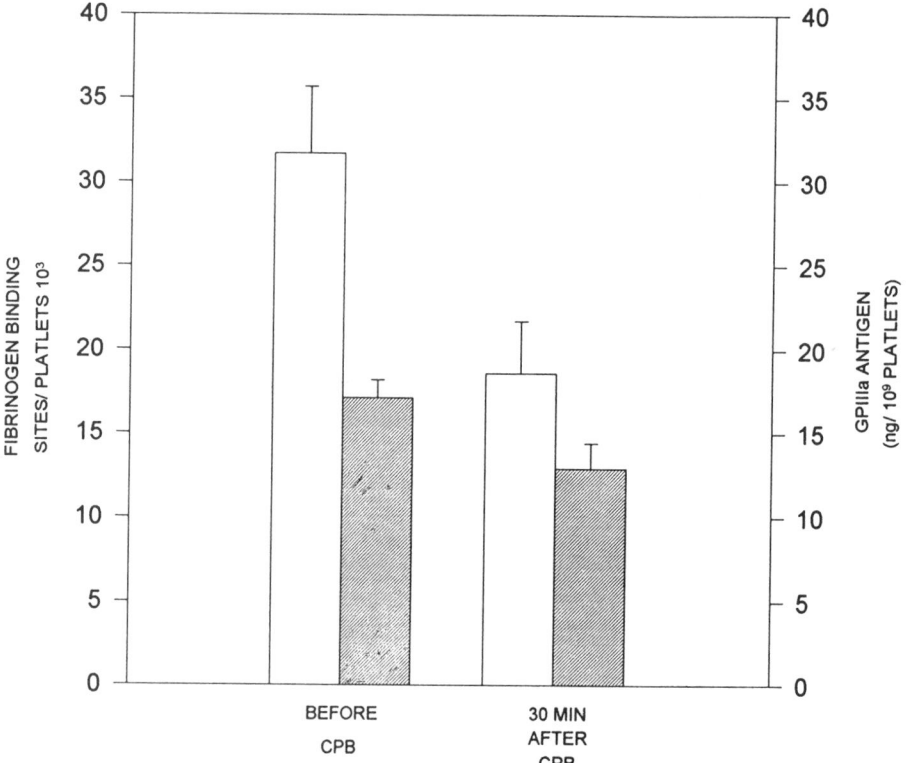

**FIGURE 2.** Mean number of fibrinogen binding sites per platelet (*open bars*) and GPIIIa antigen (*cross-hatched bars*) before and 30 minutes after the start of CPB in 10 patients. Error bars indicate SEM. (Adapted from Wenger RK, Lukasiewicz H, Mikuta BS, et al: Loss of platelet fibrinogen receptors during clinical cardiopulmonary bypass. J Thorac Cardiovasc Surg 97:235–239, 1989.)

fragments and resealed platelets. The majority of the reduced numbers of platelets appear morphologically normal.[139]

The functional state of the circulating intact platelet during and early after CPB is reduced, but it is not clear whether this functional defect is intrinsic or extrinsic to the platelet. Heparin increases bleeding times,[75] but bleeding times remain prolonged for several hours after protamine is given following CPB. Analysis of shed blood from bleeding time wounds shows reduced platelet sensitivity to agonists and reduced concentrations of plasma thromboxane $B_2$.[75] Using immunochemistry, Wenger and colleagues[135] found reduced numbers of GPIIb/IIIa receptors per platelet; using flow cytometry, Kestin and coinvestigators[75] found little change in mean numbers of platelet membrane receptors. More recently, Ferraris et al.[51] found evidence of temporary down-regulation of platelet thrombin receptors during CPB. The relative contributions of extrinsic platelet inhibition and intrinsic change of the circulating platelets during CPB are under active investigation.[98] Regardless of the cause, the end result is an increase in bleeding times during and immediately after CPB.[43,137] Bleeding times usually return to the normal range within 4–12 hours.

**Neutrophils.** During CPB, leukocyte counts decrease in response to dilution and then increase moderately after operation. Only a few neutrophils attach to synthetic surfaces and platelets. Several agonists activate circulating neutrophils during CPB: C3a, C5a,[61] kallikrein, factor XIIa, and, less strongly, neutrophil-activating peptide 2 (NAP-2) from platelets. The Mac-1 receptor, which is a cell adhesive protein, is also upregulated during CPB[73,96] and probably is involved in site-directed inflammation. Mac-1 (CD11b/18CR3) receptors also bind various coagulation proteins and may have a role in thrombogenesis.[73]

Neutrophils contain a variety of enzymes and cytotoxic substances and are responsible for much of the inflammatory response of CPB. During CPB, neutrophils release elastase and myeloperoxidase from azurophilic granules and lactoferrin and from specific granules.[49,132] In a "respiratory burst," activated neutrophils produce and release highly cytotoxic reactive oxygen molecules that include hydroxyl radicals, hydrogen peroxide, and hypobromous and hypochlorous acids.[24] Neutrophils also produce, store, and release several lysosomal enzymes and neutral proteases that are cytotoxic. CPB induces activated neutrophils to accumulate in the lungs, where they increase capillary permeability and interstitial edema.[33,106]

**Monocytes.** Monocytes are also activated during CPB. Monocytes produce and release cytokines which increase during and after extracorporeal perfusion. Interleukin-8 (IL-8) increases during CPB,[52] and IL-1, IL-2, IL-4, and IL-6 all increase after bypass.[60,117] Plasma concentrations of tumor necrosis factor (TNF) vary between studies after CPB: some studies show an increase, but others do not.[60,117] Generation of complement C3b may be a mechanism by which monocytes are activated.

Monocytes also express tissue factor and upregulate Mac-1 receptors during simulated extracorporeal perfusion of human blood.[72] Tissue factor is the procoagulant protein that initiates the extrinsic coagulation pathway. Monocytic tissue factor expression has not been demonstrated during clinical CPB, possibly because expression by activated monocytes is delayed for 2 or more hours.

**Endothelial Cells.** Endothelial cells are the fourth "blood cell" activated by CPB. Endothelial cells, of course, do not circulate but are in constant contact with blood over a surface area estimated to be between 1000–5000 m² in an adult.[69] Endothelial cells maintain the fluidity of blood, influence vascular tone, and maintain the integrity of the vascular system by active metabolic processes.[69] Endothelial cells produce prostacyclin, heparan sulfate (which accelerates AT-III), thrombomodulin and protease nexin 1 (both of which bind and remove thrombin), protein S (which accelerates the natural anticoagulant protein C), tissue factor pathway inhibitor (which inhibits the tissue factor–factor VIIa complex), and tissue plasminogen activator (tPA). Endothelial cells produce vasoactive substances, such as nitrous oxide and endothelin-1,[124] and inactivate others, such as histamine, norepinephrine, and bradykinin.[69] During CPB, endothelial cells produce tPA, probably in response to thrombin.[88] Plasminogen activator inhibitor increases only slightly. CPB causes a sharp increase in prostacyclin at the beginning of perfusion; thereafter, plasma concentrations of this short-acting eicosanoid decrease.[48] CPB also increases plasma concentrations of endothelin-1, which peak approximately 4 hours after bypass.[63] There is also evidence that platelet-activating factor (PAF) increases during and after CPB.[66]

**Lymphocytes.** CPB decreases the total number of lymphocytes and specific subsets of lymphocytes. CPB increases plasma concentrations of prostaglandin $E_2$, which is an inhibitor of certain T-cell lymphocytic functions and the ability of monocytes to present antigen and to synthesize IL-1.[94] CPB decreases B lymphocytes, natural killer cells, T-helper cells, and T-suppressor lymphocytes for 3–7 days.[37] Responses to various agonists and mitogens are depressed; IL-2, gamma-interferon production, and expression of CD4+ and IL-2 receptors by T lymphocytes are reduced.[37] Changes in lymphocytes, cytokines, complement proteins, and immunoglobulins and reduced white cell phagocytosis after CPB increase the susceptibility of postoperative patients to infection.

## Consequences of Blood Activation during CPB

### Bleeding

Nonsurgical bleeding complications associated with CPB are related to heparin, platelets, and fibrinolysis. Deficiency of soluble coagulation factors is a rare cause of bleeding during and after open heart surgery. Priming fluids dilute soluble coagulation factors in proportion to the decrease in hematocrit, but none of the soluble coagulation factors reaches concentrations that are likely to cause bleeding if plasma concentrations were normal before operation.[62] Bleeding due to reduced plasma coagulation proteins is most likely seen in patients with congenital or acquired coagulation protein deficiencies, uremia, or severe cachexia and in infants or children with deep cyanosis, polycythemia, and reduced plasma volumes.

Several CPB-related bleeding problems are related to heparin, including AT-III deficiency, heparin-induced thrombocytopenia, and inadequate heparin neutralization.

Healthy newborns have about one-half of the adult concentrations of AT-III. Infants with liver disease, cathectic babies, and prematures have even less. AT-III covalently binds with thrombin and is consumed, but heparin is not. Plasma thrombin–AT-III complexes increase progressively during CPB in direct proportion to the duration of perfusion.[16,20] If the standard dose of heparin (3 mg/kg) prior to

CPB in a cachectic patient fails to increase the activated clotting to over 400 s (750 s if aprotinin is used with celite[68]), AT-III deficiency may be the cause. Likewise, if the activated clotting time falls below 400 s during CPB despite addition of heparin, AT-III concentrations may be inadequate. Fresh frozen plasma is all that is required.

Heparin-induced thrombocytopenia occurs in 2–5% of the population.[77] In these patients, exposure to heparin, even as little as 5 mg/day in "heparin flushes" induces IgG antibodies against the Fc receptor of the platelet membrane.[74] Continued or subsequent exposure to heparin activates platelets and produces thrombocytopenia with platelet counts below 50,000/$\mu$l, usually 5–10 days after the exposure. The major concern is bleeding; the condition should be distinguished from heparin-induced thrombocytopenia and thrombosis, which may or may not be related. Treatment of heparin-induced thrombocytopenia requires stopping heparin and giving platelet transfusions to prevent internal bleeding.

At the end of CPB, heparin is neutralized by protamine. The heparin–protamine complex formed by the ionic bond between the large negatively-charged heparin molecule and the small positively-charged protamine peptide strongly activates complement.[78] The anaphylatoxins C3a, C4a, and C5a are produced and, in approximately 50% of patients, cause transient hypotension and reduced cardiac output.[110] Anaphylatoxins also cause vasodilation, cardiac dysfunction,[35] and an increase in capillary permeability and stimulate mast cells and basophils to release histamine. In rare instances, protamine causes anaphylaxis in diabetics who have taken protamine insulin or in those who have fish allergies. In even rarer instances, administration of protamine causes synthesis and release of thromboxane $A_2$ from platelets and severe pulmonary vasoconstriction.[91]

Following CPB, protamine may not be given in sufficient amounts to neutralize heparin fully. Heparin is cleared from the circulation by the reticuloendothelial system, but rates of clearance vary widely between patients and are influenced by many other factors (e.g., hypothermia). Different schemes are used to estimate the protamine dose required to neutralize heparin, but the simplest is to give 1 mg of protamine for each milligram of heparin given during the entire operation. The activated clotting time is remeasured, and if prolonged, an additional 50 mg of protamine is given. In very high doses, protamine is a weak anticoagulant; however, this is not a clinical concern.[137] Therefore, if "heparin rebound" is suspected, additional protamine doses can be given safely in the early postoperative period without laboratory verification.[70]

The deficiency in platelet numbers and function after CPB is a major cause of postoperative bleeding. Thrombocytopenia is due to dilution, platelet adhesion to circuit surfaces, aggregation, and activation and removal of damaged platelets by the reticuloendothelial system. At the end of CPB, platelet counts are usually above 100,000 platelets/$\mu$l but are 30–50% lower than preoperative values.[43,139] Bleeding times are approximately double the pre-bypass values. Over the next few hours, platelet counts do not change consistently, but bleeding times shorten progressively as new platelets enter the circulation.[84] Bleeding times return to normal within 4–12 hours; platelet counts reach the normal range in 3–7 days.

During CPB, endothelial cells produce tPA, which primarily converts fibrin-bound plasminogen to plasmin.[59] Although most plasmin is bound, production of D-dimer,[59] a marker fragment from lysed fibrin, indicates that plasmin also circulates. Whether plasmin circulates or not is less important than lysis of bound fibrin, which tends to increase bleeding. The success of antifibrinolytic agents in reducing postoperative blood losses in groups of patients suggests that fibrinolysis contributes

**TABLE 1.**  Causes of Emboli in CPB

| | |
|---|---|
| Gas (nitrogen, oxygen) | Leukocyte aggregates |
| Fibrin | Red cell debris |
| Fat (free fat, denatured lipoproteins, chylomicrons) | Foreign material (calcium, tissue debris, fibrin, clot, fat, etc.) |
| Denatured protein | Spallated material (primarily roller pumps) |
| Platelet aggregates | |

to bleeding. To be effective, antifibrinolytic agents must be given at the beginning of surgery to prevent binding of plasminogen to fibrin.[65]

## Emboli and Thrombi

CPB produces a variety of large and small emboli that can be reduced but not totally prevented by present technology[45] (Table 1). A 40-$\mu$m (pore size) arterial line filter removes macroemboli; filters with smaller pore sizes increase the pressure difference across the filter and interfere with pump flow. During CPB, arterioles, precapillaries, and capillaries are bombarded with microemboli, but the architecture and redundancy of the microcirculation tend to minimize the damage. Macroemboli (40–400 $\mu$m) cause more ischemic damage than microemboli ($< 40$ $\mu$m). The number of vessels $< 40$ $\mu$m in diameter is incalculable; thus cell death produced by microemboli is diffusely distributed and involves relatively few cells in any one location. For the most part, microembolization during CPB is not detected but can be documented histologically. Some of the observed optic and central nervous system dysfunction early after CPB is probably due to microembolization.[15]

Despite large doses of heparin and activated clotting times over 400 s, thrombin and fibrin are produced during CPB. The amounts of both are directly proportional to the duration of CPB.[16] Rough surfaces, areas of turbulence and cavitation, and recesses of stagnant flow within the perfusion system enhance fibrin formation. Fibrin emboli can be found in the brain by histologic methods after CPB.[64]

Gas microemboli are common during CPB but are less common in centrifugal pump and membrane oxygenator systems. Oxygen and carbon dioxide microbubbles are most commonly produced during *cooling* for deep hypothermia. Because nitrogen is poorly soluble in blood, air is more dangerous than oxygen or carbon dioxide. Air may enter the perfusion system via the cardiotomy sucker system or through partially opened stopcocks. Loose connections or pursestring sutures are another source of venous air emboli. Massive air embolism is a rare but catastrophic event.

Fat emboli, denatured protein material, and platelet and leukocyte aggregates can also block the microcirculation.[45] Fat emboli consist of denatured lipoproteins, aggregates of chylomicrons, or free fat composed of cholesterol or triglycerides. Platelet and leukocyte aggregates may or may not dissociate in the microcirculation; the amount of ischemic damage caused by these particles is unknown.

There are numerous sources of foreign emboli.[45] Blood aspirated from the surgical field by the cardiotomy sucker system may contain fat, fibrin, calcium, bits of muscle, tissue debris, powder, bone wax, or even suture material. Donor blood, even after filtration, contains microemboli of platelet and leukocyte aggregates, lysed red cells, and fibrin and lipid precipitates. Even washed cells aspirated from the surgical field may contain small amounts of fat, fibrin, and cellular debris. Emboli are also generated from the perfusion system. Antifoam compounds used in bubble oxygenators and industrial dusts produced during manufacture may become emboli. Lastly, spallation from tubing compressed by roller pumps can produce both macro and microemboli.

Thrombosis during CPB can occur if the heparin dose is inadequate. In patients with septicemia, additional heparin may be advisable, because uncontrolled infection is a powerful thrombotic stimulus. There is no rationale for giving inadequate doses of heparin (activated clotting times < 400 s) to reduce bleeding; such practice risks catastrophic thrombosis and is more likely to increase bleeding than to decrease it.

Heparin-induced thrombocytopenia and thrombosis is a rare condition wherein arterial and/or venous thrombosis develops upon exposure to heparin. These patients usually have a history of a thrombotic event with exposure to heparin. When suspected, the diagnosis in the presence of heparin-induced platelet antibodies can be determined by measuring serotonin release or platelet aggregation when the patient's plasma is incubated with donor platelets.[71] Plasma from patients with heparin-induced thrombocytopenia (HIT) and heparin-induced thrombocytopenia and thrombosis (HITT) both contain heparin-induced antiplatelet antibodies, but it is unclear whether the latter disorder is a severe manifestation of the former. Patients with heparin-induced antibodies to platelets who require open heart surgery should receive full doses of heparin and one of several strategies to inhibit platelet activation during CPB.[71]

## Vasoactive Substances and Endotoxin

CPB initiates a massive defense reaction that results in the production and release of a host of vasoactive hormones, autacoids, and cytokines[39] (Table 2). Most of these potent substances do not normally circulate but act only on local, specific cellular receptors. However, during CPB, vasoactive chemicals circulate[39] and alter blood pressure and distribution, vascular permeability, fluid balance, and myocardial contractility. The massive production and release of vasoactive molecules during CPB mediate the whole-body inflammatory response[12] and much of the morbidity associated with open heart surgery.

Endotoxins are structural fragments of bacteria that, like CPB, trigger the body's defense reaction. Lipopolysaccharides derived from the walls of gram-negative bacteria are particularly powerful agonists. Endotoxins have been detected during CPB using the sensitive but nonspecific lumulus amebocyte lysate test.[102] However, at present, the role of endotoxins in the defense reaction associated with CPB is not clearly defined.[102]

**TABLE 2.** Vasoactive Substances Altered during Extracorporeal Perfusion

| Hormones | Autacoids |
| --- | --- |
| Epinephrine, norepinephrine | Platelet activating factor |
| Renin, angiotensin II | Prostacyclin, thromboxane $A_2$, |
| Vasopressin, aldosterone | prostaglandin $E_2$ |
| Atrial natriuretic factor | Endothelin-1, nitric oxide, serotonin, |
| Bradykinin | histamine |
| Glucagon | Leukotrienes B4, C4, D4 |
| Thyroid hormones (triiodothyronine, | Proteases |
| thyroxine) | Free oxygen radicals |
| Complement: C3a, C4a, C5a | Lysosomal enzymes |
| Electrolytes: $Ca^{2+}$, $Mg^{2+}$, $K^+$ | Interleukins 1, 2, 4, 6, 8 |

## Fluid Balance

Although blood flow during CPB is essentially pulseless, blood distribution to major organs and tissues is minimally, if at all, affected.[18] In animals, pulseless blood flow provided by an artificial heart is compatible with survival for several weeks.[57] Despite numerous and careful studies, no conclusive evidence of the superiority of pulsatile CPB has been demonstrated.[44]

CPB, however, causes massive fluid retention and intercompartmental fluid shifts. Many factors contribute to fluid retention. Intermittent or sustained increases in systemic venous pressure raise capillary filtration pressure. Hemodilution dilutes plasma protein concentrations and decreases colloid osmotic pressure. Capillary permeability increases due to circulating vasoactive substances such as bradykinin, complement anaphylatoxins, leukotrienes, histamine, free oxygen radicals, proteases, cytokines, lysosomal enzymes, and other chemicals.[39] These molecules contract endothelial cells and widen intercellular junctions. The coefficient for Starling's law of fluid exchange across capillaries increases,[116] enabling water, electrolytes, and small molecules to pour into the extracellular compartment. As compared to normothermic perfusions, hypothermia tends to reduce fluid accumulation. CPB does not alter intracellular fluid balance.[21]

The increase in interstitial fluid is restrained by dilution of interstitial proteins and by increases in interstitial fluid pressure. Interstitial fluid pressure is influenced by the rapidity of lymph flow and by the compliance of the interstitial space,[97] which varies for different organs and tissues.

Renal function during CPB has little immediate effect on overall fluid balance, but it has important prognostic significance for later fluid management. The need to optimize cardiac filling pressures and cardiac performance focuses attention on intravascular pressures. Colloids and blood products necessary to control bleeding preempt concerns about the swollen interstitial compartment, which may increase by 18–33%.[104] Diuresis begins with restoration of a normal Starling's coefficient, a good cardiac output, and control of bleeding.

## Organ Dysfunction

It is difficult to separate cardiac dysfunction due to CPB from that due to the disease being treated, operative manipulations, and the early consequences of surgery on ventricular mechanics and myocyte metabolism. However, CPB does produce the negative inotrope C3a[35] and endothelin-1, which constricts coronary arteries. Cardioplegic hearts release neutrophil chemotactic factors[46] and intracardiac neutrophils release hydrogen peroxide[80] during and after aortic cross-clamping. Myocardial stunning is inevitable during aortic cross-clamping,[6] and in patients with diseased coronary vessels, areas of regional ischemia are likely. Both myocardial edema and distention of the flaccid cardioplegic heart[40] reduce contractility. When the heart contracts poorly, the high afterload produced by CPB during the weaning process increases wall stress and myocardial oxygen consumption.[7] The final performance of the heart depends upon many variables, and the damage caused directly by CPB is probably minor as compared to other causes.

CPB temporarily impairs lung function. Activation of complement and neutrophils causes sequestration of neutrophils in the pulmonary microvasculature.[136] Pulmonary interstitial edema increases as a result of increased pulmonary capillary permeability. Alveolar surfactant composition changes[95] and becomes less effective in maintaining alveolar stability. Atelectasis develops after CPB ends and continues to be a problem during the first 48 hours. Functional residual volume and pulmonary compliance decrease.[115] The work of breathing increases. The physiologic shunt and alveolar arterial oxygen difference increase. In occasional patients, blood extravasates into alveoli to produce the acute respiratory distress syndrome. Reduced compliance, increased atelectasis, increased work of breathing, increased shunting, and interstitial edema contribute to postoperative pulmonary dysfunction.

CPB is associated with a significant incidence of stroke and other neurologic problems. The incidence of stroke ranges between 1–5%[121] and is higher in older patients, those with severe atherosclerotic disease of the ascending aorta,[14] and patients with symptomatic carotid arterial disease.[27] The majority of strokes are embolic and related to cannulation, surgical manipulations, and CPB.[27] Ischemic brain injuries are associated primarily with operations that involve the aortic arch or circulatory arrest.

Careful neuropsychologic tests demonstrate subtle neurologic injuries in up to 50% of patients.[108,111] In some patients, deficits are temporary, but in as many as one-third of these patients, neuropsychologic deficits are still present at 1 year.[108] The etiology of CPB-related neuropsychologic deficits is believed to be primarily microemboli.

Deep hypothermia and circulatory arrest are associated with a significant number of postoperative neurologic injuries. The major causes of injury are ischemia and emboli, but excessive cooling below brain temperatures of 10–12°C may also cause postoperative neurologic dysfunction.[36]

A number of variables affect renal function during CPB, including hemodilution, circulating hormones, low perfusion pressure, prolonged perfusion, diuretics, hypothermia, microemboli, and hemolysis. Preoperative renal status and periods of low cardiac output after CPB are the most important predictors of postoperative renal insufficiency.[1] Reduced renal perfusion pressure stimulates renin release and angiotensin II production, which decreases renal blood flow. Aldosterone and vasopressin both increase to raise sodium and water resorption. Excessive hemolysis that saturates binding plasma proteins precipitates in renal tubules. Because of high renal blood flow, kidneys are bombarded with microemboli. Without hemodilution, renal blood and plasma flow, creatinine clearance, free water clearance, and urine volume decrease.[123]

Hemodilution attenuates most of the detrimental effects of CPB on renal function. Hemodilution improves outer cortical and total renal blood flow; increases creatinine, electrolyte, and water clearances; and increases glomerular filtration and urine volume.[123] After CPB, renal function, which is so important for restoration of fluid balance, largely reflects preoperative renal function, microembolic and possible ischemic injuries produced during CPB, toxic drugs, and postoperative cardiac output.

The liver, pancreas, and intestinal tract are subjected to vasoactive substances and microemboli, but clinical manifestations of damage are few. Some liver enzymes increase slightly during and early after CPB, and mild jaundice appears in 10–20% of patients.[29] The connection between CPB and occasional patients who develop severe jaundice and hepatic failure is unclear. Many patients develop a slight increase in blood amylase, but < 1% of patients develop clinical pancreatitis.[50] Gastrointestinal complications, particularly ulcers and bleeding, are postoperative concerns but are not directly related to CPB. Rare patients may develop a vasculitis of mesenteric vessels that produces severe and often fatal intestinal ischemia postoperatively; this problem may be a late manifestation of a CPB injury.[86]

## Control of the Complications of CPB

Two strategies have been developed to control the interaction of blood and synthetic surfaces of extracorporeal perfusions systems: discover or create surfaces that do not activate blood constituents, or temporarily and selectively inhibit key blood elements during the period of CPB to prevent activation by surface contact. The rationale is that reduced production of vasoactive substances and microemboli during CPB will reduce the bleeding and thrombotic complications, fluid retention, and temporary organ dysfunction associated with extracorporeal perfusion.

The endothelial cell is the only known nonthrombogenic surface and maintains the fluidity of blood by active metabolic processes. No other cell or surface is nonthrombogenic. Endothelial cells maintain a delicate balance between thrombin production and thrombin inhibition. Efforts to produce synthetic, nonthrombogenic surfaces for CPB have not succeeded, although a number of "thromboresistant" materials have been developed. Beyond the need for smoothness, no general guidelines for thromboresistance have been developed. Recent work has focused on attachment of specific chemicals (including heparin, prostaglandins, and urokinase) to synthetic materials in the hope that these chemicals will interact with flowing blood to impair coagulation.[76,83]

Heparin can be attached to certain plastic materials by ionic or covalent bonds and has been studied extensively since it was introduced in 1963.[58] Heparin-bonded plastic surfaces for catheters and entire basic CPB perfusion circuits are commercially available. The Duraflo II heparin coating (Baxter Health Care, Inc.) ionically binds standard heparin using a proprietary process that greatly retards heparin leaching into the circulation. The competing Carmeda (Medtronic, Inc.) heparinized surface covalently binds partially degraded heparin attached to "spacer arms" that are about 100 Angstroms long. Although the presence of thrombin domains 2 and 3 of bound heparin can be detected by an in vitro "thrombin inhibition test," it is not proved that the reactive sites of bound heparin are in contact with flowing blood after plasma proteins are adsorbed. Because heparin carries a strong negative charge, it is possible that the beneficial effects of surface-bound heparin are primarily due to favorable adsorbed protein topography and a paucity of exposed negative charges needed to activate factor XII. If the surface presents an attenuated stimulus to plasma contact proteins, activation of both the intrinsic coagulation pathway and complement C1 by factor XIIf (classical pathway) would be reduced. This mechanism would decrease both the amount of thrombin and C3a produced.

When heparin-coated circuits are used for several hours or for up to 7 days in animal perfusions,[11,99] macroscopic clotting does not occur and plasma fibrinogen concentrations do not fall. In vitro exposure of heparin-bound surfaces adsorbs AT-III which, in turn, binds activated factor X and thrombin.[81] Recirculation of fresh human blood containing 1 U of heparin/ml (one-fifth usual dose) through a membrane oxygenator perfusion circuit coated with Duraflo II heparin attenuates platelet adhesion and loss of function, suppresses B-thromboglobulin release, and prevents thromboxane $A_2$ synthesis as compared to an uncoated circuit and 5 U of heparin/ml.[118] In vitro studies using a different covalently bound heparin surface reduce reactivity of platelets to the surface.[90] With full-dose heparin, Carmeda-coated perfusion circuits reduce complement activation during clinical CPB for myocardial revascularization.[128]

Carmeda heparin-coated perfusion circuits have been used for treatment of trauma victims, certain operations on the descending thoracic aorta, postoperative circulatory assistance, and long-term perfusions for respiratory insufficiency.[3] More recently, Duraflo II circuits have been used with one-half doses of systemic heparin for clinical myocardial revascularization operations.[17,129] In view of the fact that thrombin is formed during every operation with full doses of heparin, a risk of catastrophic clotting exists.[26] Reduced systemic heparin is not recommended until the ability of surface-bound heparin has been shown to reduce concentrations of circulating thrombin.

The alternative strategy to control activation of blood elements during CPB by selective inhibition of key blood elements is closest to fruition with platelets. Several reversible platelet inhibitors are available to prevent platelet interaction with the CPB circuit during operations. Dipyridamole weakly inhibits platelet function and can partially preserve platelets during CPB,[120] but it is not quickly reversible because of a long plasma half-life.[53] The prostaglandins are effective, quickly reversible platelet inhibitors but are also powerful vasodilators and must be used with continuous infusion of a vasoconstrictor to maintain blood pressure.[71] The disintegrins are reversible, platelet fibrinogen receptor antagonists that inhibit the platelet GPIIb/IIIa receptor to prevent platelet adhesion and aggregation.[100] These compounds all contain an RGD (Arg-Gly-Asp) amino acid sequence that recognizes the platelet receptor. Studies with both a natural peptide[112] or a peptidomimetic[22] inhibit platelet aggregation and adhesion but are not as effective in suppressing thrombin activation.[9] However, prostanoids and disintegrins act synergistically, and combinations may prove effective in protecting platelets during CPB without side effects.[9]

In 1989, Bidstrup and colleagues[10] introduced **aprotinin** for cardiac surgery and demonstrated a 50% reduction in postoperative bleeding and a similar reduction in the need for blood and blood product transfusions. They observed that the drug reduced postoperative bleeding times but had no effect on platelet count. Many others have confirmed these findings.[13,87]

Aprotinin is a natural serine protease inhibitor that strongly inhibits plasmin ($K_i = 2.3 \times 10^{-10}$ mol/L), weakly inhibits kallikrein ($K_i = 3.0 \times 10^{-8}$ mol/L),[54] and even more weakly inhibits factor XIIa[85] and factor VIIa–tissue factor complex.[23] Plasma concentrations of 4–10 kIU of aprotinin completely inhibit plasmin, but 250–400 kIU are required to completely inhibit kallikrein.[54] The high-dose (Hammersmith) protocol (4 mg/kg load, 4 mg/kg in prime, and 2 mg/kg/hr)[10] achieves an initial plasma concentration of approximately 180 kIU/ml and decreases over 1 hour to 80–100 kIU/ml.[125] Thus clinical doses of aprotinin only partially inhibit kallikrein. If aprotinin is given with the incision, the potency of the drug is sufficient to inhibit plasmin generated by wound-produced thrombin before it attaches to fibrin. Numerous studies have shown that aprotinin reduces fibrinolysis during and after CPB.[13,92] Despite low potency, the drug partially inhibits kallikrein-mediated activation of the intrinsic coagulation pathway, complement, and neutrophils[131] and thus attenuates the "whole-body inflammatory response."

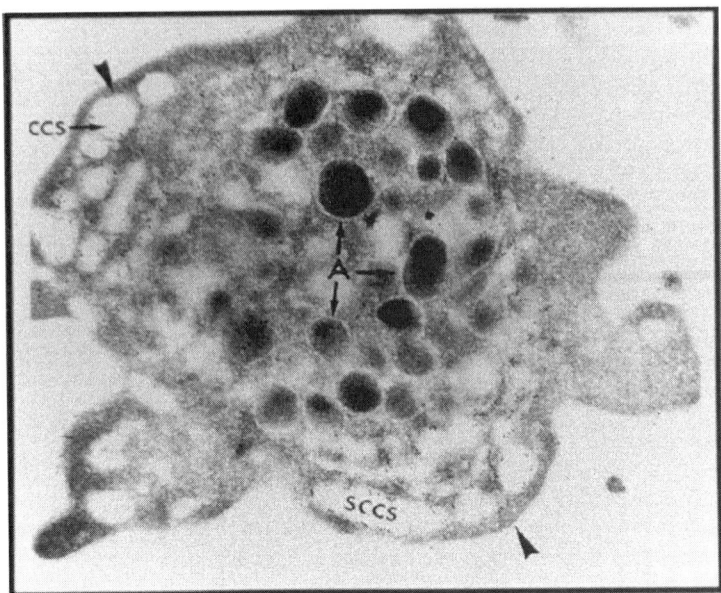

**FIGURE 3.** Plasmin stimulation of platelets performed at 37°C induced shape change and pseudopod formation as well as granule centralization. Immunolabeling for GPIb (*tiny black dots*) shows that it is virtually cleared from the plasma membrane (*arrowheads*) and that it is redistributed into the channels of the surface-connected canalicular system (secs). Alpha granules are negative for GPIb. (Original magnification × 26, 150). (From Cramer EM, Lu H, Caen JP, et al: Differential redistribution of platelet glycoproteins Ib and IIb–IIIa after plasmin stimulation. Blood 77:894–899, 1991; with permission.)

Depending upon concentration and temperature, plasmin either inhibits or stimulates platelets.[93,101] At 37°C, high concentrations of plasmin activate platelets and low concentrations inhibit. At 22°C, low concentrations of plasmin activate platelets.[93] At 37°C plasmin also causes an infolding of GPIb receptors but not GPIIb/IIIa receptors.[34] Inhibition of plasmin by aprotinin, therefore, prevents infolding of GPIb receptors (Fig. 3) and thus makes these receptors available for participation in hemostatic plug formation in wounds. Thus aprotinin attenuates the increase in bleeding times observed after CPB. Because plasmin does not affect GPIIb/IIIa receptor expression or degrade platelet membrane receptors,[34] platelet adhesion is not affected. Aprotinin also attenuates platelet alpha granule release[13,131] and thromboxane $A_2$ synthesis.[13] The drug is not known to have procoagulant activity, but it is not yet entirely clear whether the drug alters the early patency rates of coronary arterial bypass grafts.[31,87]

Nearly all of the enzymatic proteins of the coagulation and fibrinolytic systems are serine proteases. A large number of reversible and irreversible serine protease inhibitors are known (Table 3), and one or more of these or other inhibitors may prove more efficacious than heparin in controlling the activation of blood elements during CPB. These inhibitors of factor XIIa, factor XII fragments, factor IXa, factor Xa, kallikrein, C1s, tPA, plasmin, thrombin, and neutrophil elastase have different rate and binding constants for each target protease. The most inviting targets for selective inhibition are factors XIIa, kallikrein, and factor Xa. Complete inhibition of these three serine proteases offers good prospects for attenuating activation of blood elements and the production of vasoactive substances and microemboli during CPB.

**TABLE 3.** Some Inhibitors of Serine Proteases

| Thrombin inhibitors | Other inhibitors |
|---|---|
| R-hirudin and derivatives (hirulog, hirugen) | Arg-15 aprotinin |
| Argipidine | Ala-357, Arg-358, alpha$_1$-antitrypsin |
| Boroarginine peptide thrombin inhibitor | Nafamostat mesilate (FUT-175) |
| Low-molecular weight heparins | Boroarginine peptide kallikrein |
| Heparinoids (Dermatan, Lomoparin) | inhibitor |
| Benzamidine compounds | Kunitz protease inhibitors |
| Chloromethyl ketones | Corn trypsin, soybean trypsin, eglin |
| Factor Xa inhibitors | |
| Ecotin | |
| R-tick anticoagulant peptide | |
| R-anitstasin | |

# References

1. Abel RM, Buckley MJ, Austen WG, et al: Etiology, incidence and prognosis of renal failure following cardiac operations: Results of a prospective analysis of 500 consecutive patients. J Thorac Cardiovasc Surg 71:32–43, 1976.
2. Addonizio VP Jr, Strauss JF III, Chang L-F, et al: Release of lysosomal hydrolases during simulated extracorporeal circulation. J Thorac Cardiovasc Surg 84:28–34, 1982.
3. Anderson HL III, Delius RE, Sinard JM, et al: Early experience with adult extracorporeal membrane oxygenation in the modern era. Ann Thorac Surg 53:553–563, 1992.
4. Baier RE, Dutton RC: Initial events in interactions of blood with a foreign surface. J Biomed Mater Res 3:191–206, 1969.
5. Baier RE: The organization of blood components near interfaces. In Vroman L, Leonard E (eds): The Behavior of Blood and Its Components in Interfaces. Ann NY Acad Sci 17–36, 1977.
6. Bavaria JE, Furakawa S, Kreiner G, et al: Myocardial oxygen utilization after reversible global ischemia. J Thorac Cardiovasc Surg 100:210–220, 1990.
7. Bavaria JE, Ratcliffe MB, Gupta KB, et al: Changes in left ventricular systolic wall stress during biventricular circulatory assistance. Ann Thorac Surg 45:526–532, 1988.
8. Bernabei A, Rao AK, Niewiarowski S, et al: R-hirudin as a substitute for heparin during cardiopulmonary bypass. J Thorac Cardiovasc Surg 108:381–382, 1994.
9. Bernabei A, Gikakis N, Niewiarowski S, Edmunds LH Jr: Protection of platelets by combination of Iloprost and fibrinogen receptor antagonists during simulated cardiopulmonary bypass (submitted).
10. Bidstrup BP, Royston D, Sapsford RN, Taylor KM: Reduction in blood loss and blood use after cardiopulmonary bypass with high dose aprotinin (Trasylol). J Thorac Cardiovasc Surg 97:364–372, 1989.
11. Bindslev L, Gouda I, Inacio J, et al: Extracorporeal elimination of carbon dioxide using a surface-heparinized veno-venous bypass system. Trans Am Soc Artif Intern Organs 32:530–533, 1986.
12. Blackstone EH, Kirklin JW, Stewart RW, Chenoweth DE: The damaging effects of cardiopulmonary bypass. In Wu KK, Roxy EC (eds): Prostaglandins in Clinical Medicine: Cardiovascular and Thrombotic Disorders. Chicago, Yearbook Medical Publishers, 1982, pp 355–369.
13. Blauhut B, Klima U, Bettelheim P, et al: Comparison of the effects of aprotinin and tranexamic acid on blood loss and related variables following cardiopulmonary bypass. J Thorac Cardiovasc Surg (in press).
14. Blauth CI, Cosgrove DM, Webb BW, et al: Atheroembolism from the ascending aorta. J Thorac Cardiovasc Surg 103:1104–1112, 1992.
15. Blauth CI, Smith PL, Arnold JV, et al: Influence of oxygenator type on the prevalence and extent of microembolic retinal ischemia during cardiopulmonary bypass. J Thorac Cardiovasc Surg 99:61–69, 1990.
16. Boisclair MD, Lane DA, Philippou H, et al: Thrombin production, inactivation and expression during open heart surgery measured by assays for activation fragments including a new ELISA for prothrombin fragment F1+2. Thromb Haemost 70:253–258, 1993.
17. Borowiec J, Thelin S, Bagge L, et al: Decreased blood loss after cardiopulmonary bypass using heparin-coated circuit and 50% reduction of heparin dose. Scand J Thorac Cardiovasc Surg 26:177–185, 1992.

18. Boucher JK, Rudy LW, Edmunds LH Jr: Organ blood flow during pulsatile cardiopulmonary bypass. J Appl Physiol 36:86–90, 1974.
19. Brash JL, Scott CF, ten Hove P, et al: Mechanism of transient adsorption of fibrinogen from plasma to solid surfaces: Role of the contact and fibrinolytic systems. Blood 71:932–939, 1988.
20. Brister SJ, Ofosu FA, Buchanan MR: Thrombin generation during cardiac surgery: Is heparin the ideal anticoagulant? Thromb Haemost 70:259–262, 1993.
21. Canale SD, Fiacadori E, Medici D, et al: Effects of low flux-low pressure cardiopulmonary bypass on intracellular acid-base and water metabolism. Scand J Thorac Cardiovasc Surg 20:167–170, 1986.
22. Carteaux J-P, Roux S, Kuhn H, et al: Ro 44-9883, a new non-peptidic GPIIb-IIIa antagonist, prevents platelet loss during experimental cardiopulmonary bypass. J Thorac Cardiovasc Surg 106:834–841, 1993.
23. Chabbat J, Porte P, Tellier M, Steinbuch M: Aprotinin is a competitive inhibitor of the factor VIIa-tissue factor complex. Thromb Res 71:205–215, 1993.
24. Chenoweth DE, Cooper SW, Hugli TE, et al: Complement activation during cardiopulmonary bypass: Evidence for generation of C3a and C5a anaphylatoxins. N Engl J Med 304:497–503, 1981.
25. Chenoweth DE, Hugli TE: Demonstration of specific C5a receptor on intact human polymorphonuclear leukocytes. Proc Natl Acad Sci USA 75:3943, 1978.
26. Cheung AT, Levin SK, Weiss SJ, et al: Intracardiac thrombus: A risk of incomplete anticoagulation for cardiac operations. Ann Thorac Surg 58:541–542, 1994.
27. Clark RE, Davis DA, Lovell MR, et al: Microemboli during CABG: Genesis and effect on outcome. J Thorac Cardiovasc Surg (in press).
28. Cleland J, Pluth JR, Tauxe WN, Kirklin JW: Blood volume and body fluid compartment changes soon after closed and open intracardiac surgery. J Thorac Cardiovasc Surg 52:698–705, 1966.
29. Collins JD, Ferner R, Murray A, et al: Incidence and prognostic importance of jaundice after cardiopulmonary bypass surgery. Lancet 1:1119–1123, 1983.
30. Colman RW: Surface-mediated defense reactions. The plasma contact activation system. J Clin Invest 73:1249–1253, 1984.
31. Cosgrove DM III, Heric B, Lytle BW, et al: Aprotinin therapy for reoperative myocardial revascularization: A placebo-controlled study. Ann Thorac Surg 54:1031–1038, 1992.
32. Coughlin SR, Vu T-K H, Hung DT, Wheaton VI: Characterization of a functional thrombin receptor. J Clin Invest 89:351–355, 1992.
33. Craddock PR, Fehr J, Brigham KL, et al: Complement and leukocyte-mediated pulmonary dysfunction in hemodialysis. N Engl J Med 296:769–774, 1977.
34. Cramer EM, Lu H, Caen JP, et al: Differential redistribution of platelet glycoproteins Ib and IIB-IIIa after plasmin stimulation. Blood 77:894–899, 1991.
35. Del Balza UH, Levi R, Polley MJ: Cardiac dysfunction caused by purified human C3a anaphylatoxin. Proc Natl Acad Sci USA 82:886–890, 1985.
36. DeLeon S, Ilbawi M, Arcilla R, et al: Choreoathetosis after deep hypothermia without circulatory arrest. Ann Thorac Surg 50:714–719, 1990.
37. DePalma L, Yu M, McIntosh CL, et al: Changes in lymphocyte subpopulations as a result of cardiopulmonary bypass. J Thorac Cardiovasc Surg 101:240–244, 1991.
38. Didisheim P, Tirrell MV, Lyons CS, et al: Relative role of surface chemistry and surface texture in blood-material interactions. Trans Am Soc Artif Intern Organs 29:169–176, 1983.
39. Downing SW, Edmunds LH, Jr: Release of vasoactive substances during cardiopulmonary bypass. Ann Thorac Surg 54:1236–1243, 1992.
40. Downing SW, Savage EB, Streicher JS, et al: The stretched ventricle: Myocardial creep and contractile dysfunction after acute nonischemic ventricular distention. J Thorac Cardiovasc Surg 104:996–1005, 1992.
41. Dutton RC, Edmunds LH Jr: Measurement of emboli in extracorporeal perfusion systems. J Thorac Cardiovasc Surg 65:523–530, 1973.
42. Edgington TS, Mackman N, Brand K, Ruf W: The structural biology of expression and function of tissue factor. Thromb Haemost 66:67–79, 1991.
43. Edmunds LH Jr, Ellison N, Colman RW, et al: Platelet function during open heart surgery: Comparison of the membrane and bubble oxygenators. J Thorac Cardiovasc Surg 83:805–812, 1982.
44. Edmunds LH Jr: Pulseless cardiopulmonary bypass. J Thorac Cardiovasc Surg 84:800–804, 1982.

45. Edmunds LH Jr, Williams W: Microemboli and the use of filters during cardiopulmonary bypass. In Utley JR (ed): Pathophysiology and Techniques of Cardiopulmonary Bypass, vol II. Baltimore, Williams & Wilkins, 1983, pp 101–114.
46. Elgebaly SA, Hashmi FH, Houser SL, et al: Cardiac-derived neutrophil chemotactic factors: Detection in coronary sinus effluents of patients undergoing myocardial revascularization. J Thorac Cardiovasc Surg 103:952–959, 1992.
47. Ellison N, Edmunds LH Jr, Colman RW: Platelet aggregation following heparin and protamine administration. Anesthesiology 48:65–68, 1978.
48. Faymonville ME, Deby-Dupont G, Larbuisson R, et al: Prostaglandin E$_2$, prostacyclin, and thromboxane changes during nonpulsatile cardiopulmonary bypass in humans. J Thorac Cardiovasc Surg 91:858–866, 1986.
49. Faymonville ME, Pincemail J, Duchateau MD, et al: Myeloperoxidase and elastase as markers of leukocyte activation during cardiopulmonary bypass in humans. J Thorac Cardiovasc Surg 102:309–317, 1991.
50. Fernandex-del Castillo C, Harringer W, Warshaw AL, et al: Risk factors for pancreatic cellular injury after cardiopulmonary bypass. N Engl J Med 325:382–387, 1991.
51. Ferraris VA, Rodriquez E, Ferraris SP, et al: Platelet aggregation abnormalities after cardiopulmonary bypass. Blood 83:299–300, 1994.
52. Finn A, Naik S, Klein N, et al: Interleukin-8 release and neutrophil degranulation after pediatric cardiopulmonary bypass. J Thorac Cardiovasc Surg 105:234–241, 1993.
53. FitzGerald GA: Dipyridamole. N Engl J Med 316:1247–1257, 1987.
54. Gallimore MJ, Fuhrer G, Heller W, Hoffmeister HE: Augmentation of kallikrein and plasmin inhibition capacity by aprotinin using a new assay to monitor therapy. Adv Exp Med Biol 247B:55–60, 1989.
55. George JN, Pickett EB, Sauderman S, et al: Platelet surface glycoproteins: Studies on resting and activated platelets and platelet membrane microparticles in normal subjects, and observations in patients during adult respiratory distress syndrome and cardiac surgery. J Clin Invest 78:340–348, 1986.
56. Gluszko P, Rucinski B, Musial J, et al: Fibrinogen receptors in platelet adhesion to surfaces of extracorporeal circuit. Am J Physiol 252:H615–H621, 1987.
57. Golding LR, Jacobs G, Murakami T, et al: Chronic non-pulsatile blood flow in an alive, awake animal:34 days' survival. Trans Am Soc Artif Intern Organs 26:251–255, 1980.
58. Gott VL, Whiffen JD, Dutton RC: Heparin bonding on colloidal graphite surfaces. Science 142:1297–1298, 1963.
59. Gram J, Janetzko T, Jespersen J, Bruhn HD: Enhanced effective fibrinolysis following the neutralization of heparin in open heart surgery increases the risk of post-surgical bleeding. Thromb Haemost 63:241–245, 1990.
60. Haeffner-Cavaillon N, Roussellier N, Ponzio O, et al: Induction of interleukin-1 production in patients undergoing cardiopulmonary bypass. J Thorac Cardiovasc Surg 98;1100–1106, 1989.
61. Hammerschmidt DE, Stroncek DF, Bowers TK, et al: Complement activation and neutropenia during cardiopulmonary bypass. J Thorac Cardiovasc Surg 81:370–377, 1981.
62. Harker LA, Malpass TW, Branson HE, et al: Mechanism of abnormal bleeding in patients undergoing cardiopulmonary bypass: Acquired transient platelet dysfunction associated with selective alpha granule release. Blood 56:824–834, 1980.
63. Hashimoto K, Horikoshi H, Miyamoto H, et al: Mechanisms of organ failure following cardiopulmonary bypass: The role of elastase and vasoactive mediators. J Thorac Cardiovasc Surg 104:666–673, 1992.
64. Hill JD, Aguilar MJ, Baranco A, et al: Neuropathological manifestations of cardiac surgery. Ann Thorac Surg 7:409–417, 1969.
65. Horrow JC: Management of coagulopathy associated with cardiopulmonary bypass. In Gravlee GP, Davis RE, Utley JR (eds): Cardiopulmonary Bypass. Baltimore, Williams & Wilkins, 1993, pp 436–466.
66. Hoshikawa-Fujimura AY, Auler JOC Jr, DaRocha TRF, et al: PAF-acether, superoxide anion and beta-glucuronidase as parameters of polymorphonuclear cell activation associated with cardiac surgery and cardiopulmonary bypass. Braz J Med Biol Res 22:1077–1082, 1989.
67. Howard RJ, Crain C, Franzini DA, et al: Effects of cardiopulmonary bypass on pulmonary leukostasis and complement activation. Arch Surg 123:1496–1501, 1988.
68. Hunt BJ, Yacoub M: Guidelines for monitoring heparin by the activated clotting time when aprotinin is used during cardiopulmonary bypass. J Thorac Cardiovasc Surg 104:211–212, 1992.

69. Jaffe EA: Endothelial cell structure and function. In Hoffman R, Benz EJ Jr, Shattil SJ, et al: Hematology: Basic Principles and Practice. New York, Churchill Livingstone, 1991, pp 1198–1213.
70. Jobes DR, Schwartz AJ, Ellison N: Heparin rebound. J Thorac Cardiovasc Surg 82:940–941, 1981.
71. Kappa JR, Fisher CA, Bell P, et al: Intraoperative management of patients with heparin-induced thrombocytopenia. Ann Thorac Surg 49:713–723, 1990.
72. Kappelmayer J, Bernabei A, Edmunds LH Jr, et al: Tissue factor is expressed on monocytes during simulated extracorporeal circulation. Circ Res 72:1075–1081, 1993.
73. Kappelmayer J, Bernabei A, Gikakis N, et al: Upregulation of Mac-1 surface expression on neutrophils during simulated extracorporeal circulation. J Lab Clin Med 121:118–126, 1993.
74. Kelton JG, Sheridan D, Santos A, et al: Heparin-induced thrombocytopenia: Laboratory studies. Blood 72:925–930, 1988.
75. Kestin AS, Valeri CR, Khuri SF, et al: The platelet function defect of cardiopulmonary bypass. Blood 82:107–117, 1993.
76. Kim SW, Feijen J: Surface modification of polymers for improved blood compatibility. CRC Crit Rev Biocompatibility 1:229–260, 1985.
77. King DJ, Kelton JG: Heparin-associated thrombocytopenia. Ann Intern Med 100:535–540, 1984.
78. Kirklin JK, Chenoweth DE, Naftel DC, et al: Effects of protamine administration after cardiopulmonary bypass on complement, blood elements, and the hemodynamic state. Ann Thorac Surg 41:193–199, 1986.
79. Kirklin JK, Westaby S, Blackstone EH, et al: Complement and the damaging effects of cardiopulmonary bypass. J Thorac Cardiovasc Surg 86:845–857, 1983.
80. Ko W, Hawes AS, Lazenby WD, et al: Myocardial reperfusion injury. J Thorac Cardiovasc Surg 102:297–308, 1991.
81. Kodama K, Pasche B, Olsson P, et al: Antithrombin III binding to surface immobilized heparin and its relation to F Xa inhibition. Thromb Haemost 58:1064–1067, 1987.
82. Kurusz M, Butler BD: Embolic events and cardiopulmonary bypass. In Gravlee GP, Davis RE, Utley JR (eds): Cardiopulmonary Bypass. Baltimore, Williams & Wilkins, 1993, pp 267–290.
83. Larm O, Larsson R, Olsson P: A new non-thrombogenic surface prepared by selective covalent binding of heparin via a modified reducing terminal residue. Biomat Med Dev Artif Organs 11:161–173, 1983.
84. Laufer N, Merin G, Grover NB, et al: The influence of cardiopulmonary bypass on the size of human platelets. J Thorac Cardiovasc Surg 70:727–731, 1975.
85. Laurel M-TP, Ratnoff OD, Everson B: Inhibition of the activation of Hageman factor (factor XII) by aprotinin (Trasylol). J Lab Clin Med 119:580–585, 1992.
86. Leitman IM, Paull DE, Barie PS, et al: Intra-abdominal complications of cardiopulmonary bypass operations. Surg Gynecol Obstet 165:251–254, 1987.
87. Lemmer JH Jr, Stanford W, Bonney SL, et al: Aprotinin for coronary bypass operations: Efficacy, safety, and influence on early saphenous vein graft patency. J Thorac Cardiovasc Surg 107:543–553, 1994.
88. Levin EG, Marzec U, Anderson J, Harker LA: Thrombin stimulates tissue plasminogen activator from cultured human endothelial cells. J Clin Invest 74:1988–1995, 1984.
89. Lindon JN, McManama G, Kushner L, et al: Does the conformation of released adsorbed fibrinogen dictate platelet interactions with artificial surfaces? Blood 68:355–362, 1986.
90. Lindon JN, Salzman EW, Merrill EW, et al: Catalytic activity and platelet reactivity of heparin covalently bonded to surfaces. J Lab Clin Med 105:219–226, 1985.
91. Lowenstein E. Johnston WE, Lappis DG, et al: Catastrophic pulmonary vasoconstriction associated with protamine reversal of heparin. Anesthesiology 59:470–473, 1983.
92. Lu H, Soria C, Commin P-L, et al: Hemostasis in patients undergoing extracorporeal circulation: The effect of aprotinin (Trasylol). Thromb Haemost 66:633–637, 1991.
93. Lu H, Soria C, Cramer EM, et al: Temperature dependence of plasmin-induced activation or inhibition of human platelets. Blood 77:996–1005, 1991.
94. Markewitz A, Faist E, Lang S, et al: Successful restoration of cell-mediated immune response after cardiopulmonary bypass by immunomodulation. J Thorac Cardiovasc Surg 105:15–24, 1993.
95. McGowan FX, del Nido PJ, Kurland G, et al: Cardiopulmonary bypass significantly impairs surfactant activity in children. J Thorac Cardiovasc Surg 106:968–977, 1993.

96. Menasche P, Le Deist F, Tronc F, et al: Patterns of changes in neutrophil adhesion molecules during normothermic cardiopulmonary bypass—a clinical study. J Thorac Cardiovasc Surg (in press).
97. Menninger FJ III, Rosenkranz ER, Utley JR, et al: Interstitial hydrostatic pressure in patients undergoing CABG and valve replacement. J Thorac Cardiovasc Surg 79:181–187, 1980.
98. Michelson AD, Benoit SE, Barnard MR, et al: Platelet aggregation abnormalities after cardiopulmonary bypass. Blood 83:300–301, 1994.
99. Mottaghy K, Oedekoven B, Poppel K, et al: Heparin free long-term extracorporeal circulation using bioactive surfaces. Trans Am Soc Artif Intern Organs 35:635–637, 1989.
100. Musial J, Niewiarowski S, Rucinski B, et al: Inhibition of platelet adhesion to surfaces of extracorporeal circuits by disintegrins. Circulation 82:261–273, 1990.
101. Niewiarowski S, Senyi AF, Gilles P: Plasmin-induced platelet aggregation and platelet release reaction. J Clin Invest 52:1647–1659, 1973.
102. Nilsson L, Kulander L, Nystrom S-O, Eriksson O: Endotoxins in cardiopulmonary bypass. J Thorac Cardiovasc Surg 100:777–780, 1990.
103. Olson ST, Bjork I: Predominant contribution of surface approximation to the mechanism of heparin acceleration of the antithrombin-thrombin reaction. J Biol Chem 266:6353–6362, 1991.
104. Pacifico AD, Digerness S, Kirklin JW: Acute alterations of body composition after open intracardiac operations. Circulation 41:331–341, 1970.
105. Parker DJ, Karp RB, Kirklin JW, Bedard P: Lung water and alveolar and capillary volumes after intracardiac surgery. Circulation 45(Suppl I):139–146, 1972.
106. Ratliff NB, Young WG Jr, Hackel D, et al: Pulmonary injury secondary to extracorporeal circulation: An ultrastructural study. J Thorac Cardiovasc Surg 65:425–432, 1973.
107. Rinder CS, Bonan JL, Rinder HM, et al: Cardiopulmonary bypass induces leukocyte-platelet adhesion. Blood 79:1201–1205, 1992.
108. Rogers AT, Newman SP, Stump DA, Prough DS: Neurologic effects of cardiopulmonary bypass. In Gravlee GP, Davis RE, Utley JR (eds): Cardiopulmonary Bypass. Baltimore, Williams & Wilkins, 1993, pp 542–576.
109. Salzman EW, Lindon J, Brier D: Surface-induced platelet adhesion, aggregation and release. In Vroman L, Leonard E (eds): The Behavior of Blood and Its Components in Interfaces. Ann NY Acad Sci 114–117, 1977.
110. Shapira N, Schaff HV, Piehler JM, et al: Cardiovascular effects of protamine sulfate in man. J Thorac Cardiovasc Surg 84:505–514, 1982.
111. Shaw PJ, Bates D, Aartidge NEF, et al: Neurologic and neuropsychological morbidity following major surgery: Comparison of coronary artery bypass and peripheral vascular surgery. Stroke 18:700–707, 1987.
112. Shigeta O, Gluszko P, Downing SW, et al: Protection of platelets during long-term extracorporeal membrane oxygenation in sheep with a single dose of a disintegrin. Circulation 86(Suppl II):II-398–II-404, 1992.
113. Shuman MA: Thrombin-cellular interactions. Ann NY Acad Sci 485:228–239, 1986.
114. Sims PJ: Plasma proteins: Complement. In Hoffman R, Benz EJ Jr. (eds): Hematology.
115. Sladen RN, Berkowitz DE: Cardiopulmonary bypass and the lung. In Gravlee GP, Davis RE, Utley JR (eds): Cardiopulmonary Bypass. Baltimore, Williams & Wilkins, 1993, pp 468–487.
116. Smith EEJ, Naftel DC, Blackstone EH, Kirklin JW: Microvascular permeability after cardiopulmonary bypass. J Thorac Cardiovasc Surg 94:225–233, 1987.
117. Steinberg JB, Kapelanski DP, Olson JD, Weiler JM: Cytokine and complement levels in patients undergoing cardiopulmonary bypass. J Thorac Cardiovasc Surg 106:1008–1016, 1993.
118. Stenach N, Korn RL, Fisher CA, et al: The effects of heparin bound surface modification (Carmeda bioactive surface) on human platelet alterations during simulated extracorporeal circulation. J Am Soc Extracorpor Technol 24:97–102, 1992.
119. Tabuchi N, de Haan J, Boonstra PW, van Overen W: Activation of fibrinolysis in the pericardial cavity during cardiopulmonary bypass. J Thorac Cardiovasc Surg 106:828–833, 1993.
120. Teoh KH, Christakis GT, Weisel RD, et al: Dipyridamole preserved platelets and reduced blood loss after cardiopulmonary bypass. J Thorac Cardiovasc Surg 96:332–341, 1988.
121. Tuman KJ, McCarthy RJ, Najafi H, Ivankovich AD: Differential effects of advanced age on neurologic and cardiac risks of coronary artery operations. J Thorac Cardiovasc Surg 104:1510–1517, 1992.

122. Uniyal S, Brash JL: Patterns of adsorption of proteins from human plasma onto foreign surfaces. Thromb Haemost 47:285–290, 1982.

123. Utley JR: Renal function and fluid balance with cardiopulmonary bypass. In Gravelee GP, Davis RE, Utley JR (eds): Cardiopulmonary Bypass. Baltimore, Williams & Wilkins, 1993. pp 488–508.

124. Vane JR, Anggard EE, Botting RM: Regulatory functions of the vascular endothelium. N Engl J Med 323:27–36, 1990.

125. van Oeveren W, Jansen NJG, Bidstrup VP, et al: Effects of aprotinin on hemostatic mechanisms during cardiopulmonary bypass. Ann Thorac Surg 44:640–645, 1987.

126. Vane JR, Anggard EE, Botting RM: Regulatory functions of the vascular endothelium. N Engl J Med 323:27–36, 1990.

127. van Oeveren W, Jansen NJG, Bidstrup VP, et al: Effects of aprotinin on hemostatic mechanisms during cardiopulmonary bypass. Ann Thorac Surg 44:640–645, 1987.

128. Videm V, Svennevig JL, Fosse E, et al: Reduced complement activation with heparin-coated oxygenator and tubings in coronary bypass operations. J Thorac Cardiovasc Surg 103:806–813, 1992.

129. von Segesser LK, Weiss BM, Garcia E, Turina MI: Risk and benefit of low systemic heparinization during open heart surgery. Ann Thorac Surg 58:391–398, 1994.

130. Wachtfogel YT, Musial J, Jenkin B, et al: Loss of platelet alpha 2-adrenergic receptors during simulated extracorporeal ciirculation: Prevention with prostaglandin E1. J Lab Clin Med 105:601–607, 1985.

131. Wachtfogel YT, Kucich U, Hack CE, et al: Aprotinin inhibits the contact, neutrophil, and platelet activation systems during simulated extracorporeal perfusion. J Thorac Cardiovasc Surg 106:1–10, 1993.

132. Wachtfogel YT, Kucich U, Greenplate J, et al: Human neutrophil degranulation during extracorporeal circulation. Blood 69:324–330, 1987.

133. Wachtfogel YT, Harpel PC, Edmunds LH Jr, Colman RW: Formation of C1s–C1-inhibitor, kallikrien–C1-inhibitor and plasmin-alpha 2–plasmin inhibitor complexes during cardio-pulmonary bypass. Blood 73:468–471, 1989.

134. Weitz JI, Hudoba M, Massel D, et al: Clot-bound thrombin is protected from inhibition by heparin-antithrombin III but is susceptible to inactivation by antithrombin III-independent inhibitors. J Clin Invest 86:385–391, 1990.

135. Wenger RK, Lukasiewicz H, Mikuta BS, et al: Loss of platelet fibrinogen receptors during clinical cardiopulmonary bypass. J Thorac Cardiovasc Surg 97:235–239, 1989.

136. Westby S: Complement and the damaging effects of cardiopulmonary bypass. Thorax 38:321–325, 1983.

137. Woodman RC, Harker LA: Bleeding complications associated with cardiopulmonary bypass. Blood 76:1680–1697, 1990.

138. Ziats NP, Pankowsky DA, Tierney BP, et al: Adsorption of Hageman factor (factor XII) and other plasma proteins to biomedical polymers. J Lab Clin Med 116:687–696, 1990.

139. Zilla P, Fasol R, Groscurth P, et al: Blood platelets in cardiopulmonary bypass operations. J Thorac Cardiovasc Surg 97:379–388, 1989.

David C. McGiffin, MD
James K. Kirklin, MD

# 3

## Complement and the Damaging Effects of Cardiopulmonary Bypass

Intracardiac surgery has been possible only because of the development of cardiopulmonary bypass (CPB) using the pump-oxygenator. Despite the success of Lillehei's bold application of cross-circulation[29] as a means of cardiopulmonary support during correction of cardiac defects, this technique inevitably was replaced by a more widely applicable, but less physiologic machine. Over the next 40 years of open-heart surgery, the basic circuitry of the pump-oxygenator changed little, but oxygenator design, monitoring systems, and circuit materials have advanced. Development of CPB was accompanied by surgical advances for correction or palliation of the full spectrum of congenital and acquired heart disease.

Despite the fact that the vast majority of patients who undergo cardiac surgery convalesce normally, a considerable amount of morbidity and even some degree of mortality can be attributed to the unphysiologic circumstances of CPB. However, in an era when the mortality rate for routine operations for acquired heart disease is a few percent, it is easy to underestimate the damaging effects of CPB. As patients undergoing cardiac surgery become older, requiring more complex intracardiac repairs in the presence of more preoperative subsystem dysfunction, the damaging effects of CPB may become more prominent in the postoperative course.

Considerable information has accumulated about the systemic effects of CPB, which are best conceptualized as a whole-body inflammatory reaction. In the past the clinical manifestations of the damaging effects of CPB have gone by terms such as "postperfusion syndrome" and "pump lung." The whole body inflammatory response is associated with changes in microvascular permeability, fluid shifts, activation of humoral amplification systems, changes in the immune system, and secondary organ dysfunction. This chapter focuses on one of these systems—the complement system—and outlines its biology, the evidence for its participation in the response to CPB, and possible means of ameliorating the damaging effects of CPB by modulation of the complement system.

## The Clinical Syndrome

The spectrum of clinical manifestations ranges from subtle changes to serious sequelae such as pulmonary and renal dysfunction, bleeding diathesis, increased interstitial fluid, leukocytosis, fever, vasoconstriction, hemolysis, and susceptibility to infection. The hallmark of the damaging effects of CPB is increased capillary permeability. A study by Cleland[9] in 1966 found that increases in extravascular fluid after CPB were directly related to the duration of CPB. Direct evidence of increased capillary permeability came from Smith and colleagues,[54] who used an experimental model to detect movement of macromolecules from the small intestinal microvasculature into lymph. Clinical studies, however, have not been able to demonstrate increased pulmonary epithelial[56] or endothelial[31] permeability after CPB.

### Inflammatory Response to CPB

The whole-body inflammatory response to CPB is highly complex, and complement appears to be just one component. The responses with a putative role include catecholamine release (epinephrine from the adrenal medulla and norepinephrine from sympathetic nerve terminals),[25,46,47] activation of the humoral amplification systems, and release of cytokines and proteolytic enzymes. The humoral amplification systems include the kallikrein-bradykinin cascade,[44] coagulation cascade,[10,20] fibrinolytic cascade,[4] complement cascade,[8] and arachidonic acid cascade.[14,62,63] The factors that may initiate cascade system activation include exposure of blood to unphysiologic (nonendothelial) surfaces, generation of shear stresses in the pump-oxygenator and tubing, and incorporation of abnormal substances (microemboli) during CPB, such as air bubbles, tissue debris, and fibrin. The complement system is but one of a number of potentially injurious responses, and the interactions are complex.

## The Biology of the Complement System

Complement is a system of 20 plasma proteins which are capable of altering the function of cells that participate in the inflammatory and immune responses. The proteins are involved in activation and regulation of complement and function as enzymes, enzyme inhibitors, or enzyme cofactors; several circulate as inactive precursors[3] (Table 1). In addition, the membrane-bound proteins act as receptors for biologically active proteolytic complement fragments and as regulators of complement activation; they also protect host cells from damage by complement-mediated lysis[3] (Table 2).

The pivotal complement protein is C3, the precursor for many of the products of the complement system with diverse biologic activities.[61] Activation of the system occurs by one of two possible pathways—the classic pathway or the alternate pathway, both of which result in the production of a C3-convertase (Fig. 1). The C3-convertase produced by the classic pathway is generated after activation by IgG or IgM antibodies complexed to their respective antigens.[61] Certain viruses and gram-negative organisms also may activate this pathway. Recognition takes place through a circulating complex of plasma proteins called C1, which consists of various components—Cq, Cr, Cs (see Table 1). After a series of further steps, one of which results in the generation of the anaphylotoxin C4a (produced only in the classic pathway), C3a convertase is produced.

**TABLE 1.** Serum-soluble Proteins of the Complement System

| Activation | Regulation |
|---|---|
| First component (C1)—C1q, C1r, C1s | Factor I |
| Second component (C2) | Factor H |
| Third component (C3) | C4-binding protein (C4-bp) |
| Fourth component (C4) | C1 inhibitor (C1inh) |
| Fifth component (C5)* | Vitrorectin (S-protein) |
| Sixth component (C6)* | C3a/C5a inhibitor (C3a/C5a inh) |
| Seventh component (C7)* | Factor P (properdin) |
| Eighth component (C8)* | |
| Ninth component (C9)* | |
| Factor B, factor D | |

* Cytolytic enzymes
Adapted from Barnum SR: Biosynthesis and regulation of complement by cells of the central nervous system. Complement Profiles 1:76–95, 1993, with permission.

The alternative pathway results in the generation of C3-convertase after activation by a number of mechanisms, including contact with nonendothelial surfaces[8] and the cellular surfaces of certain bacteria, viruses, fungi, and parasites.[15] C3-convertase is produced after a series of steps that also incorporates an amplification loop to increase the amount of C3-convertase produced.[61] C3-convertase cleaves C3 into C3a and C3b, and some of the resulting C3b binds with C3-convertase (derived from classic or alternative pathway) to form a C5-convertase. C5-convertase cleaves C5 to form two fragments—C5a and C5b. C5b initiates the construction of a large protein complex known as the membrane attack complex (MAC).[61] The MAC consists of the C5b fragment together with components 6, 7, 8, and 9. By a series of reactions on the cell membrane, the complex becomes inserted into the lipid bilayer, forming a transmembrane channel that results in cell death.[61]

The complement cascade is controlled by a number of processes, including the intrinsic decay of various enzyme complexes, labile reactive sites, dissociation of incompletely assembled MAC from cell membranes, and regulatory proteins that either circulate in the serum or are membrane-bound.[45] The regulating proteins prevent uncontrolled activation and consumption of complement proteins. For example, the serum-soluble regulating protein H leads to the decay of the C3-convertase and C5-convertase produced by the alternative pathway. The membrane-bound regulating proteins membrane inhibitor of reactive lysis (CD59) and homologous recognition factor (HRF) inhibit the attachment of the MAC to host cells.[61] It is likely that endothelial cells are kept in a state that is unable to activate complement by regulators such as decay accelerating factor (DAF), membrane cofactor protein (MCP), HRF, and CD59 (see Table 2). Down-regulation of these proteins may allow complement activation and attachment of the MAC.[61]

**TABLE 2.** Membrane-bound Proteins of the Complement System

| Regulation | Receptors |
|---|---|
| Membrane inhibitor of reactive lysis (CD59) | Complement receptor type I (CR1) |
| Decay-accelerating factor (DAF) | Complement receptor type II (CR2) |
| Membrane cofactor protein (MCP) | Complement receptor type III (CR3) |
| Homologous recognition factor (HRF) | C3a/C4a receptor |
| | C5a receptor |

Adapted from Barnum SR: Biosynthesis and regulation of complement by cells of the central nervous system. Complement Profiles 1:76–95, 1993, with permission.

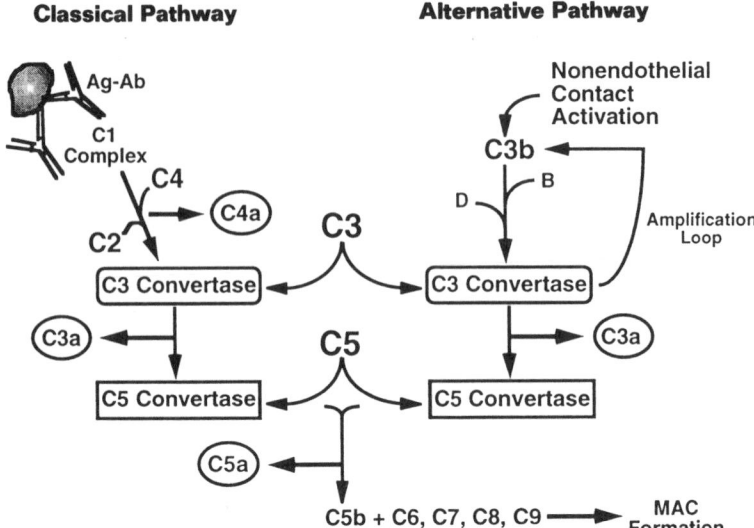

**FIGURE 1.** Schematic representation of the complement pathway. MAC, membrane attack complex; Ag-Ab, antigen-antibody complex. (From McGiffin DC, Kirklin JK: Cardiopulmonary bypass for cardiac surgery. In Sabiston DC, Spencer FC (eds): Surgery of the Chest, 6th ed. Philadelphia, W.B. Saunders [in press], with permission.)

Over 90% of serum complement, along with the great majority of components of the complement system, is produced by hepatocytes.[1] A number of extrahepatic sites also synthesize complement, including monocyte/macrophage cells, fibroblasts, and endothelial/epithelial cells. The regulation of the syntheses of each component of the complement system is component- and cell-specific.[3] The range of complement components and quantities produced by the extrahepatic sites is limited compared with that produced by hepatocytes. However, with stimulation the quantity can be significantly increased.

The complement cascade is intimately involved in the acute inflammatory response, regardless of the cause. The principal reactions of the acute inflammatory response are changes in the microvasculature and accumulation of myelomonocytic cells. Products of the activation of the complement system that are involved in changes in the microvasculature are C3a, C5a, and C5b-9 (MAC).[61] The effects of C4a are similar to those of C3a at nonphysiologic concentrations.[61] C3a is an anaphylotoxin that interacts with mast cells and basophils, resulting in the release of vasoactive substances such as histamine and leukotrienes and causing smooth muscle contraction. C5a has similar anaphylotoxin effects as C3a, but in addition C5a is chemotactic for myelomonocytic cells and acts as a secretogogue for myelomonocytic cells, mast cells, and basophils. The interaction of the complement system with leukocytes and monocytes as part of the inflammatory response is mediated by complement receptors (CR), which are cell type-specific glycoprotein receptors on the cell surface. For example, CR1 is found on erythrocytes, lymphocytes, monocytes, and granulocytes,[10] whereas CR2 is found on B-lymphocytes and follicular dendritic cells[49] and CR3 is found on mononuclear phagocytes, neutrophilis, natural killer cells, and antibody-dependent, cell-mediated cytotoxicity (ADCC) effector lymphocytes.[57] When receptors are engaged by complement fragments, CR1 and CR3 on myelomonocytic cells are upregulated. The affinity of the CR3 receptor for its counter-receptor on vascular endothelium, the intracellular adhesion molecule-1 (ICAM-1), is greatly enhanced, resulting in leukocyte-endothelial cell interaction.[61]

Of particular interest is the fact that CR1, as well as being bound to the cell surface, also is detected in the serum as a soluble molecule[64] and possibly functions as a natural complement inhibitor.[37]

## Evidence for the Role of Complement in the Damaging Effects of CPB

### Clinical Evidence

Various studies report high circulating levels of various autocoids and metabolic byproducts of the humoral amplification systems after CPB. In most studies, however, either the inflammatory response byproducts were not related to morbidity after CPB, or no conclusion was reached. This underscores the difficulty of interpreting such findings, particularly since the vast majority of patients undergoing CPB recover without obvious sequelae attributable to a whole-body inflammatory response.

Circumstantial evidence that complement activation may play a role in the damaging effects of CPB is increasing. Although no information directly implicates complement fragments as responsible for tissue injury during CPB, the evidence for involvement of the complement cascade seems compelling. The first evidence was the demonstration by Chenoweth and colleagues in 1981 that the C3a level increases after initiation of CPB and remains elevated throughout the duration of CPB (Fig. 2). A study by Kirklin and colleagues[28] found that C3a did not rise in patients undergoing cardiac surgical operations without CPB but rose significantly in patients

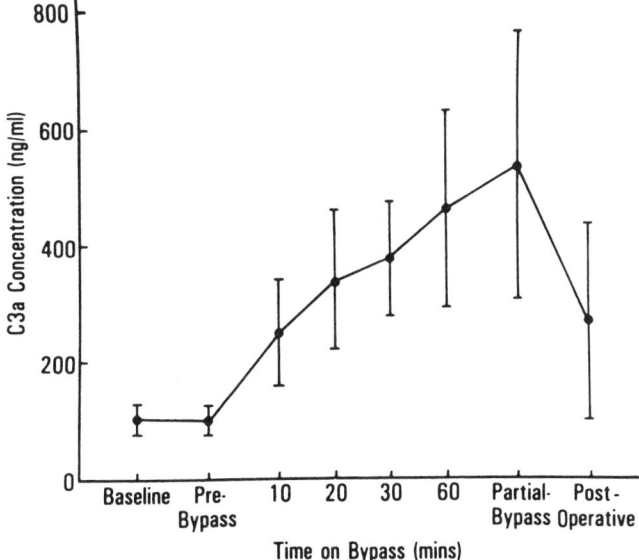

**FIGURE 2.** Plasma levels of C3a in patients undergoing CPB. (From Chenoweth DE, Cooper SW, Hugli TE, et al: Complement activation during cardiopulmonary bypass: Evidence for generation of C3a and C5a anaphylatoxins. N Engl J Med 304:497–503, 1981, with permission.)

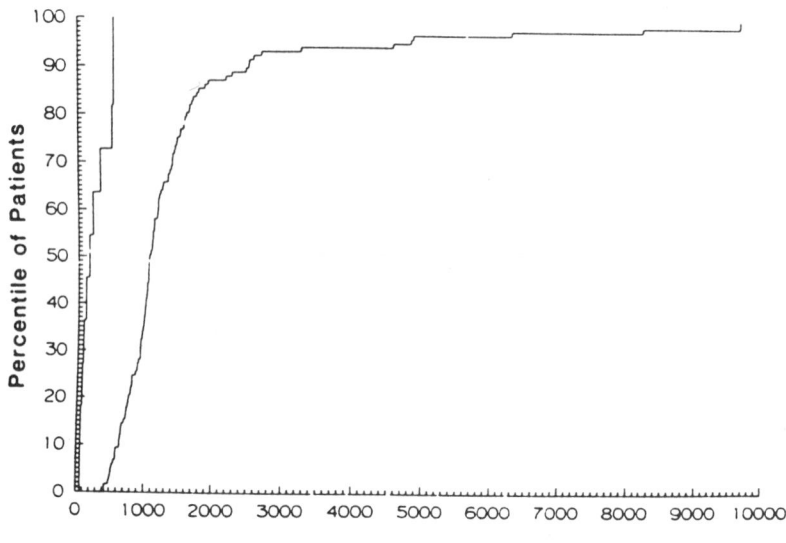

**C3a (ng·ml$^{-1}$) at End of CPB (or operation)**

**FIGURE 3.** C3a levels (ng/ml) at the end of CPB, expressed as a cumulative percentile plot. The steep line on the left represents closed-heart patients, 100% of whom had near-normal or normal levels. The curve on the right represents open-heart patients, virtually all of whom had increased levels; 50% of patients had levels above 1000 ng • ml$^{-1}$ and 25% had levels above 1600 ng • ml$^{-2}$. (From Kirklin JK, Chenoweth DE, Naftel DC, et al: Effects of protamine administration after cardiopulmonary bypass on complement, blood elements, and the hemodynamic state. Ann Thorac Surg 41:193–199, 1986, with permission.)

undergoing CPB; levels of C3a were still elevated above normal 3 hours after CPB (Fig. 3). The investigators performed a multivariable analysis to identify risk factors associated with cardiac, pulmonary, and renal dysfunction after CPB (Table 3-5). Higher levels of C3a, longer duration of CPB, and younger age at operation were risk factors associated with postoperative cardiac and pulmonary dysfunction; except for longer duration of CPB, the same risk factors were associated with postoperative renal dysfunction. The important effect of increasing levels of C3a on the probability of postoperative pulmonary dysfunction is illustrated in the nomogram solution to the multivariable equation (Fig. 4). An overall index of morbidity related cardiac, pulmonary, and renal dysfunction and abnormal bleeding to increasing levels of C3a 3 hours after CPB (Fig. 5). The results of this study emphasize the fact that neonates and infants are more likely to manifest the damaging effects of CPB than

**TABLE 3.** Cardiac Dysfunction after Open Operations

| Incremental Risk Factor | Logistic Coefficient ± SD | p Value |
|---|---|---|
| Higher C3a level | 0.0010 ± 0.00042 | 0.02 |
| Longer CPB time | 0.014 ± 0.0058 | 0.02 |
| Younger age | −0.06 ± 0.138 | ≤0.0001 |

n = 116; 27 patients had events.
SD = standard deviation, CPB = cardiopulmonary bypass.
From Kirklin JK, Westaby S, Blackstone EH, et al: Complement and the damaging effects of cardiopulmonary bypass. J Thorac Cardiovasc Surg 86:845–847, 1983, with permission.

**TABLE 4.**   Pulmonary Dysfunction after Open Operations

| Incremental Risk Factor | Logistic Coefficient ± SD | p Value |
|---|---|---|
| Higher C3a level | 0.0025 ± 0.00094 | 0.008 |
| Longer CPB time | 0.025 ± 0.0111 | 0.02 |
| Younger age | −1.17 ± 0.183 | 0.0001 |

n = 116; 41 patients had events.
SD = standard deviation, CPB = cardiopulmonary bypass.
From Kirklin JK, Westaby S, Blackstone EH, et al: Complement and the damaging effects of cardiopulmonary bypass. J Thorac Cardiovasc Surg 86:845–847, 1983, with permission.

**TABLE 5.**   Renal Dysfunction after Open Operations

| Incremental Risk Factor | Logistic Coefficient ± SD | p Value |
|---|---|---|
| Higher C3 level | 0.0009 ± 0.00036 | 0.02 |
| Younger age | −0.17 ± 0.183 | <0.0001 |

n = 116; 24 patients had events.
SD = standard deviation, CPB = cardiopulmonary bypass.
From Kirklin JK, Westaby S, Blackstone EH, et al: Complement and the damaging effects of cardiopulmonary bypass. J Thorac Cardiovasc Surg 86:845–847, 1983, with permission.

other patients. Furthermore, the association of longer duration of CPB with increased morbidity confirms a longstanding surgical impression.

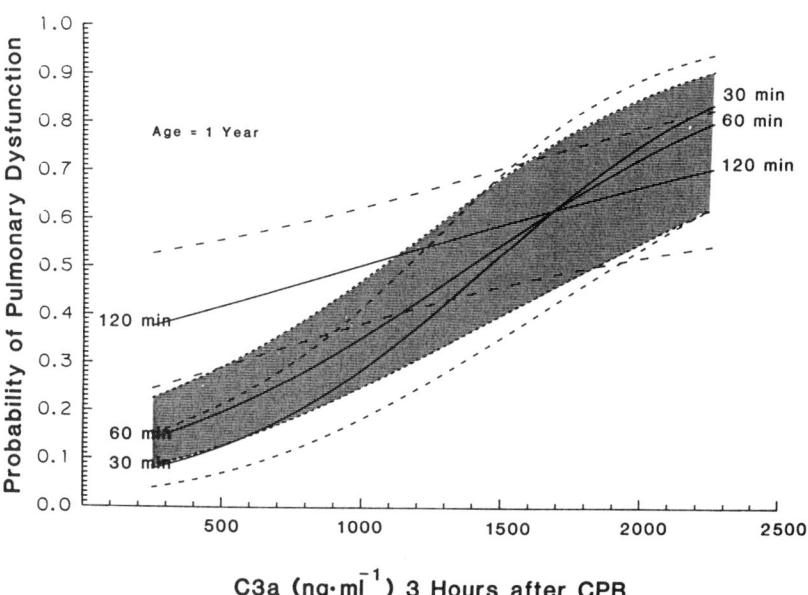

**FIGURE 4.**   Nomogram solution to the multivariable equation of probability of pulmonary dysfunction. The relationship of C3a levels 3 hours after CPB and CPB time to the probability of pulmonary dysfunction for a patient aged 1 year. The dashed lines enclose the 70% confidence limits, and the shaded area indicates the 70% confidence limits for 60 minutes of CPB. (From Kirklin JK, Chenoweth DE, Naftel DC, et al: Effects of protamine administration after cardiopulmonary bypass on complement, blood elements, and the hemodynamic state. Ann Thorac Surg 41:193–199, 1986, with permission.)

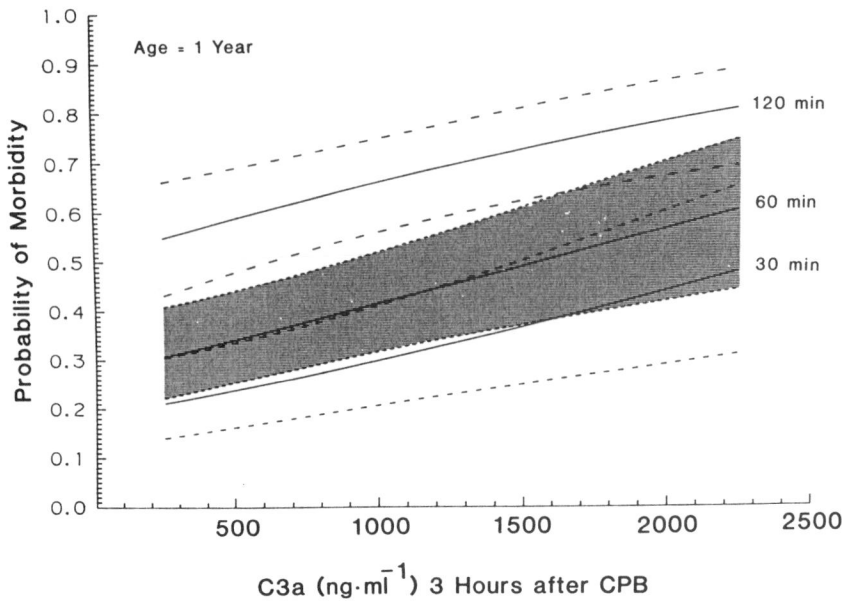

**FIGURE 5.** The nomogram solution to the multivariable equation for important postoperative morbidity. The relationship of C3a levels 3 hours following CPB and duration of CPB to the probability of important morbidity after CPB. The dashed lines enclose the 70% confidence limits, and the shaded area indicates the 70% confidence limits for 60 minutes of CPB. (From Kirklin JK, Chenoweth DE, Naftel DC, et al: Effects of protamine administration after cardiopulmonary bypass on complement, blood elements, and the hemodynamic state. Ann Thorac Surg 41:193–199, 1986, with permission.)

C5a is also generated during CPB, but this anaphylatoxin has been difficult to detect in vivo[8,23,33] because of its rapid binding to specific neutrophil receptors; hence C5a has a half-life in vivo of only 1 minute. In the past, C5a activation was inferred from its biologic activities[8] or from radioimmunoassay that required a precipitation step to remove C5. This requirement presents a significant limitation[51] because of incomplete separation and the risk of in vitro activation.

A recently developed method detects C5a/C5adesArg, based on a monoclonal antibody specific for a neoepitope that is exposed in C5a upon activation.[43] C5adesAug is a natural inactive product of C5a. This assay has demonstrated that significant amounts of C5a are generated during CPB.[36] C3a and C5a appear to be activated mostly via the alternative pathway,[38] but some activation of the classic pathway has been detected by the production of C4a at blood/air interfaces[8] and by the formation of heparin/protamine complexes.[16]

## Complement and Tissue Injury

The mechanism by which complement may participate in actual tissue injury during CPB is speculative. Various metabolic products and products of the humoral amplification system are produced during CPB and may have similar downstream effects. Consequently, determining the relative importance of the downstream effects of complement fragments compared with other humoral amplification systems in vivo becomes problematic. Nevertheless, some information suggests that generation of complement fragments is closely associated with neutrophil activation.

For neutrophils to exert their effect they must bind to vascular endothelium through the interaction of adhesion molecules. The primary neutrophil adhesion molecule (called an integrin) is a glycoprotein complex termed CD11b/CD18 (CR3).[58] Ligands of CR3 include ICAM-1 and complement fragment C3bi.[48] Furthermore, the generation of the anaphylatoxin C5a is a source of potent chemotaxis for neutrophils and an initiator of neutrophil activation. C5a has been shown to cause upregulation of neutrophil adhesion molecules, leading to a respiratory burst with release of superoxide radicals and neutrophil degranulation with release of proteolytic enzymes.[50] Further evidence of the cooperative roles of complement and neutrophil activation in mediating the damaging effects of CPB comes from Gillinov[19] who exposed C3-deficient dogs to CPB. Although CPB-associated lung injury was no different in the experimental and control groups, the C3-deficient animals had less accumulation of neutrophils in the lung and less expression of CD18 (a subunit of the neutrophil adhesion molecule) in circulating neutrophils. C3-deficient animals had no deposition of C3 in the lung, whereas C3 deposition was demonstrated in normal animals. A study by Moat and colleagues[35] provided further evidence for the nexus between complement activation and upregulation of neutrophil adhesion molecules. Using a simulated CPB circuit primed with normal human blood, the investigators demonstrated a progressive increase in plasma C3a and MAC (C5b-9) with increasing duration of CPB (maximal duration: 120 min). Concurrent with the generation of C3a and MAC was a linear rise in neutrophil surface expression of CD11b (a component of CD11b/CD18) compared with a static, nonflowing circuit (Fig. 6). The

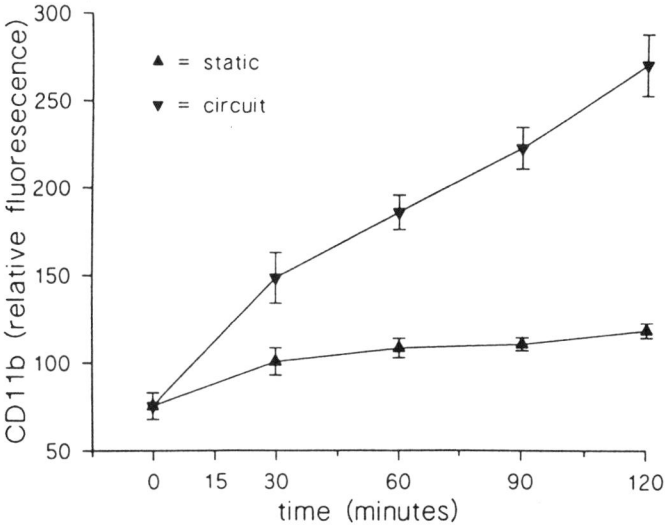

**FIGURE 6.** Depiction of the effect of a simulated extracorporeal circuit on neutrophil surface expression of CD11b. There was an increase in CD11b expression in the static loops over the 120-minute experimental protocol ($p < 0.05$). The marked and progressive increase in CD11b expression in the extracorporeal circuit was greater than the change seen in the static loop ($p < 0.05$). Data are shown as mean $\pm$ standard error of the mean; n = 5 for each group. (From Moat NE, Rebuck N, Shore DF, et al: Humoral and cellular activation in a simulated extracorporeal circuit. Ann Thorac Surg 58:1509–1514, 1993, with permission.)

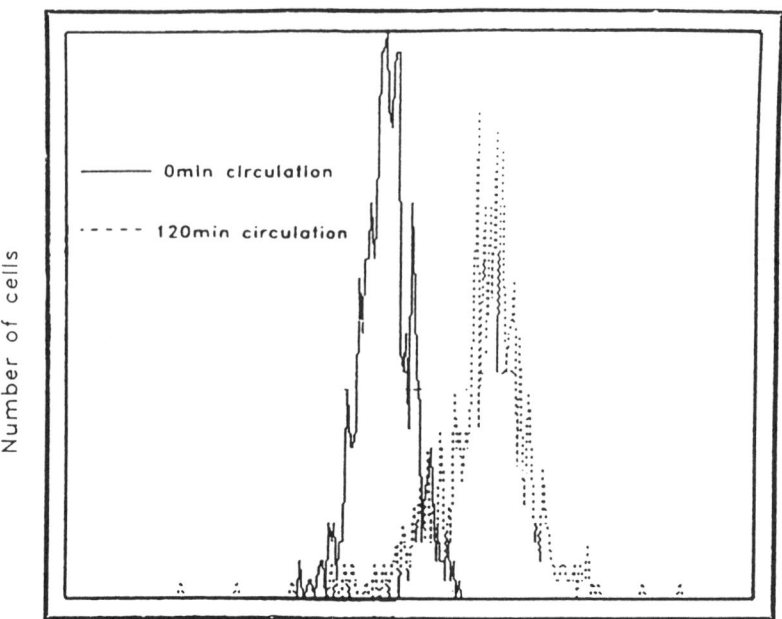

**FIGURE 7.** Effect of a simulated extracorporeal circuit on neutrophil surface expression of CD11b depicted on a fluorescence frequency histogram taken from one experiment. On the horizontal axis is fluorescence, and on the vertical axis is number of cells. The histogram in the solid line represents the population of cells expressing CD11b at baseline, and the dashed line represents the population of cells expressing CD11b at 120 minutes of CPB. The shift to the right reflects a homogeneous increase in CD11b expression throughout the population of neutrophils. (From Moat NE, Rebuck N, Shore DF, et al: Humoral and cellular activation in a simulated extracorporeal circuit. Ann Thorac Surg 58:1509–1514, 1993, with permission.)

unique design of the simulated circuit allowed the expression of neutrophil adhesion molecules to be examined in a "captive" population of neutrophils (unlike an in vivo CPB circuit). The fluorescence frequency histogram demonstrates that the increased expression of CD11b is in fact due to an increase in receptor expression (Fig. 7). This information is supported by the finding of increased CR3 expression on neutrophils obtained from patients undergoing CPB. CR3 expression increased 5 minutes after the onset of CPB.[21]

Available evidence suggests that, once activated and adherent to the endothelium during CPB, neutrophils possess the capacity to injure tissue. Neutrophils release significant quantities of hydrogen peroxide when adherent to endothelial cell monolayers[53] and isolated canine myocytes.[13] Release of neutrophil elastase has been demonstrated in a series of neonates undergoing CPB[52] and adult patients undergoing coronary bypass surgery.[5,33] However, none of these clinical series found direct evidence to implicate neutrophil enzyme release in clinically apparent injury. Neutrophil adherence to endothelium as a result of complement activation and neutrophil activation and enzyme release are a possible explanation for the damaging effects of CPB (Fig. 8), but the release of numerous other molecules and the fact that clinically apparent injury is not routine underscore the difficulty in interpreting such information.

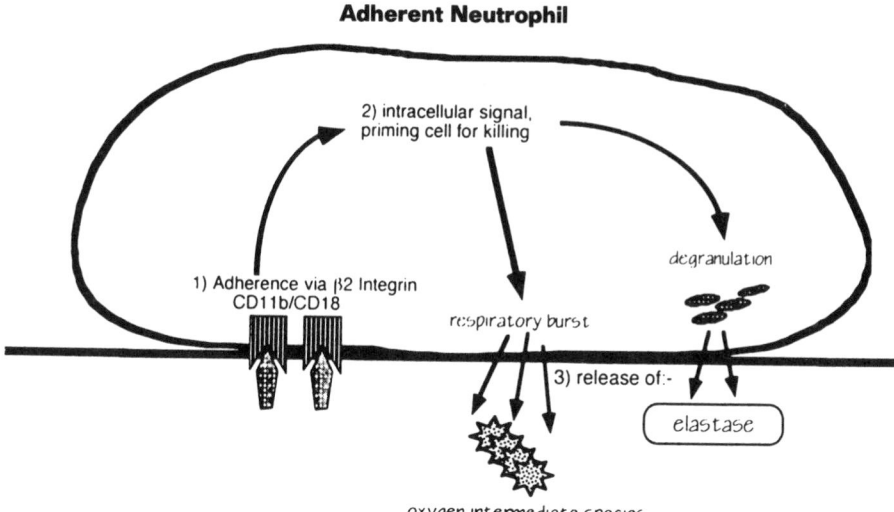

**FIGURE 8.** Possible role of CD11b/CD18-mediated endothelial adhesion in the intracellular signalling of degranulation with release of elastase and a respiratory burst with release of superoxide radicals. (From Elliott MJ, Finn AHR: Interaction between neutrophils and endothelium. Ann Thorac Surg 56:1503–1508, 1993, with permission.)

## Interaction between Protamine and Complement

A phenomenon occasionally observed after the administration of protamine at the conclusion of CPB is severe hemodynamic derangement associated with an elevation of pulmonary vascular resistance and a decrease in systemic vascular resistance.[30,41,42] The precise mechanisms have not been elucidated, but evidence suggests that the complement cascade may be involved. A study by Cavarocchi and colleagues[7] demonstrated that the protamine-heparin complex activates the complement cascade by the classic pathway, as evidenced by the generation of C4a. A study by Kirklin and colleagues[28] found that human serum containing heparin alone or protamine sulfate alone does not activate complement. However, human serum containing heparin and protamine sulfate markedly activates the classic pathway with the generation of C3a, C4a, and C5a (Fig. 9). In a series of patients undergoing coronary artery bypass surgery, elevated levels of C3a and nearly normal levels of C4a were found at the end of CPB. Administration of protamine sulfate resulted in marked elevation of C3a and C4a, indicating activation of the classic pathway[28] (Fig. 10). Unusually vigorous activation of the classic complement pathway may be responsible for the severe hemodynamic derangements occasionally seen with administration of protamine after CPB.

## Ameliorating the Damaging Effects of CPB

It seems highly unlikely that any one intervention can ameliorate the clinically apparent damaging effects of CPB, given the number of diverse cascade systems and metabolic products involved in the process. Clinical experience indicates that the duration and extent of the damaging effects of CPB are ameliorated with robust

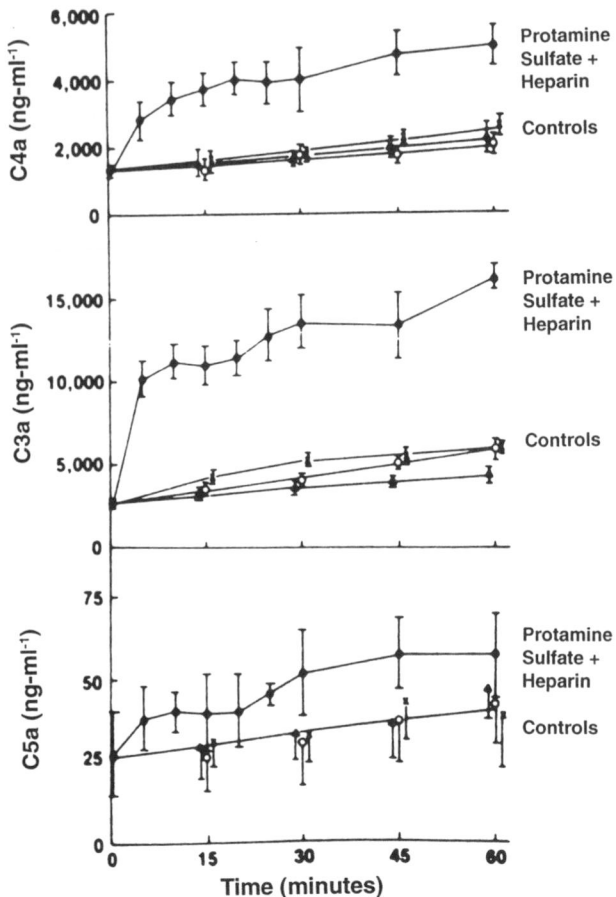

**FIGURE 9.** Levels of C4a, C3a, and C5a in normal human serum incubated with a mixture of protamine sulfate (●). The controls consisted of human serum alone (▲), serum containing heparin (○), or serum containing protamine sulfate (x). The vertical bars represent the 70% confidence limits. (From Kirklin JK, Chenoweth DE, Naftel DC, et al: Effects of protamine administration after cardiopulmonary bypass on complement, blood elements, and the hemodynamic state. Ann Thorac Surg 41:193–199, 1986, with permission.)

postoperative cardiac performance. At one time, pretreatment with corticosteroids was believed, among other effects, to reduce complement-induced neutrophil aggregation[24]; however, no in vivo evidence supports this assumption. Three interventions involving amelioration through the complement cascade are discussed below.

1. **Modification of the CPB circuit.** The use of membrane oxygenators may reduce the inflammatory response compared with bubble oxygenators. Cavarocchi and colleagues[6] found less generation of C3a with a membrane oxygenator and a significant increase in transpulmonary sequestration of leukocytes, together with increased elaboration of C3a, with a bubble oxygenator. Tamiya and colleagues[55] also found greater C3a and C5a production with bubble than with membrane oxygenators. This finding, however, has not been universal. A study by Oeveren and colleagues[59] found no difference in complement activation, and Gillinov and

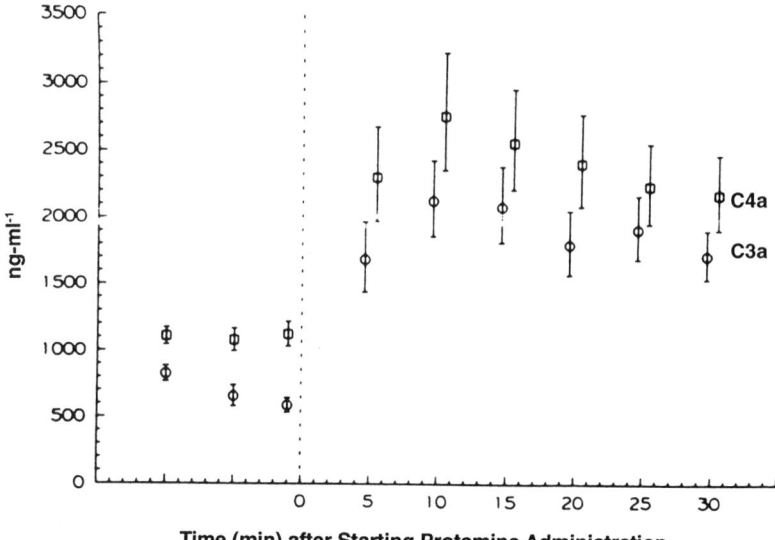

Time (min) after Starting Protamine Administration

**FIGURE 10.**  Levels of C3a (○) and C4a (□) after CPB and the beginning of protamine sulfate administration. Time 0 and the broken vertical line indicate the beginning of protamine administration, which was 10 minutes after discontinuation of CPB. Protamine was infused over 5 minutes. The vertical bars represent the 70% confidence limits. The mean normal value of C3a is 76 ng • ml$^{-1}$ and for C4a, 1200 ng • ml$^{-1}$. (From Kirklin JK, Chenoweth DE, Naftel DC, et al: Effects of protamine administration after cardiopulmonary bypass on complement, blood elements, and the hemodynamic state. Ann Thorac Surg 41:193–199, 1986, with permission.)

colleagues[17] reported similar degrees of upregulation of the neutrophil adhesion molecules CD11b and CD18 neutrophil degranulation, and complement activation with both oxygenators.

The use of heparin-coated CPB circuit tubing has been shown to reduce the production of anaphylatoxins. In a study by Gu and colleagues,[21] generation of C3a was significantly lower in patients with a heparin-coated circuit compared with controls, but the lower production of C3a became apparent only after administration of protamine. Videm and colleagues[60] found a reduction in maximal concentration of C3a and MAC in the heparin-coated compared with the uncoated circuit. No direct evidence, however, indicates that these phenomena translate into a reduction in clinically apparent injury.

2. **Ultrafiltration after CPB.** The use of ultrafiltration after CPB in infants may remove extravascular fluid that has accumulated as a result of increased capillary permeability. This process has been shown not only to reduce accumulated fluid but also to improve immediate postbypass hemodynamics and to reduce pulmonary vascular resistance.[11,39,40] A study by Andreasson and colleagues[2] demonstrated that hemofiltration reduced the high levels of C3a and C5a in infants at the end of CPB. Furthermore, high concentrations of C3a and C5a were found in the filtrate, suggesting that part of the efficacy of ultrafiltration may be due to removal of anaphylatoxins.

3. **Specific pharmacologic manipulations directed against the complement cascade.** A study by Gillinov and colleagues[18] using a porcine model of CPB demonstrated that in vitro treatment of pig plasma with recombinant soluble

human complement receptor type I (sCR1) inhibited activation of complement. However, the pulmonary dysfunction induced by CPB was only partially ameliorated (decreased pulmonary hypertension but no improvement in post-CPB oxygenation). This finding reinforces the concept that multiple pathways are involved in the post-CPB inflammatory response and elimination of the damaging effects of CPB cannot be achieved by inhibition of the complement pathway alone.

Our knowledge of the biologic repercussions of CPB has dramatically increased over the last 10 years, particularly in regard to the biology of the complement system and its putative role in the damaging effects of CPB. However, our knowledge needs to be expanded if we are to implicate directly complement activation and other cascade systems in tissue injury and to develop specific inhibitors that ultimately eliminate the damaging effects of CPB.

## References

1. Alper CA, Rosen FS: Genetics of the complement system. Adv Hum Genet 71:141–188, 1976.
2. Andreasson S, Gothberg S, Berggren H, et al: Hemofiltration modifies complement activation after extracorporeal circulation in infants. Ann Thorac Surg 56:1515–1517, 1993.
3. Barnum SR: Biosynthesis and regulation of complement by cells of the central nervous system. Complement Profiles 1:76–95, 1993.
4. Blauhut B, Gross C, Necek S, et al: Effects of high-dose aprotinin on blood loss, platelet function, fibrinolysis, complement, and renal function after cardiopulmonary bypass. J Thorac Cardiovasc Surg 101:958–967, 1991.
5. Butler J, Pillai R, Rocker GM, et al: Effect of cardiopulmonary bypass on systemic release of neutrophil elastase and tumor necrosis factor. J Thorac Cardiovasc Surg 105:25–30, 1993.
6. Cavarocchi NC, Schaff HV, Orszulak TA, et al: Evidence for complement activation by protamine-heparin interaction after cardiopulmonary bypass. Surgery 98:525–530, 1985.
7. Cavarocchi NC, Pluth JR, Schaff HV, et al: Complement activation during cardiopulmonary bypass. J Thorac Cardiovasc Surg 91:252–258, 1986.
8. Chenoweth DE, Cooper SW, Hugli TE, et al: Complement activation during cardiopulmonary bypass: Evidence for generation of C3a and C5a anaphylatoxins. N Engl J Med 304:497–503, 1981.
9. Cleland J, Pluth JR, Tauxe WN, Kirklin JW: Blood volume and body fluid compartment changes soon after closed and open intracardiac surgery. J Thorac Cardiovasc Surg 52:698–705, 1966.
10. Davies GC, Sobel M, Salzman EW: Elevated plasma fibrinopeptide A and thromboxane $B_2$ levels during cardiopulmonary bypass. Circulation 61:808–814, 1980.
11. Elliott MJ: Ultrafiltration and modified ultrafiltration in pediatric open heart operations. Ann Thorac Surg 56:1518–1522, 1993.
12. Elliott MJ, Finn AHR: Interaction between neutrophils and endothelium. Ann Thorac Surg 56:1503–1508, 1993.
13. Entman ML, Youker K, Shappell SB, et al: Neutrophil adherence to isolated adult canine myocytes: Evidence for a CD18-dependent mechanism. J Clin Invest 85:1497–1506, 1990.
14. Faymonville ME, Deby-Dupont G, Larbuisson R, et al: Prostaglandin $E_2$ prostacyclin, and thromboxane changes during nonpulsatile cardiopulmonary bypass in humans. J Thorac Cardiovasc Surg 91:858–866, 1986.
15. Fearon DT, Austen KF: The alternative pathway of complement: A system for host defense of microbial infection. N Engl J Med 303:259–263, 1980.
16. Fehr J, Rohr H: In vivo complement activation by polyanion-polycation complexes: Evidence that C5a is generated intravascularly during heparin-protamine interaction. Clin Immunol Immunopathol 29:7–14, 1983.
17. Gillinov AM, Redmond JM, Winkelstein JA, et al: Complement and neutrophil activation during cardiopulmonary bypass: A study in the complement-deficient dog. Ann Thorac Surg 57:345–352, 1994.
18. Gillinov AM, Bator JM, Zehr KJ, et al: Neutrophil adhesion molecule expression during cardiopulmonary bypass with bubble and membrane oxygenators. Ann Thorac Surg 56:847–853, 1993.

19. Gillinov AM, DeValeria PA, Winkelstein JA, et al: Complement inhibition with soluble complement receptor type 1 in cardiopulmonary bypass. Ann Thorac Surg 55:619–624, 1993.
20. Gravlee GP, Haddon WS, Rothberger HK,et al: Heparin dosing and monitoring for cardiopulmonary bypass. J Thorac Cardiovasc Surg 99:518–527, 1990.
21. Gu YJ, van Oeveren W, Boonstra PW, et al: Leukocyte activation with increased expression of CR3 receptors during cardiopulmonary bypass. Ann Thorac Surg 53:839–843, 1992.
22. Gu YJ, van Oeveren W, Akkerman C, et al: Heparin-coated circuits reduce the inflammatory response to cardiopulmonary bypass. Ann Thorac Surg 55:917–922, 1993.
23. Haeffner-Cavaillon N, Roussellier N, Ponzio O, et al: Induction of interleukin-1 production in patients undergoing cardiopulmonary bypass. J Thorac Cardiovasc Surg 98:1100–1106, 1989.
24. Hammerschmidt DE, Harris PD, Wayland JH, et al: Complement induced granulocyte aggregation in vivo. Am J Pathol 102:146–150, 1981.
25. Hirvonen J, Huttunen P, Nuutinen L, Pekkarinen A: Catecholamines and free fatty acids in plasma of patients undergoing cardiac operations with hypothermia and bypass. J Clin Pathol 31:949–955, 1978.
26. Hugli TE: The structural basis for anaphylatoxin and chemotactic functions of C3a, C4a and C5a. CRC Crit Rev Immunol 1:321–366, 1981.
27. Kirklin JK, Westaby S, Blackstone EH, et al: Complement and the damaging effects of cardiopulmonary bypass. J Thorac Cardiovasc Surg 86:845–857, 1983.
28. Kirklin JK, Chenoweth DE, Naftel DC, et al: Effects of protamine administration after cardiopulmonary bypass on complement, blood elements, and the hemodynamic state. Ann Thorac Surg 41:193–199, 1986.
29. Lillehei CW: Historical development of cardiopulmonary bypass. In Gravlee GP, Davis RF, Utley JR (eds): Cardiopulmonary Bypass: Principles and Practice. Baltimore, Williams & Wilkins, 1993, pp 1–26.
30. Lowenstein E, Johnston WE, Lappas DG, et al: Catastrophic pulmonary vasoconstriction associated with protamine reversal of heparin. Anesthesiology 59:470–473, 1983.
31. Macnaughton PD, Braude S, Hunter DN, et al: Changes in lung function and pulmonary capillary permeability after cardiopulmonary bypass. Crit Care Med 20:1289–1294, 1992.
32. Mair P, Mair J, Seibt I, Furtwaengler W, et al: To the editor: Plasma elastase concentrations and pulmonary function after cardiopulmonary bypass. J Thorac Cardiovasc Surg 108:183–185, 1994.
33. Mastroroberto P, Chello M, Marchese AR: Plasma C3a and C5a concentrations during cardiopulmonary bypass [letter]. Ann Thorac Surg 57:781–786, 1994.
34. McGiffin DC, Kirklin JK: Cardiopulmonary bypass for cardiac surgery. In Sabiston DC, Spencer FC (eds): Surgery of the Chest, 6th ed. Philadelphia, W.B. Saunders, in press.
35. Moat NE, Rebuck N, Shore DF, et al: Humoral and cellular activation in a simulated extracorporeal circuit. Ann Thorac Surg 56:1509–1514, 1993.
36. Mollnes TE, Videm V, Gotze O, et al: Formation of C5a during cardiopulmonary bypass: Inhibition of precoating with heparin. Ann Thorac Surg 52:92–97, 1991.
37. Moore FD Jr: Therapeutic regulation of the complement system in acute injury states. Adv Immunol 56:267–299, 1994.
38. Muller-Eberhard HJ: Complement. Ann Rev Biochem 44:697–724, 1975.
39. Naik S, Balaji S, Elliott MJ: Modified ultrafiltration improves hemodynamics after cardiopulmonary bypass in children [abstract]. J Am Coll Cardiol 19:37A, 1992.
40. Naik SK, Knight A, Elliott M: A prospective randomized study of a modified technique of ultrafiltration during pediatric open-heart surgery. Circulation 84(Suppl III):422–431, 1991.
41. Nordstrom L, Fletcher R, Pavek K: Shock of anaphylactoid type induced by protamine: A continuous cardiorespiratory record. Acta Anaesthesiol Scand 22:195–201, 1978.
42. Olinger GN, Becker RM, Bonchek LI: Noncardiogenic pulmonary edema and peripehral vascular collapse following cardiopulmonary bypass: Rare protamine reaction? Ann Thorac Surg 29:20–25, 1980.
43. Oppermann M, Schulze M, Gotze O: A sensitive enzyme-immunoassay for the quantitation of human C5a/C5a(desArg) anaphylatoxin using a monoclonal antibody with specificity for a neoepitope. Complement Inflamm 8:13–24, 1991.
44. Pang LM, Stalcup SA, Lipset JS, et al: Increased circulating bradykinin during hypothermia and cardiopulmonary bypass in children. Circulation 60:1503–1507, 1979.
45. Perlmutter DH, Strunk RC, Colten HR: Complement. In Crystal RG, West JB (eds): The Lung: Scientific Foundations, vol. 1. New York, Raven Press, 1991, pp 511–525.
46. Reed HL, Chernow B, Lake CR, et al: Alterations in sympathetic nervous system activity with intraoperative hypothermia during coronary artery bypass surgery. Chest 95:616–622, 1989.

47. Reves JG, Karp RB, Buttner EE, et al: Neuronal and adrenomedullary catecholamine release in response to cardiopulmonary bypass in man. Circulation 66:49–55, 1982.
48. Root RK: Leukocyte adhesion proteins: Their role in neutrophil function. Trans Am Clin Climatol Assoc 101:207–224, 1989.
49. Ross GD, Medof ME: Membrane complement receptors specific for bound fragments of C3. Adv Immunol 37:217–267, 1985.
50. Sacks T, Moldow CF, Craddock PR, et al: Oxygen radicals mediate endothelial cell damage complement-stimulated granulocytes. J Clin Invest 61:1161–1167, 1978.
51. Schulze M, Gotze O: A sensitive ELISA for the quantitation of human C5a in blood plasma using a monoclonal antibody. Complement 3:25–39, 1986.
52. Seghaye MC, Duchateau J, Grabitz RG, et al: Complement, leukocytes, and leukocyte elastase in full-term neonates undergoing cardiac operation. J Thorac Cardiovasc Surg 108:29–36, 1994.
53. Shappell SB, Toman C, Anderson DC, et al: Mac-1 (CD11b/CD18) mediates adherence-dependent hydrogen peroxide production by human and canine neutrophils. J Immunol 144:2702–2711, 1990.
54. Smith EEJ, Naftel DC, Blackstone EH, Kirklin JW: Microvascular permeability after cardiopulmonary bypass. J Thorac Cardiovasc Surg 94:225–233, 1987.
55. Tamiya T, Yamasaki M, Maeo Y, et al: Complement activation in cardiopulmonary bypass, with special reference to anaphylatoxin production in membrane and bubble oxygenators. Ann Thorac Surg 46:47–57, 1988.
56. Tennenberg SD, Clardy CW, Bailey WW, Solomkin JS: Complement activation and lung permeability during cardiopulmonary bypass. Ann Thorac Surg 50:597–601, 1990.
57. Todd RF III, Freyer DR: The CD11/CD18 leukocyte glycoprotein deficiency. Hematol Oncol Clin North Am 2:13–31, 1988.
58. Tonneson MG: Neutrophil-endothelial cell interactions: Mechanisms of neutrophil adherence to vascular endothelium. J Invest Dermatol 93:53s–58s, 1989.
59. van Oeveren W, Kazatchkine MD, Descamps-Latscha B, et al: Deleterious effects of cardiopulmonary bypass. J Thorac Cardiovasc Surg 89:888–899, 1985.
60. Videm V, Svennevig JL, Fosse E, et al: Reduced complement activation with heparin-coated oxygenator and tubings in coronary bypass operations. J Thorac Cardiovasc Surg 103:806–813, 1992.
61. Volanakis JE, Fearon DT: The molecular biology of the complement system. In McCarty DJ, Koopman WJ (eds): Arthritis and Allied Conditions, 12th ed. Philadelphia, Lea & Febiger, 1993, pp 455–467.
62. Watkins WD, Peterson MB, Kong DL, et al: Thromboxane and prostacyclin changes during cardiopulmonary bypass with and without pulsatile flow. J Thorac Cardiovasc Surg 84:250–256, 1982.
63. Ylikorkala O, Saarela E, Viinikka L: Increased prostacyclin and thromboxane production in man during cardiopulmonary bypass. J Thorac Cardiovasc Surg 82:245–247, 1981.
64. Yoon SH, Fearon DT: Characterization of a soluble form of the C3b/C4b receptor (CR1) in human plasma. J Immunol 134:3332–3338, 1985.

William C. Oliver, Jr., MD
Gregory A. Nuttall, MD

# 4

## Platelet Function and Cardiopulmonary Bypass

Patients who undergo cardiac surgery and cardiopulmonary bypass (CPB) are at risk for serious postoperative bleeding that is associated with disease transmission[1] and increased costs[2] due to transfusion of allogeneic blood and blood products. The causes of postbypass bleeding are inadequate surgical hemostasis,[3,4] acquired defects of coagulation, or both.[5] The distinction is not always obvious. Acquired defects of coagulation include reduced clotting factors, inadequate heparin reversal, fibrinolysis, complement activation, and platelet dysfunction.[4] Platelet dysfunction is considered the major cause of postbypass hemorrhage, although the mechanism is not completely understood. A generalized ooze in the surgical field frequently suggests platelet dysfunction.

This chapter includes a discussion of normal platelet function as well as the effect of CPB. Knowledge of normal platelet function is important, because it provides the basis for understanding platelet activity in abnormal physiologic situations such as extracorporeal circulation (EC).

### Normal Platelet Function

Successful hemostasis involves the vasculature, coagulation cascades, and platelets. Platelets have a complex and important role in hemostasis. Platelet response in hemostasis may be divided into four components: adhesion, aggregation, secretion, and procoagulation. Once vascular injury has occurred, the response by the platelets is rapid and localized to the injured area. Platelets act as a catalyst in the hemostatic process. Specific substances that appear at the site cause vasoconstriction and attract additional platelets. The result is the formation of a "plug." The plug is fortified with fibrin strands within minutes of the injury. Eventually it is dissolved by the fibrinolytic system. New vascular endothelial cells complete the repair process.

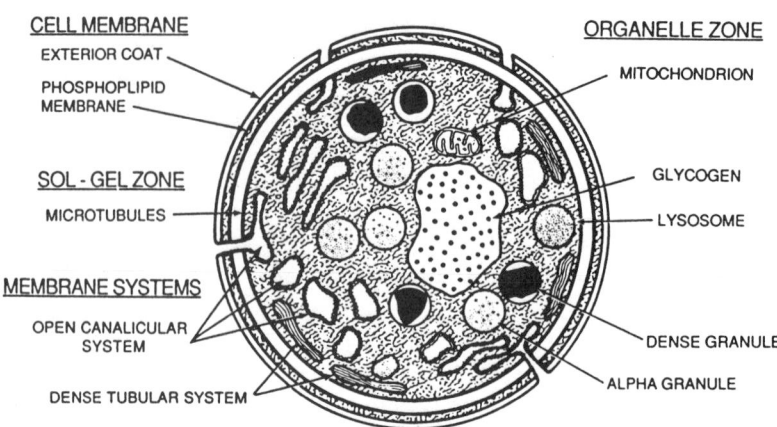

**FIGURE 1.** Anatomy of the platelet. (Adapted from Gravlee GP, Davis RF, Utley JR: Cardiopulmonary Bypass: Principles and Practice. Baltimore, Williams & Wilkins, 1993, with permission.)

## Platelet Morphology

Platelets are membrane-encapsulated fragments of megakaryocyte cytoplasm that consist of a nonuniformly constructed, trilaminar phospholipoprotein membrane[6] (Fig. 1). The external membrane is composed primarily of neutral phospholipids, whereas the inner membrane is more negatively charged. The external membrane becomes more negative when the platelet is activated because the distribution of the phospholipids is altered. The negatively charged outside membrane enhances the activation of other coagulation processes that increase the platelet's procoagulant activity. The surface of the platelet is particularly suited for involvement in various aspects of coagulation (Table 1). The platelet membrane is also a major source of arachidonic acid, which is necessary for synthesis of prostaglandin and platelet-activating factor (PAF). Both compounds are important for normal platelet function.

In the unstimulated state, the platelet is disc-shaped with a diameter of 2–3 $\mu$m. The lack of a nucleus to synthesize protein accounts for the platelet's brief lifespan of 10–14 days. Platelets contain an array of specialized structures that include microtubules, organelles, and an internal network of canaliculi (Fig. 1). The organelles include mitochondria, Golgi bodies, ribosomes, and granules. The four types of granules are lysosomes, alpha-granules, dense granules, and microperoxisomes.[7] Lysosomes contain acid hydrolyses, whereas microperoxisomes contain peroxidases such as catalase. The alpha-granules contain fibronectin, von Willebrand factor (vWF)/factor VIII, fibrinogen, platelet factor 4 (PF4), beta-thromboglobulin (BTG), factor V, and thrombospondin, along with other secretory proteins.[6] Dense granules contain adenosine diphosphate (ADP), serotonin, adenosine triphosphate (ATP),

**TABLE 1.** Platelet Functions Involved in Coagulation

| |
|---|
| Prothrombin catalyzed to thrombin by platelet receptors |
| GP IIb–IIIa thrombin-induced receptor for vWF |
| Enhanced activation of factor X |
| Receptors for factor XII and XI |
| Inhibited inactivation of factors Va, Xa, and VIIIa and thrombin |

histamine, and calcium. The alpha-granules and dense granules are important for normal platelet function. Congenital deficiencies result in mild bleeding tendencies.

Besides secretory granules and organelles, the platelet has an extensive system of microtubules to communicate with the external environment and to maintain internal access to enzymes and ions. The open and elaborate canalicular system increases the number of receptor sites that are available and facilitates granule secretion.[8]

Actin is an important component of the platelet structure. Actin polymerization and cytoskeleton reorganization are responsible for changes in platelet shape in response to stimuli.[8] Pseudopodia that gradually become noticeable during activation are formed from highly organized bundles of filaments. These calcium-mediated, actin-catalyzed myosin components contract, which changes the platelet's shape. The change in shape is important for effective platelet adhesion.

## Platelet Activation

Normally the vascular endothelium is a "neutral" surface for the blood and its formed elements. Platelets circulate primarily in a nonactivated state. Once the integrity of the vascular endothelium is disrupted, the subendothelial connective tissue is exposed to the blood and platelets. The subendothelium contains collagen, vWF, fibronectin, and proteins that recruit additional platelets to the damaged site. The initial and crucial step in the formation of the platelet plug and hemostasis is platelet adhesion to the subendothelial molecules (Fig. 2). The subendothelial compounds have a specific protein sequence (tripeptide) that interacts with the

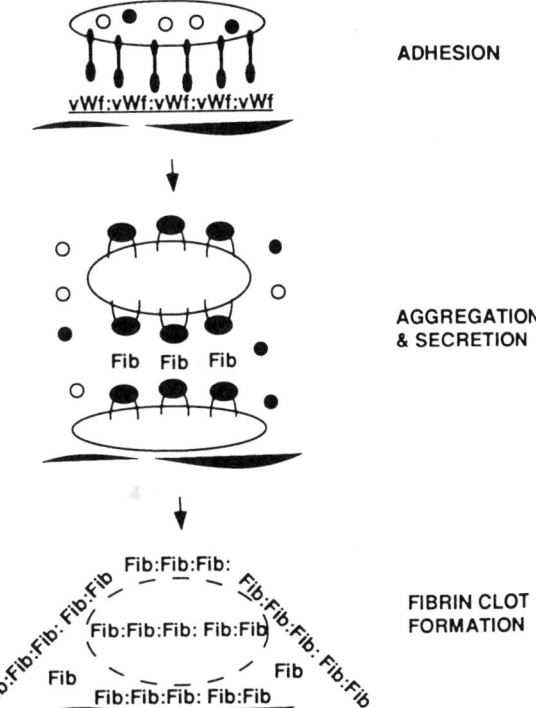

**FIGURE 2.** Platelet function. The stages of adhesion, aggregation, secretion, and fibrin clot formation. Rod with nodules at letter end = GPIb/IX; vWF = von Willebrand factor; wavy lines = extracellular matrix (subendothelium); o = alpha granule; ● = dense granule; nodule with two arms = GP IIb/IIIa; Fib = fibrinogen; Fib:Fib:Fib: = fibrin; dashed ovals = platelets undergoing autolysis. (Adapted from Bennett DA, Evans DA: Disorders of platelet function. Dis Mon 38:577–631, 1992, with permission.)

platelets.[9] The most common tripeptide sequence is arginine–glycine–aspartic acid. Specific glycoprotein receptors recognize the sequence and bind the platelet to the subendothelial compounds.[10] The characteristics of the blood flow determine which subendothelial matrix molecule will bind to a specific platelet receptor.[7] Under conditions of low blood flow (venous), glycoprotein Ia (GPIa) receptor[9] binds to collagen, whereas GPIc/IIa[8] receptors bind to fibronectin. During high blood flow and increased shear (arterial), the attachment of platelets with collagen or fibronectin is inadequate. Therefore platelets bind to vWF (Fig. 3). The unique origin and multimeric composition of vWF sustain platelet–vessel wall interactions in conditions of high blood flow.[11] VWF is found in plasma, platelets, and endothelium. The vWF that binds the platelets is not the circulating vWF but originates in the subendothelium. The platelets bind to the subendothelial vWF primarily through the attachment of either GPIb or GPIIb/IIIa receptors. However, GPIb is the major vWF-binding protein.[9] This complex of vWF and GPIb plays a critical role in platelet adhesion. An abnormality in this receptor complex may result in bleeding tendencies; vWF has no interaction in unstimulated platelets.

Platelet adhesion is a prerequisite for platelet aggregation and formation of a platelet plug in vivo. Once platelets begin to adhere to the injured site, their discoid shape becomes more spherical through centralization of cytoplasmic organelles and extension of pseudopods (Fig. 4). This stage of the platelet response involves primary platelet aggregation in conjunction with platelet adhesion. Primary aggregation is reversible and essentially reflects the affinity of platelets for one another.[12]

If the platelet plug is to develop, platelet activation and aggregation must continue. The platelets are activated by means of stimulus-response coupling. Activation

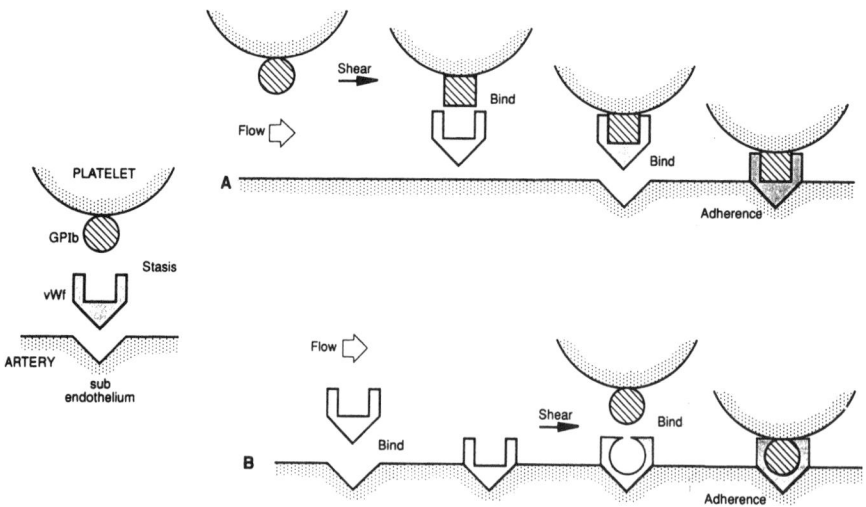

**FIGURE 3.** Mechanisms of adhesion. In the venous state of low blood flow, no interaction occurs between vWF and GPIb. With arterial blood (high flow and high shear), a change occurs in the GPIb or vWF or both. *A,* With shear, platelet GPIb undergoes a conformational change that allows attachment of vWF. *B,* vWF binds to the subendothelium and undergoes a conformational change secondary to shear, which results in the binding of circulating GPIb. (From Roth GJ: Developing relationships: Arterial platelet adhesion, glycoprotein 1b, and leucine-rich glycoproteins. Blood 77:5–19, 1991, with permission.)

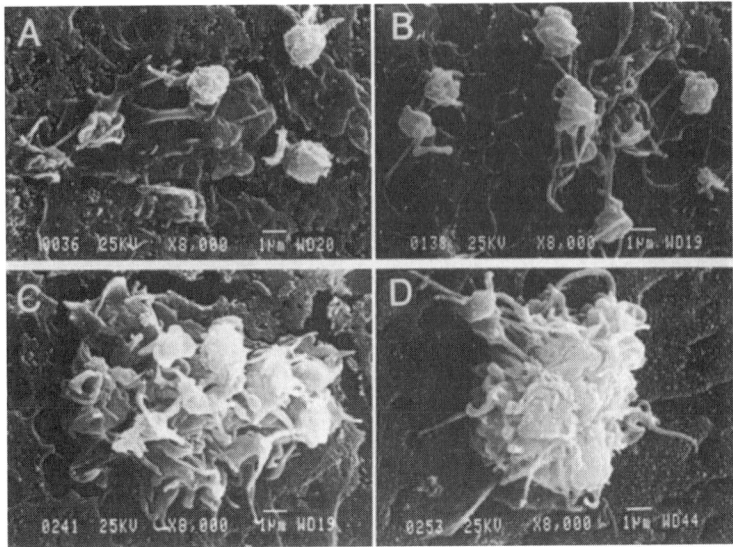

**FIGURE 4.** Scanning electron micrographs of four aggregation grades of platelets on the extracellular matrix. *A*, Platelets are discoid; no pseudopodia. *B*, Initial signs of activation with slight signs of pseudopodia. *C*, Prominent signs of aggregation. Platelets spread, multiple pseudopodia, and clustering. *D*, Aggregate. No individual platelets can be identified (× 8000). (From Golan M, Modan M, Lavee J, et al: Transfusion of fresh whole blood stored (4°C) for short period fails to improve platelet aggregation on extracellular matrix and clinical hemostasis after cardiopulmonary bypass. J Thorac Cardiovasc Surg 99:354–360, 1990, with permission.)

requires the presence of proteins, known as G-proteins, which are found in the platelet membrane. The G-proteins are involved in the complicated enzymatic pathways to produce change in platelet shape, granule secretion, or prostaglandin synthesis. G-proteins require guanine triphosphate (GTP) to activate the platelet. Platelets are activated at a rate that depends on the eliciting thrombogenic stimuli. If the stimulus becomes stronger, irreversible changes in the platelets may occur and the platelets degranulate. If the stimulus is insufficient, the platelets revert to the unstimulated state and assume a discoid shape. The shape and membrane changes associated with platelet activation and aggregation make the platelet surface more sticky (Fig. 4). Once irreversible platelet aggregation has occurred, a more solid and dense collection of platelets and fibrin is formed. The ability of the platelet to return from primary aggregation to the unstimulated state is protection against a full hemostatic response to a minor stimulus.

## Granule Secretion

An important aspect of platelet response to injury is the release of granules. Degranulation occurs in response to many stimuli, such as epinephrine, ADP, and thrombin. The alpha-granules are released at low levels of stimulation. Thrombin is a potent stimulus for dense granule secretion. Arachidonic acid metabolites are also usually necessary to stimulate granule secretion, except in the presence of strong platelet agonist. Degranulation is a calcium-dependent, active process that requires ATP. Agonists affect the cytoplasmic calcium concentration. Granule contents attract platelets to the injured site to form platelet thrombi. This aggregate of platelets incorporates fibrin and stabilizes the platelet plug. Besides recruitment of additional platelets to the injured area, degranulation causes acceleration of the coagulation cascade, local vasoconstriction, and increased vascular permeability.

## Platelet Aggregation

In contrast to platelet adhesion, platelet aggregation requires platelet stimulation and active platelet metabolism. Aggregation is initiated in several ways. It may occur after platelet activation by one of several agonists, such as thrombin, ADP, or collagen. Agonists bind to a specific platelet membrane receptor during activation.[10] A second messenger system transfers information to the platelet membrane so that the receptors can be prepared.[13,14] The preparation involves a conformational change in the receptor that exposes the fibrinogen-binding site.[15] The receptor must be altered to bind with fibrinogen and thus to achieve normal platelet activity. The receptor-specific relocation that occurs after stimulation[8] not only prepares platelet receptors to bind with fibrinogen but also increases intracellular calcium. The increased cytosolic calcium facilitates activation of phospholipase $A_2$ and mobilizes free arachidonic acid so that thromboxane $A_2$ ($TxA_2$) is produced[13] (Fig. 5). The synthesis of $TxA_2$ is important for platelet function.

The potential for platelet activation and aggregation depends on the potency of the platelet agonists, which varies. Collagen and thrombin are potent platelet activators. Weaker platelet agonists are ADP, epinephrine, prostaglandin endoperoxides, $TxA_2$, PAF, and serotonin.[16] Some of the weaker agonists can potentiate the effect of stronger agonists, such as thrombin and collagen.

Platelet aggregation results from a calcium-dependent fibrinogen binding between cells and attachment of platelet receptors to adhesive proteins[9] (see Fig. 2). The major platelet receptor for aggregation is GPIIb/IIIa.[17] Once the GPIIb/IIIa receptor has been prepared, it facilitates platelet spreading and aggregation. Although fibrinogen is important, it is not the only compound involved in aggregation; vWF also binds with GPIIb/IIIa receptors when platelets are activated by thrombin, ADP, or collagen.

The generation of $TxA_2$ is an important part of the normally functioning platelet. $TxA_2$, a vasoconstrictor and platelet aggregator, has a very short half-life and is metabolized rapidly. Various platelet agonists (thrombin, ADP, epinephrine) stimulate formation of $TxA_2$ at the platelet membrane. $TxA_2$ synthesis begins with the release of arachidonic acid from the platelet membrane by one or more phospholipases (Fig. 6). Arachidonic acid is mobilized and converted to labile endoperoxides by the enzyme cyclooxygenase. Thromboxane synthetase converts most of the endoperoxides into $TxA_2$.

Although $TxA_2$ is important for platelet activation, platelet activation is not dependent on the arachidonic pathway. Another pathway for initiation of platelet aggregation involves the agonists thrombin and collagen. Both compounds increase the level of free cytoplasmic calcium, which ultimately leads to platelet degranulation. Platelets also may be activated independently by release of PAF, which is derived from the platelet membrane through the action of membrane phospholipases.

Besides the ability of platelets to adhere, aggregate, and form a plug, the platelet surface activates the intrinsic coagulation pathway.[18] On the platelet surface,

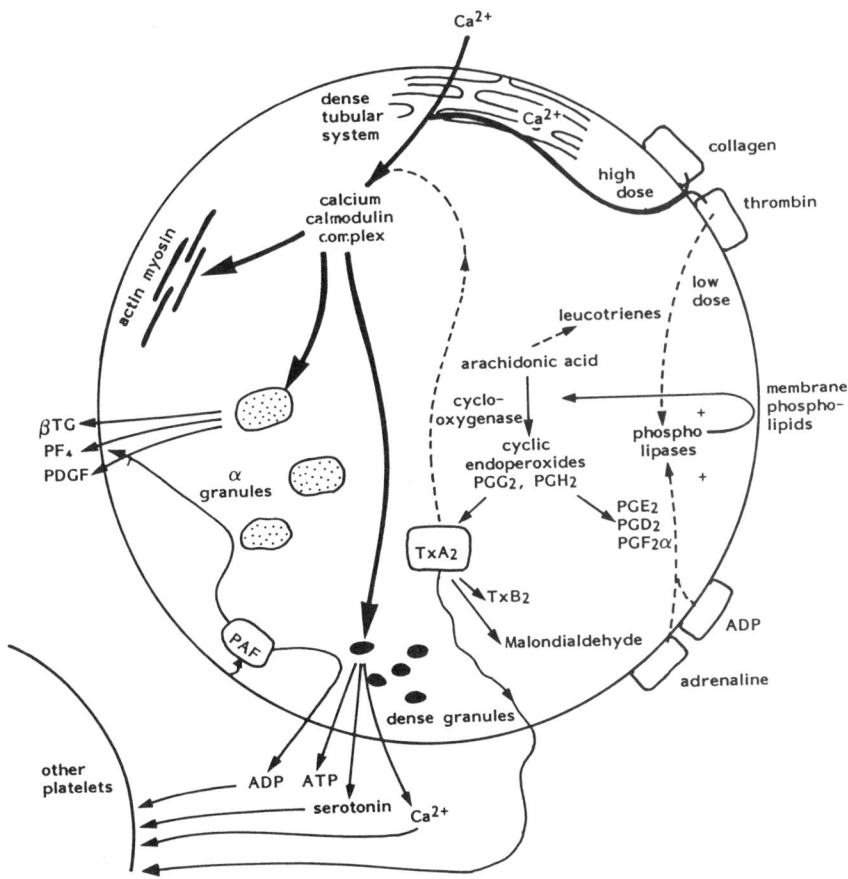

**FIGURE 5.** Representation of the pathways for platelet activation. $Ca^{++}$ = calcium ions; $PGG_2$, $H_2$, $E_2$, $D_2$, and $F_{2a}$ = prostaglandin $G_2$, $H_2$, $E_2$, $D_2$, and $F_{2a}$, respectively. $TxA_2$ = thromboxane $A_2$; $TXB2$, $\beta TG$ = beta-thromboglobulin; $PF_4$ = platelet factor 4; PDGF = platelet-derived growth factor; ADP = adenosine diphosphate; ATP = adenosine triphosphate. (From Yardumian DA, Mackie IJ, and Machin SJ: Laboratory investigation of platelet function: A review of methodology. J Clin Pathol 39:702, 1986, with permission.)

factor XI is converted to factor XIa, thus localizing the conversion of factors IX and X. Factor Xa is bound to the platelet by factor V and platelet factor 3. Because factor Va is present on the platelet surface, large amounts of thrombin may be generated.[9] Thrombin then cleaves fibrinogen into fibrin monomers that polymerize nonenzymatically to provide a solid gel network and to stabilize the platelet plug. Thrombin has a pivotal role in the formation and strengthening of the platelet plug. Involvement of the platelet in this reaction affirms its broad procoagulant activities.

## Regulation of Platelet Activity

Overall platelet response is regulated more easily at the local level of the individual platelet. An example of local control is activation of the intrinsic pathway on the

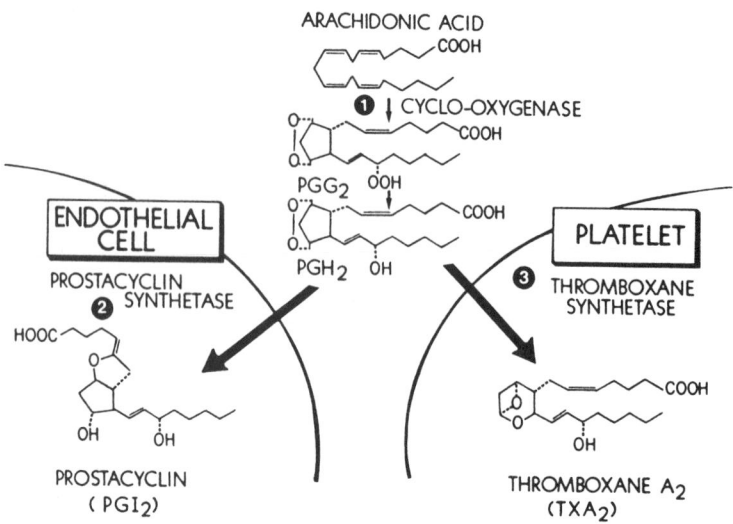

**FIGURE 6.** Arachidonate metabolism. Arachidonic acid conversion to prostacyclin and thromboxane $A_2$. (From Rossi EC, Simon TL, Moss GS: Principles of Transfusion Medicine. Baltimore, Williams & Wilkins, 1991, p 184, with permission.)

platelet surface. The mechanisms that inhibit platelet activation are found at the vascular endothelium, which manufactures prostacyclin, a potent platelet inhibitor. Prostacyclin does not circulate continuously but is released in response to local stimulation.[6] It acts by binding to adenylate cyclase in the cell membrane to increase the amount of cyclic adenosine monophosphate (cAMP), which is an inhibitor of platelet activation.[16] Platelet adenylate cyclase generates cAMP from ATP. Increased cAMP lowers the intracellular calcium concentration. Intracellular calcium is critical to platelet activity. Changes in calcium level affect the synthesis of cyclooxygenase and phospholipase $A_2$ as well as other calcium-dependent activities necessary for platelet function. The endothelial production of prostacyclin provides a balance between thrombosis and platelet inhibition.

Calcium has widespread effects on many aspects of platelet function. The resting calcium concentration in platelets is low, and most of it is in the dense granules. However, calcium is involved in practically every facet of platelet function and regulation.[13] Calcium mobilization and changes in the calcium flux affect the activation of enzymes, reactions in the cytoskeleton, changes in shape, and expression of binding sites. Furthermore, extracellular calcium is required for cell-to-cell interaction during aggregation.

### Platelet Membrane Glycoproteins

Six major glycoproteins have been characterized on the platelet surface: GPIb, GPIc, GPIIb, GPIa, GPIIa, and GPIIIa. Three of these receptors (GPIIb/IIIa, GPI/cIIa, and GPIa/IIa) have been classified as integrins. The integrins are a family of immunologically and structurally related glycoproteins that have a strong affinity for fibrinogen, vWF, fibronectin, or vibronectine.[15] As mentioned previously, the GPIIb/IIIa receptor is important in the cohesion of platelets with fibrinogen[11]; it is considered the fibrinogen receptor.[9] Although fibrinogen is the primary mediator of platelet bridging with the GPIIb/IIIa receptor in normal plasma, in the absence of fibrinogen following GPIIb/IIIa conformational change other compounds may be substituted, such as fibronectin, vitronectin, and vWF.[10]

GPIb is bound to smaller protein, GPIX, to form a noncovalent complex, which is the primary receptor for binding with vWF. The binding of vWF to GPIb-IX leads to platelet activation, attraction, and attachment.

P-selectin (platelet activation-dependent, granule-external membrane, or granule membrane protein 140), an important receptor in the alpha-granules, is expressed on the platelet surface after platelet activation by thrombin.[19] It is a marker for platelet activation.

## Effect of Cardiopulmonary Bypass

Initiation of EC exposes the blood to extensive contact with a synthetic, nonbiologic surface that is associated with major hemostatic defects.[20,21] Of the extracorporeal circuit components (oxygenator, roller pumps, plastic tubing, cardiotomy suction, and filters), the oxygenator is considered a major contributor to coagulation abnormalities. However, cardiotomy suction, hypothermia, hemodilution, medications, and duration of CPB are also factors in postbypass bleeding. Because the synthetic surface of extracorporeal circuit is a potent stimulus for clotting, full anticoagulation with heparin is necessary during CPB to prevent major thrombosis. Because heparin prevents activation only at the end of the coagulation cascade, however, platelets are adversely affected.

Platelet dysfunction is considered the most important hemostatic alteration associated with CPB.[5,21] Platelet transfusions are frequently administered in response to excessive postbypass bleeding. The platelet defect associated with CPB is both qualitative and quantitative.

### Thrombocytopenia

During the first 5 minutes of CPB, the predictable decrease in the platelet count approximates 30–50%.[4,22–24] Thrombocytopenia is due to hemodilution, liver sequestration, platelet adhesion to synthetic surfaces, formation of platelet aggregates,[24] and platelet trauma.[25] Although hemodilution is the major factor responsible for the decrease in platelet count, the decrease is sometimes more than expected from hemodilution alone.[4,26] Furthermore, the platelet count decreases regardless of the type of oxygenator.[20] The initial decrease may be greater with a membrane oxygenator, but the count continues to decrease with the bubble oxygenator throughout the duration of CPB.[27]

CPB-associated thrombocytopenia is not the critical factor in bleeding and overall platelet function. The platelet count usually remains above $100,000/\mu l$ during CPB in adults—a level that normally is adequate for hemostasis. Moreover, the platelet count correlates poorly with postoperative bleeding.[20,28] In contrast, platelet function correlated well with postbypass bleeding in several studies.[21,28] The combination of thrombocytopenia and platelet dysfunction may contribute to excessive bleeding and increased bleeding time (BT),[24] although a correspondingly good correlation with blood loss and transfusion requirements has not been demonstrated consistently.[29]

## Platelet Dysfunction

It has been established that the onset of CPB results in a prolongation of the BT that indicates platelet dysfunction.[30] The progressive nature of platelet dysfunction is demonstrated by the progressive increase in the BT as a function of CPB duration.[21,30] Platelet dysfunction usually persists 1–2 hours after CPB. The BT shortens to approximately 15 minutes in the immediate postbypass period and frequently normalizes within 2–4 hours.[30] Platelet dysfunction may persist in patients that bleed excessively.[31] Blood loss and transfusion requirements correlate with the BT 2 hours after CPB.[21] Another indication of platelet dysfunction is reduced aggregation in the presence of both weak (ADP and epinephrine) and potent (collagen and thrombin) agonists[4,26] at initiation of CPB.[32] Such defects in aggregation persist for several hours after CPB, although the reason is not clear. In a recent study that used aggregation tests as a measure of platelet function, impairment associated with CPB correlated with excessive bleeding in the immediate postbypass period.[28] Furthermore, the use of preoperative platelet aggregation studies identified patients who were most likely to bleed excessively after CPB.[28] A fourfold increase in the risk of bleeding was associated with an abnormal platelet aggregation study. This investigation is evidence for the relationship between platelet dysfunction and bleeding after CPB. The precise nature of the CPB-induced platelet function defect is not clear. A reduced ADP content has been proposed as the mechanism for the persistent dysfunction, although it is considered a minor cause. Current knowledge suggests that after CPB many circulating platelets have reduced function, whereas only a few are irreversibly activated. This phenomenon would account for the temporary platelet dysfunction.

Exposure of the blood to the large synthetic surface area of extracorporeal circuit is believed to be a considerable factor in bleeding after CPB.[33] Many of the detrimental effects of EC are attributed directly to the activation of platelets and factor XII,[34,35] which may occur during the first few minutes of CPB.[27] When the blood is exposed to the artificial surface, a layer of protein, primarily fibrinogen, is deposited on the extracorporeal circuit surface. This layer of fibrinogen permits exposure of GPIIb/IIIa receptors on activated platelets, which thus adhere to the fibrinogen more easily. Subsequent degranulation attracts additional platelets as well as a host of coagulation proteins. Platelets accumulate on the artificial surface in association with fibrin and red blood cells. As accumulation continues, the number of circulating platelets is reduced and overall platelet function is compromised.[36] Platelets are continuously removed and added during this period. The heterogenous population of new and old platelets may affect the potential for bleeding after CPB. Younger and larger platelets are considered more hemostatically active.[32] A larger mean platelet volume (MPV) has been correlated with platelet aggregation[33] and reduced postbypass bleeding.[32] The platelet count may be similar between two patients, but the lower MPV is associated with more postbypass bleeding.[32] MPV usually increases over a 2–24-hour period after CPB in conjunction with the arrival of larger platelets and improved BT.[4,21]

## Platelet Activation and Cardiopulmonary Bypass

Although platelet activation is regarded as an important factor in postbypass bleeding, the association has not been demonstrated conclusively. Harker et al.[30] found a rise in plasma and urine levels of PF4 and BTG in humans and baboons during CPB in association with an increased BT. The progressive rise of both platelet secretory products in the plasma has been cited as evidence for ongoing platelet activation during CPB.[35] However, PF4 and BTG are less specific for release of alpha-granules than P-selectin. Studies with P-selectin as the marker for release of alpha-granules support ongoing platelet activation during CPB[37] (Fig. 7) and suggest

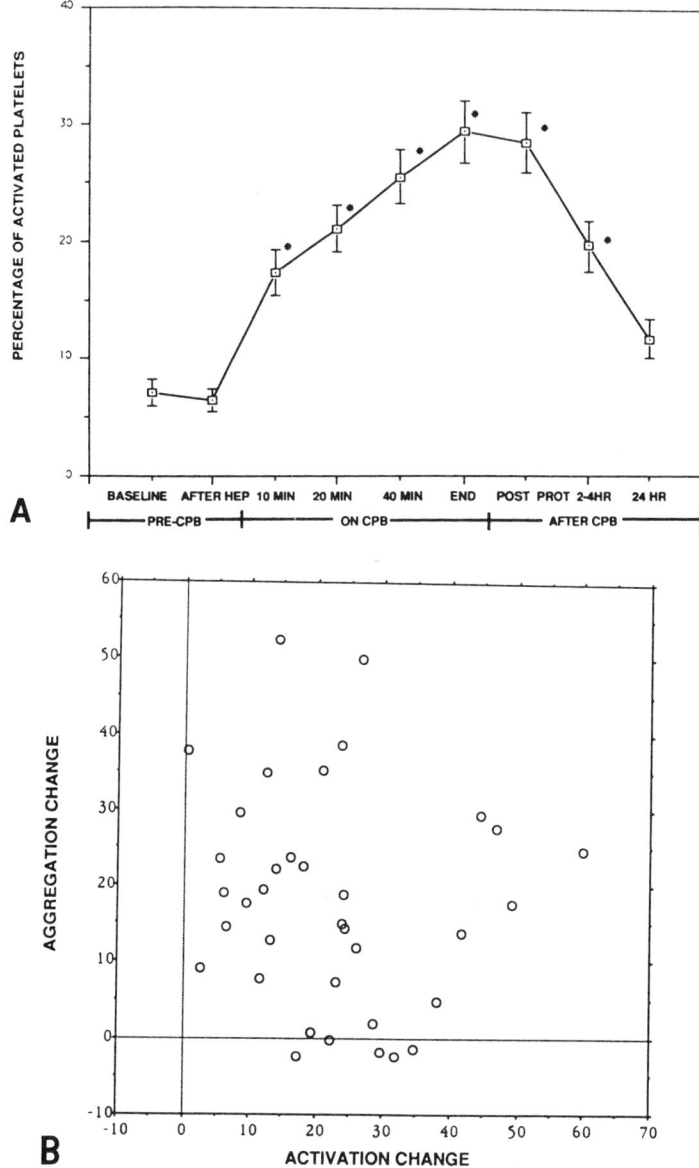

**FIGURE 7.** *A,* Percentage of circulating activated platelets in whole blood before, during, and after CPB. Data are means ± SEM. HEP = heparin; PROT = protamine. Samples are compared to baseline by ANOVA (*$p < 0.05$. *B,* Correlation between change in activation and change in aggregation (absolute value) between baseline and end of CPB. No correlation was observed at r = 0.03. (From Rinder CS, Bohnert J, Rinder HM, et al: Platelet activation and aggregation during cardiopulmonary bypass. Anesthesiology 75:388–393, 1991, with permission.)

that postbypass coagulopathy is related to platelet activation and subsequent loss of functioning platelets. However, if platelet aggregation is used as an indication of platelet function, the period of poorest aggregation does not coincide with the period of peak activation, and the change in activation does not correlate with the change in aggregation (Fig. 7).[37] Furthermore, neither peak activation nor peak aggregation of platelets predicted postoperative bleeding in a recent investigation, although the sample was small.[37] However, investigations in patients who received agents that inhibit platelet activation, such as prostacyclin, have demonstrated an improved platelet count, decreased plasma levels of PF4 and BTG during CPB, and reductions in chest tube drainage compared with controls.[36] Although inhibitory agents may partially preserve platelet function by preventing activation and aggregation during CPB, the CPB-induced platelet defect appears to involve more than activation.

Others have questioned the association between platelet activation and postbypass bleeding.[38] Zilla et al. believe that platelet activation is not sustained throughout CPB despite elevated plasma levels of PF4 and BTG. They found minimal PF4 and BTG in the plasma at initiation of CPB, and only 3.4% of the available PF4 remained in the plasma at the end of CPB.[39] They view previous reports of increased plasma levels of PF4 and BTG[30] as of minimal importance in comparison with the potential for granule release. Other studies of the actual platelet content of alpha-granules do not support significant degranulation during CPB.[27] Elevated plasma levels of alpha-granules may be attributed to platelet trauma and lysis without necessarily representing activation. An association between bleeding, platelet dysfunction, and release of alpha-granules is further strained by the knowledge that the BT normalizes several hours after discontinuation of CPB despite a continuing deficiency in PF4 and BTG. This suggests that depletion of alpha-granules and platelet dysfunction may be independent events.

The claim of Zilla et al. that activation of platelets during CPB is minimal is based also on ultrastructural analysis. Platelets change shape with activation, which may either proceed to an irreversible state of aggregation or revert to an unstimulated state.[39] Because it detects the reversible component, ultrastructural analysis is a more sensitive method of detecting activation. The release of alpha-granules and dense granules in the plasma usually represents irreversible aggregation but not necessarily platelet activation. Zilla et al. found that although nearly one-half of the platelets are activated at the beginning of CPB (based on shape changes), granular secretory products did not rise[39] (Fig. 8). Therefore, the initial exposure of platelets to CPB is sufficient to induce a change in shape but not sufficient to cause irreversible secondary aggregation. As CPB continues, the morphology of the platelets continues to improve, yet the aggregability is still poor.[39] This finding contradicts evidence of continual platelet activation.

Causes of platelet activation during CPB other than artificial surface contact include release of PAF and generation of plasmin. Plasmin activation of platelets during CPB renders them less useful for hemostasis after CPB.

## Platelet Membrane Receptors

Platelet adhesion and aggregation are crucial to the formation of the platelet plug. The role of the platelet glycoprotein receptors is established in normal hemostasis. The effect of CPB and EC on glycoprotein receptors and on postbypass hemorrhage is still uncertain.

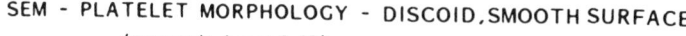

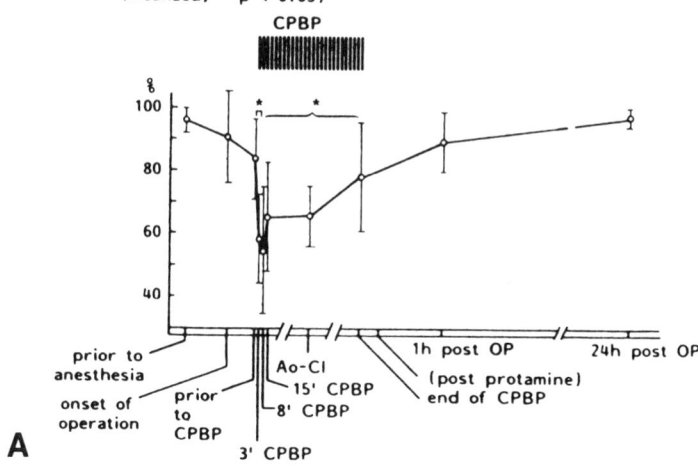

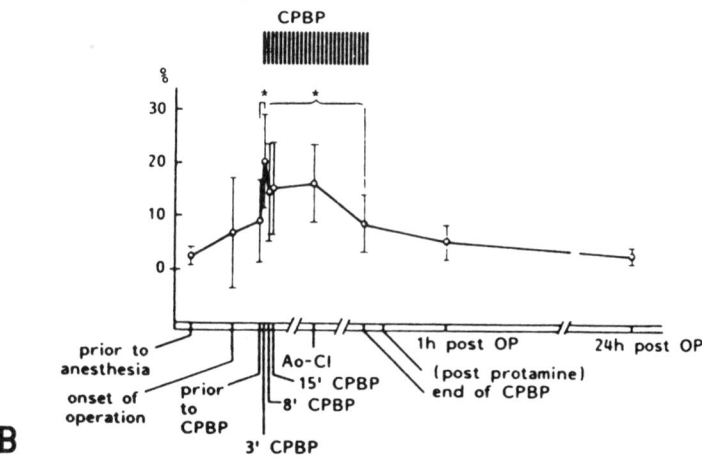

**FIGURE 8.** Schematic presentation of quantitatively measured parameters. Significant changes ($p < 0.05$) are indicated by the asterisk. *A*, Platelet morphology—discoid, smooth surface. *B*, Platelet morphology—shape changed. (From Zilla P, Fasol R, Groscurth P, et al: Blood platelets in cardiopulmonary bypass operations. Recovery occurs after initial stimulation, rather than continual activation. J Thorac Cardiovasc Surg 97:382, 1989, with permission.)

An essential step in the formation of a platelet plug is the binding of platelets to one another with fibrinogen as the bridge. The platelet receptor that binds fibrinogen is GPIIb/IIIa. A reduction in the GPIIb/IIIa receptors during and after CPB has been reported in some studies[40,41] and not in others.[42] The decrease in GPIIb/IIIa receptors may be due to detachment of membrane receptors from previously activated platelets that have separated from aggregates.[40] However, the reduction in GPIIb/IIIa receptor during CPB may not be the result of shear forces alone, because the GPIV receptor for thrombospondin stabilization of the platelet aggregate increases simultaneously with the decrease in GPIIb/IIIa.[41] Loss of the GPIIb/IIIa receptors, which may impair platelet-to-platelet interactions, has been postulated as a cause for platelet dysfunction after CPB. The 20–30% reduction in GPIIb/IIIa receptors after CPB is unlikely to impair hemostasis significantly (Fig. 9). However, the number of destroyed receptors varies greatly from patient to patient. The actual reduction in membrane receptor loss may not be appreciated, because

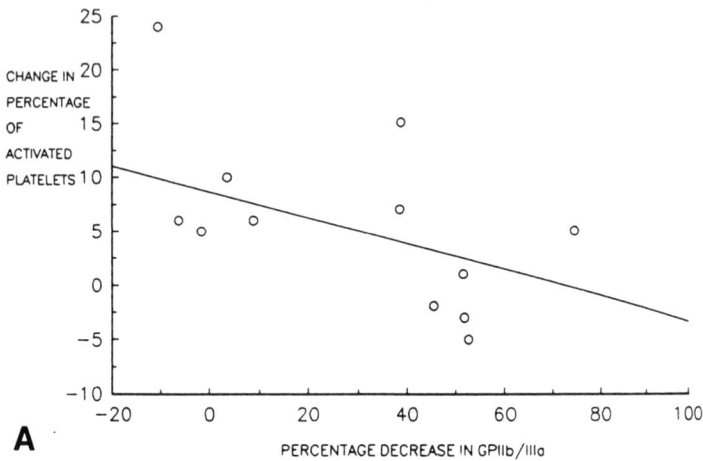

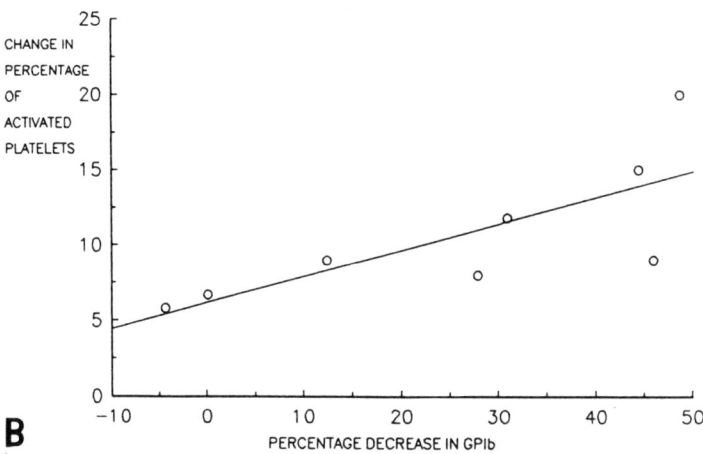

**FIGURE 9.** *A*, Correlation between the change in the percentage of activated platelets and the percentage decrease in GPIIb/IIIa in samples of whole blood taken after heparinization and at the end of CPB. ($r = 0.6$; $p < 0.05$). *B*, Correlation between platelet activation and percentage of decrease in GPIb. The x axis is the percentage of decrease in the GPIb in samples of whole blood taken after heparinization and 2–4 hours after the end of CPB. The y axis is the increase in the numbers of circulating activated platelets between the same time points ($r = 0.76$; $p < 0.05$). (From Rinder CS, Mathew JP, Rinder HM, et al: Modulation of platelet surface adhesion receptors during cardiopulmonary bypass. Anesthesiology 75:388–393, 1991.)

new platelets enter the circulation and are not absorbed onto the protein-coated EC surface. At the end of CPB, the platelet population becomes heterogenous as the damaged platelets are replaced. This process may offset any CPB-associated reduction in platelet function secondary to receptor loss. It also may explain the lack of correlation in some patients between bleeding and receptor loss. A newly discovered nonpeptide that acts as an antagonist to GPIIb/IIIa receptors has been shown in dogs to prevent the significant drop in platelet count that usually accompanies the onset of CPB.[43] The antagonist prevents platelet attachment to the synthetic surfaces as well as membrane fragmentation. This finding supports the importance of GPIIb/IIIa receptors during EC.

The adhesive receptor GPIb also has been reported to decrease during CPB.[41,44] Rinder et al. found a 28% decrease in the GPIb only at the end of CPB. Some patients had GPIb levels as low as 41% (Fig. 9b). The loss of GPIb was greatest in patients with the greatest platelet activation, but platelet activation is not the only reason for decreased GPIb receptor. Plasmin reduces the GPIb receptor in association with a reduction in the ADP-induced platelet aggregation in vitro and in vivo.[45,46] Van Oeveren et al.[44] found a 50% decrease in GPIb in the initial 5 minutes of CPB in patients who were not treated with aprotinin, an inhibitor of proteinase. Patients who received aprotinin did not experience a decrease in the GPIb. Administration of aprotinin and preservation of GPIb also correlated with significant reductions in transfusion requirements and postoperative chest tube drainage. In contrast, Kestin et al. found no reduction in GPIb receptors associated with CPB.[42] The results concerning postbypass blood loss after administration of aprotinin support the important role of plasmin and the adhesive receptor GPIb in hemostasis and CPB, although other factors may become more important in the future.[42]

Two other receptor abnormalities are associated with CPB. In vitro preparations with CPB in a recirculation system have demonstrated reduced fibrinogen binding.[47] Moreover, within 2 minutes of initiation of CPB, the number of alpha-2-adrenergic receptors decreases significantly.[24] The clinical significance of such abnormalities has not been established with certainty.

## Heparin Inhibition of Platelet Function

The mechanism for CPB-induced platelet dysfunction includes extrinsic defects of platelet function.[42] Recently, Kestin et al. found a lack of degranulating platelets, no loss of GPIb/IX and GPIIb/IIIa complexes, and normal platelet reactivity in vitro in patients undergoing CPB. They attributed platelet dysfunction after CPB to heparin-induced inhibition of thrombin. Heparin-induced platelet dysfunction is not completely new. The effect of heparin on platelet function has been assessed with platelet aggregometry, platelet morphology, and BT.[48] A mechanism for platelet dysfunction due to heparin has not been established. Some evidence suggests that direct binding of heparin to activated platelets may inhibit adenylate cyclase or release of intracellular calcium through a platelet membrane interaction.[48] Hemostatometry, a new method of assessing platelet function that does not require the use of anticoagulated blood, showed a mild platelet inhibition after administration of heparin in 58.6% of cardiac patients.[49] Another assessment with hemostatometry in cardiac surgical patients attempted to correlate clinical indices of bleeding with platelet dysfunction and heparin.[48] The investigators found that patients who exhibited severe platelet inhibition with heparin also experienced significantly greater chest tube drainage at 4, 12, and 18 hours after bypass. These findings suggest that heparin affects platelet function significantly in some patients. The role of heparin in postbypass hemorrhage is not yet completely defined.

The interaction of thrombin with platelets during and after CPB may have implications for hemostasis apart from the indirect effect of thrombin inhibition by heparin. Recent work with platelet aggregation in response to various agonists, such as thrombin, suggests that the thrombin receptor may be temporarily unavailable after CPB.[50] Heparin and thrombin may continue to be explored as major factors in the pathogenesis of CPB-induced platelet dysfunction.

### Other Platelet Inhibitors

Among the additional causes of bypass-induced platelet dysfunction is hypothermia,[51] which causes abnormal platelet morphology and activation and reduces platelet aggregation.[52] Platelet aggregation is greatly affected by a temperature less than 33°C in vitro and continues to worsen as the temperature is lowered. Hypothermia may affect platelets by inhibiting synthesis of $TxA_2$

Certain medications also are known for their platelet inhibitory actions, such as nitroglycerin, nitroprusside,[53] calcium channel blockers, and aspirin. The effect of aspirin on platelet function may be significant, delaying the return of platelet function by as much as 24 hours. Blood loss[54] and transfusion requirements[55] in patients taking aspirin have been significantly higher in some studies.

Hemodilution and cell salvage technology also may be factors in platelet dysfunction. Boldt et al. recently demonstrated that platelet aggregation was diminished more markedly in patients who had red blood cell salvage than in patients who had hemofiltration.[26] The additional trauma related to washing and centrifuging the red blood cells was postulated as the cause. It is also possible that some type of circulating platelet inhibitor has not been identified.[5]

The bubble oxygenator causes platelet dysfunction secondary to the air-blood interface,[27] at which many platelets are destroyed. Studies have been divided concerning any advantage to the use of the bubble oxygenator vs. the membrane oxygenator.[21,27,56] One major difference is the fact that the bubble oxygenator apparently destroys the platelets, whereas the membrane oxygenator recirculates a certain number. Platelets may be less damaged with a membrane oxygenator than with a bubble oxygenator, although this assumption has not translated into less postoperative blood loss.[56]

Cardiotomy suction also involves platelet damage secondary to the air-blood interface[27] and may adversely affect platelet function.[27] The amount of aspirated blood correlates directly with platelet loss. The effect of cardiotomy suction during many cardiac procedures may reduce the potential advantage of a membrane oxygenator. In addition, filters may affect platelet function (Fig. 10).

### Conclusion

Normal platelet function is a highly complex physiologic process and an essential part of successful hemostasis. CPB causes a temporary platelet dysfunction. Although much is understood about some of the causes and mechanisms, many questions still need to be answered. Once such areas have been investigated, newer and more advanced therapeutic alternatives may become available to prevent bleeding associated with platelet dysfunction and CPB.

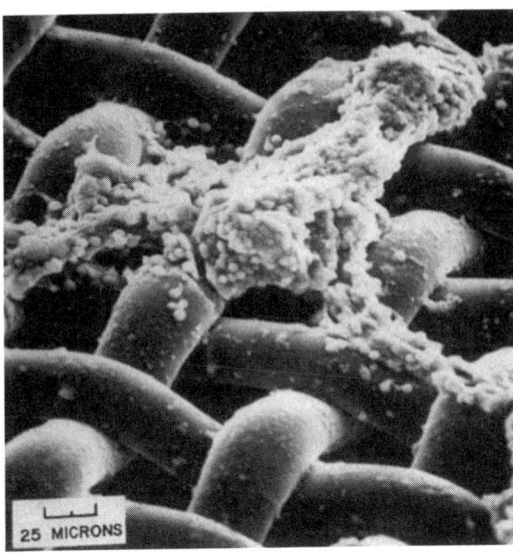

**FIGURE 10.** Platelet aggregate emboli trapped on a 40-micron arterial line filter during CPB. (From Edmunds LH: Blood surface interactions during cardiopulmonary bypass. J Cardiovasc Surg 8:404–410, 1993, with permission.)

## References

1. Jett JR, Kuritsky JN, Katzmann JA, Homburger HA: Acquired immunodeficiency syndrome associated with blood-product transfusions. Ann Intern Med 99:621–624, 1983.
2. Nightingale CH, Robotti J, Deckers PJ, et al: Quality care and cost-effectiveness: An organized approach to problem solving. Arch Surg 122:451–456, 1987.
3. Bachmann F, McKenna R, Cole ER, Najafi H: The hemostatic mechanism after open-heart surgery: I. Studies on plasma coagulation factors and fibrinolysis in 512 patients after extracorporeal circulation. J Thorac Cardiovasc Surg 70:76–85, 1975.
4. Mammen EF, Koets MH, Washington BC, et al: Hemostasis changes during cardiopulmonary bypass surgery. Semin Thromb Hemost 11:281–292, 1985.
5. Harker LA: Bleeding after cardiopulmonary bypass. N Engl J Med 314:1446–1448, 1986.
6. Yardumian DA, Mackie IJ, Machin SJ: Laboratory investigation of platelet function: A review of methodology. J Clin Pathol 39:701–712, 1986.
7. Bennett JS, Kolodziej MA: Disorders of platelet function [review]. Dis Mon 38:577–631, 1992.
8. Kieffer N, Guichard J, Breton-Gorius J: Dynamic redistribution of major platelet surface receptors after contact-induced platelet activation and spreading. An immunoelectron microscopy study. Am J Pathol 140:57–73, 1992.
9. Harker LA: Acquired disorders of platelet function. Ann NY Acad Sci 509:188–204, 1987.
10. Khaspekova SG, Vlasik TN, Byzova TV, et al: Detection of an epitope specific for the dissociated form of glycoprotein IIIa of platelet membrane glycoprotein IIb-IIIa complex and its expression on the surface of adherent platelets. Br J Haematol 85:332–340, 1993.
11. Hantgan RR, Hindriks G, Taylor RG, et al: Glycoprotein Ib, von Willebrand factor, and glycoprotein IIb:IIIa are all involved in platelet adhesion to fibrin in flowing whole blood. Blood 76:345–353, 1990.
12. Barrer MJ, Ellison N: Platelet function. Anesthesiology 46:202–211, 1977.
13. Rao GHR: Signal transduction, second messengers, and platelet function [editorial; comment]. J Lab Clin Med 121:18–20, 1993.
14. Peerschke EIB: Glycoprotein IIB and IIIa retention on fibrinogen-coated surfaces after lysis of adherent platelets. Blood 82:3358–3363, 1993.

15. Lewis JC, Hantgan RR, Stevenson SC, et al: Fibrinogen and glycoprotein IIb/IIIa localization during platelet adhesion. Localization to the granulomere and at sites of platelet interaction. Am J Pathol 136:239–252, 1990.
16. Krishnamurthi S, Westwick J, Kakkar VV: Regulation of human platelet activation—analysis of cyclooxygenase and cyclic AMP-dependent pathways. Biochem Pharmacol 33:3025–3035, 1984.
17. Hynes RO: The complexity of platelet adhesion to extracellular matrices. Thromb Haemost 66:40–43, 1991.
18. Walsh PN: Platelet-mediated coagulant protein interactions in hemostasis. Semin Hematol 22:178–186, 1985.
19. George JN, Pickett EB, Saucerman S, et al: Platelet surface glycoproteins: Studies on resting and activated platelets and platelet membrane microparticles in normal subjects, and observations in patients during adult respiratory distress syndrome and cardiac surgery. J Clin Invest 78:340–348, 1986.
20. Bick RL: Hemostatic defects associated with cardiac surgery, prosthetic devices, and other extracorporeal circuits. Semin Thromb Hemost 11:249–280, 1985.
21. Khuri SF, Wolfe JA, Josa M, et al: Hematologic changes during and after cardiopulmonary bypass and their relationship to the bleeding time and nonsurgical blood loss. J Thorac Cardiovasc Surg 104:94–107, 1992.
22. Addonizio VP: Platelet function in cardiopulmonary bypass and artificial organs. Hematol Oncol Clin North Am 4:145–155, 1990.
23. Holloway DS, Summaria L, Sandesara J, et al: Decreased platelet number and function and increased fibrinolysis contribute to postoperative bleeding in cardiopulmonary bypass patients. Thromb Haemost 59:62–67, 1988.
24. Wachtfogel YT, Musial J, Jenkin B, et al: Loss of platelet $\alpha_2$-adrenergic receptors during simulated extracorporeal circulation: Prevention with prostaglandin $E_1$. J Clin Lab Med 105:601–607, 1985.
25. Martin JF, Daniel TD, Trowbridge EA: Acute and chronic changes in platelet volume and count after cardiopulmonary bypass induced thrombocytopenia in man. Thromb Haemost 57:55–58, 1987.
26. Boldt J, Zickmann B, Czeke A, et al: Blood conservation techniques and platelet function in cardiac surgery. Anesthesiology 75:426–432, 1991.
27. Edmunds LHJ, Ellison N, Colman RW, et al: Platelet function during cardiac operation: Comparison of membrane and bubble oxygenators. J Thorac Cardiovasc Surg 83:805–812, 1982.
28. Ray MJ, Hawson GAT, Just SJE, et al: Relationship of platelet aggregation to bleeding after cardiopulmonary bypass. Ann Thorac Surg 57:981–986, 1994.
29. Simon TL, Aki RF, Murphy W: Controlled trial of routine administration of platelet concentrates in cardiopulmonary bypass surgery. Ann Thorac Surg 37:359–364, 1984.
30. Harker LA, Malpass TW, Branson HE, et al: Mechanism of abnormal bleeding in patients undergoing cardiopulmonary bypass: Acquired transient platelet dysfunction associated with selective $\alpha$-granule release. Blood 56:824–834, 1980.
31. Czer LS, Bateman TM, Gray RJ, et al: Treatment of severe platelet dysfunction and hemorrhage after cardiopulmonary bypass: Reduction in blood product usage with desmopressin. J Am Coll Cardiol 9:1139–1147, 1987.
32. Mohr R, Golan M, Martinowitz U, et al: Effect of cardiac operation on platelets. J Thorac Cardiovasc Surg 92:434–441, 1986.
33. Boldt J, Zickmann B, Benson M, et al: Does platelet size correlate with function in patients undergoing cardiac surgery? Intensive Care Med 19:44–47, 1993.
34. Edmunds LH Jr: Blood-surface interactions during cardiopulmonary bypass. J Cardiovasc Surg 8:404–410, 1993.
35. Stratta P, Canavese C, Costa P, et al: Biological stress induced by extracorporeal circulation: Comparison between cardiopulmonary bypass, hemodialysis and plasma exchange. Trans Am Soc Artif Intern Organs 30:502–507, 1984.
36. Aren C, Feddersen K, Radegran K: Effects of prostacyclin infusion on platelet activation and postoperative blood loss during coronary bypass. Ann Thorac Surg 36:49–54, 1983.
37. Rinder CS, Bohnert J, Rinder HM, et al: Platelet activation and aggregation during cardiopulmonary bypass. Anesthesiology 75:388–393, 1991.
38. Zilla P: Blood platelets and bypass [letter]. J Thorac Cardiovasc Surg 98:797–800, 1989.
39. Zilla P, Fasol R, Groscurth P, et al: Blood platelets in cardiopulmonary bypass operations. Recovery occurs after initial stimulation, rather than continual activation. J Thorac Cardiovasc Surg 97:379–388, 1989.

40. Wenger RK, Lukasiewicz H, Mikuta BS, et al: Loss of platelet fibrinogen receptors during clinical cardiopulmonary bypass. J Thorac Cardiovasc Surg 97:235–239, 1989.
41. Rinder CS, Mathew JP, Rinder HM, et al: Modulation of platelet surface adhesion receptors during cardiopulmonary bypass. Anesthesiology 75:563–570, 1991.
42. Kestin AS, Valeri CR, Khuri SF, et al: The platelet function defect of cardiopulmonary bypass. Blood 82:107–117, 1993.
43. Carteaux J-P, Roux S, Kuhn H, et al: Ro 44-9883, a new nonpeptide glycoprotein IIb/IIIa antagonist, prevents platelet loss during experimental cardiopulmonary bypass. J Thorac Cardiovasc Surg 106:834–841, 1993.
44. Van Oeveren W, Harder MP, Roozendaal KJ, et al: Aprotinin protects platelets against the initial effect of cardiopulmonary bypass. J Thorac Cardiovasc Surg 99:788–797, 1990.
45. Adelman B, Michelson AD, Loscalzo J, et al: Plasmin effect on platelet glycoprotein IB-von Willebrand factor interactions. Blood 65:32–40, 1985.
46. Woodman RC, Harker LA: Bleeding complications associated with cardiopulmonary bypass [review]. Blood 76:1680–1697, 1990.
47. Musial J, Niewiarowski S, Hershock D, et al: Loss of fibrinogen receptors from the platelet surface during simulated extracorporeal circulation. J Lab Clin Med 105:514–522, 1985.
48. John LCH, Rees GM, Kovacs IB: Inhibition of platelet function by heparin. An etiologic factor in postbypass hemorrhage. J Thorac Cardiovasc Surg 105:816–822, 1993.
49. John LCH, Rees GM, Kovacs IB: Effect of heparin on in vitro platelet reactivity in cardiac surgical patients: A comparative assessment by whole blood platelet aggregometry and haemostatometry. Thromb Res 66:649–656, 1992.
50. Ferraris VA, Rodriguez E, Ferraris SP, et al: Platelet aggregation abnormalities after cardiopulmonary bypass [letter]. Blood 83:299–300, 1994.
51. Valeri C, Feingold H, Cassidy G, et al: Hypothermia-induced reversible platelet dysfunction. Ann Surg 205:175–181, 1987.
52. Golan M, Modan M, Lavee J, et al: Transfusion of fresh whole blood stored (4°C) for short period fails to improve platelet aggregation on extracellular matrix and clinical hemostasis after cardiopulmonary bypass. J Thorac Cardiovasc Surg 99:354–360, 1990.
53. Hines R, Barash PG: Infusion of sodium nitroprusside induces platelet dysfunction in vitro. Anesthesiology 70:611–615, 1989.
54. Boldt J, Knothe C, Zickmann B, et al: The effects of preoperative aspirin therapy on platelet function in cardiac surgery. Eur J Cardiothorac Surg 6:598–602, 1992.
55. Sethi GK, Copeland JG, Goldman S, et al: Implications of preoperative administration of aspirin in patients undergoing coronary artery bypass grafting. J Am Coll Cardiol 15:15–20, 1990.
56. Boers M, van den Dungen JJAM, Karliczek GF, et al: Two membrane oxygenators and a bubbler: A clinical comparison. Ann Thorac Surg 35:455–462, 1983.

**Sylvia Haas, MD**
**Günther Blümel, MD**

# 5

# Effect of Aprotinin on Bleeding Complications in Noncardiac Surgery: Experimental Studies and Clinical Trials

Bleeding complications may counteract the success of any type of surgery. The major causes are vascular disorders or dysfunctions of platelets, blood coagulation, or fibrinolysis. Vascular bleeding complications are congenital and cannot be influenced by drugs. Bleeding complications due to platelet dysfunction or imbalances of blood coagulation or fibrinolysis, however, may be either congenital or acquired and may occur systemically or locally. Especially in surgery, the acquired bleeding disorders play an important role; thus, it is of clinical significance to develop preventive and therapeutic strategies.

Numerous research studies at the Institute of Experimental Surgery of the Technical University of Munich have been designed to determine whether the risk of postoperative bleeding may be reduced by administration of the proteinase inhibitor, aprotinin. This chapter describes the results of selected experiments and clinical trials.

As early as 1960, Benzer and Blümel examined the effect of a precursor of aprotinin on blood coagulation. They incubated different concentrations of this trypsin inhibitor with native blood in vitro. The kinetic of blood coagulation was assessed by various parameters of thromboelastography (TEG) (Fig. 1). The reaction time (r) needed for the beginning of blood coagulation in the TEG cup was prolonged by the trypsin inhibitor on a dose-dependent basis, whereas the k-value, which is the time needed for the development of a predefined clot strength and thus describes the velocity of thrombus formation, was retarded. The maximal amplitude of the TEG, which is influenced mainly by the concentration and quality of fibrinogen as well as by platelet count and reactivity, was significantly lowered.[2] All three effects could be repeated in vitro with aprotinin and also were observed in patients treated with high doses of Trasylol.

In further studies, Benzer and Blümel examined whether the procoagulant and profibrinolytic effect of brain tissue can be influenced by aprotinin. The authors had observed frequent secondary hemorrhages in neurosurgical patients despite fast repair of the primary wound. The r-time in the TEG after incubation of brain

Effect of Trypsin Inhibitor (Precursor of Aprotinin) on Thromboelastography

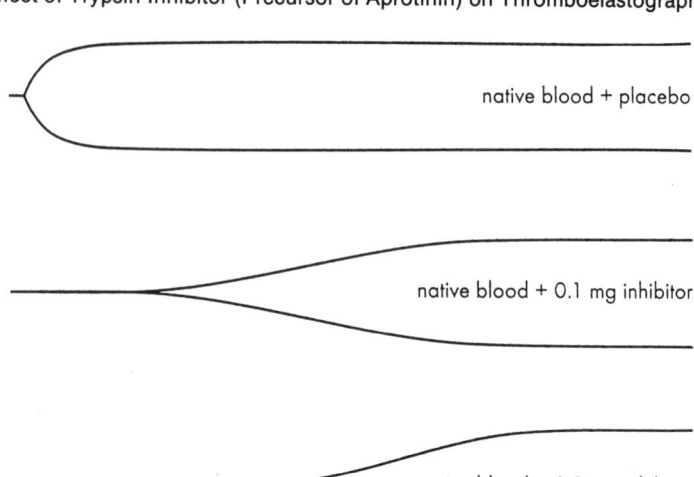

native blood + placebo

native blood + 0.1 mg inhibitor

native blood + 1.0 mg inhibitor

**FIGURE 1**

tissue extract with native blood was extremely shortened. Brain tissue extract also showed a significant profibrinolytic effect. Both procoagulant and fibrinolytic effects could be inhibited by adding Trasylol to the mixture of native blood and brain tissue extract[1] (Fig. 2).

Based on these findings in the early 1960s, further experimental and clinical studies were performed to answer the following questions:

1. Is tissue-type plasminogen activator (tPA) affected by aprotinin? If so, are the effects different from those of the synthetic inhibitor, tranexamic acid?

2. Can the risk of hemorrhage during surgery be reduced by local application of aprotinin in organs containing high amounts of tPA?

3. What is the influence of aprotinin on platelets?

4. Can the bleeding risk of patients undergoing total hip replacement be reduced by aprotinin without increasing the risk of deep venous thrombosis?

## Effect of Aprotinin and Tranexamic Acid on Tissue-type Plasminogen Activator of the Lung

Treatment with antifibrinolytic agents involves the risk of deposition of nonlysable clots in vital organs, especially in clinical conditions associated with impaired fibrinolysis, such as shock, trauma, and major surgical interventions. On the other hand, treatment with aprotinin may help to reduce the bleeding risk in the same conditions. Therefore, it is of great clinical interest to investigate whether aprotinin affects the activity of tPA and whether its effect is different from that of tranexamic acid.

Experiments were carried out in rats, because their fibrinolytic system appears to be similar to that of humans. Anesthetized rats were randomly divided into three

Effect of Trasylol on the Procoagulant and Fibrinolytic Effect
of Brain Tissue in Vitro

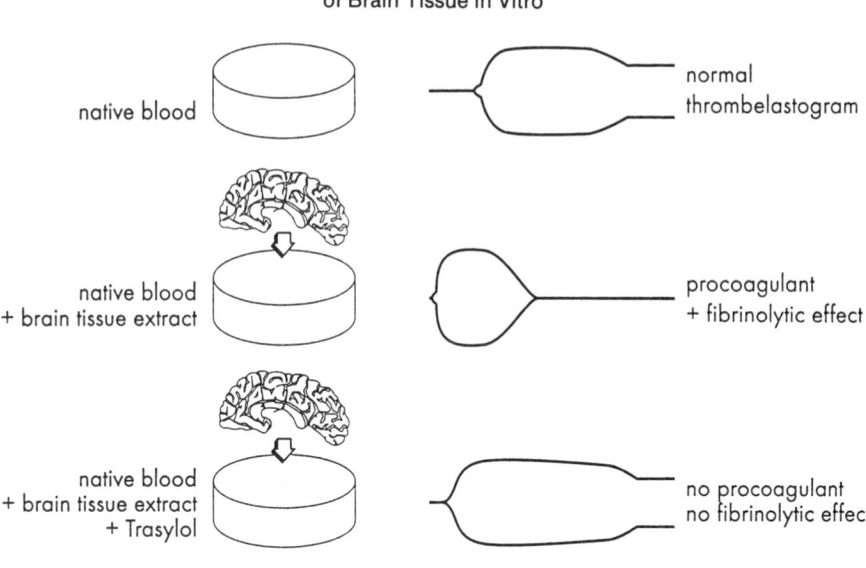

**FIGURE 2**

groups that were treated with (1) 1 ml of saline intravenously, (2) 20,000 KIU/kg body weight of aprotinin (Trasylol), or (3) 40 mg/kg body weight of tranexamic acid (Ugurol). Sixty minutes later the lungs were perfused with saline, and lung specimens were snap frozen. The tPA activity of the lung tissue was assessed by a modified technique of fibrinolysis autography, according to Todd.[31] Although aprotinin had no inhibitory effect, tranexamic acid significantly inhibited tPA activity.[8]

This finding was confirmed by another series of experiments in which the rats were treated as described above. The antiplasmin activity of the lung tissue specimen was examined by the so-called sandwich-slide technique of Noordhoek-Hegt.[26] As expected, aprotinin had no effect on tPA but strongly inhibited the activity of plasmin, whereas the opposite results were seen in the group of rats treated with tranexamic acid.[11] In addition, antiplasmin activity in the blood was determined by the use of a chromogenic substrate method. Antiplasmin activity increased significantly in the aprotinin-treated group, whereas no increase was observed after treatment with tranexamic acid.

In addition, further clinical trials have provided evidence that aprotinin does not affect tPA; therefore, its use does not seem to be contraindicated in clinical conditions that involve activated blood coagulation and/or impaired fibrinolysis.[30] Tranexamic acid and other synthetic fibrinolysis inhibitors, however, should not be given.

## Local Application of Aprotinin

To determine whether topical application of aprotinin reduces the risk of local hemorrhage, the effect of aprotinin on wound healing after experimental dissection of nerves and experimentally induced thermic skin lesions was examined.

Fibrin, the end product of plasmatic coagulation, plays a specific role in wound repair and is produced during the exudative phase; therefore, it appears to be a promising hemostyptic agent. Previous attempts failed, however, because the applied fibrin could not be protected against premature lysis, which resulted in undesired secondary hemorrhages and wound dehiscences. Thus three series of experiments were carried out to examine whether the applied fibrin could be stabilized for a longer period by addition of an antifibrinolytic agent.

## Study I: Material, Methods, and Results

The sciatic nerve, which consists of three fascicles, was exposed and dissected in anesthetized rats. The fascicle groups were adapted so that both components of the fibrin glue, thrombin and fibrinogen cryoprecipitate, could be dropped on the perineurium tube. Then the nerve stumps were exposed for about 1 more minute until fibrin polymerization was achieved. At the end of the operation the nerve stumps were completely joined. Twenty-four hours after the operation, however, many dehiscent anastomoses were observed. With addition of fibrinolysis inhibitors to the glue mixture, the anastomoses were stabilized visibly. To quantitate the efficacy of different inhibitors, the maximal mechanical strength of the anastomosed nerves was examined 24 hours postoperatively with and without the addition of inhibitors.

Figure 3 shows the measurements of mechanical strength at the end of the operation (0.5 hr) and 24 hours after anastomosis. In the group without the inhibitor the immediate postoperative measurement of 32.9 p was reduced to 8.6 p on the following day. This highly significant decrease in mechanical strength cannot be counteracted even by the local addition of factor XIII (84 plasma units/ml of thrombin solution) to the glue. The loss of mechanical strength can be reduced

Effect of Fibrin and Various Doses and Administration Schemes of Factor XIII and Tranexamic Acid (AMCA) on the Mechanical Strength of Injured Nerves

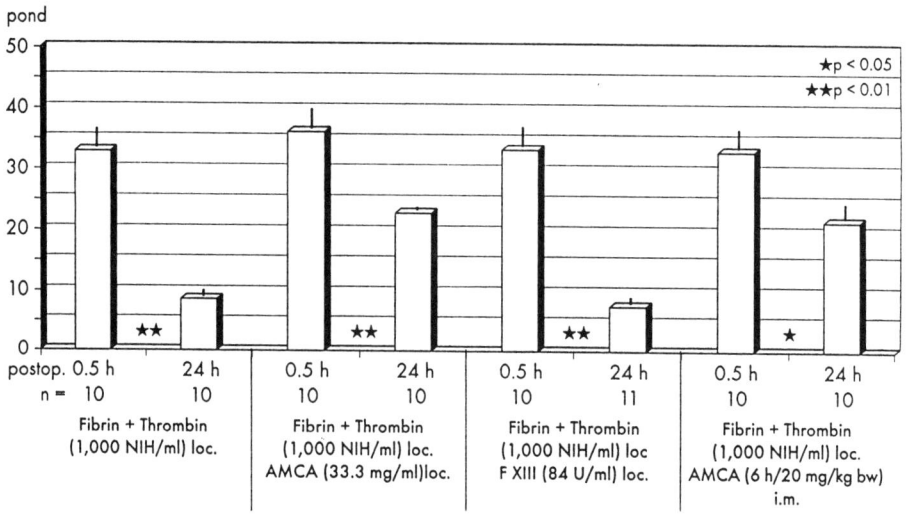

**FIGURE 3**

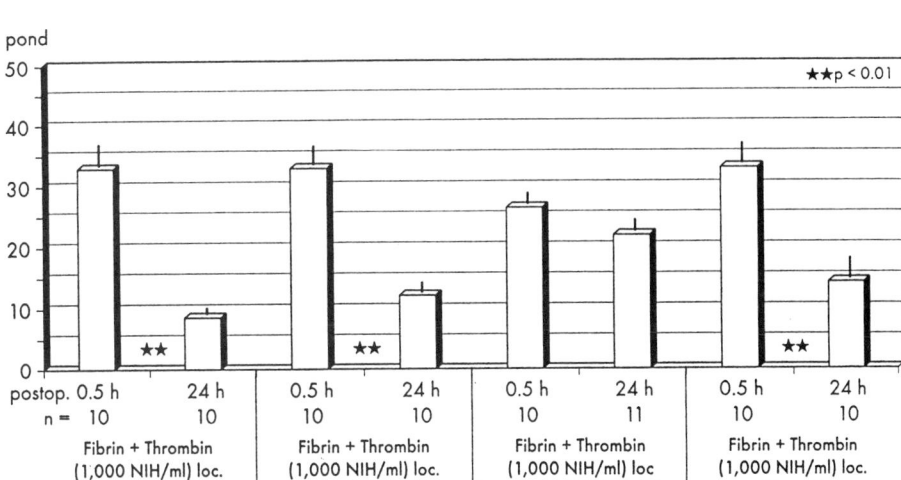

Effect of Fibrin and Various Doses and Administration Schemes of Trasylol on the Mechanical Strength of Injured Nerves

**FIGURE 4**

slightly 24 hours postoperatively by local addition of tranexamic acid (33.3 mg/ml of thrombin solution). However, the loss is still highly significant. A significant reduction in mechanical strength also was seen after intramuscular administration of tranexamic acid (20 mg/kg body weight) every 6 hours.

Sufficient stabilization of the anastomosis could be achieved only by local addition of aprotinin (6667 KIU/ml of thrombin solution) to the glue mixture (Fig. 4). Parenteral administration of Trasylol every 4 hours, even in concentrations of 40,000 KIU/kg body weight, could not prevent a highly significant decrease in mechanical strength 24 hours postoperatively.

## Study II: Material, Methods, and Results

In another series of studies the inhibitors aprotinin (Trasylol), tranexamic acid (Ugurol), C1 inactivator (Immuno GmbH), and Foy (Sanol-Schwarz GmbH) were compared by using the model of neural anastomosis with fibrin glue. The sciatic nerve of the rat was dissected and treated under the microscope with fibrin and various inhibitors. The following glue components were used:

Human fibrin glue, deep-frozen (Tissucol; Immuno GmbH, Heidelberg)
Topostasin (Hoffmann-LaRoche), 500 NIH/ml of thrombin
Ringer lactate
Aprotinin, 6670 KIU
Tranexamic acid, 32 mg
Aprotinin, 6670 KIU, and tranexamic acid, 32 mg
C1 inactivator, 305 plasma units
Foy, 13.4 mg
C1 inactivator, 305 plasma units, and Foy, 13.4 mg

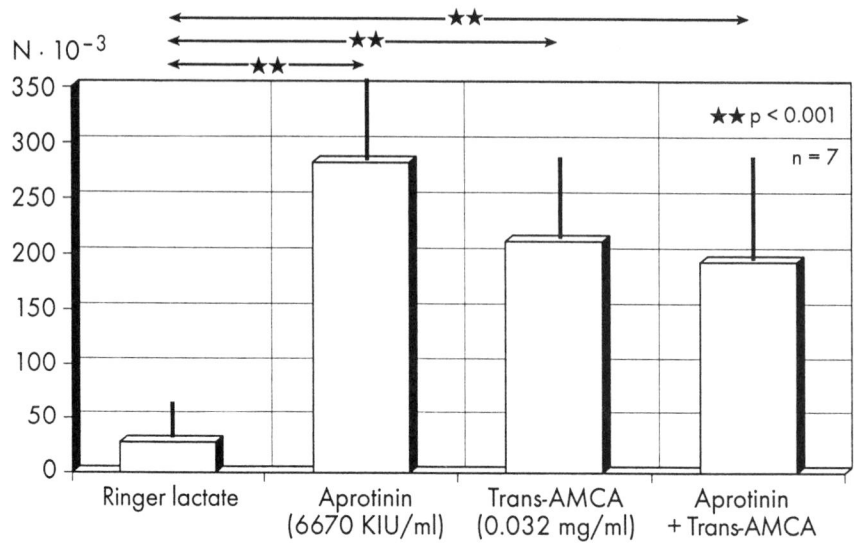

Effect of Fibrin and Various Inhibitors
on the Mechanical Strength of Injured Nerves

**FIGURE 5**

Twenty-four hours after the initial anastomosis of the sciatic nerve the rats were reanesthetized and the treated nerves were excised. Figures 5 and 6 show the effect of fibrin and various inhibitors on the mechanical strength of the injured nerves. A highly significant increase in the strength of the glued nerves was achieved with aprotinin or tranexamic acid. Of special interest is the relatively high mechanical strength of the nerve anastomoses after the application of C1 inactivator, despite a highly significant inhibition of proteases in the tissue and a partial inhibition of thrombin. Foy was applied to the polymerized fibrin film only after the start of coagulation, because its thrombin-inhibiting activity interferes with the polymerization of fibrin. In comparison with the control group (Ringer lactate), the improvement in mechanical strength was slight.

Among the tested inhibitors, aprotinin was superior for stabilization of topically applied fibrin because of its strong inhibition of locally generated plasmin; mixtures of aprotinin plus tranexamic acid or C1 inactivator and Foy did not improve the mechanical strength of nerves treated with fibrin glue.

## Study III: Material, Methods, and Results

To examine the effects of fibrin on wound healing, a standardized thermic lesion of the skin was induced in anesthetized rats, and both glue components, fibrinogen and thrombin, were applied to the wound in various compositions. The studies were carried out in male Wistar rats with a body weight of 400–450 grams. Under general anesthesia, a metal stamp heated to 200° C with a diameter of 1 cm was applied for 15 minutes in the region of the thoracic and lumbar vertebrae after the back was shaved. Fifteen minutes later the necrotic skin within the burnt area was

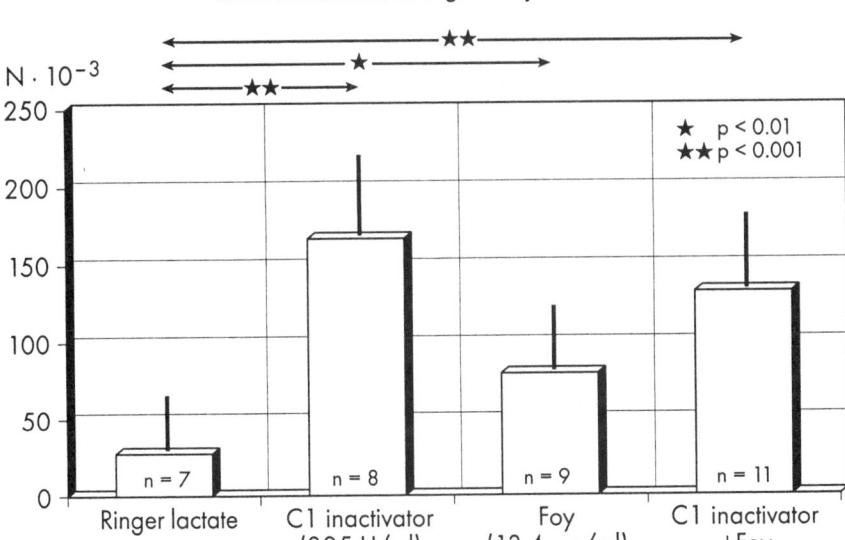

Effect of Fibrin and Various Inhibitors
on the Mechanical Strength of Injured Nerves

**FIGURE 6**

excised down to the fascia with a punch of the same diameter. Immediately afterward, the rats were allocated randomly to five different groups that received various kinds of treatment. In two control groups, no burns were inflicted; only a punch of the skin was performed. One of the control groups received treatment with fibrin, whereas the other did not.

Photographic documentation and planimetric evaluation of the wound areas were performed on the day of operation and on the ninth day postoperatively. In addition, the wound areas were excised for micromorphologic examination on the ninth day postoperatively. The rats were allocated to the following treatment groups:

Group 1: Fifteen minutes after production of the thermic skin lesion and necrectomy by skin punch, a highly concentrated fibrinogen solution (Tissucol; Immuno GmbH, Heidelberg) and a highly concentrated thrombin solution (3000 NIH/ml) were applied simultaneously, with no inhibitor of fibrinolysis.

Group 2: As group 1, with the addition of 3000 KIU/ml of aprotinin to the thrombin solution.

Group 3: As group 1, with application of a low concentration of thrombin solution (4 NIH/ml).

Group 4: As group 1, with application of a low concentration of thrombin solution (4 NIH/ml) and a low concentration of aprotinin (300 KIU/ml).

Group 5: As group 1, with application of a low concentration of thrombin solution (4 NIH/ml) and 3000 KIU/ml of aprotinin.

Group 6: Necrectomy 15 min after thermic skin lesion without fibrin treatment.

Group 7: Skin punch without thermic skin lesion, followed by necrectomy but no treatment.

Group 8: Skin punch without thermic skin lesion but with wound care as in group 2.

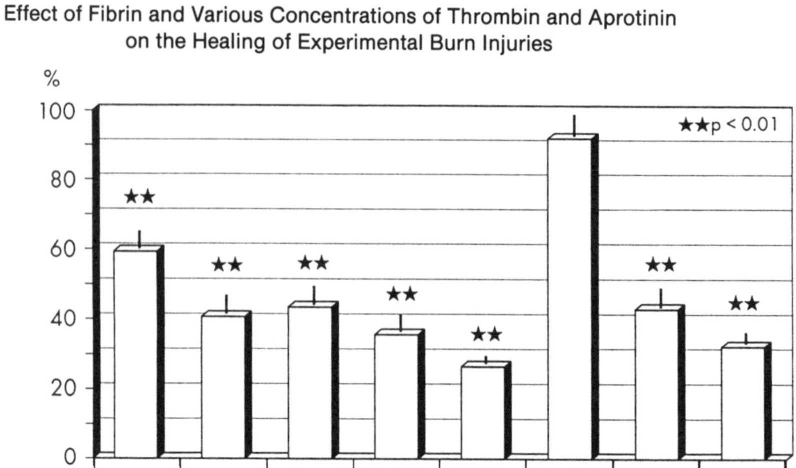

Effect of Fibrin and Various Concentrations of Thrombin and Aprotinin
on the Healing of Experimental Burn Injuries

| Group | 1 | 2 | 3 | 4 | 5 | 6 | 7 | 8 |
|---|---|---|---|---|---|---|---|---|
| n | 12 | 10 | 7 | 6 | 12 | 12 | 4 | 7 |
| Burn injury | + | + | + | + | + | + | Ø | Ø |
| Punch | + | + | + | + | + | + | + | + |
| Fibrin + Thrombin [NIH/ml] | 3,000 | 3,000 | 4 | 4 | 4 | Ø | Ø | 3,000 |
| Aprotinin [KU/ml] | Ø | 3,000 | Ø | 300 | 3,000 | Ø | Ø | 3,000 |

**FIGURE 7**

The planimetric examination of the wound areas on the ninth day postoperatively showed that the healing of burn injuries was significantly accelerated by
fibrin (Fig. 7). Addition of aprotinin to the glue mixture seems to increase the
favorable effects on wound repair, whereas the concentration of the thrombin
solution seems to be of secondary importance. The areas of the burnt punch
wounds were approximately the same in groups 1–6; it is striking that the groups
without addition of aprotinin (groups 1, 3, and 6) showed the least regression of the
burnt area. Apart from group 6, all groups showed a highly significant difference in
wound size on the ninth day postoperatively compared with the original size on the
day of operation.

## Discussion

The first two series of experiments show that local applications of aprotinin play a
significant role in the prevention of postoperative wound dehiscences due to local
fibrinolytic activity. Inhibition of locally generated plasmin may be the underlying
mechanism in its prevention of secondary hemorrhagic complications after surgery
in tissues containing high amounts of plasminogen activators. Furthermore, the
experiments provide evidence that the concentration of locally applied aprotinin
may be of clinical significance; extremely high concentrations may interfere with
posttraumatic nerve regeneration despite a successful primary nerve anastomosis.
This observation also was made by Kuderna et al., who recommend a dosage of 50
KIU of aprotinin/ml of fibrin glue. The authors also conclude that aprotinin is

superior to tranexamic acid.[20] Thus it seems to be of clinical significance to balance maximal mechanical strength with optimal nerve regeneration.

The third series of experiments was carried out to investigate whether aprotinin has beneficial effects on wound repair. The process of wound healing appears to be stimulated by aprotinin, and even higher concentrations do not hamper regression of the wound area. The inhibition of fibrinolysis seems to have a stabilizing effect on the wound covering, which possibly enhances regression. The results of these experiments are discussed in detail by Haas et al.[13]

## Influence of Aprotinin on Platelets

Platelets play a specific role in peri- and postoperative bleeding complications. In major surgery—for example, total hip replacement—an immediate stimulation of platelet function has been described.[12,14] Pulmonary complications may result from circulating platelet aggregates and especially from the release reaction of aggregated platelets, which produces mainly adenosine diphosphate (ADP), serotonine, cate-cholamines, prostaglandins, and platelet factors 3 and 4. Thus several reactions are initiated: vasoconstriction, increased permeability of the vessel wall, and procoag-ulant activity.[3] Modig et al. reported that major bone surgery can lead to pulmonary complications similar to those of "shock lung." Acute pulmonary dysfunction with increased vascular resistance in the lung, constriction of the bronchioli, and a decrease in $PaO_2$ has been seen in patients with total hip replacement.[24] Hyper-reactive platelets may be responsible for such pulmonary complications. Therefore, substances that affect certain platelet functions without increasing the risk of bleeding are of great clinical interest. One of these substances seems to be aprotinin (Trasylol; Bayer Pharma, Leverkusen, Germany), which has a stabilizing effect on platelets in vitro.[19,18] On the basis of these observations the following series of experiments were performed.

### Study I: Material, Methods, and Results

Two groups of patients with osteosynthesis were treated at the beginning of surgery with 20,000 (group 1) or 10,000 (group 2) KIU/kg body weight of aprotinin; the control group (group 3) received the same volume of saline. Citrated blood was drawn before and at 5, 15, 30, 60, 120, and 180 minutes after the above treatments. To control the in vitro effect, the "before" samples from groups 1 and 2 were incubated in saline with 200 and 100 KIU/ml of aprotinin, respectively, for 20 minutes at 37° C. All blood samples were evaluated as follows:

1. Platelet adhesiveness was assessed according to Morris.[25] One milliliter of citrated blood was rotated with 0.5 gm of unsiliconized glass beads for 1 minute at a temperature of 37° C. The percentage of platelet retention was determined by calculation of the platelet number before and after contact with the glass.

2. Platelet aggregability was assessed according to Born.[6] Aggregation was induced by collagen, ADP, and epinephrine.

3. Activated partial thromboplastin time (aPTT) was assessed with reagents from Merz & Dade, Munich.

4. Thromboelastographic parameters were assessed with the thromboelasto-graph from Hellige, Freiburg.

5. Results were evaluated statistically with Student's t-test.

Platelet Adhesion in Major Bone Surgery (left)
in Comparison with the Initial Value.
In Vitro Incubations (right)

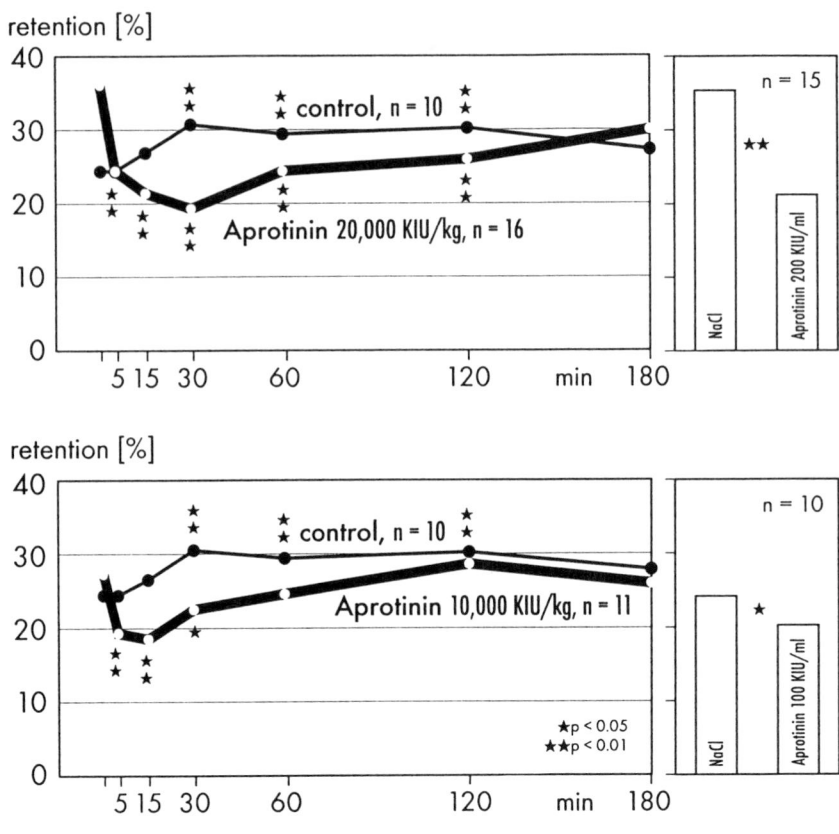

**FIGURE 8**

Platelet adhesiveness was significantly increased in the saline group, whereas a significant decrease was seen after treatment with aprotinin (Fig. 8). The lower dose of 10,000 KIU/kg was less effective. The decreasing effect of aprotinin on platelet adhesion is also evident in the in vitro incubations (Fig. 8). Platelet aggregation induced by ADP was increased in the control group, whereas the opposite effect occurred after aprotinin treatment (Figs. 9 and 10). The alpha angle and the maximal amplitude of the curve were significantly reduced by aprotinin, especially when the higher dose was used. The same effect was seen in vitro. Similar effects were obtained after induction of platelet aggregation by collagen and epinephrine.

The aPTT was significantly shortened in the placebo group, whereas a significant prolongation was seen in both aprotinin-treated groups (Fig. 11). The reaction time of the thromboelastogram was affected by aprotinin only initially. As soon as 15 minutes after application of 20,000 KIU/kg of aprotinin, the r-time was normalized.

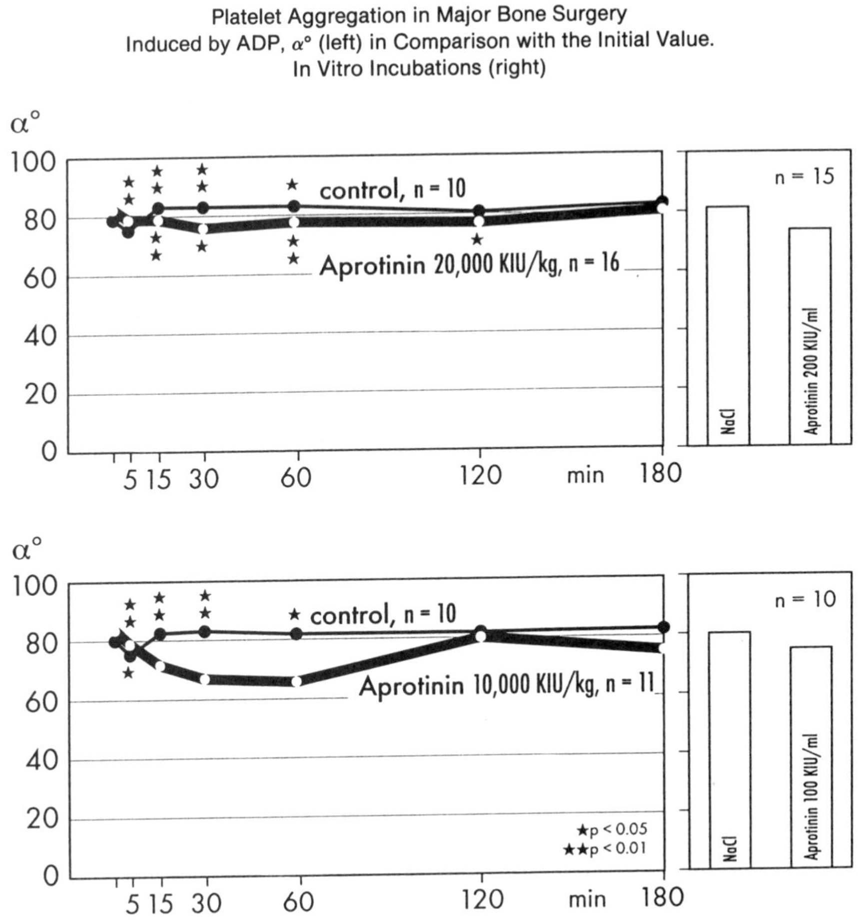

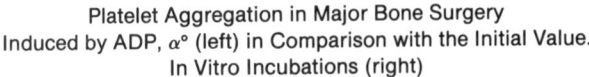

Platelet Aggregation in Major Bone Surgery
Induced by ADP, $\alpha°$ (left) in Comparison with the Initial Value.
In Vitro Incubations (right)

**FIGURE 9**

## Study II: Material, Methods, and Results

Two groups of patients with total hip replacement were studied postoperatively: one group without and the other group with aprotinin treatment. Samples of citrated blood were drawn at the following intervals:

1. Induction of anesthesia
2. Arthrostomy
3. Preparation of the acetabulum
4. Polymerization of the bone cement in the acetabulum
5. Preparation of the bone marrow in the femur shaft
6. Implantation of the prosthesis shaft
7. Two hours postoperatively

The second group received 20,000 KIU/kg of aprotinin after induction of anesthesia. Platelet function was assessed by the following methods:

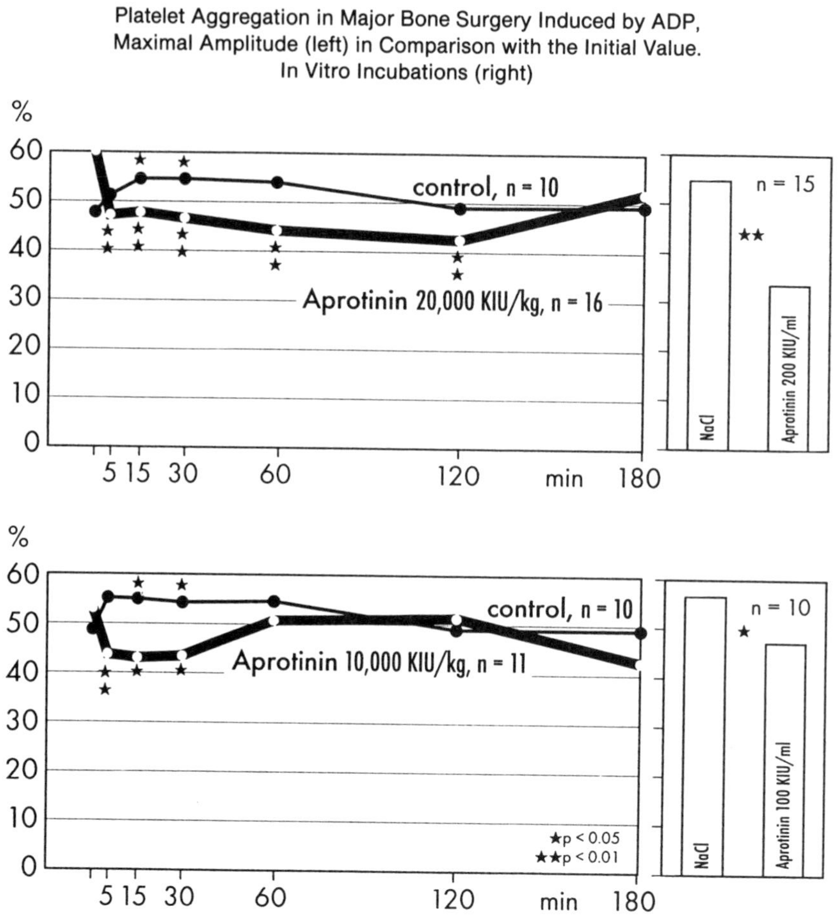

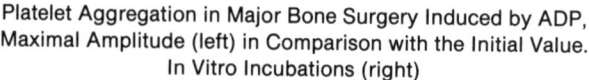

Platelet Aggregation in Major Bone Surgery Induced by ADP,
Maximal Amplitude (left) in Comparison with the Initial Value.
In Vitro Incubations (right)

**FIGURE 10**

1. The shape change of thrombocytes, according to Krzywanek and Breddin[19]
2. The Morris test (see study 1)
3. The Born Test (see study 1)
4. Spontaneous platelet aggregation, according to Breddin et al.[7]

The statistical evaluation of the results was performed with Student's t-test. The number of thrombocytes that changed shape increased significantly with the time of operation; the largest number was found when the bone marrow was prepared in the femur shaft. After treatment with aprotinin, the morphology of platelets was markedly less affected (Fig. 12). The number of nonaggregated platelets was correlated inversely with the number of thrombocytes that changed shape. The minimal platelet count coincided with the largest number of platelets that changed shape (Fig. 13). In the aprotinin-treated group, the decrease in platelets was less distinct. Preparation of the bone marrow in the femur shaft seemed to be the critical moment for increased adhesiveness of the thrombocytes, whereas no increase was seen in the aprotinin-treated group (Fig. 14). After induction of

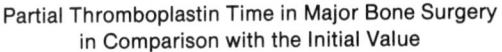

Partial Thromboplastin Time in Major Bone Surgery
in Comparison with the Initial Value

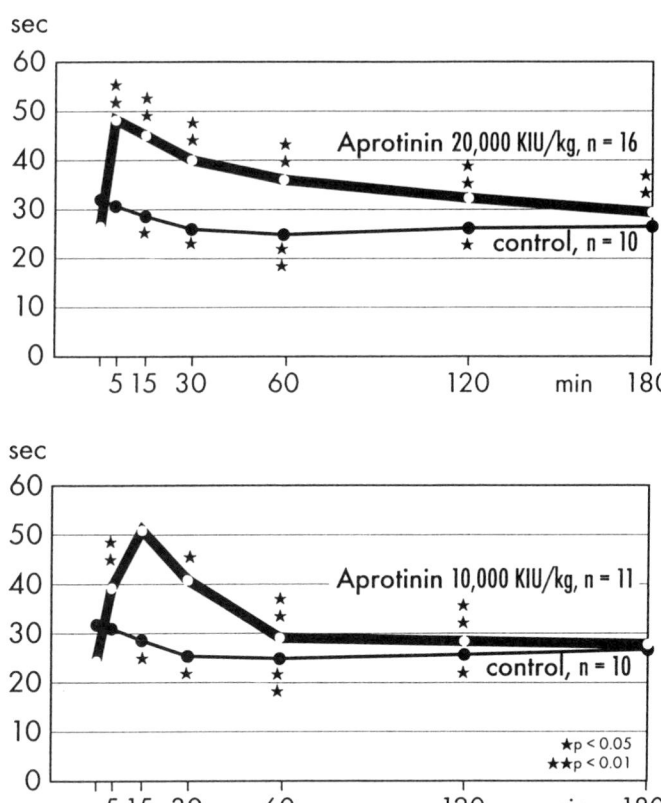

**FIGURE 11**

platelet aggregation with collagen, a characteristic shortening of the lag phase and an increase in maximal amplitude of the curve were found in the control group. Again, the maximal deviations were seen at preparation of the bone marrow. A significant prolongation of the lag phase and a significant decrease in the maximal amplitude were observed after treatment with aprotinin (Figs. 15 and 16). Similar results were obtained from the test for spontaneous aggregation, which was significantly enhanced in the saline group and significantly reduced by aprotinin.

## Study III: Material, Methods, and Results

The third study consisted of 32 patients of either gender, aged 60–75 years, with normal metabolism. All patients underwent an alloarthroplastic total hip replacement with cemented prostheses and were assigned to treatment with aprotinin or placebo on a blinded, random basis. All patients received low-dose heparin (5000 IU/day) as prophylaxis against venous thromboembolism. After the induction of anesthesia, the first blood sample was taken as a control value; an intravenous

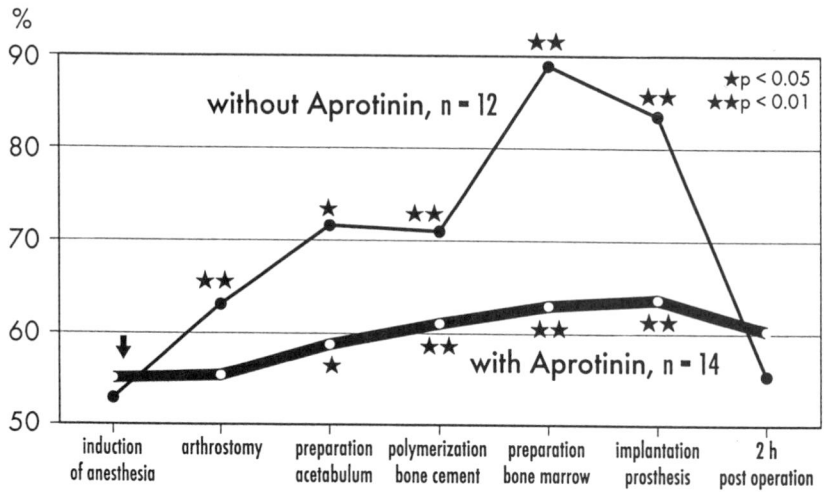

Platelet Morphology in Total Hip Replacement
after Application of Aprotinin and without Aprotinin Treatment
in Comparison with the Initial Value

**FIGURE 12**

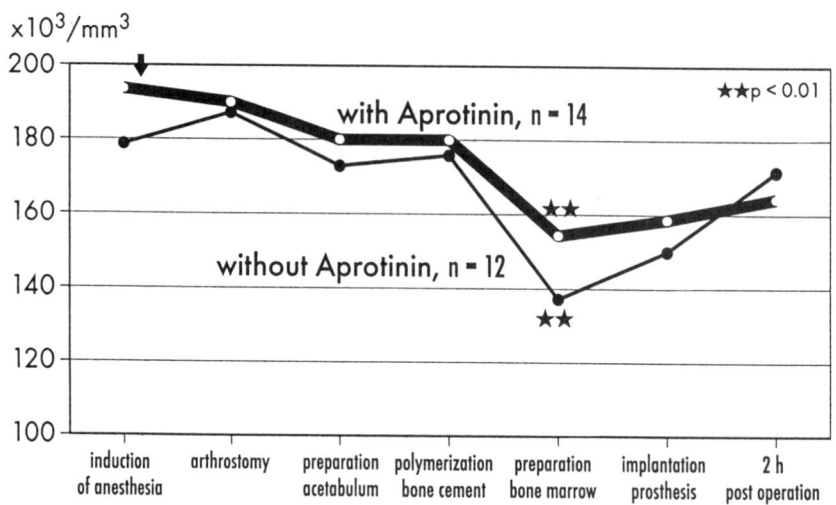

Number of Platelets in Total Hip Replacement
after Application of Aprotinin and without Aprotinin Treatment
in Comparison with the Initial Value

**FIGURE 13**

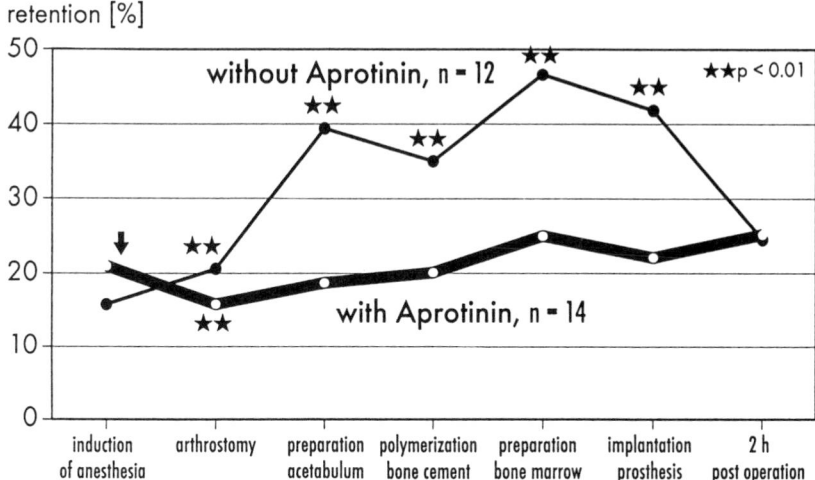

**FIGURE 14**

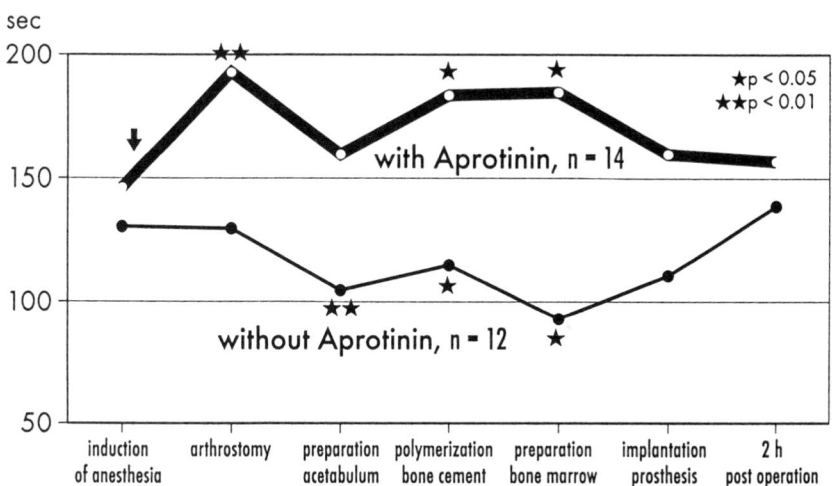

**FIGURE 15**

Platelet Aggregation in Total Hip Replacement Induced by Collagen, Maximal Amplitude, after Application of Aprotinin and without Aprotinin Treatment in Comparison with the Initial Value

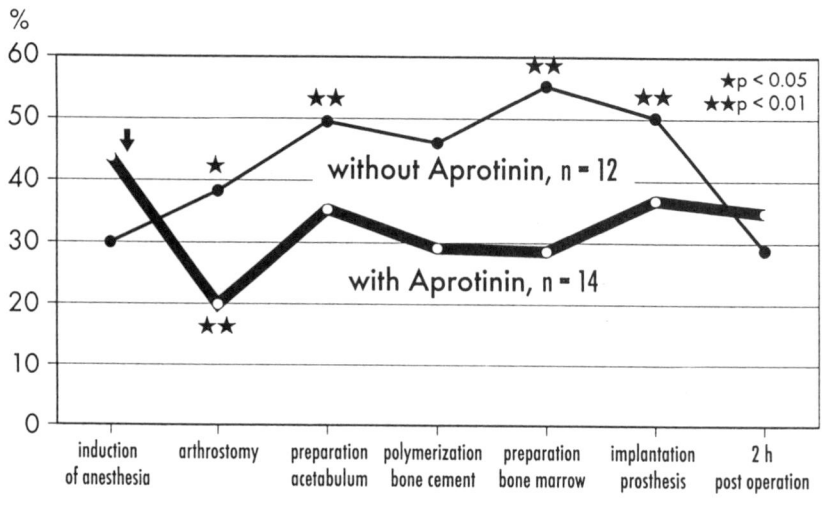

**FIGURE 16**

infusion of 20,000 KIU/kg of Trasylol A or B was performed within 15 minutes. Further blood samples were taken 10 minutes after infusion, at the moment of preparation of the femoral shaft, and 1, 2, 6, and 24 hours after infusion of Trasylol A or B. All blood samples were evaluated as follows:

1. Thromboelastogram (Hellige, Freiburg)
2. Availability of factor Xa after activation of the endogenous clotting cascade (chromogenic substrate S-2222; Deutsche Kabi Vitrum, Munich)
3. Partial thromboplastin time (PTT) (reagents from Merz & Dade, Munich)
4. Platelet number (TOA platelet counter; Colora Meβtechnik, Lorch, Germany)
5. Ratio of platelet aggregates, according to Wu and Hoak[33]
6. Platelet adhesiveness, according to Morris[25]
7. Platelet aggregability, according to Born[6]
8. Spontaneous platelet aggregation, according to Breddin et al.[7]
9. Blood lactate (reagents from Boehringer, Mannheim)

Figure 17 shows the shortened r-time in the control group and a significant prolongation after treatment with aprotinin. The k-values were affected accordingly. The maximal amplitude of the thromboelastogram was significantly expanded in the placebo group and diminished in the Trasylol-treated group (Fig. 18). The availability of factor Xa after activation of the endogenous clotting cascade was unchanged in the placebo group and strongly reduced in the Trasylol-treated group, probably because of the inactivation of plasma kallikrein (Fig. 19). The PTT, which describes the activity of the endogenous blood clotting cascade after activation of factor XII, followed the same pattern. The consumption of platelets during surgery was far more pronounced in the placebo group (Fig. 20). The ratio of platelet aggregates, which indicates the amount of circulating platelet aggregates, ranges

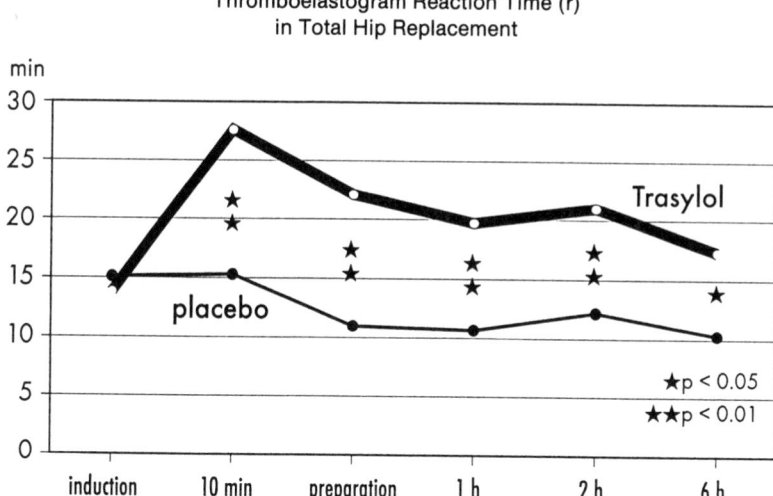

**FIGURE 17**

between 1 (no aggregation) and 0 (100% of platelets in the form of aggregates). Thus 0.5 indicates that 50% of circulating platelets are aggregated. The normal range is between 0.8 and 1. During surgery the fraction of circulating platelet aggregates was elevated in the placebo group, whereas the opposite was seen in the Trasylol-treated group (Fig. 21).

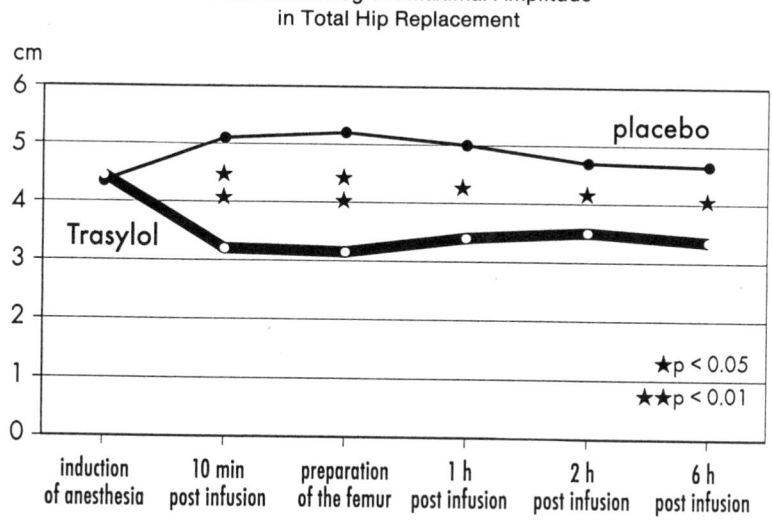

**FIGURE 18**

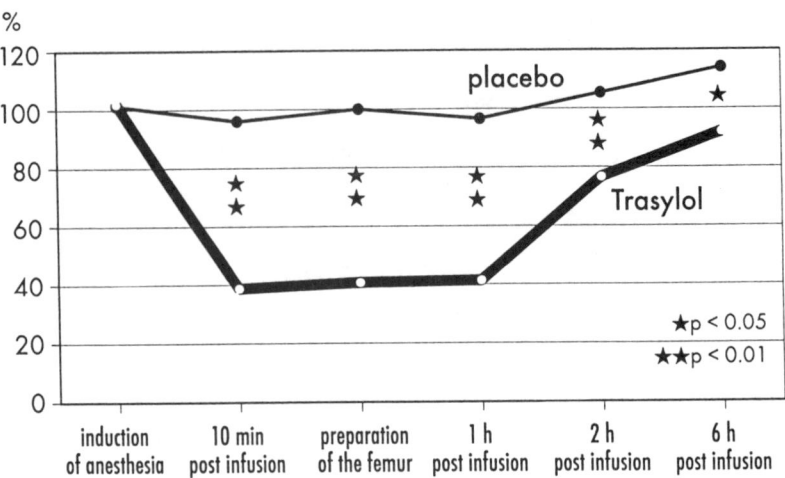

**FIGURE 19**

Platelet retention upon contact with glass beads peaks intraoperatively, indicating an increased reactivity in the placebo group. In contrast, shortly after treatment with Trasylol a marked decrease occurs and lasts throughout surgery, with a tendency toward normalization after 6 hours (Fig. 22). The maximal amplitude of the ADP-induced platelet aggregation, according to Born, corresponds to the amount and sizes of platelet aggregates. In comparison with starting values, the placebo group showed

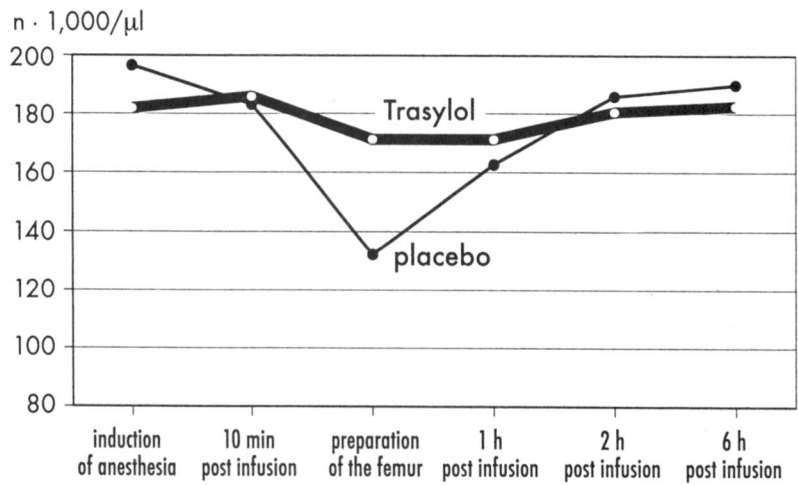

**FIGURE 20**

Ratio of Platelet Aggregates in Total Hip Replacement

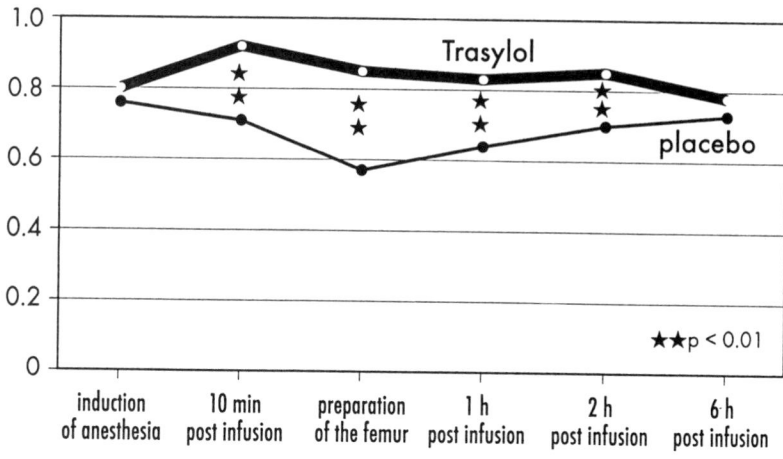

**FIGURE 21**

enhanced reactivity of platelets upon contact with ADP, whereas the number of reacting platelets was considerably lower in the aprotinin-treated group (Fig. 23).

Similar effects were obtained with the test for spontaneous aggregation, which was significantly enhanced in the saline group and significantly reduced by aprotinin. The blood lactate content—descriptive of the quality of microcirculation—was observed over 24 hours. In the placebo group the lactate level showed a highly significant tendency to normalize even after 24 hours. In contrast, the pattern of the Trasylol-treated group looked rather like that of a nonoperated control group.

Platelet Adhesivity in Total Hip Replacement

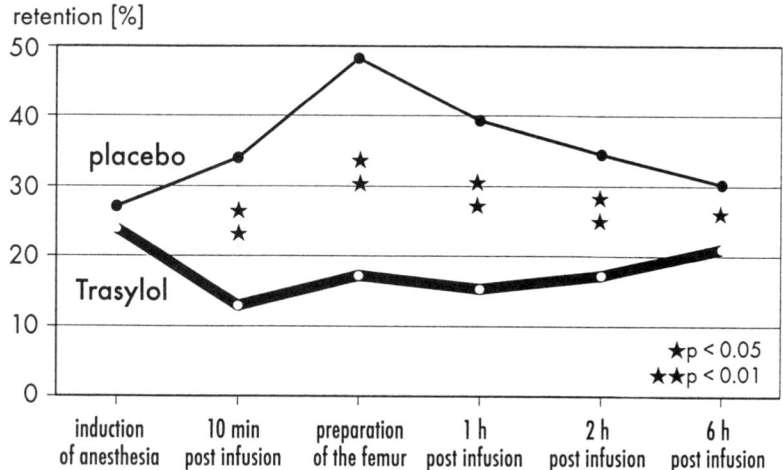

**FIGURE 22**

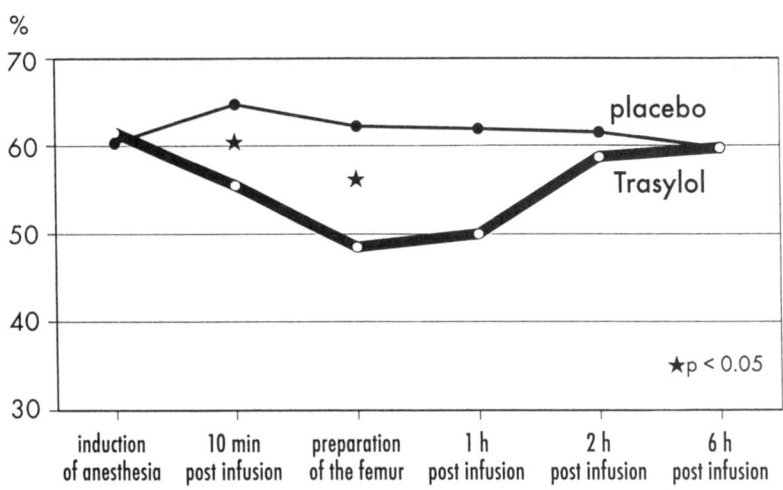

ADP-induced Platelet Aggregation
Maximal Amplitude in Total Hip Replacement

**FIGURE 23**

## Discussion

The critical moment in total hip replacement seems to be preparation of the bone marrow in the femur shaft, when platelet count is minimal and platelet adhesiveness and aggregability are maximal. Aprotinin in high doses reduces the activation of platelet function. In addition, aprotinin affects the endogenous system of blood coagulation, as evidenced by the prolonged aPTT. This effect may be due to inhibition of plasma kallikrein, a potent activator of the contact phase of intrinsic blood coagulation. The protective effect of aprotinin on platelets is also supported by several studies in the literature. McMichan et al. showed that pulmonary insufficiency in patients with multiple trauma is associated with a distinct and critical fall in platelet count, which can be prevented to a certain extent by aprotinin.[23] The important role of the lung as a filter for platelet aggregates after multiple trauma was shown by Peer and Schwartz.[27] Experimental studies in animals indicate that aprotinin diminishes the trapping of thrombocytes in the lung after polytrauma and burn injury.[4,5,22]

Of clinical importance, the effect of aprotinin is reversible, as demonstrated by Harke and Gennrich[17] and Reuter.[28] The underlying principle seems to be an interaction between aprotinin and membrane-bound enzymes. Therefore, aprotinin does not act like other antiaggregating agents and can be given without increasing the risk of bleeding.

## Risk of Postoperative Thrombosis

Deep venous thrombosis (DVT) occurs in 60–70% of patients undergoing surgery for total hip replacement and in up to 40% of patients treated with heparin, in part because fibrinolytic activity is decreased or inhibited after major surgical procedures. Thus it is of great clinical interest to determine whether perioperative administration of high doses of aprotinin is associated with an increased risk of DVT, particularly in patients at high risk of thromboembolic complications despite prophylaxis with low-dose heparin. A clinical trial was designed to answer this question.

## Patients, Material, Methods, and Results

A randomized, double-blind, parallel-group trial was conducted in 1983 at the Garmisch-Partenkirchen Hospital, the teaching hospital of the Technical University of Munich.[15,16] The protocol and informed consent forms were approved by the local institutional review board. Men and women who were 50 years or older and scheduled for elective hip replacement surgery (with cement implantation; no revision procedures) were included. The criteria for exclusion were allergic diathesis, manifest metabolic dysfunction, and renal insufficiency. All patients received 5000 IE of heparin as routine DVT prophylaxis in a fixed combination with 0.5 mg of dihydroergotamine, given subcutaneously twice daily. Within 15 minutes after the induction of anesthesia, 150 ml of Trasylol, which corresponds to 1.5 million KIU, was administered in the test group and 150 ml of saline in the control group. Blood loss and transfusion requirements were determined intra- and postoperatively. The number of patients with wound hematomas and reduced hemoglobin ($< 10 gm/dl$) was also determined postoperatively.

DVT was diagnosed by the radio-labeled fibrinogen uptake test (RFUT), which was performed daily on postoperative days 1–7 at each of 11 measuring points on the lower extremities. Because all data from the RFUTs were recorded with electronic data processing, it was possible to evaluate the results by using several algorithms. In version 1, the assessment points 0 (area of the groin) on both legs and 0–2 on the operated leg were omitted from the evaluation to exclude nonspecific results due to accumulation of radioactivity in the bladder or wound hematoma. In version 2, the mean value of two adjacent measuring points was used as the basis for the evaluation to ensure that artifacts were excluded. The chi-squared test was used to compare the frequencies of thromboses, wound hematomas, and transfusions with the distribution of gender. Blood loss was evaluated by means of the Mann-Whitney test.

The homogeneity of the two groups in terms of age, body weight and size, and duration of surgery was assessed by Student's t-test. The groups were sufficiently homogeneous in age ($p < 0.43$), body weight ($p < 0.64$), and height ($p < 0.73$). The mean values in the aprotinin-treated group were 65.5 years, 71.0 kg, and 167.9 cm; in the placebo group, 66.6 years, 71.8 kg, and 167.3 cm, respectively. The male-to-female ratios were also relatively parallel: 24 to 36 in the aprotinin-treated group and 20 to 38 in the placebo group. The mean duration of operation was 55 minutes in both groups. Some patients were excluded from analysis of the RFUT results because of transfer to other hospitals or missing data due to technical problems with the test. Fifty-five patients remained in the aprotinin-treated group and 52 in the placebo group for statistical evaluation.

Version 1 analysis of the RFUTs revealed positive thrombotic findings in 25 patients (45%) in the aprotinin-treated group and 20 patients (38%) in the placebo group. The low percentage of difference may be dismissed as random ($p < 0.45$). The results of version 5 were similar. Although the total number of thromboses was significantly lower in the version 2 analysis, the ratio between the aprotinin-treated

Frequency of Thrombosis (Versions 1 and 2)

| version | thrombosis | Aprotinin | placebo |
|---------|-----------|-----------|---------|
| V1 | yes | 25 = 45 % | 20 = 38 % |
|    | no  | 30 = 55 % | 32 = 62 % |
| V2 | yes | 15 = 27 % | 15 = 29 % |
|    | no  | 40 = 73 % | 37 = 71 % |
| total |   | 55 | 52 |

**FIGURE 24**

group (15 patients with thrombosis, or 27%) and the placebo group (15 patients with thrombosis, or 29%) changed only slightly (Fig. 24).

In the aprotinin-treated group 7 patients (12%) received transfusions—3 intraoperatively and 4 postoperatively. In comparison, the frequency in the placebo group was significantly higher ($p < 0.01$): 19 patients (32%) received transfusions—1 intraoperatively and 18 postoperatively (Fig. 25). In the aprotinin-treated group 8 patients (13%) had a postoperative reduction in hemoglobin $< 10$ gm/dl compared with 22 patients (38%) in the placebo group. The difference was statistically significant (Fig. 26). The number of wound hematomas (15% vs. 28%) and the postoperative drainage volumes (580 ml vs. 800 ml) were also significantly lower in the aprotinin-treated group ($p < 0.05$) than in the placebo group (Figs. 27 and 28).

## Discussion

The results indicate that perioperative administration of aprotinin reduces both blood loss and transfusion requirements in patients undergoing total hip replacement without increasing the risk of DVT. Such findings are of major clinical significance. Perioperative hyperfibrinolysis is followed by a marked postoperative inhibition of fibrinolysis in patients undergoing elective hip replacement; maximal inhibition was observed on the third postoperative day[16] because of the concomitant increase in antiplasmin. Because antiplasmin is an acute-phase reactant, its increase correlates

Transfusions (Intra- and Postoperative)

|  | total | Aprotinin |  | placebo |
|---|---|---|---|---|
| I only intraoperative | 4 | 3 | | 1 |
| II only postoperative | 16 | 2 | $p \le 0.01$ | 14 |
| III intra- and postoperative | 6 | 2 | | 4 |
| total | 26 = 21 % | 7 = 12 % | $p \le 0.01$ | 19 = 32 % |
| total group | 118 | 60 | | 58 |

**FIGURE 25**

Postoperative Reduction in Hemoglobin

| Hb ≤ 10 g/dl | postop. transfusion | Aprotinin | | placebo |
|---|---|---|---|---|
| yes | yes | 4 | | 17 |
| | no | 4 | | 5 |
| | total | 8 = 13 % | p < 0.01 | 22 = 38 % |
| no | yes | 0 | | 1 |
| | no | 52 | | 35 |
| | total | 52 = 87 % | | 36 = 62 % |

**FIGURE 26**

with the intensity of surgical trauma. Because of the short half-life of aprotinin, however, perioperative treatment does not interfere with the postoperative shutdown of fibrinolysis. Therefore, the high perioperative dose of aprotinin does not lead to a postoperative predisposition to DVT. These findings may be transferred without restriction to the use of aprotinin in cardiac surgery, in which hyperproteolysis also is seen in the immediate postoperative period and high doses of aprotinin are administered only during the perioperative period. Thus, the perioperative administration of aprotinin does not increase the risk of postoperative thrombosis. This conclusion, however, applies only to direct plasmin inhibitors and not to synthetic inhibitors that interfere with the release and activity of tPA.

The association of both orthopedic and cardiovascular surgery with significant postoperative blood loss indirectly indicates that the endogenous proteinase inhibitors are not sufficient to restore the physiologic balance between activators and inhibitors in the postoperative period. Therefore, it seems logical to administer therapeutic doses of proteinase inhibitors. In cardiovascular surgery this treatment has proved highly successful for many years; both blood loss and transfusion requirements are reduced significantly by perioperative administration of high doses of aprotinin.[29] The effect is particularly striking in patients at high risk of bleeding. The clinical trial in patients undergoing total hip replacement indicates that aprotinin also may be considered as a blood-conserving therapy in orthopedic surgery.

Wound Hematoma

| | no | | yes | total |
|---|---|---|---|---|
| Aprotinin | 51 | | 9 = 15 % | 60 |
| placebo | 42 | p ≤ 0.05 | 16 = 28 % | 58 |
| total | 93 | | 25 | 118 |

**FIGURE 27**

Blood Loss

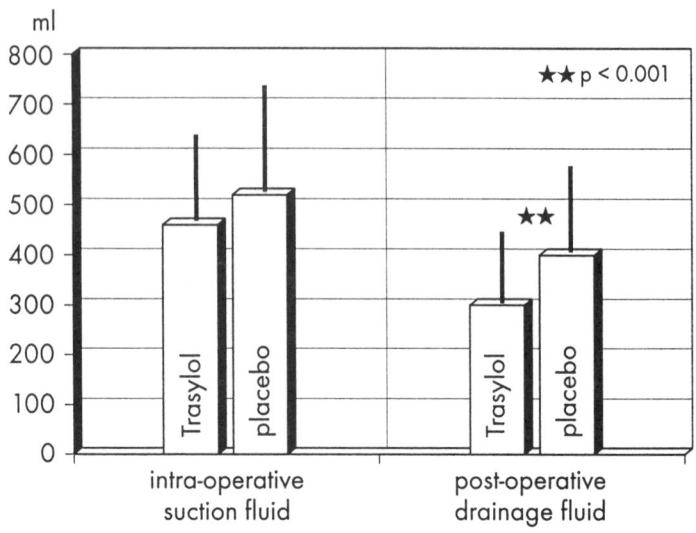

**FIGURE 28**

## Conclusion

Aprotinin, which has a molecular weight of 6512, is a nonspecific inhibitor of several serine proteases, including trypsin, plasmin, and kallikrein. Although the inhibitory profile of aprotinin has been described in detail, its mode of action in various clinical conditions remains unclear. Various experimental and clinical trials were performed at the Technical University of Munich to investigate (1) the different effects of aprotinin and the synthetic inhibitor tranexamic acid on tPA; (2) the mode of action of aprotinin in preventing local bleeding; (3) the influence of aprotinin on platelets; and (4) the potential prothrombotic effect of aprotinin in patients at high risk of DVT and bleeding complications.

The results indicate that the main difference between aprotinin and tranexamic acid lies in their mechanism of action: aprotinin inhibits antiplasmin, whereas tranexamic acid strongly inhibits tPA. This difference is of utmost clinical interest. Aprotinin is the treatment of choice in all conditions associated with hyperplasminemia, whereas tranexamic acid results in the formation of clots resistant to further fibrinolysis because of its strong affinity for plasminogen and its inhibition of tPA. Histomorphologic examinations of lung and muscle specimens from patients in traumatic shock have confirmed the finding that aprotinin does not affect the activity of tPA.[9]

Two experimental models—the measurements of mechanical strength of dissected nerves and the induced thermic skin lesions in rats—showed that proteolytic activity may interfere with the process of wound repair. The results also indicate that topical application of aprotinin may be an effective treatment to prevent secondary local hemorrhages in surgical procedures involving organs that contain high amounts of tPA. The effect is particularly striking in patients undergoing neurosurgery, as shown in several clinical trials.[21,32] The beneficial effect of aprotinin can be attributed to its strong inhibition of locally generated plasmin. On the basis of these experiments, aprotinin has become an essential component of the so-called fibrin glue that is widely used in all situations associated with local bleeding complications.

Systemic bleeding complications play a major role in cardiovascular surgery that requires the use of CPB. Because the pathophysiology of such complications is highly complex, it is not known whether the preventive effect of aprotinin is due to its inhibition of plasmin or plasma kallikrein (via activated factor XII) or to its protective effects on platelets. The normalization of platelet dysfunction with high doses of aprotinin has been demonstrated in several experimental and clinical trials; the clinical significance, however, remains unclear. If platelet function is conserved until the end of surgery, nonactivated platelets may be responsible for the initial wound repair, thereby reducing blood loss and other bleeding complications.

Because the potential risk of thrombogenicity due to high doses of aprotinin had not been ruled out, a controlled clinical trial was initiated in patients at high risk of DVT. The results provide firm evidence that the postoperative risk of DVT is not increased by perioperative treatment with aprotinin. The simultaneous discovery that aprotinin shows remarkable efficacy in reducing bleeding in orthopedic surgery was truly by chance; the drug was intended to address prothrombotic concerns.[16] However, treatment with aprotinin should not continue beyond the perioperative period or after neutralization of heparin in extracorporeal bypass surgery to avoid interference with the physiologic decrease in fibrinolysis.

The final question is whether the effect of aprotinin on blood coagulation counteracts its beneficial effects on blood preservation in cardiac surgery. As shown by the early experiments of Benzer and Blümel, the reaction time of the thromboelastogram is significantly prolonged by the addition of aprotinin in vitro; this finding was confirmed by experimental and clinical trials in vivo. The prolongation of the reaction time correlates with a prolongation of the aPTT, indicating that aprotinin affects the intrinsic pathway of coagulation through its inhibition of plasma kallikrein, which interferes with the positive feedback mechanism in the contact phase of intrinsic blood coagulation. The extrinsic pathway of blood coagulation, however, is not affected by aprotinin; therefore, the bleeding risk is not increased. It may be misleading to use the term anticoagulant agent; for example, in cardiac surgery an intraoperative prolongation of the aPTT and ACT due to high doses of aprotinin must not be corrected by lowering the dose of heparin. Otherwise a prothrombotic state may occur.

# References

1. Benzer H, Blümel G, Brenner H, Piza F: Über Blutgerinnungsstörungen nach Hirnverletzungen und Hirnoperationen. Wien Med Wochenschr 41/42:725, 1963.
2. Benzer H, Blümel G, Piza F: Einflüsse von Trypsininhibitoren auf die Blutgerinnung. Wien Med Wochenschr 28/29:609, 1960.
3. Bergentz SE, Lewis D, Ljungquist U: Die Lunge in der Schock: Thrombozytenanhäufung nach Polytrauma and intravasale Gerinnung. Langenbecks Arch Klin Chir 329:658, 1971.
4. Blaisdell FW, Lim RC, Stallone RJ: The mechanism of pulmonary damage following traumatic shock. Surg Gynecol Obstet 130:15, 1970.
5. Blaisdell FW, Schlobohm RN: The respiratory distress syndrome: A review. Surgery 74:251, 1973.

6. Born GVR, Cross UJ: The aggregation of platelets. J Physiol 168:178, 1963.
7. Breddin K, Grun H, Krzywanek HJ, Schremmer WP: Zur Messung der spontanen Thrombozytenaggregation. Plättchenaggregationstest II. Methodik. Klin Wochenschr 53:81, 1975.
8. Denk S, Blümel G, Kujat R, v. Sommoggy S: The different effects of natural and synthetic proteinase inhibitors on tissue plasminogen activators and blood coagulation. In Cantin M, Haberland GL, et al (eds): New Aspects of Trasylol Therapy. FK Schattauer, Stuttgart, 1975, pp 49–59.
9. Denk S, Kujat R, Schlag G, et al: Das Verhalten gewebeständiger Plasminogenaktivatoren nach Polytrauma. Med Welt 18:876, 1976.
10. Haas-Denk S, Kaunzner W, v. Sommoggy S: Beeinflussung der Thrombozytenfunktion und der Gerinnung von Konservenblut durch Azetylsalizylsäure und Aprotinin. Med Welt 28:912, 1977.
11. Haas S, v.d. Goltz A, Wriedt-Lübbe I, et al: Unterschiedliche Wirkung von natürlichen Proteinasen- und synthetischen Fibrinolyseinhibitoren auf die gewebeständigen Plasminogenaktivatoren und Plasmininhibitoren nach Polytrauma. In Mayrhofer-Krammel O, Schlag G, et al (eds): Akutes Progressives Lungenversagen. Thieme, Stuttgart, 1979, p 102.
12. Haas S, Ketterl R, Landauer B, et al: Platelet function and proteinase inhibition. In McConn RM (ed): The Role of Chemical Mediators in the Pathophysiology of Acute Illness and Injury. New York, Raven Press, 1982, pp 219–228.
13. Haas S, Stemberger A, Erhardt W, et al: Einfluß lokal applizierter Gerinnungsfaktoren (Fibrinkleber) auf die Wundheilung. Hämostaseologie 3:1, 1983.
14. Haas S, Ketterl R, Stemberger A, et al: The effect of aprotinin on platelet function, blood coagulation, and blood lactate level in total hip replacement—A double blind clinical trial. In Hörl WR, Heidland A (eds): Proteases—Potential Role in Health and Disease. New York, Plenum Press, 1984, pp 287–297.
15. Haas S, Müller-Esterl W, Fritsche H-M, et al: Effects of aprotinin on the incidence of thrombosis and postoperative bleeding [abstract P587]. Thromb Haemost 54:99, 1985.
16. Haas S, Fritsche H-M, Ritter H, et al: Is the risk of postoperative thrombosis increased after perioperative therapy with the plasmin inhibitor aprotinin? In Hartel W, et al (eds): Chirurgisches Forum 1991 für Experimentelle und Klinische Forschung. Berlin-Heidelberg, Springer, 1991, pp 371–374.
17. Harke H, Gennrich M: Aprotinin-ACD-Blut. Experimentelle Untersuchungen über den Einfluss von Aprotinin auf die plasmatische und thrombozytäre Gerinnung. Anaesthesist 29:266, 1980.
18. Harke H: Beeinflussung der Mikroaggregation in lagernden Blutkonserven. Anaesthesist 25:347, 1976.
19. Krzywanek HJ, Breddin K: Primary shape change of thrombocytes and platelet aggregation after administration of acetylsalicylic acid. Thromb Haemost 38:251, 1977.
20. Kuderna H: Ergebnisse und Erfahrungen in der klinischen Anwendung des Fibrin-Klebers bei der Wiederherstellung durchtrennter peripherer Nerven. In Cotta H, Martini AK (eds): Implantate und Transplantate in der Plastischen Wiederherstellungschirurgie. Springer, Berlin, 1981, p 96.
21. Leheta F, Lenz C, Weichenmeier I, et al: Die Beeinflussung der Fibrinolyse am traumatisierten Rattenhirn durch lokale Applikation von Aprotinin, Wasserstoffperoxid und physiologischer NaCl-Lösung. Med Welt 33:1802, 1982.
22. Loew D, Breddin K, Flenker H, Schnells G: Blutplättchen, Gerinnungsfaktoren und morphologische Organveränderungen nach Verbrühungsschock beim Rhesus-Affen. Med Welt 25:2118, 1974.
23. McMichan DS, Rosengarten J, McNeur C, Philipp E: Das posttraumatische Lungen-Syndrom. Definition, Diagnose und Therapie. Med Welt 27:2331, 1976.
24. Modig J, Olerud S, Malmberg P: Sudden pulmonary dysfunction in hip replacement surgery. Acta Anaesthiol Scand 17:276, 1973.
25. Morris CDW: Observations on the effect of glass beads on platelet aggregation and its relation to platelet stickiness. Thromb Diathes Haemorrh 20:345, 1968.
26. Noordhoek-Hegt V, Brakman P: Histochemical study of an inhibitor of fibrinolysis in the human arterial wall. Nature 248:75–76, 1974.
27. Peer RM, Schwartz SI: Development and treatment of post-traumatic pulmonary platelet trapping. Ann Surg 181:447, 1975.
28. Reuter HD: The stabilizing effect of Trasylol on platelet membranes. Thromb Haemost 42:298, 1979.

29. Royston D, Bidestrup BP, Taylor KM, Sapsford RM: Effect of aprotinin on need for blood transfusion after repeat open-heart surgery. Lancet ii:1289, 1987.
30. Schlag G, Haas-Denk S, Wriedt-Lübbe I, Blümel G: Untersuchungen der fibrinolytischen Aktivität im Gewebe bei polytraumatisierten Patienten Unfallheilkunde 80:269, 1977.
31. Todd AS: The histological localisation of fibrinolytic activator. J Pathol Bacteriol 78:281, 1959.
32. Trappe A, Hafter R, Wendt P, et al: Nachweis der Fibrinolyse im chronischen subduralen Hämatom. In Dietz H (ed): Neurochirurgie. Stuttgart, Thieme, 1986, pp 67–98.
33. Wu KK, Hoak JC: Measurement of platelet aggregates in whole blood. Lancet 19:924, 1974.

Jawed Fareed, PhD
Debra Hoppensteadt, MS
Michael J. Koza, BS
Walter Jeske, BS
Jeanine M. Walenga, PhD
Roque Pifarré, MD

# 6

# Pharmacokinetics of Aprotinin and Its Relevance to Antifibrinolytic and Other Biologic Effects

Aprotinin is a low-molecular-weight, Kunitz-type, broad-spectrum protease inhibitor of mammalian origin that conventionally has been used as an antifibrinolytic agent in both physiologic and pharmacologic control of hyperfibrinolytic states,[12,21] such as pancreatitis and overdose of thrombolytic agents. More recently, aprotinin has been demonstrated to reduce postoperative bleeding during surgery, especially cardiopulmonary bypass (CPB) surgery.[7,13,19,20]

As an effective inhibitor of kallikreins, aprotinin readily prevents the generation of kinins and the conversion of profibrinolytic mediators into their active forms. Table 1 lists various sites at which aprotinin can produce its effects. During CPB surgery, contact activation and other processes lead to the complex activation of proteases such as factor XIIa, kallikrein, plasmin, and elastase. Aprotinin inhibits these enzymes to varying degrees and also produces cytostabilizing effects on platelets, presumably by inhibiting the proteolytic digestion of membrane glycoproteins. Furthermore, by inhibiting elastase, aprotinin modulates the action of the leukocytes and related cells. Thus, it produces certain therapeutic effects in a multiple fashion.

The third Kunitz domain on the newly discovered protease inhibitor, tissue factor pathway inhibitor (TFPI), is similar to aprotinin, which presumably produces a synergistic enhancement of the action of TFPI.[2] Heparin is known to release TFPI during CPB surgery. Thus, patients who receive aprotinin during surgical procedures may benefit from a synergistic interaction between TFPI and aprotinin.

## Pharmacodynamics of Aprotinin

Although aprotinin has been used clinically for over three decades, a systematic pharmacodynamic/pharmacokinetic study is not available, possibly because of the limited methods available for measurement. Of interest, although extensive studies

**TABLE 1.** Potential Mechanisms by which Aprotinin Produces Its Clinical Effects

| Action | Clinical Consequences |
| --- | --- |
| Plasmin inhibition | Control of fibrinolysis |
| Kallikrein inhibition | Control of kallikrein-mediated pathway |
| Qualitative and quantitative restoration of platelets | Restoration of hemostatic process |
| Inhibition of elastase | Control of leukocyte-mediated pathologic events |
| Inhibition of protease-mediated degradation of platelet glycoproteins | Stabilization of platelet membrane |
| Synergistic actions on heparin-releasable tissue factor pathway inhibitor | Increased inhibition of elastase-mediated pathologic responses |

of the early renal uptake and later tubular metabolism of radiolabeled aprotinin have been carried out in both humans and animals, no attempts have been made to provide valid pharmacokinetic profiles.[6,14,15]

The specific activity of various clinically used aprotinin preparations is usually designated in terms of kallikrein inhibitor units (KIU). Most preparations have a potency of 6000–8000 KIU/mg. The chemical structure of aprotinin is comparable to that of the specific thrombin inhibitor, hirudin (Fig. 1), which is isolated from the saliva of the medicinal leech, *Hirudo medicinalis*.[10] Both aprotinin and hirudin have now been characterized fully, and their recombinant forms are available commercially. The molecular weight of both agents is around 6.5 kDa.

Table 2 shows the protease inhibitory spectrums of aprotinin and hirudin. Whereas hirudin is a highly specific inhibitor of thrombin, aprotinin exhibits a wide spectrum of inhibitory actions against various enzymes. Although plasmin and kallikrein are the most strongly inhibited ($k_i \leq \mu M$), aprotinin also inhibits protein Ca, trypsin, elastase, and several other enzymes. Thus, the relative enzyme inhibitory

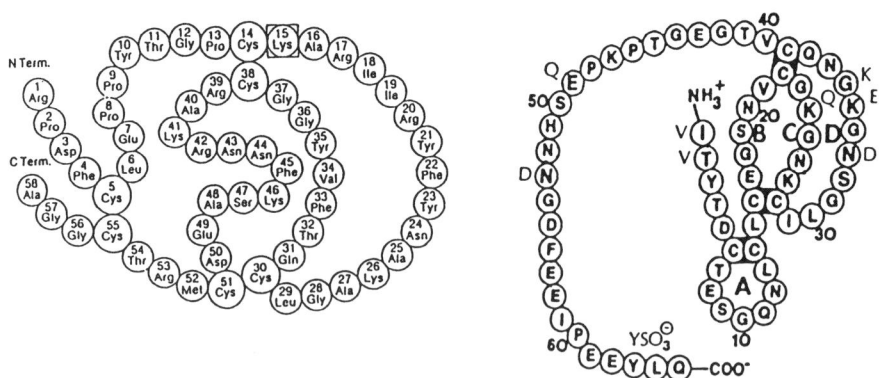

APROTININ                    HIRUDIN

**FIGURE 1.** A comparison of the primary structure of bovine aprotinin and natural hirudin. Both proteins have a molecular weight of approximately 6.5 kDa. Aprotinin is usually obtained from mammalian lungs, whereas hirudin is obtained from the salivary gland of the medicinal leech, *Hirudo medicinalis*.

**TABLE 2.** Serine Protease Inhibitory Spectrums of Aprotinin and Hirudin as Measured by Amidolytic Methods

| Serine Protease | Aprotinin | Hirudin |
|---|:---:|:---:|
| Glandular kallikrein | + + + | − |
| Plasma kallikrein | + + | − |
| Factor XIIa | + | − |
| Factor Xa | − | − |
| Thrombin | − | + + + + |
| Tissue-type plasminogen activator | ± | − |
| Urokinase | ± | − |
| Plasmin | + + + + | − |
| Trypsin | + + | − |
| Protein Ca | + + | − |

actions of hirudin and aprotinin can be used to measure their circulating level in blood. Both the plasmin and kallikrein inhibitory functions can be used to estimate circulating functional levels of aprotinin.[8]

Table 3 lists potential methods of measuring the levels of aprotinin in blood. Activated partial thromboplastin time (aPTT), the conventional method for monitoring heparin, is also prolonged by aprotinin. This effect is relatively weak, however, and the aPTT is not useful for monitoring aprotinin levels in the presence of heparin. Antiprotease assays such as anti-factor Xa and anti-factor IIa are not affected by aprotinin, whereas they are strongly affected by heparin. Biochemically defined assays for inhibitors of kallikrein and plasmin are useful for monitoring the functional levels of aprotinin in circulating blood. Enzyme immunoassays for both hirudin and aprotinin have been developed. For aprotinin, such assays may be useful but do not distinguish between the functional and immunologic levels of aprotinin when aprotinin is complexed with kallikrein and plasmin. Because radiolabeled aprotinin can be used only in animal studies, its usefulness in the measurement of pharmacokinetics is rather limited.

Unfortunately, valid data about the pharmacodynamic and pharmacokinetic profile of aprotinin were not available until recently.[9,17,18] However, because of the widespread use of aprotinin for various clinical indications and it simultaneous administration with other drugs, additional information about its pharmacokinetics and pharmacodynamics is crucial for clinical purposes.

In a recent study, Levy and coworkers used a sandwich-linked immunosorbent assay to measure the antigen levels of aprotinin in human plasma.[9] The authors noted a shortened half-life for aprotinin in cardiac surgical patients compared with

**TABLE 3.** Methods to Measure Aprotinin Blood Levels

| Method | Feasibility |
|---|---|
| Prothrombin time | Relatively insensitive |
| aPTT | Limited sensitivity |
| Heptest | Insensitive; of limited use |
| Anti-factor Xa | Not sensitive |
| Anti-factor IIa | Not sensitive |
| Antikallikrein | Sensitive and reliable method for functional aprotinin levels |
| Antiplasmin | Sensitive and reliable method for functional aprotinin levels |
| Enzyme immunoassay | Measurement of total amount of aprotinin (both free and complexed) |
| Radiolabeled aprotinin | Not readily available; can be used only in animal studies |

the half-life reported in control studies of normal volunteers. Effective inhibition of both kallikrein and plasmin was noted with a 2 million-KIU loading dose of aprotinin. With a 1 million-KIU loading dose, however, only plasmin was inhibited. Because plasmin is the main fibrinolytic enzyme, the authors speculated that the effectiveness of the half dosage is due to the inhibition of plasmin. The pharmacokinetic data in this study, however, were based on approximations.

In two previous studies, Schall and coworkers studied the pharmacokinetic profile of high dosages of aprotinin in patients undergoing primary elective hysterectomy.[17,18] The results of these studies suggest that aprotinin, when administered intravenously over a period of 30 minutes, exhibits a dose-dependent pharmacokinetic effect over a wide dose range. The authors also suggest that plasma concentrations of aprotinin decrease in a biphasic manner. The total urinary excretion of the intact drug is rather low but appears to increase with the injected dosage. In contrast, hirudin is excreted in its intact form.[10] The authors reported that no age-dependent differences in the pharmacokinetics of aprotinin were evident.

A study that simultaneously measures the absolute level of aprotinin and functional inhibition of kallikrein and plasmin is not available. Such a study in the clinical setting would provide useful data in the management of patients undergoing different surgical procedures and medical treatment.

During CPB surgery, various methods have been used to administer aprotinin. Generally, a total of 4–5 million KIU equivalents (600–700 mg) is administered in various phases, including the bolus loading dose ($\simeq$ 2 million KIU), a continuous infusion (0.5 million KIU/hr), and a pump-priming dose (2 million KIU total dose). Thus a very high dosage of aprotinin is given to heparinized patients, whose blood is fully anticoagulated. Routinely performed coagulation tests cannot determine the level of anticoagulation for the circulating levels of aprotinin. Although enzyme-linked immunoassays can be used to quantitate the aprotinin levels, they are not readily available. Furthermore, the measurement of aprotinin levels may provide no clinically useful information during CPB surgery.

For the optimal development of any drug, its pharmacokinetic and pharmacodynamic actions should be known. The pharmacokinetic profile of aprotinin may provide useful information for monitoring, determining optimal dosage, and controlling wasteful use. Most commonly, high-dose aprotinin has been used in CPB surgery. However, effective control of bleeding has been achieved with half of the dosage in noncompromised patients. In most studies, patient weight has not been taken into consideration for dosing.

## Experimental and Clinical Observations on the Pharmacokinetics of Aprotinin

At present a specific approach to selecting a proper dosage of aprotinin is not available. The dosage is based largely on empirical observations, regardless of the patient's weight or other considerations. Although aprotinin has a high safety index, various adverse reactions have been reported.[3,11,16,22] Dosage considerations for overweight patients, elderly patients, and women are important. To obtain information about the pharmacokinetics of aprotinin, a systematic investigation was undertaken at Loyola University Medical Center, with both experimental and clinical protocols.

## Validation of Methodology

Aprotinin was added to citrated, pooled human plasma in a concentration range of 0–100 μg/ml to validate the coagulation methods routinely used to assess its effect, including prothrombin time (PT), aPTT, Heptest time, thrombin time, tissue factor clotting time (TFCT), and anti-factor Xa and anti-factor IIa assays. Because measurements of aprotinin are usually performed in the presence of heparin, the relative contribution of the heparin–antithrombin III complex was also measured in the antikallikrein and antiplasmin assays.

Supplementation of aprotinin at a concentration range of 0–100 μg/ml produced no progressive increase in the prothrombin time or Heptest (Fig. 2). A doubling of the aPTT assay was noted at levels of 50 μg/ml, which approximate circulating levels of aprotinin during CPB surgery. Because most patients are fully heparinized and hemodiluted, however, measurement of the aPTT level is not possible. Thus none of the above tests is of value in the functional measurement of aprotinin levels.

Similarly, at concentrations as high as 100 μg/ml, aprotinin produced no effect on the thrombin time (5U) or TFCT (Fig. 3). Aprotinin produced no inhibition of factor Xa and only a very weak inhibition of thrombin at a concentration of 100 μg/ml (Fig. 4). Thus, the global clotting tests and the amidolytic anti-factor Xa and anti-factor IIa assays are not applicable for the measurement of functional aprotinin levels.

The comparative antiprotease actions of the heparin–AT-III complex and aprotinin were measured in the antikallikrein assay as performed by an amidolytic

IN VITRO PROFILE OF APROTININ IN NORMAL HUMAN POOLED PLASMA

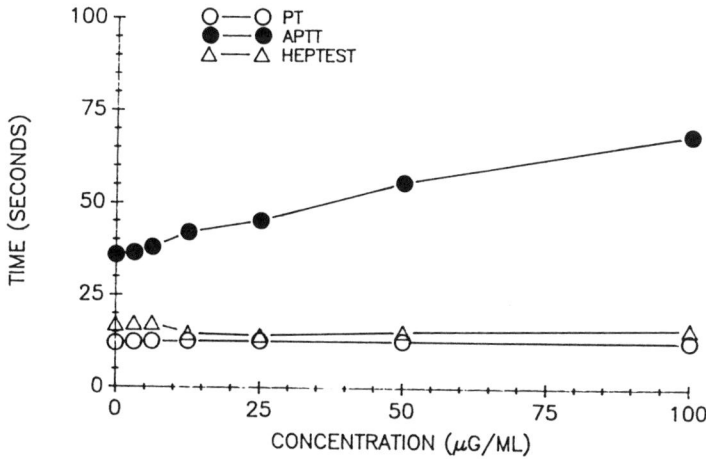

**FIGURE 2.** Effect of aprotinin on the clotting profile of pooled normal human plasma. Citrated, frozen pooled plasma prepared from 10–15 normal healthy donors was supplemented with aprotinin at a concentration range of 0–100 μg/ml. Prothrombin time was measured with thromboplastin C (Dade, Miami, FL) and partial thromboplastin time with Organon Teknika reagent (Organon Teknika, Durham, NC). Heptest (Haemachem, St. Louis, MO) measurements also were made. All results represent a mean of three individual determinations.

IN VITRO PROFILE OF APROTININ IN NORMAL HUMAN POOLED PLASMA

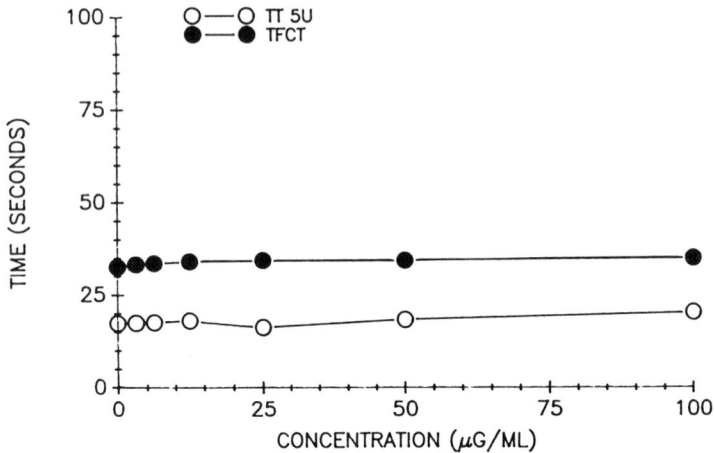

**FIGURE 3.** Effect of aprotinin on the thrombin time (TT [5U]) and tissue factor clotting time (TFCT) measured in normal human plasma. Pooled human plasma supplemented with aprotinin in a concentration range of 0–100 µg/ml was assayed with the TT (5U) and TFCT reagents. All results represent a mean of three individual determinations.

IN VITRO PROFILE OF APROTININ IN NORMAL HUMAN POOLED PLASMA

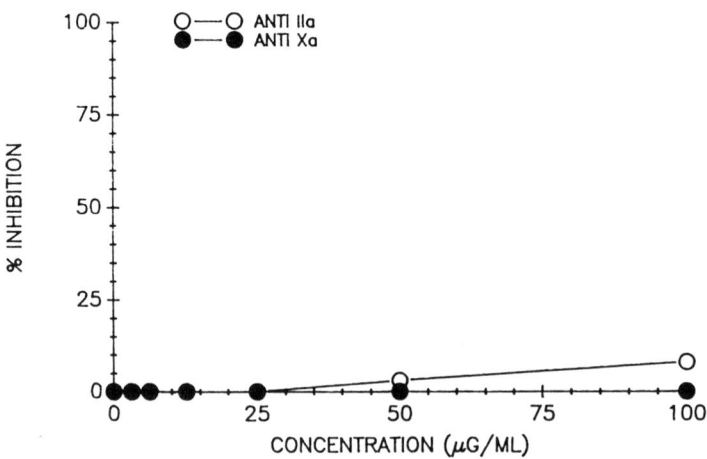

**FIGURE 4.** Effect of aprotinin on the amidolytic anti-factor IIa and anti-factor Xa assays. Pooled human plasma preparations supplemented with aprotinin were assessed for the anti-IIa and anti-Xa assays using chromogenic substrate methods. All results represent a mean of three individual determinations.

COMPARATIVE ANTIPROTEASE ACTIONS OF HEPARIN/AT III AND APROTININ
INHIBITION OF KALLIKREIN

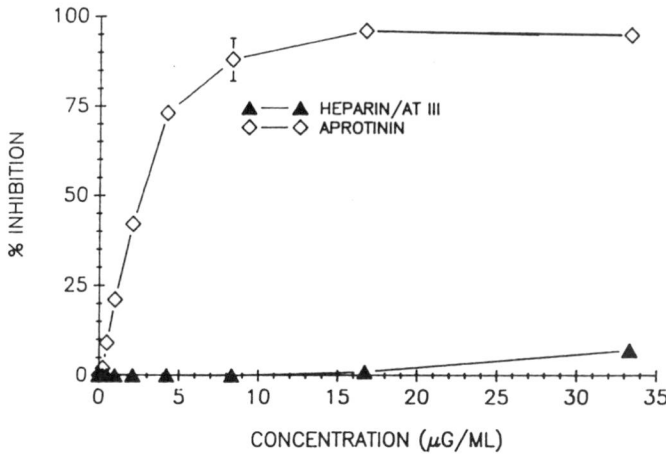

**FIGURE 5.** A comparison of the effects of the heparin–AT-III complex and aprotinin on the amidolytic actions of glandular kallikrein in defined biochemical systems. Aprotinin was diluted in saline to obtain various concentrations. The heparin–AT-III complex was prepared using human AT-III and bovine heparin. The antikallikrein activity of both inhibitors was measured by a chromogenic substrate method.

method (Fig. 5). Aprotinin produced a concentration-dependent inhibition of kallikrein with an apparent inhibitory concentration ($IC_{50}$) below 3.0 $\mu$g/ml. Because the clinical concentration of aprotinin is 10–50 $\mu$g/ml, this method can be readily modified for the measurement of circulating levels of aprotinin. The heparin–AT-III complex does not interfere with the results.

Inhibition of plasmin by aprotinin and the heparin–AT-III complex was measured by an amidolytic method (Fig. 6). Aprotinin produced a highly potent inhibition of plasmin with an $IC_{50}$ value $\leq 1.0$ $\mu$g/ml. The heparin–AT-III complex also produced a weak inhibition of plasmin with an $IC_{50}$ value $> 35$ $\mu$g/ml.

Aprotinin also produced a concentration-dependent effect on the whole blood clotting asays such as thromboelastography (TEG) and saline activated clotting time (ACT) (Fig. 7). Aprotinin prolonged the R and RK values in the TEG assay, suggesting a mild anticoagulant effect in the in vitro studies. A previous report also showed that aprotinin can affect the ACT. This may be the cause of falsely elevated values in heparinized patients.[11] In the saline ACT test, aprotinin produced an anticoagulant effect (Fig. 8) that was too weak to be used to determine its concentration in blood. Furthermore, heparinization masks the mild anticoagulant effect of aprotinin. Thus, both TEG and ACT tests are of no value in monitoring the effect of aprotinin in blood.

## Circulating Aprotinin Levels During Cardiopulmonary Bypass Surgery

One of the major mechanisms of action of aprotinin is inhibition of both plasma and glandular kallikreins. During surgical interventions such as CPB, complex

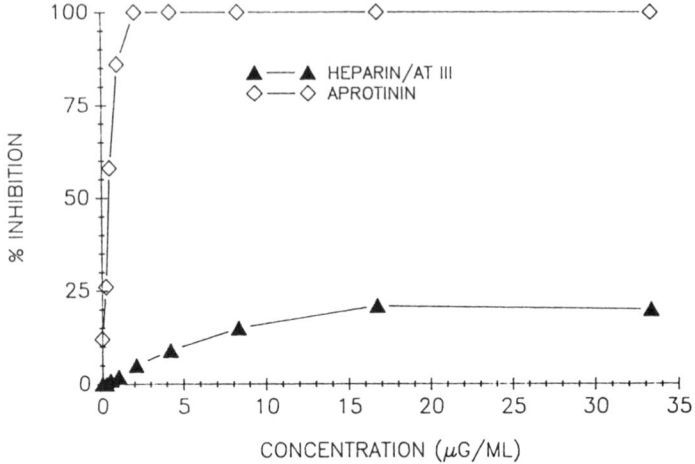

COMPARATIVE ANTIPROTEASE ACTIONS OF HEPARIN/AT III AND APROTININ
INHIBITION OF PLASMIN

**FIGURE 6.** A comparison of the heparin–AT-III complex and aprotinin on the amidolytic activity of human plasmin in defined biochemical systems. Aprotinin and heparin–AT-III complex were tested for the antiplasmin activities in a modified amidolytic assay. All results represent a mean of three individual determinations.

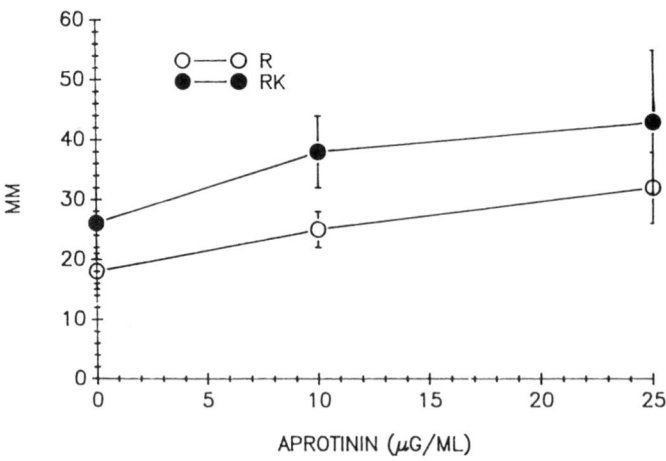

EFFECT OF APROTININ ON THE TEG PROFILE IN NORMAL HUMAN WHOLE BLOOD

**FIGURE 7.** Effect of ex vivo aprotinin supplementation on the thromboelastographic (TEG) profile of native human whole blood. Blood samples were drawn in plastic syringes containing varying amounts of aprotinin. TEG profile was immediately determined, and the R and RK times were calculated. All results represent a mean of three individual determinations.

EFFECT OF APROTININ ON SALINE ACT IN HUMAN BLOOD

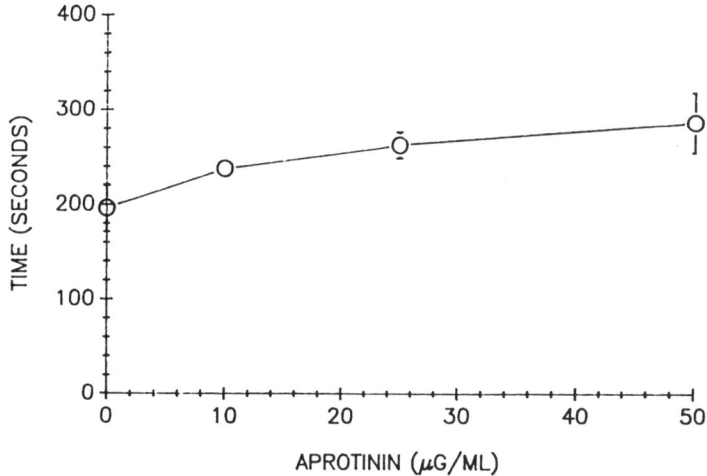

**FIGURE 8.** Effect of ex vivo aprotinin supplementation on the activated clotting time (ACT) of native human whole blood. Blood samples were drawn in plastic syringes containing varying amounts of aprotinin. ACT measurements were made with a Hemachron device. All results represent a mean of three individual determinations.

pathophysiologic activation results from the release of tissue factor, the effect of the extracorporeal circuit, and the activation of the fibrinolytic sytstem by heparin. Furthermore, several cytokines and other mediators are released. Because aprotinin inhibits plasmin and kallikrein, the ex vivo inhibition of either enzyme can be used to quantitate the functional levels of aprotinin in biologic fluids. Based on this observation, a simple method was developed to quantitate the inhibition of glandular kallikrein by blood plasma samples from patients treated with aprotinin. The relative degree of kallikrein inhibition can be related to the concentration of aprotinin in the plasma. In contrast to other approaches, this amidolytic method is rather specific for the quantitation of aprotinin in blood.[8] Furthermore, it measures the functional level of aprotinin as an inhibitor of kallikrein. This method, therefore, was used to determine the circulating levels of aprotinin in both experimental and clinical conditions.

Relativley high dosages of aprotinin are used to produce an antifibrinolytic state during CPB surgery. The total amount of aprotinin and the method of administration vary widely. Protocols are usually determined empirically on the basis of clinical outcome at individual institutions. The simple amidolytic method described above was used to determine the circulating amounts of aprotinin during CPB surgery. Because the expected levels of aprotinin were in the range of 10–50 μg/ml, a dilution step can be used to obtain results within the assay range.

Circulating levels of aprotinin were calculated in two groups of patients (Fig. 9). The first group consisted of 21 patients who underwent CPB surgery without aprotinin. The second group consisted of 18 patients treated with a loading dose of 280 mg of Trasylol brand of aprotinin. An additional 280 mg of aprotinin was administered to the circuit, followed by a continuous infusion of 70 mg/hr during

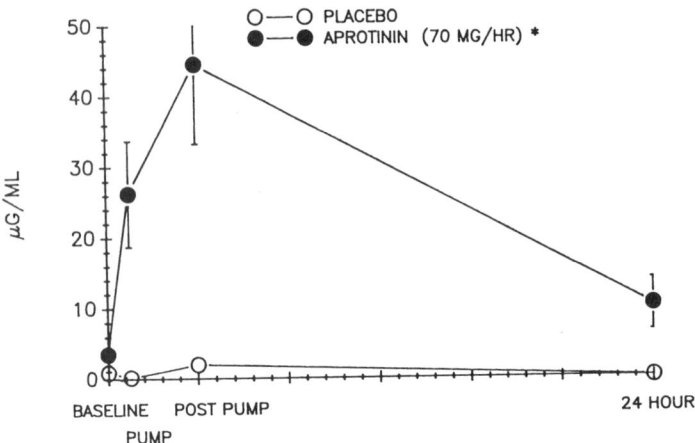

ANTI–KALLIKREIN LEVELS IN BYPASS PATIENTS GIVEN APROTININ

* LOADING DOSE 280 MG + 70 MG/HR INFUSION +280 MG ADDED TO CPB CIRCUIT

**FIGURE 9.** Antikallikrein levels in blood of patients treated with aprotinin during CPB surgery. Blood samples were obtained at baseline, on pump, after pump, and 24 hours after surgery from a placebo group (n = 21) and the aprotinin-treated group (n = 18). The antikallikrein level from each blood sample was measured with an amidolytic method. All results represent a mean of ± 1 SD.

the surgical procedure. The placebo group exhibited no significant antikallikrein activity. In the treated group, however, a 20–30-μg/ml level of aprotinin was found during CPB. Postpump blood samples revealed a high aprotinin level of ≥ 40 μg/ml, and even 24 hours after surgery the amount was sizeable (approximately 7–15 μg/ml).

Such data clearly suggest that the administration of aprotinin to heparinized patients produces a strong antiprotease action. The circulating levels of aprotinin, as calculated by an indirect enzyme inhibition method, appear to be directly correlated with the therapeutic effect. The detection of aprotinin even at 24 hours postoperatively is noteworthy.

Because aprotinin and TFPI have similar structures, levels of TFPI were also quantitated in the plasma of both groups (Fig. 10). The time course of the TFPI increase in both groups corresponded to the degree of heparinization. A marked increase in the level of TFPI was noted immediately after heparinization. However, the levels of TFPI dropped precipitously at the time of protamine neutralization. Thus, the antiprotease actions induced by aprotinin did not follow the same time course as the generation of TFPI in either group. Levels of TFPI also increased in the placebo group. Thus, aprotinin produced no alteration of the TFPI antigen levels in this study. It would be of interest to measure the functional levels of TFPI because of the various antiprotease actions that it modulates.

## Pharmacokinetic and Pharmacodynamic Studies in Primates

The pharmacokinetics and pharmacodynamics of aprotinin in current protocols are rather complex. No attempt has been made to explain its endogenous behavior.

TISSUE FACTOR PATHWAY INHIBITOR LEVELS IN BYPASS SURGERY

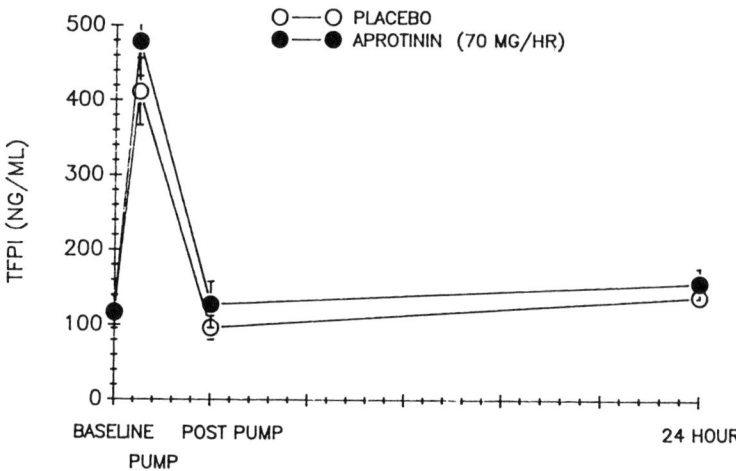

**FIGURE 10.** Levels of tissue factor pathway inhibitor (TFPI) antigen in blood of patients treated with aprotinin during CPB surgery. Blood samples were obtained at baseline, on pump, after pump, and 24 hours after surgery from the placebo group (n = 21) and the aprotinin-treated group (n = 18). TFPI antigen was measured with a commercially available kit (American Diagnostica, Greenwich, CT). All results represent a mean ± 1 SD.

A primate colony of 12 monkeys *(Macaca mulatta)* was used for this purpose because of certain similarities in the hemostatic system compared with human parameters.[4] Ex vivo inhibition of kallikrein was measured with a modified amidolytic method to determine the functional levels of aprotinin in plasma samples. Plasma containing an unknown concentration of aprotinin is first diluted in either saline or baseline plasma and incubated with a specified amount of kallikrein (Sigma Chemical Co., St. Louis, MO) for 1 minute at 37°C. After incubation, a chromogenic substrate specific for kallikrein (S-2301, Kabi Diagnostica, KibiVitrum, Stockholm, Sweden) is added, and the activity of the enzyme is determined at 405 nm on an ACL 300 Plus (Instrumentation Laboratories, Lexington, MA). The concentration of aprotinin is extrapolated from a standard curve derived from aprotinin concentrations of 0–100 μg/ml in normal human pooled plasma. Because aprotinin inhibits plasmin, the relative inhibition of plasma was also measured in an amidolytic assay. Before assaying the plasma samples of primates, both antikallikrein and antiplasmin methods were validated in pooled monkey plasma.

Figure 11 shows the effect of in vitro supplementation with aprotinin on the inhibition of glandular (pancreatic) kallikrein. Inhibition of the amidolytic activity was concentration-dependent; a linear response was observed at concentrations of up to 50 μg/ml. Because its range apparently covered the expected clinical range of aprotinin, this assay was used throughout the pharmacokinetic/pharmacodynamic studies.

In addition, aprotinin strongly inhibited the amidolytic activity of plasmin (Fig. 12). However, the concentration response curve was rather steep, and the response was linear only up to 10 μg/ml. Although this assay was used to determine

APROTININ STANDARD CURVE IN NORMAL MONKEY PLASMA
BASED ON KALLIKREIN/S−2302 ANTIPROTEASE ACTIVITY

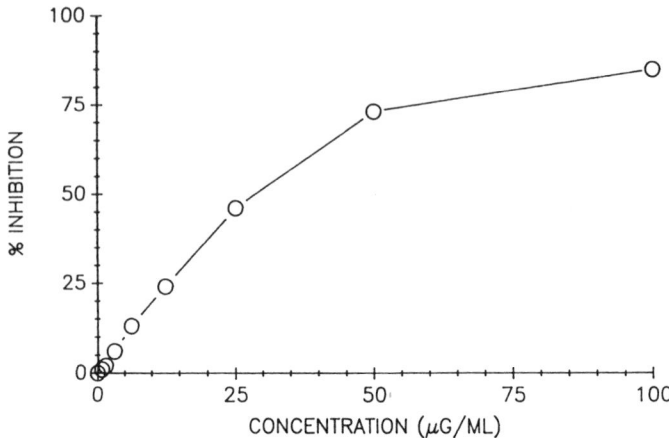

**FIGURE 11.** Calibration curve for the aprotinin-induced inhibition of kallikrein activity as measured by an amidolytic method. Freshly prepared, pooled monkey plasma was supplemented with aprotinin at concentrations of 0-100 µg/ml. The relative inhibition of kallikrein by various samples was calculated as % inhibition, and a calibration curve was constructed to determine the concentration of aprotinin in plasma obtained from treated primates.

APROTININ STANDARD CURVE IN NORMAL MONKEY PLASMA
BASED ON PLASMIN/S−2251 ANTIPROTEASE ACTIVITY

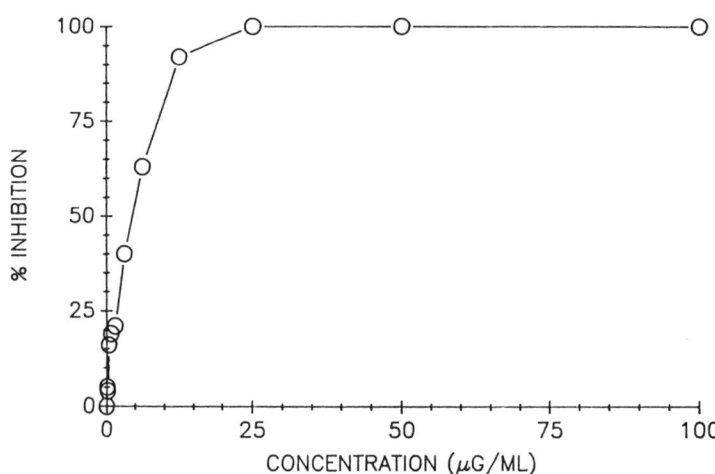

**FIGURE 12.** Calibration curve for the aprotinin-induced inhibition of human plasmin activity as measured by an amidolytic method. Freshly prepared, pooled monkey plasma was supplemented with aprotinin at concentrations of 0-100 µg/ml. The relative inhibition of plasmin by various samples was calculated as % inhibition, and a calibration curve was constructed to determine the concentration of aprotinin in plasma obtained from treated primates.

the antiplasmin activity of some of the blood samples collected from aprotinin-treated primates, the antikallikrein method was preferred to determine the concentration of aprotinin in primate plasma.

Figure 13 shows the results of antiplasmin and antikallikrein activities in plasma samples from primates (n = 4) treated with a bolus dosage of 5.0 mg/kg of aprotinin (roughly equal to 35,000 KIU/kg, the approximate dosage during the initial phase of aprotinin administration in CPB surgery). At this dosage the circulating antiplasmin activity lasted for a much longer time than the antikallikrein activity. Although the pharmacokinetics of both antikallikrein and antiplasmin activities was complex, clearance of the antikallikrein activity was much faster than clearance of the antiplasmin activity. Almost 80% of the antikallikrein activity was cleared within the first hour; however, the antiplasmin activity persisted for a much longer period. Such data suggest that aprotinin produces strong antifibrinolytic effects in the circulating blood. The circulating functional levels of aprotinin can be followed by monitoring plasmin and kallikrein. The apparent difference in the antikallikrein and antiplasmin activities may be due to the testing methodologies; it would be of interest to measure the absolute levels of aprotinin.

The elimination kinetics of aprotinin was measured with the kallikrein inhibition assay in two groups of primates (n = 3 in each group) that received a dosage of 5.0 mg/kg and 2.5 mg/kg, respectively (Fig. 14). A dose-dependent effect was observed. At a dose of 5.0 mg/kg the peak levels of aprotinin reached as high as 46 $\mu$g/ml, whereas at a dose of 2.5 mg/kg only 30 $\mu$g/ml of aprotinin was detected 5 minutes after administration. Both dosages exhibited a time-dependent and biphasic clearance. At 120 minutes, the equivalent of only 3–7 $\mu$g/ml was detected in the group treated with 5.0 mg/kg; in the group treated with 2.5 mg/kg, no aprotinin

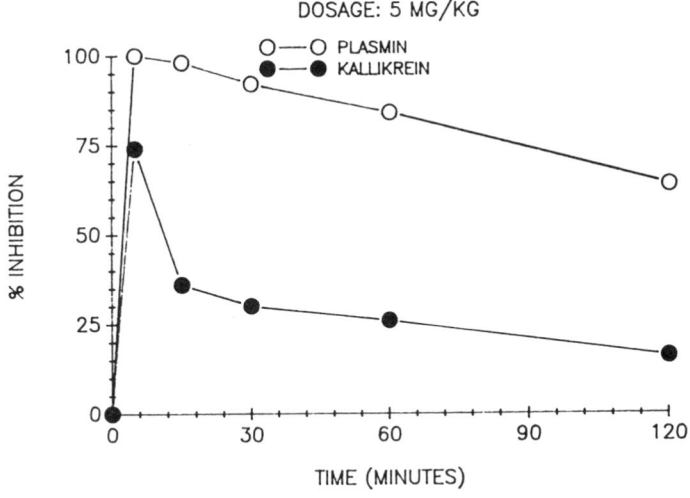

RELATIVE KINETICS OF THE KALLIKREIN AND PLASMIN INHIBITION BY APROTININ
AS STUDIED IN PRIMATES

DOSAGE: 5 MG/KG

**FIGURE 13.** Relative kinetics of antikallikrein and antiplasmin action after aprotinin administration in primates. A group of primates (n = 3) was given 5.0 $\mu$g/kg of aprotinin intravenously. Blood samples were collected at varying periods and assayed for antikallikrein and antiplasmin activities. All results are expressed as a mean of three individual determinations.

## PHARMACOKINETICS OF APROTININ IN NON–HUMAN PRIMATES
### APROTININ LEVEL AS MEASURED BY KALLIKREIN INHIBITION

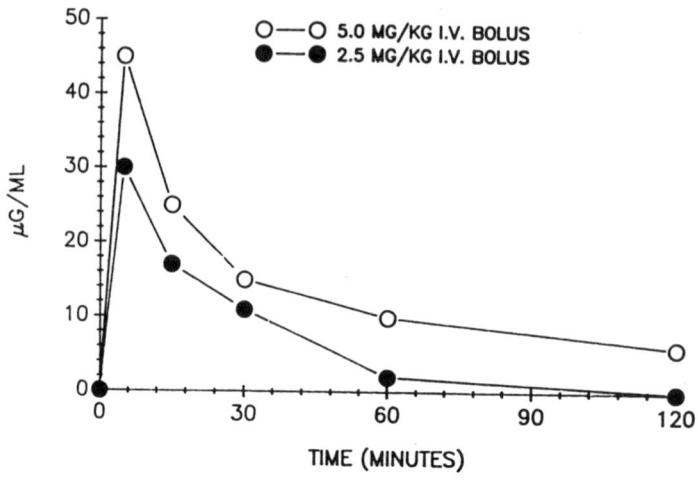

**FIGURE 14.** Pharmacokinetics of aprotinin after intravenous administration of 2.5 and 5.0 mg/kg in primates. Two groups of primates (n = 3 in each group) were treated with aprotinin, and blood samples were collected at varying periods. Antikallikrein and antiplasmin activities were measured with amidolytic methods. Aprotinin levels in each of the collected samples were calculated with an external calibration curve. All results were expressed as μg/ml and are a mean of three determinations.

was detectable at this time. The biologic half-life of the antikallikrein effects of aprotinin was independent of dosage (around 20 minutes in both groups).

The pharmacokinetic parameters of the group treated with 5.0 mg/kg were calculated by standard methods[5] (Table 4). The elimination constant was 0.035/min, and the half-life was approximated at 19 minutes. The area under the curve for the 6-hour period was approximated at 1420 μg/ml/min. The mean residence time was around 27.4 minutes, whereas system clearance was computed to be 3.1 ml/kg/min. The apparent volume of distribution was around 64 ml/kg. Pharmacokinetic parameters, however, were calculated with data from the kallikrein inhibition assay and should be interpreted with caution. The pharmacokinetics of aprotinin appears to be similar to that of other low-molecular-weight proteins and indicates no complex endogenous interactions, such as vascular uptake or target-site binding.

**TABLE 4.**   Pharmacokinetic Profile of Aprotinin in Primates as Measured by Kallikrein Inhibition

| Parameter | Result* |
| --- | --- |
| Elimination constant | 0.035/min |
| Half-life | 19 min |
| Area under the curve (0–360 min) | 1420 μg/ml/min |
| Mean residence time | 27.4 min |
| System clearance | 3.1 ml/kg/min |
| Apparent volume of distribution | 64 ml/kg |

* Based on a total dosage of 5.0 mg/kg.

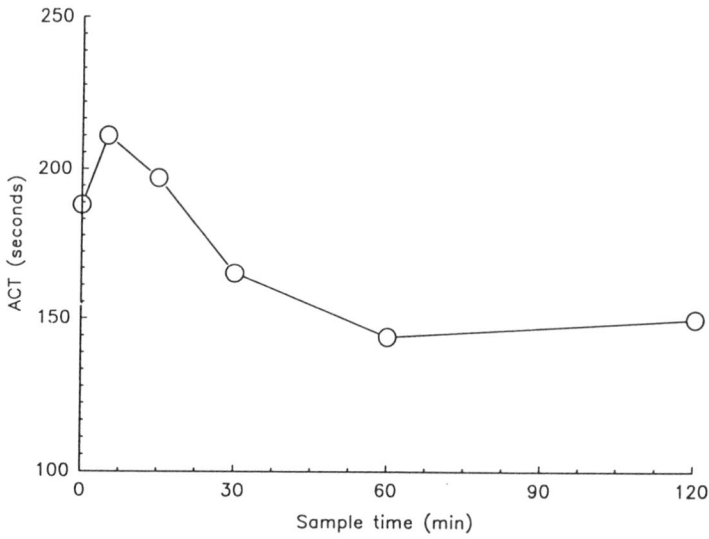

**FIGURE 15.** Effect of aprotinin on the saline ACT in primates. A group of primates (n = 3) was given 5.0 mg/kg of aprotinin intravenously. Blood samples were collected at varying periods, and saline ACT was measured. All results represent a mean of three individual determinations.

The 5.0-mg/kg dose of aprotinin produced a slight elevation of the saline ACT (Fig. 15). At 15 minutes, the ACT reverted to baseline. During CPB surgery large amounts of heparin are administered in combination with aprotinin. When drugs are administered in combined protocols, the pharmacokinetic and pharmacodynamic profile changes markedly.

Although some reports of the interaction of aprotinin and heparin have been published, the effect of heparin on the pharmacokinetics of aprotinin has not been investigated. To determine this effect, two groups of 3 primates each were treated with 5.0 mg/kg of aprotinin alone or 5.0 mg/kg of aprotinin followed by 2.5 mg/kg of heparin. Blood samples were drawn at varying periods, and aprotinin levels were measured with kallikrein inhibition tests (Fig. 16). Although preliminary, this study demonstrated that in the presence of heparin, the clearance rate of aprotinin is increased. Additional studies that measure both the absolute concentration and the functional level of aprotinin will provide insight into the mechanisms.

Data concerning the effect of repeated administrations on the circulating level of aprotinin are limited. Because aprotinin is administered repeatedly during CPB surgery, the possibility of accumulation should be considered. In one study an initial dose of 5 mg/kg of aprotinin and a second dose of 2.5 mg/kg (115 minutes later) were given intravenously to a group of primates (n = 3). This regimen resulted in a transitory elevation of the saline ACT (Fig. 17) that was proportional to the dosage of aprotinin. The anticoagulant effects produced by aprotinin returned to baseline within 30 minutes. Such data suggest that aprotinin, when administered in a bolus form, produces a dose-dependent anticoagulant effect as measured by the saline ACT. In addition, a dose-dependent increase in the aprotinin level was observed (Fig. 18). Initial analysis of the data revealed no cumulative effect after the

Effect of Heparin on the Pharmacokinetics of Aprotinin in Primates

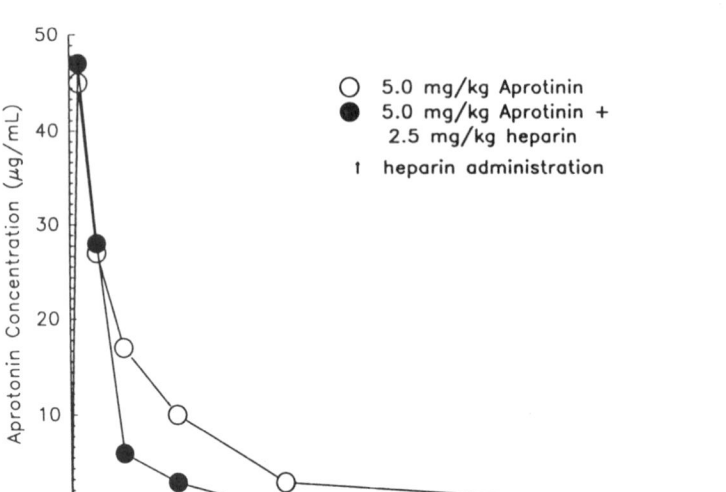

**FIGURE 16.** Effect of heparin on the pharmacokinetics of aprotinin as measured in primates. Two groups of primates (n = 3 in each group) were given 5.0 mg/kg of aprotinin alone or 5 mg/kg of aprotinin followed by 2.5 mg/kg of heparin. Blood samples were collected at varying periods, and aprotinin levels were determined with the antikallikrein method. All results represent a mean of three individual determinations.

second dosage of aprotinin; the area under the curve was proportional to the dosage. Thus aprotinin exhibited a simple pharmacokinetic and pharmacodynamic behavior that can be analyzed with pharmacokinetic modeling.

## SYNOPSIS

Aprotinin has been used for various clinical indications for over three decades. Unlike heparin, it is a pure protein and exhibits no endogenous interactions as a result of its antiprotease activities. Aprotinin was first used to control bleeding related to CPB surgery about 10 years ago in Europe. Since then aprotinin has been used globally to prevent bleeding in heart surgery.

Several mechanisms have been proposed to explain how aprotinin restores hemostasis.[1,19] During CPB surgery, contact activation, heparinization, and endogenous release of mediators contribute to a fibrinolytic state that aprotinin helps to control. It also has been suggested that aprotinin modulates cellular activation during simulated extracorporeal perfusion[1]; in particular, it prevents plasmin-mediated digestion of platelet glycoproteins.

The suggested regimen for administration of aprotinin results in circulating plasma levels that are quite high (up to 100 $\mu$g/ml [16 $\mu$m] in some protocols). Despite a large number of clinical trials, the relevance of circulating plasma levels to the observed clinical effects of aprotinin has not been established. Such

PHARMACOKINETICS OF REPEATED ADMINISTRATION OF APROTININ
IN PRIMATES

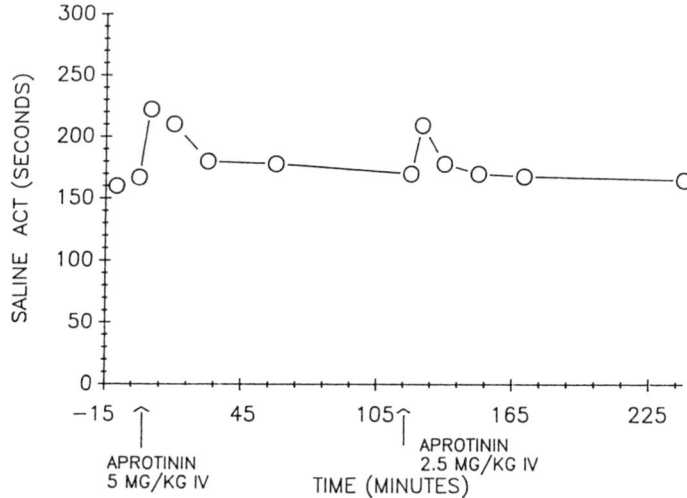

**FIGURE 17.** Effect of repeated administration of aprotinin on the saline ACT in primates. A group of primates (n = 3) was given 5.0 mg/kg of aprotinin intravenously. Blood samples were collected for varying periods. A second dose of 2.5 mg/kg was given at 2 hours, and additional blood samples were collected. Saline ACT measurements were made on each of the blood samples. All results represent a mean of three determinations.

information can be readily generated if data from the pharmacokinetic profile are provided. The pharmacokinetics of aprotinin or any related agent, such as hirudin, may be complicated during CPB surgery by hemodilution, renal compromise, and drug interactions. Thus determination of the pharmacokinetic and pharmacody-namic profile is necessary to optimize clinical use. It has been suggested that half of the commonly used dosages of aprotinin can produce a similar effect in the control of bleeding during CPB surgery (see chapter 21). If this in fact is true, one can minimize the cost—a particular advantage in the current cost-conscious climate.

The functional pharmacokinetics of protease inhibitors such as aprotinin, hirudin, and tissue factor pathway inhibitor can be readily determined by enzyme inhibition assays. Both the antiplasmin and antikallikrein assays can be used in current studies of aprotinin. Although an optimized method for measuring the antikallikrein action of aprotinin has been used to investigate its pharmacokinetics, the antiplasmin assay also is appropriate for monitoring the effects of aprotinin. Both methods can be readily adapted for clinical laboratories and provide valid data about the pharmacokinetics of aprotinin. An integrated pharmacokinetic and pharmacodynamic study that measures simultaneously the absolute levels of aprotinin and its antiprotease activities is not available at this time.

Although the clinical effects of aprotinin are polycomponent, fundamental information about its endogenous behavior will provide important insight into its actions. The available antiprotease assays can be used to obtain these important

PHARMACOKINETICS OF REPEATED ADMINISTRATION OF APROTININ
IN PRIMATES

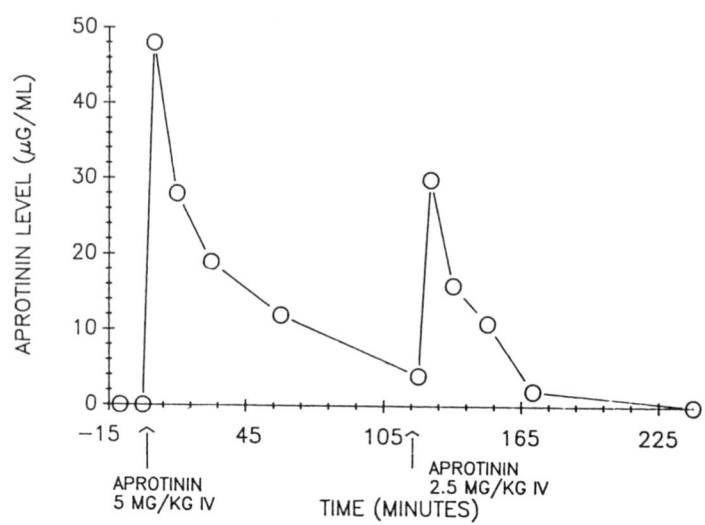

**FIGURE 18.** Effect of repeated administration of aprotinin on the circulating antikallikrein activity in primates. A group of primates ( n = 3) was given 5.0 mg/kg of aprotinin intravenously. Blood samples were collected for varying periods of time. A second dose of 2.5 mg/kg was given at 2 hours, and additional blood samples were collected. Aprotinin levels were calculated with an external calibration method for the antikallikrein activity in primate pooled plasma. All results represent a mean of three individual determinations.

data. The purpose of some of the studies reported in this chapter is to demonstrate that the antiprotease actions of aprotinin can be used to determine its pharmacokinetic behavior in both clinical and experimental settings. In patients undergoing CPB surgery, the circulating levels of aprotinin can be readily quantitated, because heparin and protamine do not interfere in the antikallikrein assay.

Although it would be of interest to measure simultaneously the absolute and functional levels of aprotinin, an immunoassay with this capability is not readily available. An absolute level of aprotinin antigen may reflect the total level of aprotinin (complexed and free forms). Simultaneous measurement of aprotinin antigen and functional aprotinin also may be useful in quantifying the proteases generated during CPB surgery and in optimizing the dosage for various indications.

The studies in primates provide preliminary data about the pharmacokinetic behavior of aprotinin, which, in controlled conditions, follows a simple profile with a fast elimination half-life as measured by available methods. Additional data about the biologic half-life of aprotinin may be useful in proper dosing. Of interest, the studies demonstrated that heparin increases the elimination of aprotinin, thereby reducing its half-life. This observation should be validated in simulated models of CPB surgery, because it may have clinical implications for clinical management.

A limited study in primates demonstrated no staircasing effect from multiple doses of aprotinin. Because aprotinin is used in a stepwise manner during CPB surgery, knowledge of its pharmacokinetic behavior may be of major value in optimizing the dosage.

This chapter clearly points to the lack of integrated pharmacokinetic and pharmacodynamic data about aprotinin, despite its widespread use. Current data suggest that simple antiprotease assays can be readily used to study the pharmacokinetics of aprotinin. It is now clear that aprotinin is useful in the control of bleeding during CPB surgery; however, the currently used dosage is based on subjective observation. A well-designed clinical trial that assesses the relationship between dosage and hemostatic efficacy will facilitate its optimal use. Additional trials to obtain complete pharmacokinetic data about aprotinin are clearly warranted.

## References

1. Blauhut B, Gross C, Necek S, et al: Effects of high-dose aprotinin on blood loss, platelet function, fibrinolysis, complement and renal function after cardiopulmonary bypass. J Thorac Cardiovasc Surg 101:958–996, 1991.
2. Broze GJ, Girard TJ, Novotny WF: Regulation of coagulation by multivalent Kunitz-type inhibitor. Biochemistry 29:7539–7546, 1990.
3. Dewachter P, Mouton C, Masson C, et al: Anaphylactic reaction to aprotinin during cardiac surgery. Anaesthesia 48:1110–1111, 1993.
4. Fareed J, Kumar A, Rock A, et al: A primate model (Macaca mulatta) to study the pharmacokinetics of heparin and its fractions. Semin Thromb Hemost 11(2):128–154, 1985.
5. Gibaldi M, Perrier D: Pharmacokinetics. New York, Marcel Dekker, 1984.
6. Haas M, deZeeuw D, Meijer DK: Quantification of renal low molecular weight protein degradation in the intact rat. Contrib Nephrol 101:78–84, 1993.
7. Havel M, Teufelsbauer H, Knobl P: Effect of intraoperative aprotinin administration on postoperative bleeding in patients undergoing cardiopulmonary bypass operation. J Thorac Cardiovasc Surg 101:968–972, 1991.
8. Kim T, Hoppensteadt D, Moran S, et al: The effects of aprotinin treatment during CABG on TFPI, tissue factor and other hemostatic parameters [abstract 2673]. Thromb Hemost 69:1290, 1993.
9. Levy JH, Bailey JM, Salmenpera M: Pharmacokinetics of aprotinin in preoperative cardiac surgical patients. Anesthesiology 80:1013–1018, 1994.
10. Markwardt F, Hauptman J, Nowak G, et al: Pharmacological studies on the antithrombotic action of hirudin in experimental animals. Thromb Haemost 47:226–229, 1982.
11. Najman DM, Walenga JM, Fareed J, Pifarre R: Effects of aprotinin on anticoagulant monitoring: Implications in cardiovascular surgery. Ann Thorac Surg 55:662–666, 1993.
12. Neuhaus P, Bechstein WO, Lefebre O, et al: Effect of aprotinin on intraoperative bleeding and fibrinolysis in liver transplantation. Lancet ii:924–925, 1989.
13. Royston D: The serine antiprotease aprotinin (Trasylol): A novel approach to reducing postoperative bleeding. Blood Coagul Fibrinol 1:55–69, 1990.
14. Rustom R, Grime JS, Maltby P, et al: Observations on the early renal uptake and later tubular metabolism of radiolabelled aprotinin (Trasylol) in man: Theoretical and practical considerations. Clin Sci 84:231–235, 1993.
15. Rustom R, Grime S, Maltby P, et al: A new method to measure renal tubular degradation of small filtered proteins in man using radiolabelled aprotinin (Trasylol). Clin Sci 83:289–294, 1992.
16. Saffitz JE, Stahl DJ, Sundt TM, et al: Disseminated intravascular coagulation after administration of aprotinin in combination with deep hypothermic circulatory arrest. Am J Cardiol 72:1080–1082, 1993.
17. Schall R, Groenewoud G, Hundt HKL, et al: Pharmacokinetic profile of aprotinin (Trasylol) in female patients undergoing primary elective hysterectomy. Drug Invest 4:292–299, 1992.
18. Schall R, Muller FO, Hundt HKL, et al: Pharmacokinetic profile of high doses of aprotinin in patients undergoing primary elective hysterectomy. A meta-analysis of two clinical trials. Drug Invest 7:200–208, 1994.
19. van Oeveren W, Jansen NJG, Bidstrup BP: Effects of aprotinin on hemostatic mechanisms during cardiopulmonary bypass. Ann Thorac Surg 44:645–650, 1987.
20. van Oeveren W, Eijsman L, Roosendaal KJ, Wildevuur CRH: Platelet preservation by aprotinin during cardiopulmonary bypass. Lancet ii:644, 1988.
21. Verstraete M: Clinical applications of inhibitors of fibrinolysis. Drugs 29:236–261, 1985.
22. Wuthrich B, Schmid P, Schmid ER, et al: IgE-mediated anaphylactic reaction to aprotinin during anesthesia. Lancet 340:173, 1992.

# Friedrich Schumann, PhD

# 7

# Developmental Aspects of Aprotinin

In January 1988 an editorial in *The Lancet* asked the question: "Can drugs reduce surgical blood loss?"[3] Five years later, in a letter to the same journal, Royston answered with an unconditional "yes."[72] The 5-year interval had seen the revival of an "oldtimer" drug for an old indication: the proteinase inhibitor and antifibrinolytic compound, aprotinin (Trasylol). Now as prominent as ever, it has become available for the largest hospital market in the world, the United States. The first part of this chapter tells—from the viewpoint of a professional in the drug industry—how the revival occurred; the second part summarizes a few lessons to be learned from this development, and the third part presents still open questions and possibilities for further clinical research with aprotinin. (For the complete history of aprotinin, starting in 1930 with the discovery of a kallikrein inactivator from bovine tissue, see the chapter by Haas and Blümel.

## Evolution of the Indication

Clinical use of aprotinin for the treatment of bleeding complications in cardiac surgery was described as early as 1963.[81] Subsequently, several other groups published their experience with aprotinin used as a treatment but not as prophylaxis.[2,23,49] Aprotinin showed no effect on the alterations in coagulation and fibrinolysis in a clinical study in which a single dose of 10,000 KIU/kg was administered at the end of cardiopulmonary bypass (CPB) before neutralization of heparin with protamine.[40] That study seemed to dispell the strong early interest in aprotinin as a potential therapeutic and prophylactic agent for hemorrhage associated with extracorporeal circulation. Nevertheless, early package inserts for Trasylol in two countries, Canada and Sweden, listed extracorporeal circulation as a clinical setting in which hyperfibrinolytic hemorrhage was an indication for the drug. The drug was launched in Germany in 1959 and became available in most European countries during the early sixties. It was introduced in Japan in 1967 and in Canada in 1974.

The antifibrinolytic property of aprotinin, which is related to the direct inhibition of plasmin, was discovered rather early. One of the first reports discusses the potential use of aprotinin as an antidote in thrombolytic therapy with streptokinase.[51] The idea of giving Trasylol to patients with severe hyperfibrinolysis and bleeding problems induced by the rough CPB equipment of the early years of modern cardiac surgery can be traced to a high-ranking German medical journal in 1961. A comprehensive paper with 169 references reviewed blood coagulation during extracorporeal circulation with the heart-lung machine and suggested Trasylol as an antifibrinolytic treatment.[25]

Despite the apparently diminishing size of the medical problem and despite the discouraging results of the study of Köstering et al.,[40] who used a rather high dosage compared with previous reports, the scientific interest in the effects of aprotinin in patients subjected to CPB did not fade completely. The interest shifted from blood loss to other potentially harmful but poorly understood consequences of extracorporeal circulation, such as the postperfusion syndrome. In an elegant investigation in 1975,[60] Nagaoka and Katori found that aprotinin significantly reduced kinin formation during extracorporeal circulation (ECC) and concluded that Trasylol "appears to be an effective counteragent for circulatory disturbances which occur during extracorporeal circulation." Their results were later confirmed by a group in Vienna,[15] which used aprotinin from a different manufacturer.

In 1980, clinicians at the Medical Academy of Wroclaw, Poland, reported results of a simple-dose comparison study of Trasylol in cardiac surgery with ECC for correction of congenital malformations. Doses ranged from 10,000 to 80,000 KIU/kg. Because this report appeared in the Polish language in a rather remote journal,[53] it received practically no attention, even when a second paper in English followed in the proceedings of an international symposium on kinin research.[52] Their findings merit review in the light of our present knowledge and experience with high-dose aprotinin.

When the author assumed responsibility for clinical research with Trasylol, he inherited a project that had grown in sometimes rather loose and sometimes close cooperation with a group at the University of Bonn. This group, directed by the hematologist Smilja Popov-Cenic, had kept a strong interest in the hemostatic effect of Trasylol. From 1977 to 1981 the group developed an empirical, quite complex protocol for the dosage and administration of Trasylol in adult and pediatric patients undergoing open heart surgery. Their results concerning blood loss and transfusion requirement were excellent.[65,67] Clinical use of higher doses of aprotinin ($>500,000$ KIU) in open-heart surgery had been investigated at other centers in Germany and abroad. The time had come for a prospective, placebo-controlled clinical trial.

Two placebo-controlled, double-blind studies were initiated, one at the University of Bonn in male patients undergoing primary elective coronary artery bypass grafting (CABG),[66] the other in patients undergoing aortic or mitral valve replacement.[26] The design of both studies, especially that of the group at Bonn, was less than optimal. In addition to the two blinded treatments with aprotinin and a matching placebo, there was a third arm in the CABG study: patients were given C1-esterase inhibitor from human plasma as a nonblinded study medication under the same protocol. The protocol also permitted treatment of patients with open-label Trasylol in addition to the study medication, when early postoperative blood loss exceeded 1 ml/kg/hr. Both studies focused more on laboratory parameters than on generation of a clinically relevant answer. In a strict sense, neither protocol was designed to test a hypothesis.

However, when biometric evaluation of the data revealed a clearcut improvement in hemostasis with the use of aprotinin, past and present investigators of aprotinin in cardiovascular surgery, together with a few well-known experts in proteolysis or inhibitor research, were invited to an international meeting. The company hoped to gauge how the "new" (i.e., revived) indication for aprotinin would be received after a decade of costly mainstream research with disappointing returns on investment. At the time the ominous description of aprotinin as "a drug in search of an indication" was going around. The meeting took place in May 1984 in Luxembourg, and the proceedings were published in 1985.[19] Unfortunately, the prevailing opinion was that the results were not of great clinical relevance. The exception was an impressive retrospective clinical evaluation of efficacy and safety in children undergoing cardiac surgery.[83]

The generally rather skeptical attitude may seem surprising from today's viewpoint. At the time, however, blood transfusions were given rather generously, and the full threat of acquired immunodeficiency syndrome (AIDS) had not reached the present degree of awareness. True or untrue, Trasylol also had the image of an expensive drug. Although the overall result was not as positive as expected, the meeting planted the germ for further clinical research, conducted by others, that resulted in the recent renewal of clinical development.

When the author prepared the scientific program for the meeting in Luxembourg, he contacted Stephen Westaby, who in an editorial published in *Thorax*,[87] had stated his views on the development of more biocompatible materials for oxygenator components:

> This is probably of limited value since, whatever the alternative material, the body's defence mechanisms will respond by means of platelet adherence, protein denaturation, or activation of the plasmin or the kallikrein or bradykinin system if not through complement activation.

Westaby obviously was in a position to appreciate a drug that inhibits both plasmin and kallikrein.

So it went. At the meeting Westaby presented a summary of the research done with John Kirklin's group on complement activation during CPB and returned to Hammersmith Hospital in London with knowledge of aprotinin and its clinical effects in patients having open-heart surgery. He approached the Bayer company in November 1984 with a proposal for studying the effect of high-dosage aprotinin on complement activation in patients undergoing cardiac surgery. It is impossible to say who made the essential contributions to the research proposal. Complement activation and the damaging effects of CPB on vascular and alveolar permeability was a research theme for several ambitious investigators, not only at the Hammersmith Hospital in London but also at the University of Groningen, Netherlands, where Charles Wildevuur's group had investigated the different effects of bubble and membrane oxygenators on exposed heparinized blood. The study was proposed to the author by the triumvirate of Westaby, Wildevuur, and Heinz Neuhof, professor of experimental medicine at the University of Giessen, Germany. Neuhof had previously expressed interest in proteinase inhibition as a potential therapy in patients with acute respiratory disease and sepsis. It was proposed that the clinical part of the study should be conducted at the Hammersmith Hospital, whereas specific tests of frozen plasma samples would be performed in Groningen and Giessen.

An essential part of the research plan was accurate measurements of the aprotinin concentration at fixed sampling times during and after surgery; the working hypothesis was that only plasma concentrations of 200 KIU/ml or above would provide efficient inhibition of plasma kallikrein. The invaluable help of the group led by Hans Fritz, professor of biochemistry and head of the Institute for Clinical Biochemistry in Munich (where the first experimental work with aprotinin was begun in the 1950s under Eugen Werle) made it possible to develop a rational dosing scheme. While the CABG study at the University of Bonn was under way, Marianne Jochum and Werner Müller-Esterl developed an enzyme-linked immunosorbent assay (ELISA) for aprotinin and validated it against a functional assay based on inhibition of porcine pancreas kallikrein.[35,36,57] The ELISA proved to be much more robust and convenient than tests based on enzyme inhibition, and with the stimulating cooperation of the group in Munich, it became possible, at least in principle, to obtain information about plasma concentrations in future clinical studies with different dosages of aprotinin. Despite the declining enthusiasm at Bayer after the Luxembourg meeting, it was possible to procure a minimal grant for the proposed study in cardiac surgery; the internal approval document was signed on March 14, 1985.

Based on information from Popov-Cenic's group and other small studies with different dosage regimens of aprotinin[36] as well as on earlier theories about inhibition of plasma kallikrein,[63] the target for the new study was a plasma level of about 200 KIU/ml during CPB. Too often in the past an ambitious experiment produced inconclusive results and had to be repeated with a higher dose. Because of the rather limited budget, we had to ensure that the study would detect any effect of aprotinin (within an acceptable dose limit) on complement activation and that no second trial would be necessary.

There was some delay in the start of the study. After Westaby left the Hammersmith Hospital, David Royston, a senior lecturer in anesthesiology, and Ben Bidstrup, then a visiting cardiac surgeon from Australia, took over his portion of the study. Wildevuur acted as the research coordinator and signed most of the correspondence with Bayer until the final results were published in December 1987 in *The Annals of Thoracic Surgery*.[84]

In the meantime, however, the company received astonishing news: at Hammersmith Hospital patients no longer bled after cardiac surgery—or, in a more moderate version, blood loss was reduced to an extent that had alarmed the nursing staff. Improved hemostasis with aprotinin was not a completely new effect, but the report appeared so exaggerated that it was just not plausible. Royston also had treated on his own a handful of patients with complex repeat cardiac surgery who were expected to have high volumes of blood loss and to require massive transfusion; the effect of aprotinin was dramatic. He was convinced to start a small prospective, randomized parallel study in patients with repeat cardiac surgery to confirm the results. The result of that trial, in which the Bayer company played only a minor role, was published almost simultaneously with the study of complement activation; it appeared in *The Lancet*[73] on December 5, 1987, to be followed a few weeks later by the editorial mentioned above.[3] Royston's lasting contribution was his immediate clear-sighted view of the relevance of improved hemostasis with high-dose aprotinin, the clinical effectiveness of which appeared to exhibit a quantum leap.

An important question had not yet been answered: were the findings at the Hammersmith Hospital reproducible? Or had some unidentified factor in surgical technique or general perioperative treatment created conditions in which the effect of the drug was magnified? Had aprotinin merely corrected some iatrogenic disorder? Answers to such questions required more clinical trials at different institutions with various conditions of open-heart surgery. Because the first results were so exciting, it was not difficult to find investigators. At the end of 1988 five double-blind studies had been concluded in primary elective CABG operations: in Amsterdam by Wildevuur,[27] in London by Royston and Bidstrup,[7] in Munich by Dietrich et al.,[18] in Freiburg by Fraedrich et al.,[21] and in Giessen by Neuhof et al.[76] These clinical trials were performed independently, with different protocols. The overall results concerning blood loss and blood transfusions confirmed the initial observation.[69]

When it became obvious that the so-called Hammersmith regimen could achieve a reproducible, clinically relevant reduction in transfusion requirements, regardless of specific institutional conditions of open-heart surgery, a major decision had to be made. In the United States, aprotinin still had the status of an experimental drug with no active, company-sponsored Investigational New Drug Application (INDA). Bayer had submitted an unsuccessful New Drug Application (NDA) in 1966 but had not tried again. Despite encouragement from well-known opinion makers who had seen the effect of aprotinin in vivo, the company hesitated. Would the investment necessary for new clinical development of an old drug generate sufficient revenue? Was it possible to predict the time frame for clinical development in the United States? Eventually Miles Inc., of West Haven, CT (the American affiliate of Bayer) decided to prepare a new INDA, the core of which formed the new European studies in open-heart surgery, and to discuss the development plan with the Food and Drug Administration (FDA).

The first meeting with the FDA took place on September 6, 1989—and it was remarkable. Stephen Fredd and Robert Temple of the FDA showed a positive interest in making the drug available for clinical use in the United States—an attitude that has continued. It was made clear to the representatives of Miles and Bayer, however, that a handsome clinical benefit in terms of reduced transfusion requirements was expected and that patients with a high medical need should be given preference in clinical trials.

Because of the long clinical experience with aprotinin in other countries and the evidence provided by the recent European studies, it was agreed that development in the United States should start at phase III. The Hammersmith regimen was accepted, but in two of the three pivotal trials a dose reduced by exactly 50% was to be used for comparison in addition to placebo. The half dosage also proved effective compared with placebo and in retrospect raised questions about whether the search for optimal dosing had been abandoned prematurely. However, data from a recent large, multicenter study in patients undergoing repeat CABG have confirmed the superior efficacy of the higher dose in patients at increased risk of perioperative hemorrhage (Miles Inc.: Trasylol package insert). Two of the three pivotal studies in the United States have been published as full papers,[13,44] whereas the third has been published only in abstract form.[14]

It was not clear whether the results of the three studies would suffice for NDA approval. The result of the multicenter study of patients undergoing cardiac valve replacement had been disappointing: significant reduction in early postoperative blood loss did not translate into reduced transfusion requirements. In addition, one study of patients undergoing repeat CABG[13] showed unfavorable trends in the incidence of perioperative myocardial infarction and postoperative renal dysfunction. The second study of both primary and repeat CABG[44]—an ambitious multicenter project that also tried to answer the crucial question of graft patency by using noninvasive, ultrafast computed tomography—had produced results that were difficult to assess and led to heavy internal dispute over the validity of the methods. Nonetheless, the efficacy data in the two CABG studies were of such clarity that, at least for repeat CABG, a favorable risk-benefit ratio could be assumed. Another meeting with the FDA proved to be helpful, and the NDA was submitted on November 23, 1992.

The FDA took about 7 months to issue a letter of approvability. Bayer worked hard to adjust manufacturing and quality-control standards to pass the FDA inspection of its German facilities. Finally, on December 29, 1993, Miles Inc. received the NDA approval for Trasylol.

It is impractical to report all of the clinical studies of Trasylol that followed the early publication in England and the Netherlands of the results of high-dose treatment in open-heart surgery. Most of these studies, which were performed in a great number of countries with and without sponsorship by the manufacturer, have been published.[1,5,9,12,16,24,28,30–33,38,42,43,45,46,48,50,55,56,58,61,71,74,79,85] A comprehensive review[70] summarizes the first 5 years of clinical experience with high-dose aprotinin.

In terms of clinical development, the large American studies were of highest priority. However, once a drug is commercially available, further clinical development can be controlled only in part by the manufacturer. Even the preparation of aprotinin study medication for a double-blind trial with saline as a placebo in intravenous infusion does not present a major problem for a well-equipped hospital pharmacy. Not infrequently clinical studies of Trasylol are performed and published with no prior notice to the manufacturer.

## Possible Detours and Short-Cuts

In the case of aprotinin, animal studies are of limited value in predicting the success of clinical trials with human patients because of interspecies differences in the quantitative and qualitative composition of mammalian serine proteinases, their precursors, and their physiologic inhibitors, the serpins.[37] Furthermore, aprotinin shows different binding constants ($K_i$ values) in bovine, porcine, canine, rodent and other mammalian target enzymes, such as plasmin and the kallikreins from plasma and tissues.[22,82] Successful treatment of a condition in experimental animals has little relevance to clinical efficacy, nor does failure in a well-designed animal experiment preclude efficacy in humans. For example, pigs are not useful for investigating the effect of aprotinin in CPB. Studies with nonhuman primates to some degree may avoid the problem of a species-specific response.

An elegant solution to this problem of uncertain transferability of results from animal experiments to the clinic appeared to be the development of simulated extracorporeal circulation (ECC) in a shortcut heart-lung machine, by which human blood is recirculated under conditions comparable with those in patients undergoing open-heart surgery. Although demonstrating significant and dose-dependent suppression of contact activation by foreign surfaces,[86] simulated ECC elucidates only part of the complex pathophysiology of disturbed hemostasis after CPB—and it may well be a minor part. Simulated ECC lacks the vascular and tissue (endothelial) components. Recent discussions of the mechanism of action in humans[10,62] have strongly favored the antiplasmin activity of aprotinin. Unfortunately, simulated ECC cannot make a significant contribution to this ongoing discussion.

Thus the first lesson is not to waste time with preclinical or ex vivo experiments when the risks and benefits of a new clinical application of aprotinin or any similar compound have to be assessed. It is the prospective, comparative clinical trial that matters. (The gathering of indispensable information about safety and toxicology before start of phase I studies in humans, of course, is not challenged by this statement.)

"The mechanism of action of aprotinin is not known." This often seen quotation is true only from a rigorous scientific viewpoint. In the complex pathomechanistic interaction between contact activation, tissue factor-derived activation of coagulation, fibrinolysis activation, and platelet dysfunction, the precise role of aprotinin has remained unclear. For this deficiency of knowledge, however, the drug cannot be blamed; improved understanding of the pathophysiology of the hemostatic defect after open-heart surgery is the only way to fill this gap. Aprotinin can help as a heuristic tool, since inhibition of a rather limited number of serine proteinases is the only relevant mechanism of the drug at the molecular level. In other words, before inventing a "new" mechanism of action for aprotinin it may be more rational to redefine the role of an enzyme within the inhibitory spectrum of the clinically relevant dosage. Thus the second lesson is that the successful clinical development of a compound does not necessarily require precise knowledge of its mechanism of action.

A striking feature of the clinical development of aprotinin, especially in the United States, has been the almost ritualized concern with potential adverse effects. Although several European trials had shown excellent tolerability and in fact had formed the basis for phase III development in the United States, internal discussions about potential side effects were led with utmost scrutiny. It was difficult to accept that hypothetical problems (e.g., inactivation of heparin, interaction with anesthetic agents, drug-induced kidney failure) should occupy a prominent place in the background information for clinical investigators. In the medical literature on aprotinin, accumulated from 35 years of clinical usage, strange reports can be found, related not only to efficacy but also to safety. In retrospect, one may be tempted to consider that negative expectations resulted in a self-fulfilling prophecy. Certainly, the double-blind protocol should exclude bias, but many investigators have admitted that they were able to "see" the effect of improved hemostasis in an aprotinin-treated patient. Thus a third lesson is that long clinical experience with a drug does not obviate a balanced risk/benefit assessment for a new clinical indication.

Many clinicians reported a "bone-dry surgical field," which we tried to document with simple assessment scales in several double-blind studies. Biometric evaluation of such ratings repeatedly produced highly significant differences, but in no protocol was this subjective criterion a primary target for assessment of efficacy. This raises the question whether the clinical benefit of aprotinin has been fully captured. The tendency to neglect so-called clinimetric information may not be justified. In addition to shortening the operation time, aprotinin may have the potential to reduce the incidence of early reoperation due to bleeding complications, not only those of diffuse nature but also those of surgical origin, because the surgeon can work in a cleaner operative site not obscured by oozing blood. However, this theory awaits clinical confirmation in a large prospective trial. Thus a fourth lesson may be the desirability of a heightened awareness of parameters based on clinical observation, provided that interobserver variation can be minimized.

## Open Questions

For the blood-saving indication in open-heart surgery, no formal dosage studies were executed. Given the empirical formation of the Hammersmith regimen, which is based on a working hypothesis of kallikrein inhibition by sufficiently high plasma levels of aprotinin, it is theoretically possible that the optimal dosage and administration scheme are yet to be found. However, because the number of possible permutations is not small, it makes no sense to test all of them in systematic fashion. Nevertheless, whether higher doses during the initial phase of ECC and discontinuance of infusion at the end of CPB would be more effective than the same total dosage given by the Hammersmith regimen remains an open question. One also can speculate on the superior effectiveness of weight-adjusted dosage compared with fixed dosage. On the other hand, other parameters may have a greater effect on plasma concentrations than body weight (e.g., renal blood flow, glomerular filtration rate). In theory, the optimal dose may depend on the type of surgery and the cardiotechnique. A question of practical interest is the efficacy of aprotinin in ECC with heparin-coated equipment. Such a study also may shed additional light on the mechanism of action.

Negative experience[80,88] with aprotinin in uncontrolled series of patients undergoing reconstruction of the thoracic aorta in total circulatory arrest with deep hypothermia has led to a warning statement in the manufacturer's product information. However, there are opposing views.[78] Only the conduct of carefully controlled clinical studies will produce a final answer.

Whether intraoperative aprotinin therapy affects the rate of early graft occlusion in patients after CABG has been addressed in three placebo-controlled, double-blind studies. Each study used a different method for the diagnosis of occluded grafts; only one study[41,64] used the gold standard of radiographic contrast angiography. Because the perception of risk associated with early recatheterization varies from institution to institution, the initial investigations of graft patency understandably used noninvasive techniques. The multicenter American study[44] used ultrafast computed tomography (CT), whereas the single-center English study[8] used magnetic resonance imaging (MRI). Both methods have been described in the literature as yielding satisfactory specificity and sensitivity. The negative trend seen in the study using ultrafast CT was absent in the study using MRI. The study with radiographic contrast angiography also showed no difference in the overall occlusion rate and tends to confirm the results of the English study with MRI. A recent publication reported the results of coronary angiography in a part of the total patient population of a controlled trial with aprotinin (although the procedure was not requested by the study protocol).[29] No difference in graft occlusion rates was seen. A large cooperative multicenter study in primary elective CABG with early postoperative coronary angiography is ongoing. This study will have sufficient statistical power to determine whether concerns about an increased rate of graft occlusions in aprotinin-treated patients are unjustified or not.

Clarifying the mechanism of action remains an incentive for many investigators seeking sponsorship for new clinical studies. However, real progress may come from more refined investigation of the complex pathophysiology of the acquired hemostatic defect associated with ECC—which is not an easy exercise—rather than from a placebo-controlled aprotinin study that adds one or two new laboratory parameters to a standard protocol. The recent challenge of the theory that attributes a predominant role to platelet dysfunction[39,54,62] is a good example.

Clearly an unresolved issue is the conflicting evidence for efficacy of aprotinin in pediatric cardiac surgery.[11,17,20] Because Dietrich discusses this subject in a separate chapter, a general comment will suffice. In the author's opinion, failure to demonstrate efficacy by the standard variables used for adult cardiac surgery (i.e., transfusion requirements based on perioperative blood loss) may not reflect lack of clinical benefit. Thus it is worthwhile to reconsider appropriate targets for the definition of clinical benefit in pediatric cardiac surgery before embarking on new clinical trials. (See also the earlier remarks about validity of clinical observations.)

As a nonhuman protein aprotinin may cause anaphylactic reactions in sensitized individuals. Signs and symptoms vary in intensity and duration and range from flush, urticaria, isolated drop in blood pressure, tachycardia or bradycardia, and airway obstruction to severe hypotension and anaphylactic shock that leads, in rare cases, to death. Hypersensitivity reactions are rare in patients with no prior exposure to aprotinin ($< 0.1\%$). However, the incidence of such reactions after second or repeat exposure may reach 5%, as documented in retrospective analyses of small series of patients with documented aprotinin treatment at the first and second (or third) operation.[6,75]

To acquire a better understanding of the conditions and/or predisposing factors that place patients at risk for an anaphylactic reaction is a challenging task. Only about 10% of patients who develop aprotinin-specific antibodies of any type (IgE has been found rarely) show signs and symptoms of hypersensitivity at a second exposure. Preventive measures, including the prophylactic administration of antihistamines of the $H_1$ and $H_2$ type, should be evaluated by prospective investigation. Currently such prophylaxis is recommended by analogy with patients treated with colloidal volume substitution, especially gelatin solutions.[47]

The most intriguing question for someone who has observed the ups and downs of medical appreciation for aprotinin for more than 20 years may be its future application in areas other than cardiac surgery. Several chapters in this book offer such perspectives. The reduction of blood loss and transfusion requirement in bone and joint surgery (e.g., total hip replacement, as demonstrated in pilot studies[34,59]) again calls for development decisions on the company's part. Aprotinin has also found successful application in liver transplantation for the prophylaxis and treatment of massive hemorrhage. Despite the lack of a prospective, placebo-controlled clinical trial, a wealth of information is already available.[68]

The option for clinical development of a recombinant aprotinin mutant with altered enzyme specificity awaits realization. Mutants with improved inhibition of human plasma kallikrein have been described.[4,77] Only then we will learn whether the initial hypothesis that inhibition of plasma kallikrein by high-dose aprotinin makes an essential contribution to the dramatic improvement in hemostasis is correct. The future will tell whether aprotinin has been only the first step toward bloodless surgery, made possible by the administration of sophisticated drugs.

## Acknowledgment

This personal account of the clinical development of aprotinin for blood conservation should not create the erroneous impression that the author played a major role. In fact, his contribution was small in comparison with that of many colleagues in the Bayer-Miles organization. To mention all of them is not feasible. There is no fresh snow; vestiges of previous travelers can always be seen.

# References

1. Alajmo F, Calamai G, Perna AM, et al: High-dose aprotinin: Hemostatic effects in open heart operations. Ann Thorac Surg 48:536–539, 1989.
2. Ambrus JL, Schimert G, Lajos TZ, et al: Effect of antifibrinolytic agents and estrogens on blood loss and blood coagulation factors during open heart surgery. J Med 2:65–81, 1971.
3. Anonymous: Can drugs reduce surgical blood loss? [editorial]. Lancet I:155–156, 1988.
4. Auerswald EA, Hörlein D, Reinhardt G, et al: Expression, isolation and characterization of recombinant [Arg-15-Glu-52]-aprotinin. Biol Chem Hoppe-Seyler 369(Suppl):27–35, 1988.
5. Baele PL, Ruiz-Gomez J, Londot C, et al: Systematic use of aprotinin in cardiac surgery: Influence on total homologous exposure and hospital cost. Acta Anaesth Belg 43:103–112, 1992.
6. Beckmann H, Mayer G: Allergic/anaphylactic reaction in patients with cardiac reoperation and Trasylol re-exposition—retrospective analysis in 2 cardiosurgical units—statistical report. Bayer Report No. PH-23223 (P), 1994.
7. Bidstrup BP, Royston D, Sapsford RN, Taylor KM: Reduction in blood loss and blood use after cardiopulmonary bypass with high dose aprotinin (Trasylol). J Thorac Cardiovasc Surg 97:364–372, 1989.
8. Bidstrup BP, Underwood SR, Sapsford RN: Effect of aprotinin (Trasylol) on aorta-coronary bypass graft patency. J Thorac Cardiovasc Surg 105;147–153, 1993.
9. Blauhut B, Gross C, Necek S, et al: Effects of high-dose aprotinin on blood loss, platelet function, fibrinolysis, complement, and renal function after cardiopulmonary bypass. J Thorac Cardiovasc Surg 101:958–967, 1991.
10. Boisclair MD, Lane DA, Philippou H, et al: Mechanisms of thrombin generation during surgery and cardiopulmonary bypass. Blood 82:3350–3357, 1993.
11. Boldt J, Knothe C, Zickmann B, et al: Comparison of two aprotinin dosage regimens in pediatric patients having cardiac operations. J Thorac Cardiovasc Surg 105:705–711, 1993.
12. Carrel T, Bauer E, Laske A, et al: Low-dose aprotinin also allows reduction of blood loss after cardiopulmonary bypass. J Thorac Cardiovasc Surg 102:801–802, 1991.
13. Cosgrove DM III, Heric B, Lytle BW, et al: Aprotinin therapy for reoperative myocardial revascularization: A placebo-controlled study. Ann Thorac Surg 54:1031–1038, 1992.
14. D'Ambra MN, Akins CW, Blackstone EH, et al: Aprotinin in primary cardiac valve replacement reduces bleeding, increases creatinine. Circulation 86(Suppl I):I-495, 1992.
15. Deklerk J, Benzer H, Haider W, et al: Beeinflussung des Kininogen-Kininsystems durch einen Kallikrein-Hemmer bei Operationen am offenen Herzen in extracorporaler Zirkulation. Anaesthesist 26:639–643, 1977.
16. Deleuze P, Loisance DY, Feliz A, et al: Réduction des pertes sanguines per et postopératoires par l'aprotinine (Trasylol) au cours de la circulation extracorporelle. Arch Mal Coeur 84:1797–1802, 1991.
17. Dietrich W, Mössinger H, Spannagl M, et al: Hemostatic activation during cardiopulmonary bypass with different aprotinin dosages in pediatric patients having cardiac operations. J Thorac Cardiovasc Surg 105:712–720, 1993.
18. Dietrich W, Spannagl M, Jochum M, et al: Influence of high-dose aprotinin treatment on blood loss and coagulation patterns in patients undergoing myocardial revascularization. Anesthesiology 73:1119–1126, 1990.
19. Dudziak R, Kirchhoff PG, Reuter HD, Schumann F (eds): Proteolyse und Proteinaseninhibition in der Herz- und Gefäßchirurgie. Stuttgart, Schattauer, 1985.
20. Edmunds LH: Invited letter concerning: Aprotinin use in pediatric cardiac operations. J Thorac Cardiovasc Surg 105:757–760, 1993.
21. Fraedrich G, Engler H, Weber C, Schlosser V: Effect and potential mechanism of high-dose aprotinin regimen in open heart surgery. In Birnbaum DE, Hoffmeister HE (eds): Blood Saving in Open Heart Surgery. Stuttgart, Schattauer, 1990, pp 83–94.
22. Fritz H, Wunderer G: Biochemistry and applications of aprotinin, the kallikrein inhibitor from bovine organs. Arzneim Forsch/Drug Res 33:479–494, 1983.
23. Gans H, Castaneda AR, Subramanian V, et al: Problems in hemostasis during open heart surgery: IX. Changes observed in the plasminogen-plasmin system and their significance for therapy. Ann Surg 166:980–986, 1967.
24. Gardaz JP, Hauert J, Chassot PG, et al: Modification of hemostatic parameters during cardiopulmonary bypass (CPB): Effects of high dose aprotinin. Anesthesiology 75:A991, 1991.
25. Gross R, Holemans R: Fragen der Blutgerinnung bei extrakorporalem Kreislauf mit der Herz-Lungen-Maschine. Klin Wochenschr 39:165–173, 1961.

26. Hannekum A, Reuter HD, Dalichau H, et al: Anlage und zusammenfassendes Ergebnis einer klinischen Doppelblindstudie bei Operationen am offenen Herzen. Einfluß von Aprotinin auf Thrombozytenzahl und -funktion. In Dudziak R, Kirchhoff PG, Reuter HD, Schumann F (eds): Proteolyse und Proteinaseninhibition in der Herz- und Gefäßchirurgie. Stuttgart, Schattauer, 1985, pp 221-233.

27. Harder MP, Eijsman L, Roozendaal KJ, et al: Aprotinin reduces intraoperative and postoperative blood loss in membrane oxygenator cardiopulmonary bypass. Ann Thorac Surg 51:936-941, 1991.

28. Hardy JF, Desroches J, Belisle S, et al: Low-dose aprotinin infusion is not clinically useful to reduce bleeding and transfusion of homologous blood products in high-risk cardiac surgical patients. Can J Anaesth 40:625-631, 1993.

29. Havel M, Grabenwöger F, Schneider J, et al: Aprotinin does not decrease early graft patency after coronary artery bypass grafting despite reducing postoperative bleeding and use of donated blood. J Thorac Cardiovasc Surg 107:807-810, 1994.

30. Havel M, Owen AN, Simon P, et al: Decreasing use of donated blood and reduction of bleeding after orthotopic heart transplantation by use of aprotinin. J Heart Lung Transplant 11:348-349, 1992.

31. Havel M, Teufelsbauer H, Knöbl P, et al: Effect of intraoperative aprotinin administration on postoperative bleeding in patients undergoing cardiopulmonary bypass operation. J Thorac Cardiovasc Surg 101:968-972, 1991.

32. Heller W, Wendel HP, Hoffmeister HM: Lower troponin-T levels in patients undergoing cardiopulmonary bypass surgery and receiving high dose aprotinin therapy indicate reduction in perioperative myocardial damage. Thorac Cardiovasc Surgeon 42(Suppl I):117, 1994.

33. Huang H, Ding W, Su Z, Zhang W: Mechanism of the preserving effect of aprotinin on platelet function and its use in cardiac surgery. J Thorac Cardiovasc Surg 106:11-18, 1993.

34. Janssens M, Joris J, David JL, et al: High-dose aprotinin reduces blood loss in patients undergoing total hip replacement surgery. Anesthesiology 80:23-29, 1994.

35. Jochum M, Jonáková V, Dittmer H, Fritz H: An enzymatic assay convenient for the control of aprotinin levels during proteinase inhibitor therapy. Fresenius Z Anal Chem 317:719-720, 1984.

36. Jochum M, Müller-Esterl W: Bestimmung von Aprotinin-Plasmakonzentrationen nach therapeutischer Anwendung von Trasylol. In Dudziak R, Kirchhoff PG, Reuter HD, Schumann F (eds): Proteolyse und Proteinaseninhibition in der Herz- und Gefäßchirurgie. Stuttgart, Schattauer, 1985, pp 157-167.

37. Karges HE, Funk KA, Ronneberger H: Activity of coagulation and fibrinolysis parameters in animals. Arzneim-Forsch/Drug Res 44:793-797, 1994.

38. Kawasuji M, Ueyama K, Sakakibara N, et al: Effect of low-dose aprotinin on coagulation and fibrinolysis in cardiopulmonary bypass. Ann Thorac Surg 55:1205-1209, 1993.

39. Kestin AS, Valeri CR, Khuri SF, et al: The platelet function defect of cardiopulmonary bypass. Blood 82:107-117, 1993.

40. Köstering H, Kirchhoff PG, Völker P, et al: Untersuchungen der Blutgerinnungsveränderungen während und nach Operationen mit Hilfe der Herz-Lungen-Maschine. Thoraxchirurgie 21:534-543, 1973.

41. Lass M, Welz A, Kochs M, et al: Aprotinin in elective primary bypass surgery—graft patency and clinical efficacy. Europ J Cardiothorac Surg (in press), 1994.

42. Lavee J, Raviv Z, Smolinsky A, et al: Platelet protection by low-dose aprotinin in cardiopulmonary bypass; Electron Microscopic Study. Ann Thorac Surg 55:114-119, 1993.

43. Lavee J, Savion N, Smolinsky A, et al: Platelet protection by aprotinin in cardiopulmonary bypass: Electron microscopic study. Ann Thorac Surg 53:477-481, 1992.

44. Lemmer JH, Stanford W, Bonney SL, et al: Aprotinin for coronary bypass operations: Efficacy, safety, and influence on early saphenous vein graft patency. J Thorac Cardiovasc Surg 107:543-553, 1994.

45. Liu B, Belboul A, Al-Khaja N, et al: Effect of high-dose aprotinin on blood cell filterability in association with cardiopulmonary bypass. Coronary Artery Dis 3:129-132, 1992.

46. Liu B, Belboul A, Radberg G, et al: Effect of reduced aprotinin dosage on blood loss and use of blood products in patients undergoing cardiopulmonary bypass. Scand J Cardiovasc Surg 27:149-155, 1993.

47. Lorenz W, Duda D, Dick W, et al: Mainz/Marburg Trial Group: Incidence and clinical importance of perioperative histamine release: Randomised study of volume loading and antihistamines after induction of anaesthesia. Lancet 343:933-940, 1994.

48. Lu H, Soria C, Commin PL, et al: Hemostasis in patients undergoing extracorporeal circulation: The effect of aprotinin (Trasylol). Thromb Haemost 66:633–637, 1991.
49. Mammen EF: Natural protease inhibitors in extracorporeal circulation. Ann N Y Acad Sci 146:754–762, 1968.
50. Marx G, Pokar H, Reuter H, et al: The effects of aprotinin on hemostatic function during cardiac surgery. J Cardiothorac Vasc Anesth 5:467–474, 1991.
51. Marx R, Clemente P, Werle E, Appel W: Zum Problem eines Antidotes in der internen Thrombotherapie mit Fibrinolytika. Blut 5:367–375, 1959.
52. Masiak M: Trasylol as an inhibitor of fibrinolysis in ECC. In Fritz H, Dietze G, Fidler F, Haberland GL (eds): Recent Progress on Kinins. Basel, Birkhäuser, 1982, pp 690–699.
53. Masiak M, Bross W: Zastosowanie Trasylolu Jako Leku Hamujacego Proteazy Ukladu Fibrynolizy W Krazeniu Pozaustrojowym (ECC) [Application of trasylol as a drug inhibiting proteases of the fibrinolysis system in extracorporeal circulation (ECC)]. Folia Medica Cracoviensia 22:455–461, 1980.
54. Matzdorff AC, Green D, Cohen I, Bauer KD: Effect of recombinant aprotinin on platelet activation in patients undergoing open heart surgery. Haemostasis 23:293–300, 1993.
55. Minami K, Notohamiprodjo G, Buschler H, et al: Alpha-2 plasmin inhibitor-plasmin complex and postoperative blood loss: Double-blind study with aprotinin in reoperation for myocardial revascularization. J Thorac Cardiovasc Surg 106:934–936, 1993.
56. Mohr R, Goor DA, Lusky A, Lavee J: Aprotinin prevents cardiopulmonary bypass-induced platelet dysfunction—a scanning electron microscope study. Circulation 86(Suppl II):II-405–II-409, 1992.
57. Müller-Esterl W: Aprotinin, pancreatic basic trypsin inhibitor: Enzyme-linked immunosorbent assay. In Bergmeyer HU, Graβl M (eds): Methods of Enzymatic Analysis. Weinheim, VCH Verlagsgesellschaft, 1986, pp 246–256.
58. Murkin JM, Lux J, Shannon NA, et al: Aprotinin significantly decreases bleeding and transfusion requirements in patients receiving aspirin and undergoing cardiac operations. J Thorac Cardiovasc Surg 107:554–561, 1994.
59. Murkin JM, Shannon NA, Bourne RB, et al: Aprotinin decreases blood loss in patients undergoing revision total hip replacement surgery. Anaesth Analg (in press), 1994.
60. Nagaoka H, Katori M: Inhibition of kinin formation by a kallikrein inhibitor during extracorporeal circulation in open-heart surgery. Circulation 52:325–332, 1975.
61. Neuhof CH, Dapper F, Irle K, et al: Efficacy of aprotinin on postoperative blood loss and transfusion requirement in patients with coronary bypass surgery—Controlled dose comparison study [abstract]. Thorac Cardiovasc Surgeon 41(Suppl I):105, 1993.
62. Orchard MA, Goodchild CS, Prentice CRM, et al: Aprotinin reduces cardiopulmonary bypass-induced blood loss and inhibits fibrinolysis without influencing platelets. Br J Haematol 85:533–541, 1993.
63. Philipp E: Calculations and hypothetical considerations on the inhibition of plasmin and plasma kallikrein by Trasylol. In Davidson JF, Rowan RM, Samama MM, Desnoyers PC (eds): Progress in Chemical Fibrinolysis and Thrombolysis. New York, Raven Press, 1978, pp 291–295.
64. Philipp E, Mayer G, Schumann F: Investigation of coronary bypass occlusion rate by postoperative coronary angiography in patients after coronary artery bypass grafting (CABG) with extracorporeal circulation, following administration of Trasylol or placebo. Bayer Report No. R-6215 (P), 1994.
65. Popov-Cenic S, Kirchhoff PG, Hack G, et al: Prophylaktische Behandlung mit Antiplasmin (Aprotinin) vor, während und nach Operationen am offenen Herzen bei Erwachsenen. Klinische Bedeutung und ein neues Behandlungskonzept. In Blümel G, Haas S (eds): Mikrozirkulation und Postaglandinstoffwechsel. Stuttgart, Schattauer, 1981, pp 211–219.
66. Popov-Cenic S, Murday H, Kirchhoff PG, et al: Anlage und zusammenfassendes Ergebnis einer klinischen Doppelblindstudie bei aorto-koronaren Bypass-Operationen. In Dudziak R, Kirchhoff PG, Reuter HD, Schumann F (eds): Proteolyse und Proteaseninhibition in der Herz- und Gefäβchirurgie. Stuttgart, Schattauer, 1985, pp 171–186.
67. Popov-Cenic S, Urban AE, Noe G: Studies on the cause of bleeding during and after surgery with a heart-lung machine in children with cyanotic and acyanotic congenital cardiac defects and their prophylactic treatment. In McConn R (ed): Role of Chemical Mediators in the Pathophysiology of Acute Illness and Injury. New York, Raven Press, 1982, pp 229–242.
68. Riess H (ed): Hemostasis in liver transplantation. Semin Thromb Hemost 19:183–314, 1993.
69. Royston D: The serine antiprotease aprotinin (Trasylol): A novel approach to reducing postoperative bleeding. Blood Coag Fibrinol 1:55–69, 1990.

70. Royston D: High-dose aprotinin therapy: A review of the first
    Cardiothorac Vasc Anesth 6:76–100, 1992.
71. Royston D: Aprotinin therapy in heart and heart-lung transplantation.
    12:S19–S25, 1993.
72. Royston D: Perioperative bleeding. Drugs for surgical blood loss. Lance
73. Royston D, Bidstrup BP, Taylor KM, Sapsford RN: Effect of aprotir
    transfusion after repeat open-heart surgery. Lancet ii:1289–1291, 198
74. Schönberger JPAM, Everts PAM, Ercan H, et al: Low-dose aprotinin i
    artery bypass operations contributes to important blood saving. Ann T
    1176, 1992.
75. Schulze K, Graeter T, Schaps D, Hausen B: Severe anaphylactic sho
    application of aprotinin in patients following intrathoracic aortic
    Cardiothorac Surg 7:495–496, 1993.
76. Schumann F, Dirksen MSC: Report on a clinical double-blind study with T
    open heart surgery. Bayer Pharma-Report No. R-5124 (P), 1990.
77. Scott CF, Wenzel HR, Tschesche HR, Colman RW: Kinetics of inhibitio
    kallikrein by a site-specific modified inhibitor Arg-15-aprotinin: Evaluatio
    system and comparison with other proteases. Blood 69:1431–1436, 198
78. Smith CR, Mongero LB, DeRosa CM, et al: Safety of aprotinin in profound
    circulatory arrest. Ann Thorac Surg 58:606–607, 1994.
79. Struck E, Kalmar P, Hehrlein F-W, et al: Safety and efficacy of Trasylol^R in o
    A controlled dose comparison study in 3 German hospitals [abstract].
    Surgeon 41(Suppl I):144–145, 1993.
80. Sundt TM, Kouchoukos NT, Saffitz JE, et al: Renal dysfunction and intravascu
    with aprotinin and hypothermic circulatory arrest. Ann Thorac Surg 55:141
81. Tice DA, Reed GE, Clauss RH, Worth MH: Hemorrhage due to fibrinolysis occu
    heart operations. J Thorac Cardiovasc Surg 46:673–679, 1963.
82. Traverso LW: Effectiveness of aprotinin in blocking a hypotensive factor of panc
    from the pig, dog and monkey. Resuscitation 12:271–277, 1985.
83. Urban AE, Brecher A-M, Popov-Cenic S: Blutungen nach intrakardialen operativer
    im Säuglingsalter: Klinische Relevanz und perioperative Therapie. In Dudziak R,
    PG, Reuter HD, Schumann F (eds): Proteolyse und Proteinaseninhibition in der
    Gefäßchirurgie. Stuttgart, Schattauer, 1985, pp 273–279.
84. van Oeveren W, Jansen NJ, Bidstrup BP, et al: Effects of aprotinin on hemostatic me
    during cardiopulmonary bypass. Ann Thorac Surg 44:640–645, 1987.
85. Vedrinne C, Girard C, Jegaden O, et al: Reduction in blood loss and blood u
    cardiopulmonary bypass with high-dose aprotinin versus autologous fresh whole
    transfusion. J Cardiothorac Vasc Anesth 6:319–323, 1992.
86. Wachtfogel YT, Kucich U, Hack CE, et al: Aprotinin inhibits the contact, neutrophil, a
    platelet activation systems during simulated extracorporeal perfusion. J Thorac Cardiovas
    Surg 106:1–10, 1993.
87. Westaby S: Complement and the damaging effects of cardiopulmonary bypass. Thorax 38:321–
    325, 1983.
88. Westaby S, Forni A, Dunning J, et al: Aprotinin and bleeding in profoundly hypothermic
    perfusion. Eur J Cardiothorac Surg 8:82–86, 1994.

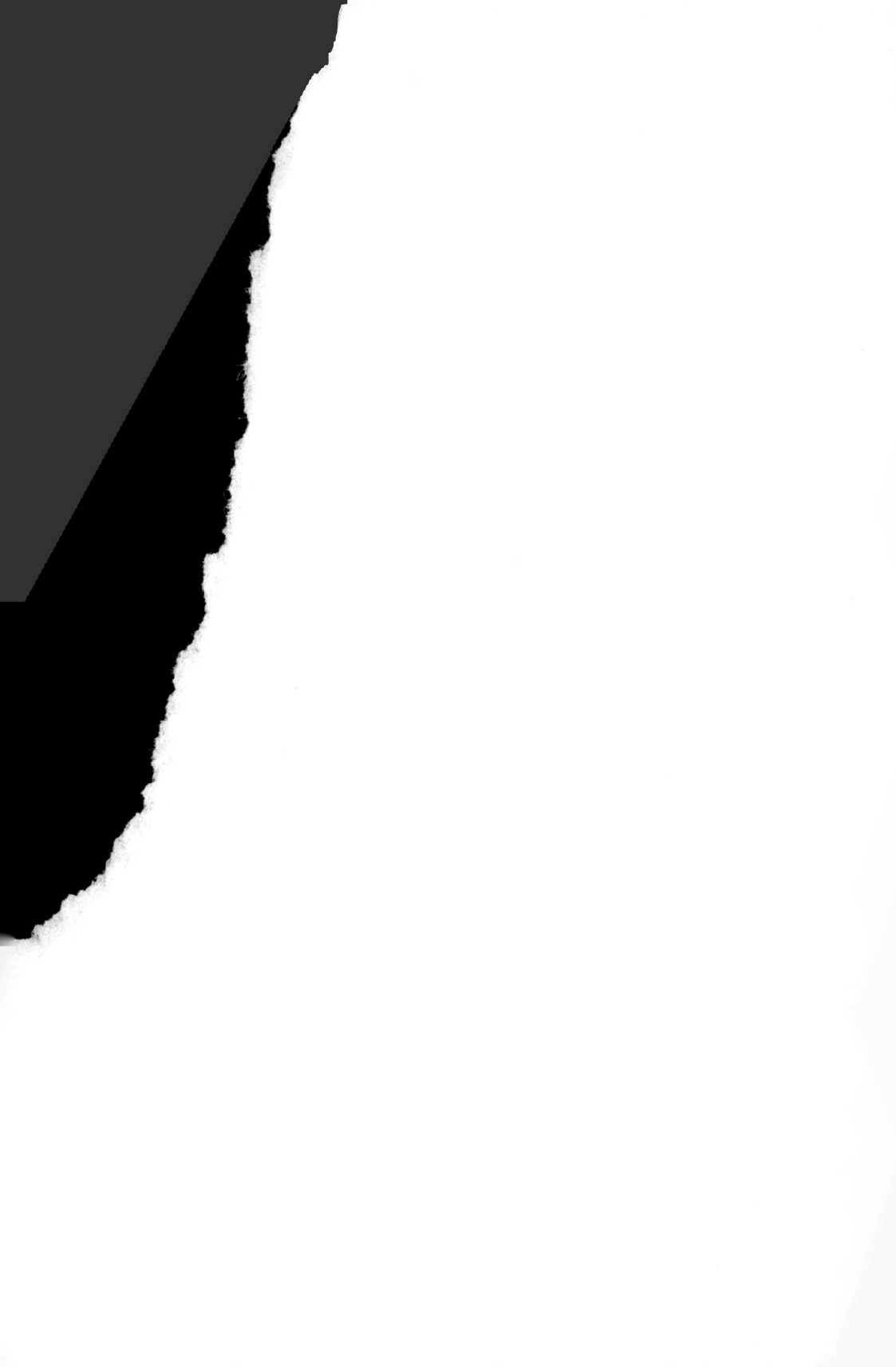

**W. Heller, PhD**
**H. P. Wendel, MSc**
**M. J. Gallimore, PhD**

# 8

# Hemostatic Restoration by Aprotinin in Cardiopulmonary Bypass: Experimental Rationale

Our interest in investigating the use of aprotinin in cardiac surgery was kindled in the early part of the 1980s when Huth and Hoffmeister reported a reduction in postoperative blood loss in aprotinin-treated patients undergoing open-heart surgery.[28] Because of the broad spectrum of inhibitory activities of aprotinin,[11] we began a series of investigations both in vitro and in vivo to ascertain the mechanism of its therapeutic action.

## Specific Effects of Cardiopulmonary Bypass on Blood

During cardiopulmonary bypass (CPB) the blood comes into contact with the artificial surfaces of the bypass machine, leading to activation of the so-called contact system. Studies by numerous research groups over the past four decades have revealed that artificial surfaces can activate the coagulation, fibrinolytic, kallikrein-kinin, and complement systems as well as affect blood and other cells.[5,13,20,21,31,44] Several proteins are involved in the activation, including factor XII (FXII, Hageman factor), prekallikrein (PKK, Fletcher factor), factor XI (FXI, plasma thromboplastin antecedent [PTA]), and high-molecular-weight kininogen (HMWK). These proteins circulate in inactive forms in blood and are converted to active enzymes or liberate active peptides after contact with artificial surfaces. The proenzymes FXII, PKK, and FXI are converted into the active serine proteases alpha-FXII (FXIIa) and beta-FXIIa (FXIIf), plasma kallikrein (KK), and FXIa.

PKK and FXI circulate as bimolecular complexes with HMWK, which has a positively charged, histidine-rich region that binds HMWK, together with complexed PKK and FXI, to negatively charged surfaces. A similar binding region is found on the FXII molecule. When blood comes into contact with an artificial surface, the four proteins of the contact system are assembled on the surface. It is believed that when FXII is bound to the surface, autoactivation occurs, followed by the rapid generation of alpha-FXIIa and beta-FXIIa. Only alpha-FXIIa binds to the surface. Both alpha-FXIIa and beta-FXIIa activate PKK to KK, whereas alpha-FXIIa is a much better activator of FXI than beta-FXIIa.

Because KK is a powerful activator of surface-bound FXII and because both alpha-FXIIa and beta-FXIIa convert PKK to KK, self-amplification of the system results in rapid activation of FXII. The resulting production of KK leads to the liberation of bradykinin from HMWK. Bradykinin enhances vascular permeability, produces hypotension, contracts smooth muscle, causes pain, and releases tissue-type plasminogen activator (tPA).[8,41] KK also converts plasminogen to plasmin,[3,14] liberates renin from prorenin,[6,47] and primes neutrophils for chemotactic activity.[57] FXII, PKK, FXI, and HMWK were discovered in studies of patients with abnormal contact coagulation[24,42,48,54]; each of these proteins participates in surface-mediated coagulation. The fact that the major inhibitor of activated protein C (protein C inhibitor) also inhibits KK and FXIa establishes a link between the contact system and the protein C pathway.[38]

## Stimulation of Fibrinolysis by the Contact System

Extensive research has shown that activation of the contact system stimulates fibrinolysis in a complex manner. Alpha- and beta-FXIIa,[19,36] FXIa,[31] and KK[3,14] have been shown to activate plasminogen directly. However, the indirect effect of contact activation may play a more significant role in fibrinolysis. Both KK and bradykinin have been shown to release large quantities of tPA when infused into pigs,[8] and alpha-FXIIa, beta-FXIIa, and KK have been shown to convert prourokinase to urokinase.[25,27] Granulocyte elastase, a powerful proteolytic enzyme released from polymorphonuclear white cells as a result of contact activation, may have a direct local effect on fibrinolysis.[35] Beta-FXIIa has been shown to activate the first component of complement.[18] The activation of FXII leads to formation of both plasmin and thrombin, which activate C1; in addition, plasmin converts C3 to C3a.[43] Thus activation of FXII may lead indirectly to activation of the complement system.

Alpha- and beta-FXIIa[30,53] and KK[4] are chemotactic for neutrophils. Recent evidence indicates that KK in fact primes neutrophils for activation.[57] KK has been shown to produce a fall in leukocytes after infusion into pigs,[9] and we have reported that both beta-FXIIA and KK release PMN elastase in vitro.[16] In the presence of PKK and HMWK, platelet membranes have been reported to serve as surfaces for activation of FXII,[55] and platelets have been shown to have receptors for FXI and FXIa.[34]

## Inhibition of Fibrinolysis by Native Inhibitors and Aprotinin

Surface activation produces a wide range of active enzymes that have various effects on cells. The generation and activities of these enzymes are controlled by inhibitors. The major inhibitor of alpha- and beta-FXIIa and plasma kallikrein is C1-esterase inhibitor.[15,45] Other important inhibitors of contact system activation include alpha-2 macroglobulin, which inhibits kallikrein[23]; alpha-1-proteinase inhibitor (alpha-1 antitrypsin), which inhibits FXIa[38]; antithrombin III, which in the presence of heparin inhibits kallikrein[49,50]; protein C inhibitor, which inhibits kallikrein and FXIa[38]; and beta-2 glycoprotein, which inhibits the conversion of prekallikrein to kallikrein by alpha-FXIIa.[46] After activation of the contact system, other important inhibitors include inhibitors of plasminogen activation[1] and alpha-2 antiplasmin.[39]

Despite the presence of inhibitors, activation of the contact system during CPB often leads to hyperfibrinolysis.[7] Aprotinin is a broad-spectrum serine protease inhibitor and has been shown to inhibit trypsin, plasmin, glandular kallikrein, plasma kallikrein,[11] and activated protein C.[10] The aprotinin molecule also has a strongly positively charged region that may allow it to bind to both artificial and natural negatively charged surfaces. Therefore, aprotinin may produce beneficial effects during CPB by several possible mechanisms.

## In Vitro Methods of Study

This chapter outlines our methods of investigating the effects of aprotinin on contact system activation and CPB and describes some of the results. Along with the routine determinations of blood cells and coagulation, we used chromogenic peptide substrate and enzyme-linked immunosorbent assays (ELISAs) to determine proenzymes, enzymes, and enzyme inhibitors. These assays were developed during the course of our studies and are now available in kit form for routine purposes. The assessed parameters, the supplier of the kits, and the type of method are outlined in Table 1. Assays that were not available to us but are vital for studies of contact system activation are shown in Table 2. The basic principles of these assays are as follows:

**Proenzymes** (e.g., FXII). Diluted plasma is mixed with a suitable specific activator and incubated for a certain time to complete activation. The active enzyme is determined by using a chromogenic peptide substrate.

**Enzyme inhibitors** (e.g., antithrombin III). Plasma diluted with either buffer or buffer containing a necessary cofactor (e.g., heparin) is mixed and incubated with a purified enzyme preparation (e.g., thrombin). Some of the enzyme is inhibited (depending on inhibitor concentration), and the residual enzyme activity is determined by using a chromogenic peptide substrate.

**Cofactors** (e.g., heparin). Plasma is diluted with buffer containing a purified inhibitor (e.g., antithrombin III) and mixed and incubated with a purified enzyme preparation (e.g., thrombin, FXa). Some of the enzyme is inhibited (depending on cofactor concentration), and the residual enzyme activity is determined by using a chromogenic peptide substrate. By using standardized plasmas for standard curve generation, the value for each parameter can be determined.

**Free enzymes or enzymes complexed to alpha-2 macroglobulin** (e.g., KK–alpha-2 macroglobulin complex). Plasma is diluted with buffer containing an inhibitor to block unwanted enzyme activities. The enzyme activity is determined by incubating the diluted plasma with a chromogenic peptide substrate.

**ELISAs for enzyme inhibitor complexes or immunologic determination of individual parameters** (e.g., thrombin–antithrombin complex, platelet factor 4). Microtiter plates are coated with antibodies directed against an epitope of the protein or enzyme–inhibitor complex to be determined, and test and standard samples are added. After washing off unbound protein, peroxidase-labeled antibodies are added, and bound antibody is detected with a peroxidase substrate.

**TABLE 1.** Parameters Assayed during Experimental Contact System Activation in In-vitro Cardiopulmonary Bypass Models and Cardiopulmonary Bypass

| | Parameter Measured | Assay Method | Kit Supplier |
|---|---|---|---|
| Proenzymes | Hageman factor (FXII) | CS | 1 |
| | Prekallikrein | CS | 1,2 |
| | Plasminogen | CS | 1,2,3,5,6 |
| | FXI | CS | 1 |
| | Protein C | CS | 1,2,3,5,6,8 |
| Inhibitors and | Alpha-FXIIa inhibition | CS | 1 |
| inhibitor assays | Beta-FXIIa inhibition | CS | 1 |
| | Kallikrein inhibition | CS | 1,2 |
| | FXIa inhibition | CS | 1 |
| | C1-esterase inhibition | CS | 1,4 |
| | Antithrombin III | CS | 1,2,3,4,5,6 |
| | Heparin cofactor II | CS | 1 |
| | Alpha-2 macroglobulin | CS | 1,2 |
| | Alpha-1 antitrypsin | CS | 1,2 |
| | Alpha-2 antiplasmin | CS | 1,2,5,6 |
| | Protein C inhibition | CS | 1 |
| | Plasminogen-activator inhibitors | CS | 2,5,6 |
| | Plasminogen-activator inhibitors | ELISA | 2,5,6,7 |
| | PMN-elastase inhibition | CS | 1 |
| | Aprotinin | CS | 1 |
| Enzymes | Plasma Kallikrein | CS | 1,2 |
| | Alpha- and beta-FXIIa | CS | 1,2 |
| | Tissue-type plasminogen activator | CS | 2,5,6 |
| | Tissue-type plasminogen activator | ELISA | 2,5,6,7 |
| | Activated protein C | CS | 1,2 |
| Cofactors | High-molecular-weight kininogen | Clotting | 8 |
| | Heparin | CS | 1,2,5,6 |
| | Dermatan sulphate | CS | 1 |
| Enzyme–inhibitor | Kallikrein–alpha-2 macroglobulin complex | CS | 1,2 |
| complexes | FXIIa–alpha-2 macroglobulin complex | CS | 1 |
| | Thrombin-antithrombin III complex | ELISA | 8 |
| | Plasmin-antiplasmin complex | ELISA | 7 |
| | PMN-elastase–alpha-1-proteinase inhibitor complex | ELISA | 1,9 |
| Other parameters | Hemolysis | Color | 8 |
| | Platelet factor 4 | ELISA | 8 |
| | Fibrinogen | Clotting | 3 |
| | D-dimers | ELISA | 2,5,6 |
| | Fibrinopeptide A | ELISA | 3 |

CS = chromogenic peptide substrate; tPA = tissue-type plasminogen activator.
Kit suppliers: 1. Unicorn Diagnostics Ltd., London. 2. Chromogenix AB, Molndal, Sweden. 3. Boehringer, Mannheim, Germany. 4. Immuno, Vienna. 5. Diagnostica-Stago, Asnieres, France. 6. Biopool, Umea, Sweden. 7. Technoclone, Vienna. 8. Behring-Werke, Marburg, Germany. 9. Merck, Darmstadt, Germany.

One of the difficulties of working with whole blood in in-vitro models is that the blood has to be anticoagulated. We used both freshly drawn citrated blood (1 part 0.11M trisodium citrate plus 9 parts blood) and transfusion blood (less than 24 hours old). Statistical analysis was performed by the SPSS statistical software package (SPSS Software, Inc., Chicago). Results were expressed as mean values $\pm$ standard deviation (SD). Differences between mean values were assessed by two-way analysis of variance and Student's t-test; $p$ values $< 0.05$ were considered significant.

**TABLE 2.** Suggested Assays for Studying Experimental Contact System Activation and Simulated Cardiopulmonary Bypass in Vitro and in Patients

| Parameters | Assay Method | References |
|---|---|---|
| Kallikrein–alpha-2 macroglobulin complex | ELISA | 32 |
| Kallikrein–C1-esterase inhibitor complex | ELISA | 33,51 |
| Kallikrein–C1-esterase inhibitor complex | RIA | 40 |
| Alpha-FXIIa–C1-esterase inhibitor complex | RIA | 40 |
| Beta-FXIIa–C1-esterase inhibitor complex | ELISA | 51 |
| C1s–C1-esterase inhibitor complex | ELISA | 33 |
| C1s–C1-esterase inhibitor complex | RIA | 22 |

RIA = radioimmunoassay.

## Simple Tube Assays

Contact system activation can be studied by using polystyrene tubes containing a known weight or size of the surface to be tested. After 8-ml volumes of fresh citrated blood were pipetted into polystyrene tubes measuring 16 × 100 mm, a pretesting sample of 1000 $\mu$l was taken from each tube. The surfaces to be studied were added to the tubes, the tubes were rotated at room temperature or in an incubator, and 1000-$\mu$l samples were taken at various intervals. The blood samples were centrifuged to collect the plasma, which can be analyzed immediately or flash-frozen and stored at –70°C for later analysis.

Results from a simple study using glass slides and plastic as activating surfaces to compare contact system activation with and without aprotinin are shown in Figures 1 and 2. All blood samples contained unfractionated heparin (5 U/ml). In the samples containing aprotinin, the aprotinin levels were 250 KIU/ml. The glass and plastic strips measured 12 × 40 mm.

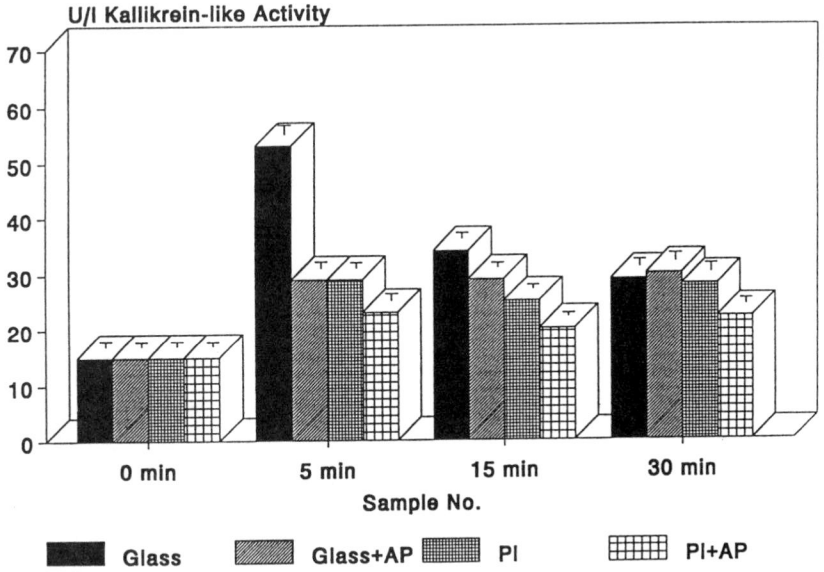

**FIGURE 1.** Kallikrein-like activities produced by glass and plastic (Pl) contact activation in the presence and absence of aprotinin (AP).

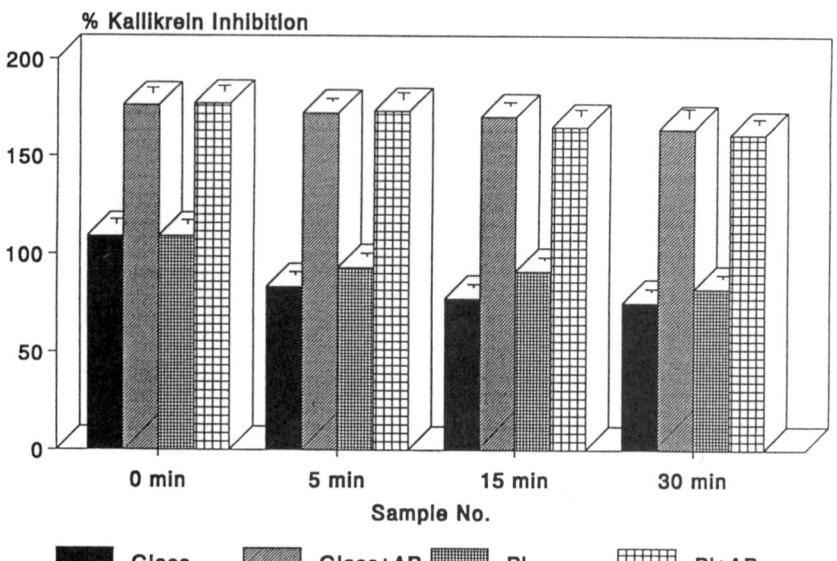

% Kallikrein Inhibition

Glass ▪ Glass+AP ▨ PI ▦ PI+AP

**FIGURE 2.** Kallikrein inhibition in glass and plastic (PI) contact-activated blood in the presence and absence of aprotinin (AP).

With glass contact, rapid activation of the contact system led to the generation of plasma kallikrein (as detected by kallikrein–alpha-2 macroglobulin complexes [KK] and free plasma kallikrein). Aprotinin markedly reduced the activation produced by glass contact. Plastic produced significantly less activation than glass, and the combination of aprotinin and plastic produced the least activation. Figure 2 shows the inhibition of kallikrein, which increased significantly in the glass and plastic samples containing aprotinin. Pronounced falls in kallikrein inhibition were observed with glass or plastic activation in the absence of aprotinin within 5 minutes of the start of contact activation. The greatest falls in inhibition were seen with glass. Other significant changes included reduced levels of FXII and prekallikrein as well as significant increases in FXIIa-like activity and levels of PMN elastase-alpha-1-proteinase inhibitor complexes following glass and plastic contact activation. These effects were partially but not completely blocked by aprotinin.

## Tuebingen Loop Model

The Tuebingen loop model is based on the well-known Chandler loop model[2] (Fig. 3). Fresh human blood is rotated in polyvinyl chloride tubing, which can be formed into a water-tight loop by closing with a larger piece of silicone tubing. The loops are rotated in temperature-controlled water that allows studies at normal body temperature, hypothermic temperature (28° C), and extreme hypothermic temperature (17° C). Four loops of exactly the same dimensions are used, each containing 20 ml of fresh blood from the same donor. Blood samples are obtained at four intervals simply by removing one loop and pouring out the contents. So far we have performed only a few studies with this model. The results (Fig. 4) show that both kallikrein-like and FXIIa-like activities increased significantly in heparinized

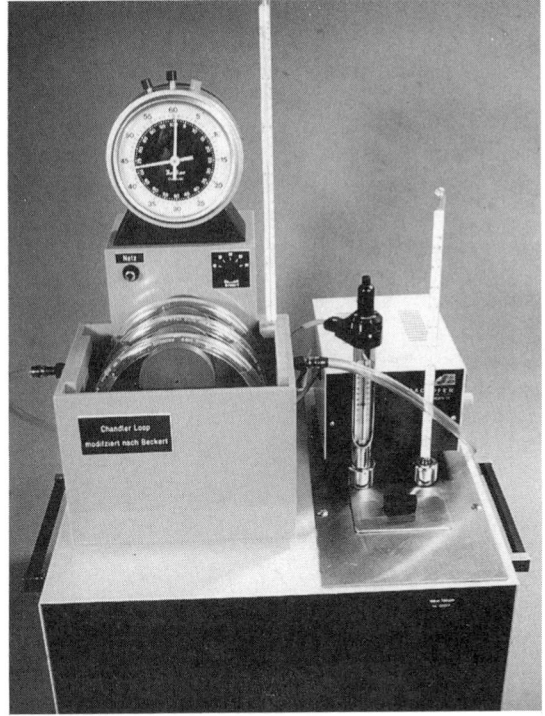

**FIGURE 3.** The Tuebingen loop model.

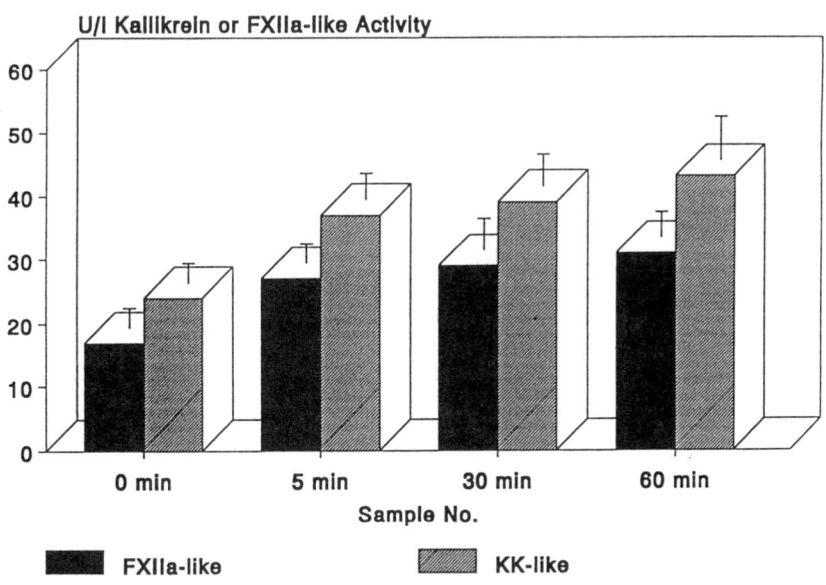

**FIGURE 4.** FXIIa-like and kallikrein-like activities produced in heparinized blood (3 U/ml) in the Tuebingen loop model.

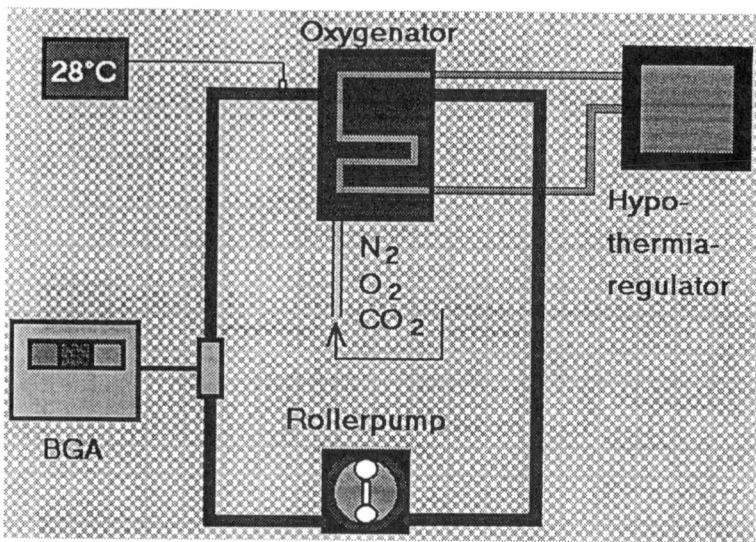

**FIGURE 5.**   In vitro CPB model.

blood that was circulated in the loop at 28° C for 60 minutes; in fact, significant increases were seen after a 5-minute rotation of the loops.

## Simulated Cardiopulmonary Bypass Model

In a typical study using the simulated CPB model (Fig. 5), 500-ml volumes of fully recalcified fresh ACD whole blood were recirculated through an oxygenator with a roller pump for periods up to 90 minutes at 28° C. Hemodilution, temperature, and gas flow were regulated in a manner similar to clinical CPB. The variables to be studied were either added before simulated CPB or immediately after commencement of circulation. The machine was primed with 50 ml of 5% glucose solution, 116 ml of Ringer lactate, and 24 ml of 10% calcium chloride. Before priming, the oxygenators and tubing were rinsed with 700 ml of Ringer lactate for 30 minutes. Eight 10-ml blood samples were taken after 0, 1, 5, 10, 20, 30, 60, and 90 minutes of circulation. After centrifugation to obtain the plasma, the heparin concentration in each sample was determined in order to antagonize the heparin with protamine chloride. All plasma samples were then shock-frozen in liquid nitrogen and stored at –20° C. Before analysis the plasma samples were thawed rapidly at 37° C. Ten runs were performed for each experiment.

### Effects of Different Types of Heparin on Contact System Activation

During 1987 a sudden increase in the volume of blood loss after CPB was observed in our clinic. It was subsequently discovered that the purchasing department had changed the supplier and type of heparin. With a return to the previous type of heparin, blood loss was reduced. This experience led us to investigate the effects of various types of heparin in the simulated CPB model. Two unfractionated heparins (A and B) were tested at 3 U/ml, and one fractionated heparin (C) was tested at 6 U/ml. Results are shown in Figures 6, 7, and 8. With all three types the contact

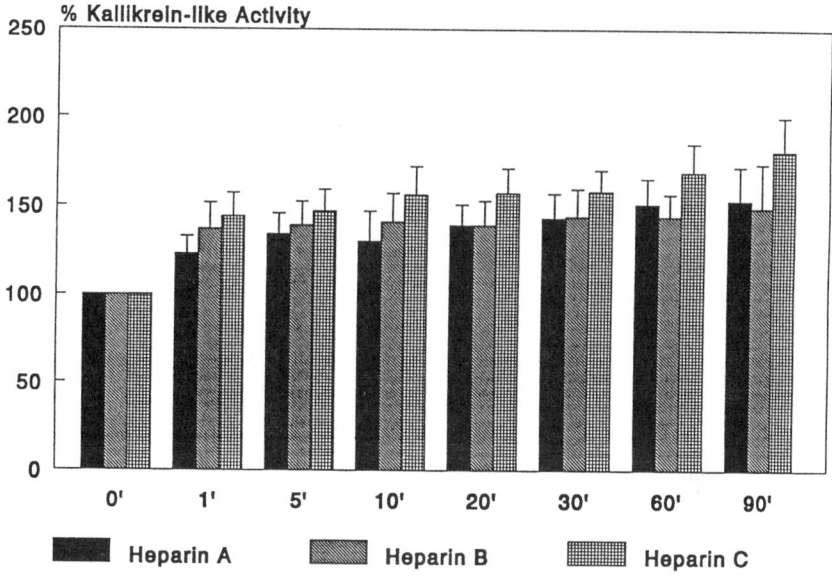

**FIGURE 6.** Kallikrein-like activities in the in vitro CPB model with blood containing three different types of heparin.

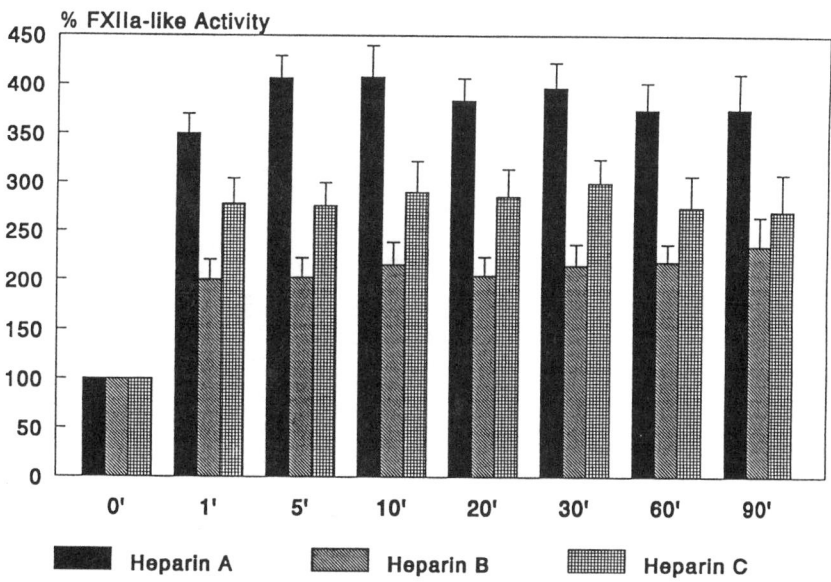

**FIGURE 7.** FXIIa-like activities in the in vitro CPB model with blood containing three different types of heparin.

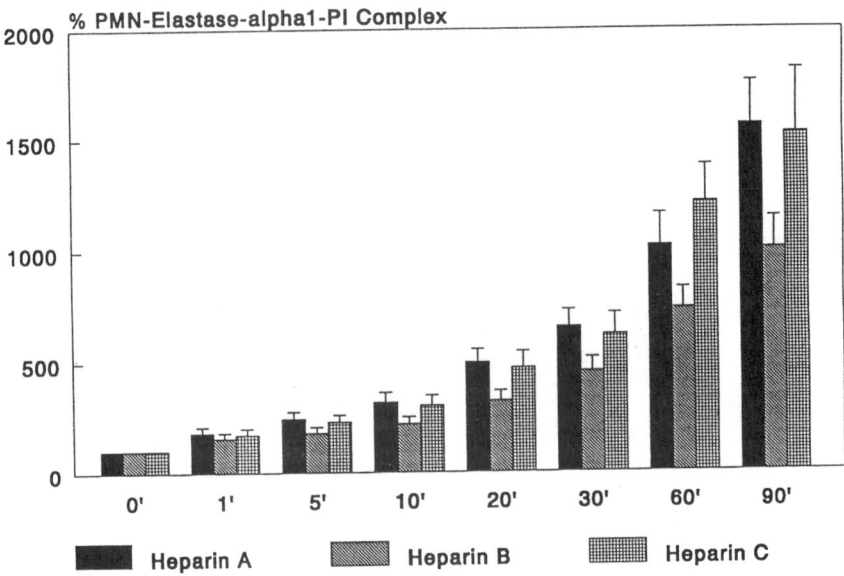

**FIGURE 8.** PMN-elastase–alpha-1-proteinase inhibitor complexes in the in vitro CPB model with blood containing three different types of heparins.

system was activated early in the simulated bypass, as exemplified by significantly increased kallikrein and FXIIa-like activities and increased levels of PMN-elastase–alpha-1-proteinase inhibitor complexes. As the period of simulated CPB lengthened, kallikrein-like activities increased with all three heparins, but the highest values were found with heparin C (Fig. 6). FXIIa-like activity was most markedly elevated with heparin A, whereas the lowest values were seen with heparin B (Fig. 7). The values for heparin B were significantly lower than those for heparin A. Levels of PMN-elastase–alpha-1-proteinase inhibitor complex were very high after 90 minutes of simulated CPB. The values were significantly lower for heparin B than for heparins A and C (Fig. 8).

### Heparin-coated Oxygenators plus Aprotinin

In the preceding figures and in published work[26] we have shown that heparin contributes to contact system activation in CPB. We also have reported that aprotinin at therapeutic doses reduces the contact system activation in heparinized blood.[17] In the study reported below we compared the effect of aprotinin in the simulated CPB model using heparin-coated oxygenators and identical uncoated oxygenators. Ten runs were performed for each variable. For the uncoated oxygenators, 3 U/ml of unfractionated heparin were used; for the coated oxygenators, 1 U/ml of the same heparin was used. Aprotinin was used at a level of 250 KIU/ml. The results for some of the parameters are shown in Figures 9, 10, 11, 12, and 13. Increases in kallikrein-like and FXIIa-like activities were significant in all groups after 1 minute of simulated CPB, and activity continued to increase throughout the study (Figs. 9 and 10). The highest values were seen in the uncoated oxygenators with and without aprotinin. With aprotinin in the uncoated oxygenators the values for kallikrein-like activity were somewhat lower (Fig. 9); for FXIIa-like activity, the

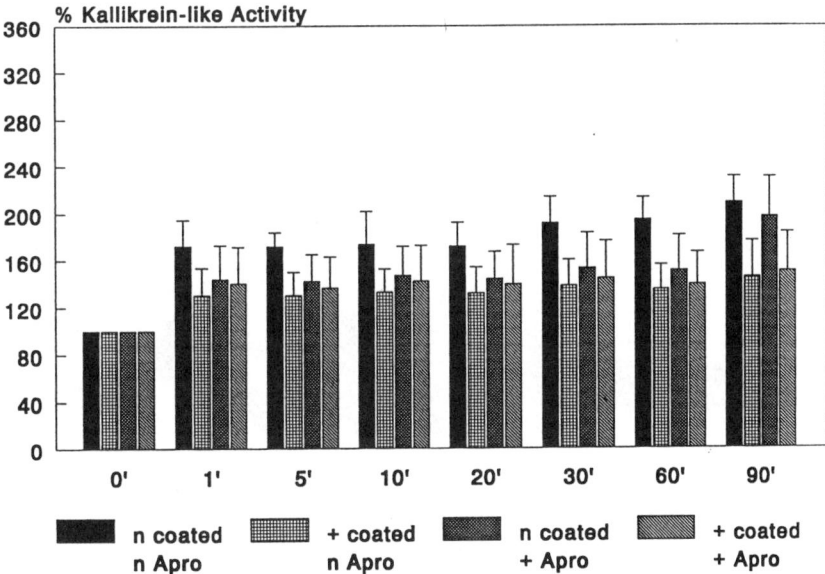

**FIGURE 9.** Kallikrein-like activities in blood samples in the in vitro CPB model using heparin-coated oxygenators with and without aprotinin and uncoated oxygenators with and without aprotinin.

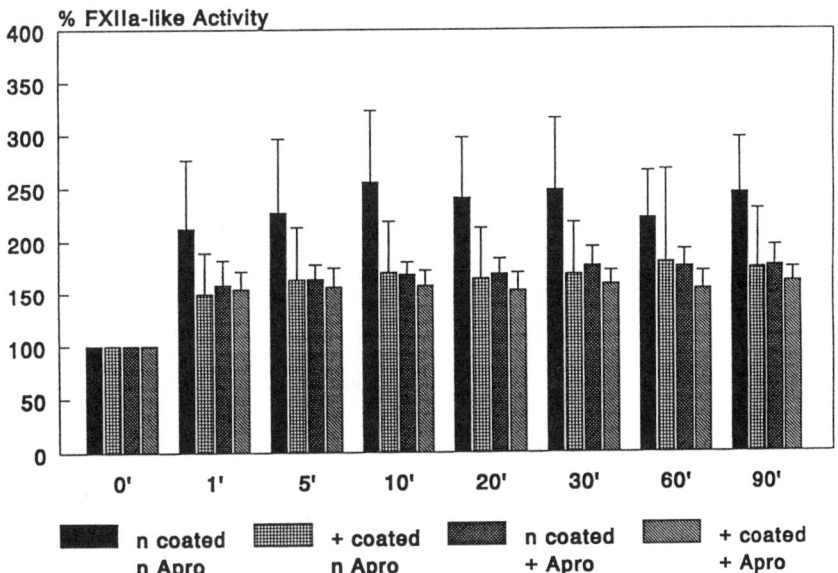

**FIGURE 10.** FXIIa-like activities in blood samples in the CPB model using heparin-coated oxygenators with and without aprotinin and uncoated oxygenators with and without aprotinin.

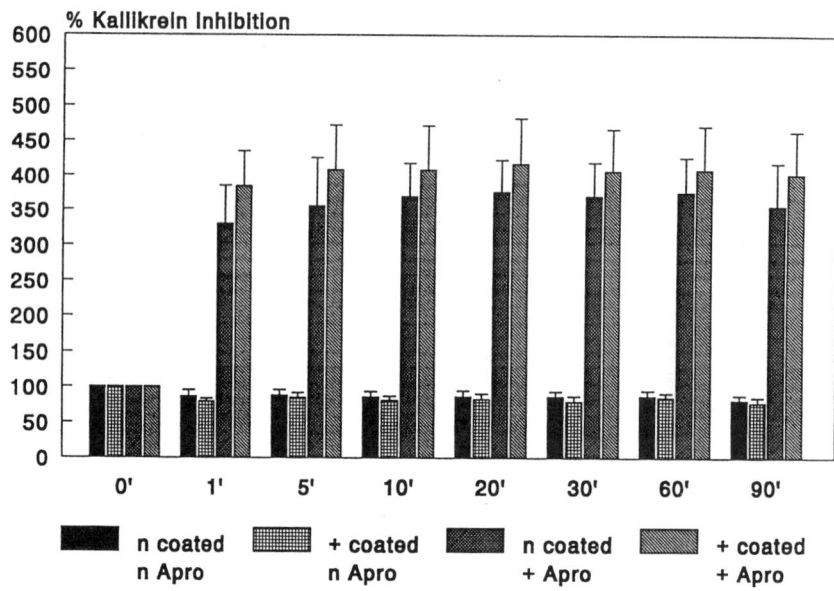

**FIGURE 11.** Kallikrein inhibition in blood samples in the CPB model using heparin-coated oxygenators with and without aprotinin and uncoated oxygenators with and without aprotinin.

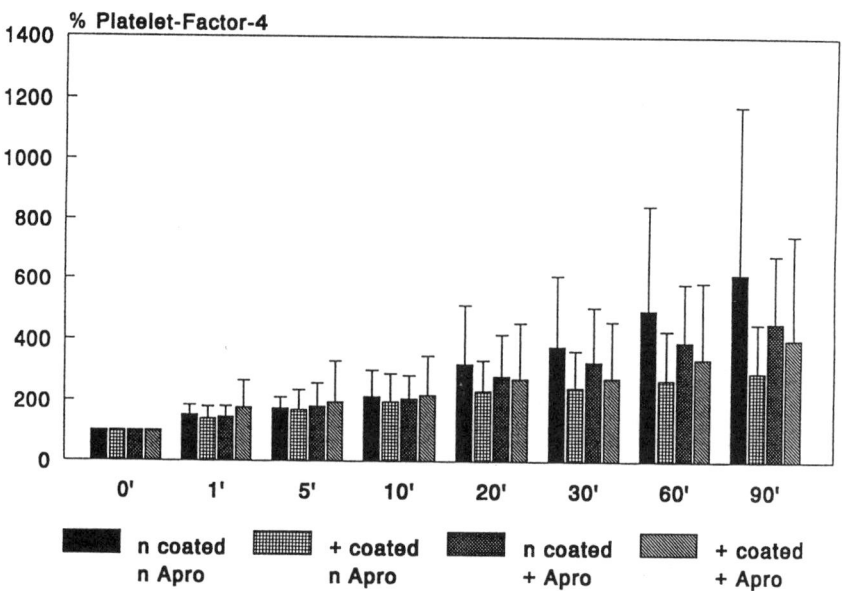

**FIGURE 12.** Platelet factor 4 levels in blood samples in the CPB model using heparin-coated oxygenators with and without aprotinin and uncoated oxygenators with and without aprotinin.

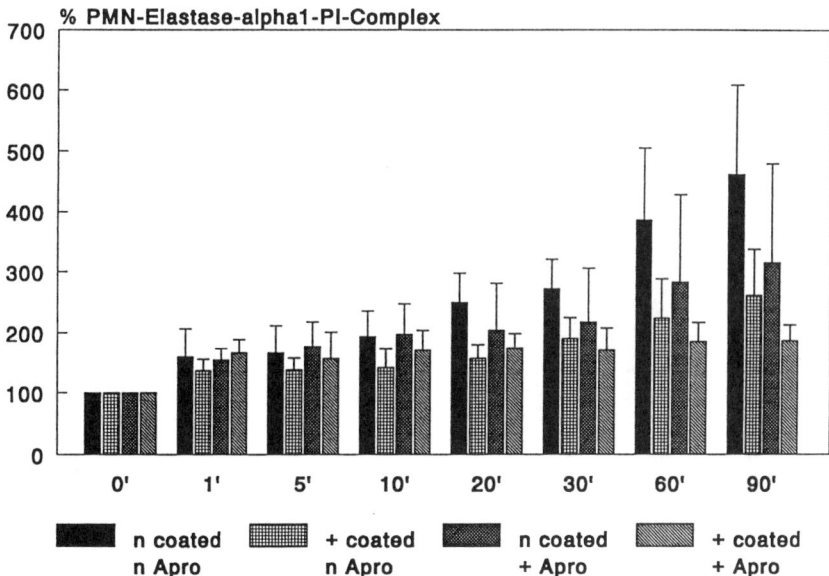

**FIGURE 13.**   PMN-elastase–alpha-1-proteinase inhibitor levels in blood samples in the CPB model using heparin-coated oxygenators with and without aprotinin and uncoated oxygenators with and without aprotinin.

values were significantly lower (Fig. 10). With the coated oxygenators significantly lower kallikrein-like and FXIIa-like activities were observed both with and without aprotinin. Kallikrein inhibition was significantly higher in the two aprotinin groups throughout the study (Fig. 11). Levels of platelet factor 4 rose significantly in all groups during simulated CPB; the lowest levels were seen in the coated oxygenators (Fig. 12). In the presence of aprotinin, values were lower in the uncoated oxygenators and higher in the coated oxygenators. Levels of PMN-elastase–alpha-1-proteinase inhibitor complex rose significantly in all groups during simulated CPB (Fig. 13). The highest values were obtained in the uncoated oxygenators without aprotinin, whereas significantly lower values were obtained in the uncoated oxygenators with aprotinin and in the coated oxygenators. The lowest values were seen in the coated oxygenators with aprotinin.

### Heparin vs. Hirudin

Because in our opinion heparin contributes to contact system activation in CPB, we performed a study in the simulated CPB model comparing unfractionated heparin (3 U/ml) and hirudin (6 $\mu$g/ml). Ten simulated CPB runs were performed with each drug (Figs. 14, 15, and 16). Kallikrein-like and FXIIa-like activities rose in both groups 1 minute after commencement of simulated CPB and continued to rise during the 90 minutes of the experiment. The hirudin group had significantly lower values than the heparin group (Figs. 14 and 15). Levels of PMN-elastase–alpha-1-proteinase inhibitor complex also rose in both groups; after 90 minutes of blood circulation in the CPB machine, however, the values were markedly lower in the hirudin group (Fig. 16).

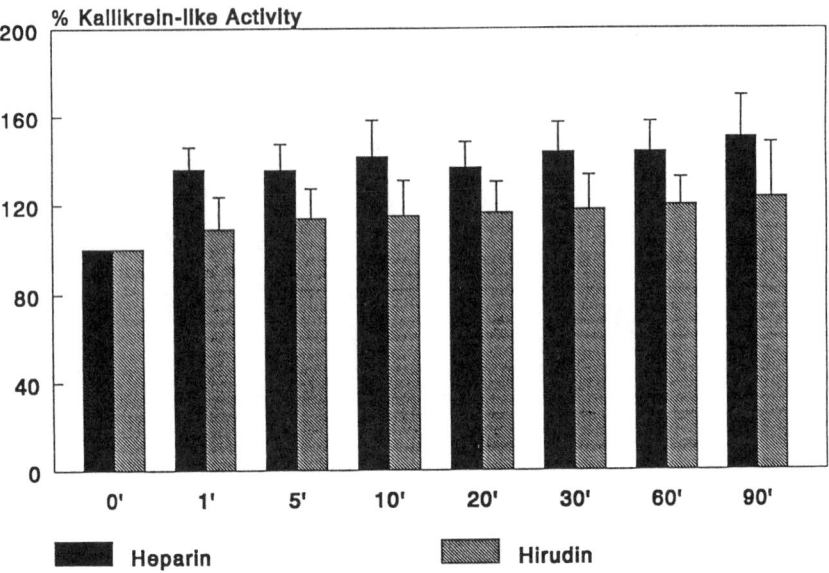

**FIGURE 14.** Kallikrein-like activities in the CPB model with either heparin or hirudin.

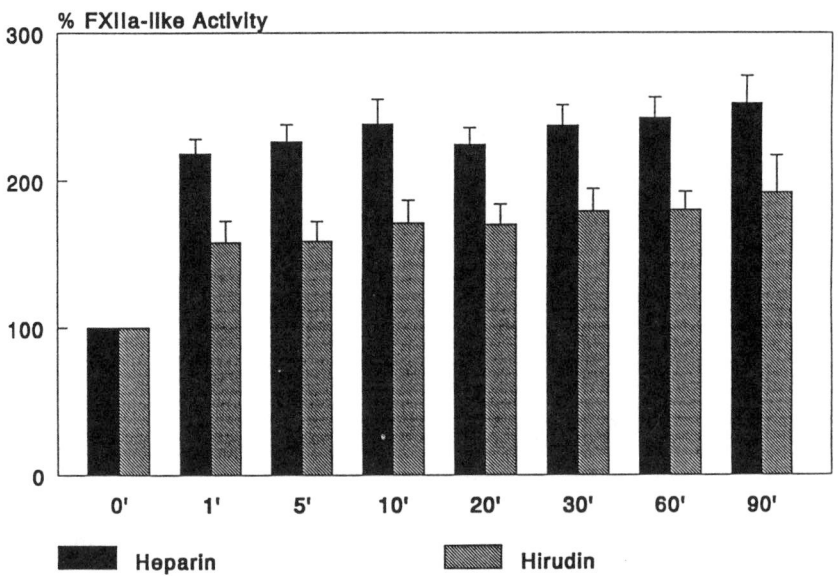

**FIGURE 15.** FXIIa-like activities in the CPB model with either heparin or hirudin.

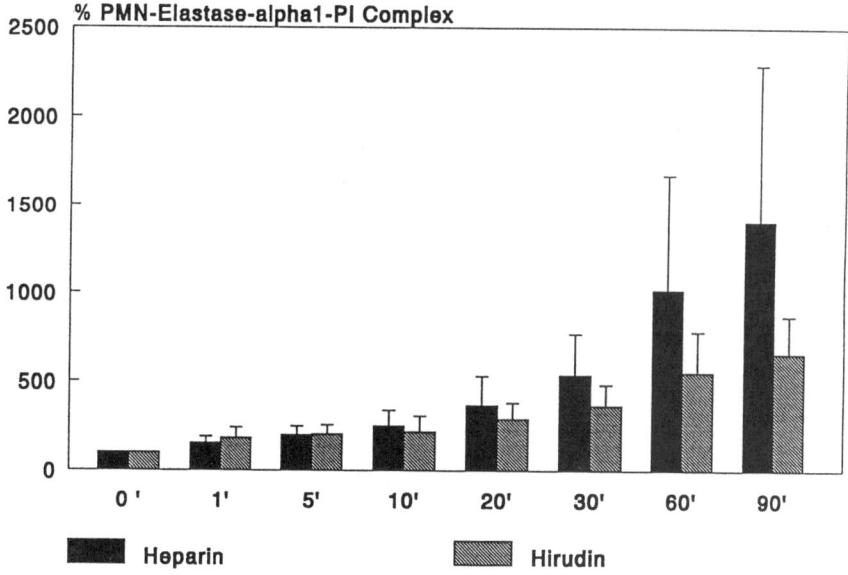

**FIGURE 16.** PMN-elastase–alpha-1-proteinase inhibitor complexes in the CPB model with either heparin or hirudin.

## Conclusion

By using in vitro models along with a battery of tests, we can predict to some extent whether a particular anticoagulant, proteinase inhibitor, or even CPB machine has an advantage over those in current use. Simple tube assays and the Tuebingen loop model determine whether a particular plastic is good or bad in terms of contact activation. Other workers have used similar tests for the same purpose.[29] It is apparent from various studies[13,52] that aprotinin inhibits activation of the contact system in simulated CPB. Our results with heparin-coated oxygenators indicate that activation of the contact system, platelet damage, and release of neutrophil enzymes are markedly reduced by reduced levels of heparin. Our results also show that some types of heparin are worse than others in both clinical and simulated CPB. The replacement of heparin by hirudin resulted in a marked reduction in activation of the contact system, platelet damage, and PMN-elastase release in the simulated CPB model. This finding indicates that the use of genetically engineered variants of this tight-binding thrombin inhibitor[12] may be of great benefit in CPB.

As mentioned previously, we already use a "good" heparin in patients undergoing CPB in our clinic, and studies are in progress to examine whether heparin-coated oxygenators give better results than uncoated oxygenators.

We have been using aprotinin in CPB in our clinic for over 15 years, and 10 years ago we reported that aprotinin inhibits the kallikrein-kinin system in CPB, as exemplified by reduced kallikrein-like activities, among other changes. [12] In a recent study in which blood levels of aprotinin during CPB were maintained at 250–350 KIU/ml, kallikrein-like activities were significantly lower, release of PMN elastase was reduced, and blood loss was markedly reduced (Figs. 17, 18, and 19). The beneficial effects of aprotinin in CPB may be due to enzyme inhibition (e.g., contact

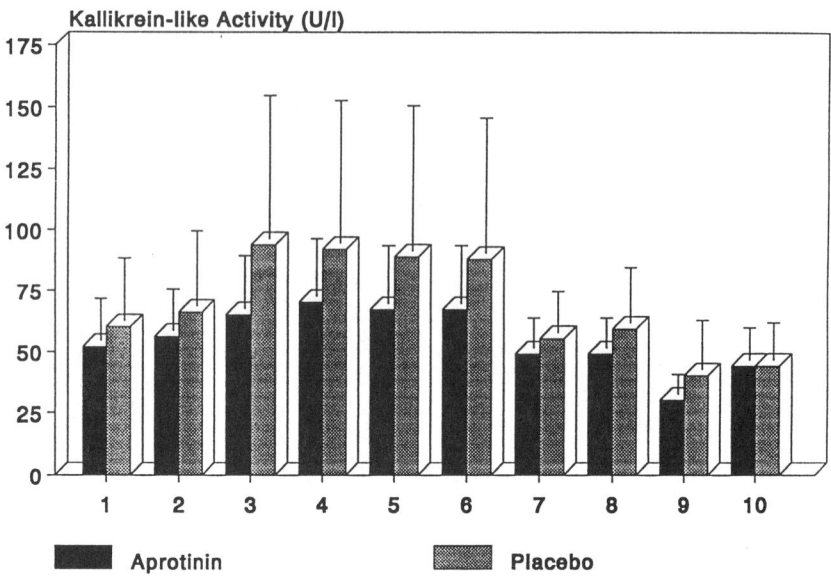

**FIGURE 17.** Kallikrein-like activities in blood samples from patients undergoing CPB with and without high-dose aprotinin.

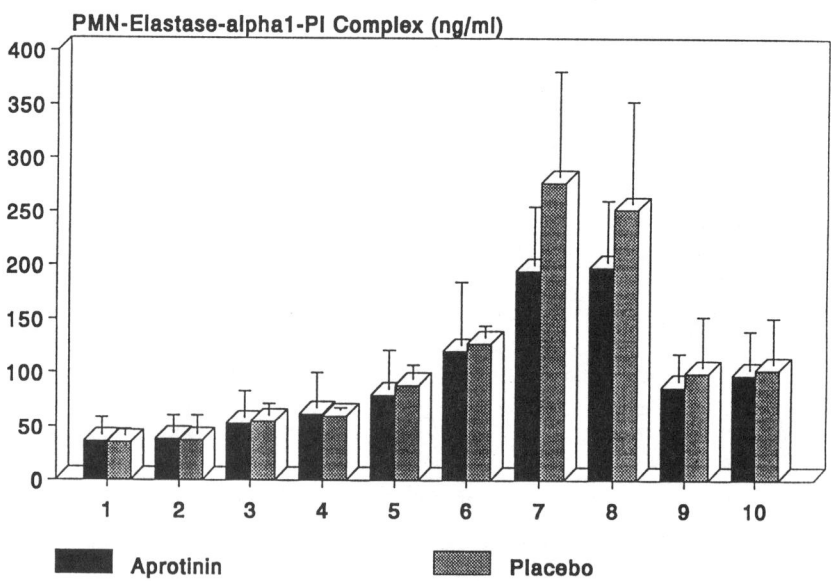

**FIGURE 18.** PMN-elastase–alpha-1-proteinase inhibitor complexes in blood samples from patients undergoing CPB with and without high-dose aprotinin.

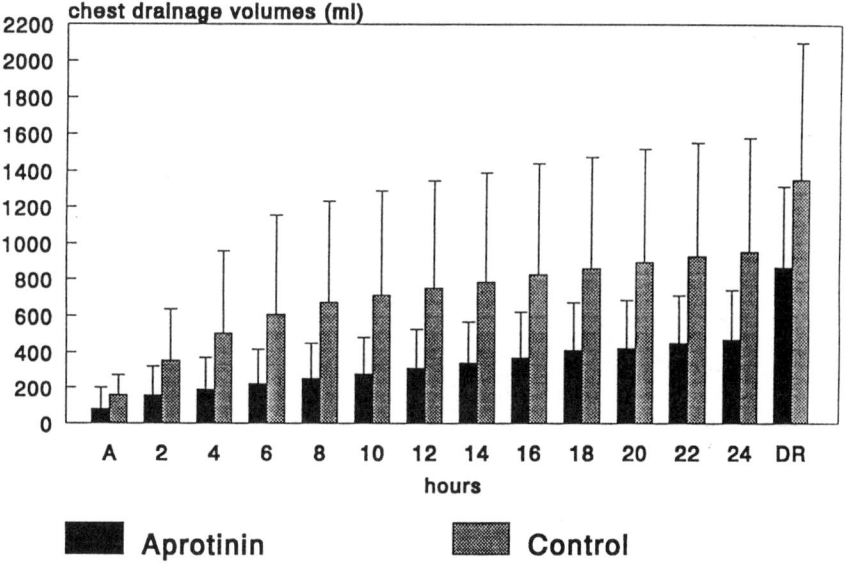

**FIGURE 19.** Chest drainage volumes (postoperative blood loss) from arrival in intensive care until 24 hours later in patients who underwent CPB with and without high-dose aprotinin.

system enzymes, plasmin, protein C), stabilization of cell membranes (aprotinin is a strongly positively charged molecule), platelet protection, antiheparin effects,[56] or other mechanisms; determination of the exact mechanism(s) will entertain the minds of numerous researchers. Whatever the outcome of such studies, we believe that inhibition of contact system activation by aprotinin has major therapeutic benefits. Perhaps the next major improvements in CPB will result from the combined use of heparin-coated oxygenators and high-dose aprotinin therapy.

## References

1. Bachman F: Fibrinolysis. In Verstraete M, Vermylen M, Iijnen R, Arnout J (eds): Thrombosis and Haemostasis. Leuven University Press, 1987, pp 227–265.
2. Chandler AB: In vitro thrombotic coagulation of blood: A method for producing a thrombus. Lab Invest 7:110–116, 1958.
3. Colman RW: Activation of plasminogen by human plasma kallikrein. Biochem Biophys Res Commun 35:273–279, 1969.
4. Colman RW, Wachtfogel YT, Kucich U, et al: Effect of the cleavage of the heavy chain of human plasma kallikrein on its functional properties. Blood 65:311–318, 1985.
5. Colman RW, Scott CF, Schmaier AH, et al: Initiation of blood coagulation at artificial surfaces. Ann N Y Acad Sci 516:253–267, 1987.
6. Derkx FHM, Bouma BN, Schalekamp MMPA, Schalekamp MADH: An intrinsic factor XII-prekallikrein-dependent pathway activates the human plasma renin-angiotensin system. Nature 280:315–316, 1979.
7. Dietrich W, Mossinger H, Spannagl M, et al: Haemostatic activation during cardiopulmonary bypass with different aprotinin dosages in paediatric patients having cardiac operations. J Thorac Cardiovasc Surg 105:712–720, 1993.
8. Egberg N, Gallimore MJ, Green K, et al: Effects of plasma kallikrein and bradykinin infusions into pigs on plasma fibrinolytic variables and urinary excretion of thromboxane and prostacyclin metabolites. Fibrinolysis 2:101–106, 1988.

9. Egberg N. Gallimore MJ, Jacobsson J: Effect of plasma kallikrein infusions into pigs on haemodynamic and haemostatic variables. Fibrinolysis 2:95–100, 1988.
10. Espana F, Estelles A, Griffin JH, et al: Aprotinin (Trasylol) is a competitive inhibitor of activated protein C. Thromb Res 56:751–756, 1989.
11. Fritz H, Wunderer G: Biochemistry and application of aprotinin, the kallikrein inhibitor from bovine organs. Drug Res 33:479–494, 1983.
12. Fuhrer G, Gallimore MJ, Heller W, Hoffmeister HE: Studies on components of the plasma kallikrein-kinin system in patients undergoing cardiopulmonary bypass. In Greenbaum LW, Margolis H (eds): KININS IV. Advances in Experimental Medicine and Biology, vol. 198. New York, Plenum Press, 1986, pp 385–391.
13. Fuhrer G, Gallimore MJ, Heller W, Hoffmeister HE: FXII. Blut 61:258–266, 1990.
14. Gallimore MJ, Fareid E, Stormorken H: The purification of a plasma kallikrein with weak plasminogen activator activity. Thromb Res 12:409–420, 1978.
15. Gallimore MJ, Amundsen E, Larsbraaten M, et al: Studies on plasma inhibitors of plasma kallikrein using chromogenic peptide substrate assays. Thromb Res 16:695–703, 1979.
16. Gallimore MJ, Fuhrer G, Heller W, Hoffmeister HE: The effects of plasma kallikrein and beta FXIIa (FXIIf) on blood components circulating in a cardiopulmonary bypass machine. Thromb Haemost 62:268, 1989.
17. Gallimore MJ, Heller W, Fuhrer G, et al: Contact activation, heparins and cardiopulmonary bypass. Thromb Haemost 68:91–92, 1992.
18. Ghebrehiwet B, Randazzo BP, Dunn JT, et al: Mechanism of activation of the classical pathway of complement by Hageman factor fragment. J Clin Invest 71:1450–1456, 1983.
19. Goldsmith G, Saito H, Ratnoff OD: The activation of plasminogen by Hageman factor (FXII) and Hageman factor fragments. J Clin Invest 62:54–60, 1978.
20. Griffin JH, Bouma BN: The contact phase of blood coagulation. In Bloom A, Thomas DP (eds): Haemostasis and Thrombosis. Edinburgh, Churchill Livingstone, 1987, pp 101–115.
21. Griffin JH, Cochrane CG: Recent advances in the understanding of contact activation reactions. Semin Thromb Haemost 5:254–273, 1979.
22. Hack CE, Hannema AJ, Eerenberg-Belmer AJM, et al: A C1-inhibitor-complex assay (INCA): A method to detect C1 activation in vitro and in vivo. J Immunol 127:1450–1453, 1981.
23. Harpel PC: Human plasma alpha-2-macroglobulin: An inhibitor of plasma kallikrein. J Exper Med 132:329–352, 1970.
24. Hathaway WE, Belhasen LP, Hathaway HS: Evidence for a new plasma thromboplastin factor: I. Case report, coagulation studies and physicochemical properties. Blood 26:521–532, 1965.
25. Hauert J, Bachmann F: Prourokinase activation in euglobulin fractions. Thromb Haemost 54:122, 1985.
26. Heller W, Wendel HP, Klaffschenkel R, Hoffmeister HE: A comparative study of fractionated and unfractionated heparins on components of the FXII–plasma kallikrein system in an in vitro cardiopulmonary bypass model. KININ 1991. Munich, EK Frey–E Werle Foundation, Limbach-Verlag, abstract PW-3,15, 227, 1991.
27. Huisveld IA, Haspers H, Van Heeswijk GMD, et al: Contribution of contact activation factors to urokinase-related fibrinolytic activity in whole human plasma. Thromb Haemost 54:102, 1985.
28. Huth CH, Hoffmeister HE: Einsatz von Proteinaseninhibitoren während der extrakorporalen Zirkulation. Wirkungsverbesserung der Dosis einer klinischen Studie. In Dudzil R (ed): Proteolyse and Proteaseninhibitoren in der Herz- und Gefäßchirurgie. Stuttgart, Schattauer, 1984, pp 243–253.
29. Irvine L, Courtney JM, Lowe GDO: Contact activation and biocompatibility assessment. Artif Organs 14(4):223–234, 1991.
30. Kaplan AP, Kay AB, Austen KF: A prealbumin activator of prekallikrein: II. Appearance of chemotactic activity for human neutrophils by the conversion of prekallikrein to kallikrein. J Exper Med 135:81–97, 1972.
31. Kaplan AP, Silverberg M: The coagulation-kinin pathway of human plasma. Blood 70:1–15, 1987.
32. Kaufman N, Page JD, Pixley RA, et al: $\alpha2$-Macroglobulin–kallikrein complexes detect contact system activation in hereditary angioedema and human sepsis. Blood 77:2660–2667, 1991.
33. Lewin MF, Kaplan AP, Harpel PC: Studies on C1 inactivator–plasma kallikrein complexes in purified systems and in plasma: Quantitation by an enzyme-linked differential antibody immunoabsorbent assay. J Biol Chem 258:6415–6421, 1983.
34. Lipscomb MS, Walsh RN: Human platelets and factor XI. Localization in platelet membranes of factor XI-like activity and its functional distinction from plasma factor XI. J Clin Invest 63:1006–1014, 1979.

35. Machovich R, Owen WG: The elastase-mediated pathway of fibrinolysis. Blood Coagul Fibrinol 1:79–90, 1990.
36. Mandle R Jr, Kaplan AP: Hageman factor substrates. Human plasma prekallikrein: Mechanism of activation by Hageman factor and participation in Hageman factor-dependent fibrinolysis. J Biol Chem 252:6097–6104, 1977.
37. Markwardt F: The development of hirudin as an antithrombotic drug. Thromb Res 74:1–23, 1994.
38. Meijer JCM, Kanters DHAJ, Vloosvik RAA, et al: Inactivation of human plasma kallikrein and factor XIa by protein C inhibitor. Biochemistry 27:4231–4237, 1988.
39. Mullertz S: The primary plasmin-inhibitor, $\alpha$2-plasmin inhibitor or $\alpha$2-antiplasmin: A review. In Collen D, Wiman B, Verstraete M (eds): The Physiological Inhibitors of Blood Coagulation and Fibrinolysis. Amsterdam, Elsevier, 1978, pp 87–101.
40. Nuijens JH, Huijbregts CCM, Cohen M, et al: Detection of activation of the contact system of coagulation in vitro and in vivo: Quantitation of activated Hageman factor–C1-inhibitor and kallikrein–C1-inhibitor complexes by specific radioimmunoassays. Thromb Haemost 58:778–785, 1987.
41. Pisaro JJ: Chemistry and biology of the kallikrein-kinin system. Proteases and biological control. Cold Spring Harbour Conference on Cell Proliferation. 2:199–207, 1975.
42. Ratnoff OD, Calopy JE: A familial hemorrhagic trait associated with a deficiency of a clot-promoting fraction from plasma. J Clin Invest 34:602–613, 1955.
43. Ratnoff OD, Naff GB: The conversion of C1s to C1 esterase by plasmin and trypsin. J Exper Med 125:337–345, 1961.
44. Ratnoff OD: A quarter century with Mr Hageman. Thromb Haemost 43:95–98, 1980.
45. Schapira M: Major inhibitors of the contact phase coagulation factors. Semin Thromb Haemost 13:69–78, 1987.
46. Schousboe I: Inositolphospholipid-accelerated activation of prekallikrein by activated FXII and its inhibition by $\beta$2-glycoprotein. Eur J Biochem 176:629–636, 1988.
47. Sealey JE, Atlas SA, Laragh JH, et al: Initiation of plasma prorenin activation by Hageman factor dependent conversion of plasma prekallikrein to kallikrein. Proc Natl Acad Sci USA 76:5914–5918, 1979.
48. Soulier J-P, Prou-Wartelle O: New data on Hageman factor and plasma thromboplastin antecedent: The role of "contact" in the initial phase of blood coagulation. Br J Haematol 6:88–101, 1960.
49. Stead N, Kaplan AP, Rosenberg RD: Inhibition of activated FXII by antithrombin III-heparin cofactor. J Biol Chem 251:6481–6488, 1976.
50. Vennerod AM, Laake K, Solberg AK, Stromland S: Inactivation and binding of human plasma kallikrein by antithrombin III. Thromb Res 9:457–466, 1975.
51. Wachtfogel YT, Harpel PC, Edmunds LH Jr, Colman RW: Formation of C1s–C1-inhibitor, kallikrein–C1 inhibitor, and plasmin–$\alpha$2-plasmin inhibitor complexes during cardiopulmonary bypass. Blood 73:468–471, 1989.
52. Wachtfogel YT, Kucich U, Hack CE, et al: Aprotinin inhibits the contact, neutrophil, and platelet activation systems during simulated extracorporeal perfusion. J Thorac Cardiovasc Surg 106:1–10, 1993.
53. Wachtfogel YT, Pixley RA, Kucich U, et al: Purified plasma FXIIa aggregates human neutrophils and causes degranulation. Blood 67:1731–1737, 1986.
54. Waldman R, Abraham JP, Rebuck JW, et al: Fitzgerald factor: A hitherto unrecognized clotting factor. Lancet i:949–951, 1975.
55. Walsh PN, Griffin JH: Contribution of human platelets to the proteolytic activation of blood coagulation factors XII and XI. Blood 57:106–118, 1981.
56. Wendel HP, Heller W, Gallimore MJ, et al: The prolonged activated clotting time (ACT) with aprotinin depends on the type of activator used for measurement. Blood Coagul Fibrinol 4:41–45, 1993.
57. Zimmerli W, Huber I, Bouma BN, Lämmle B: Purified human plasma kallikrein does not stimulate but primes neutrophils for superoxide production. Thromb Haemost 62:1121–1125, 1989.

Jeanine M. Walenga, PhD
Michael J. Koza, BS, MT(ASCP)
Debra A. Hoppensteadt, MS, MT (ASCP)
Henry J. Sullivan, MD
Alvaro Montoya, MD
Roque Pifarré, MD

# 9

# Fibrinolysis and the Antifibrinolytic Activity of Aprotinin in Cardiac Surgery

Replacement of intra- and postoperative blood loss with blood products in cardiac surgery patients may be associated with risk of infections, disease transmission, or transfusion reactions. Clinical complications such as re-exploration for bleeding, wound infection, adult respiratory distress syndrome (ARDS), hemodynamic instability, and even death may occur as a result of excessive bleeding. With current techniques, the incidence of clinically significant postoperative bleeding typically remains 3–7% for routine cardiac operations and 9–12% for special procedures. The reasons for the blood loss are varied.[3]

The fibrinolytic components of the hemostatic system are activated during cardiopulmonary bypass (CPB) surgery, as evidenced by an increase in fibrin(ogen) degradation products and plasminogen activator with a concomitant decrease in plasminogen and alpha-2 antiplasmin in the patient's plasma and a shortening of the euglobulin lysis time.[1,16] However, it is unclear whether this enhanced fibrinolysis is a major contributor to postsurgical bleeding in a significant proportion of these patients.

Two specific antifibrinolytic agents have been used in the past with CPB in an attempt to reduce blood loss. Epsilon-aminocaproic acid is a lysine analogue that inhibits plasminogen activators, plasminogen binding to fibrin and plasmin. Although it reduces blood loss in several clinical situations, its efficacy in CPB is controversial with some reports of thrombotic complications.[21] Tranexamic acid, another lysine analogue with stronger inhibitory effects against plasminogen activation and binding to fibrin, has been shown to be of no clinical benefit over epsilon-aminocaproic acid.[10] The effect of these agents, however, does demonstrate an association of blood loss with fibrinolytic activation during CPB surgery.

Aprotinin was first described for use in cardiovascular operations by D. Tice in 1964. After many years, it has finally been proven to be an attractive means to help alleviate postoperative blood loss.[2,4,21] This nonspecific protease inhibitor is isolated from bovine lung. It is a single-chain, 58-amino-acid moiety with three disulfide bridges (6512 kd). It is known to inhibit trypsin, chymotrypsin, kallikrein, plasmin, thrombin, and protein C by reversibly binding to these enzymes.[6,8,20] Tissue factor and leukocyte elastase may also be inhibited by aprotinin.[22] The mechanism through which postsurgical bleeding is reduced by aprotinin involves its antifibrinolytic effect (improved clot stability),[9,17] coupled with a platelet "protective" effect (via plasmin inhibition).[11,23] By preserving the platelet receptors glycoprotein (GP)Ib (von Willebrand factor) and GPIIb/IIIa (fibrinogen), platelet adhesion to damaged endothelium can occur.

Other studies have not been able to confirm a protective effect on platelets.[17-19] Reports on aprotinin's inhibition of the antiplatelet effect of heparin, the activation of prourokinase by platelet-bound kallikrein, and the impairment of von Willebrand factor function by plasmin strongly suggest other mechanisms for the improvement of platelet function in aprotinin therapy.[7,12,15] The role of activated protein C as a cause of bleeding during CPB surgery is unknown, but because protein C activity is decreased by aprotinin, there may be less bleeding due to the inhibition of both the anticoagulant and profibrinolytic properties of protein C.[24]

The basic mechanism of aprotinin to reduce postoperative blood loss is complex at best. For the platelet, it is most likely an indirect mechanism via inhibition of several enzymes, partially related to the fibrinolytic system, that would otherwise affect the platelet membrane. The antifibrinolytic, contact/coagulation system, and leukocyte effects play some role as well. However, no definitive proof is yet available that clearly demonstrates the exact mechanism of action of aprotinin in vivo.

In a randomized, double-blind, placebo-controlled study recently completed at Loyola University Medical Center, patients undergoing repeat CPB surgery for myocardial revascularization (CABG) were administered one of three doses of aprotinin or placebo to determine the optimal dosing regimen for efficacy (reduction of postoperative blood loss) and safety.[13] Blood samples collected pre-, intra-, and postoperatively from these patients were evaluated by state-of-the-art assays for fibrinolytic parameters to determine the association of the fibrinolytic state with postsurgical bleeding.

## Material and Methods

Of the 42 patients enrolled in this study at Loyola, blood samples were obtained from 36 for evaluation. Male and female patients over 18 years of age, requiring repeat isolated myocardial revascularization through a previous median sternotomy for myocardial revascularization, were studied. Patients who met the inclusion criteria[13] were stratified as low (stratum I) or high (stratum II) risk for perioperative myocardial infarction (MI) then randomized to receive either aprotinin or placebo. Stratification was based on patients having an MI within 30 days prior to surgery or patients having angina requiring nitroglycerin therapy within 30 days prior to surgery. Further stratification was based on aspirin consumption within 5 days prior to surgery as follows:

Stratum IA: Low risk, with aspirin
     IB: Low risk, no aspirin
    IIA: High risk, with aspirin
    IIB: High risk, no aspirin

The four treatment arms are summarized in Table 1.

**TABLE 1.** Aprotinin Treatment Arms

|  | Loading Dose | Continuous Infusion Dose | CPB Circuit Prime Dose |
|---|---|---|---|
| Group I (High-dose 4.5 MU) | Aprotinin 280 mg | Aprotinin 70 mg/hr | Aprotinin 280 mg |
| Group II (Low-dose 2.25 MU) | Aprotinin 140 mg + placebo | Aprotinin 35 mg/hr + placebo | Aprotinin 140 mg + placebo |
| Group III (2 MU, pump prime only) | Placebo | Placebo | Aprotinin 280 mg |
| Group IV (Placebo) | Placebo | Placebo | Placebo |

Treatment was begun after induction of anesthesia and continued until the patient was transferred to the intensive care unit. A loading dose of heparin of at least 300 IU/kg was administered prior to cannulation of the heart. Supplemental amounts of heparin were given during surgery to maintain the levels as determined by the Hepcon System (heparin/protamine titration).

## Blood Collection

Citrated whole blood was collected from the patients preoperatively prior to aprotinin administration (under anesthesia, after intubation), after 30 minutes on-pump, immediately post-protamine sulfate after pump, and 24 hours after surgery. Blood samples were placed on ice and immediately centrifuged at 2000 rpm (4°C). Plasma was aliquoted and frozen at –70°C until analyzed. This study was approved by the Institutional Review Board of the Loyola University Medical Center. All patients gave written informed consent prior to enrollment.

## Assays

Each patient sample was analyzed in a blinded fashion for each of the following parameters. Immunologic-based procedures included fibrinogen degradation products (FgDP) (Organon Teknika Corp., Durham, NC), fibrin degradation products (FbDP) (Organon Teknika), tissue plasminogen activator (tPA) (Diagnostica Stago, Asnières, France), and plasminogen activator inhibitor (PAI-1) (Diagnostica Stago). The chromogenic-based procedures included plasminogen and alpha-2 antiplasmin (Instrumentation Laboratory, Lexington, MA) performed on the ACL 300 + (Instrumentation Laboratory) and alpha-2 macroglobulin (Boehringer Mannheim, Mannheim, Germany) performed on a Beckman spectrophotometer.

All results are reported as a mean ± 1 SEM. Statistical analysis was performed by ANOVA using the Primer of Biostatistics (McGraw-Hill) IBM-PC compatible package.

## Results

The description of the patient groups ($n$ = 7–11; males:females 2.5:1) and adverse events for each treatment arm is given in Table 2. Only minor adverse events of

**TABLE 2.**  Study Patient Information

| Group | No. | Male | Female | Aspirin | Adverse Events* |
|---|---|---|---|---|---|
| High-dose aprotinin | 11 | 5 | 6 | 6/11 | 4/11; atrial fibrillation; post-pericardiotomy syndrome × 2; IABP |
| Low-dose aprotinin | 11 | 9 | 2 | 6/11 | 6/11; atrial fibrillation; IABP; LVAD; ARI; chest pain–no MI; tachycardia; pneumothorax with chest tube insertion |
| 2-million pump prime | 7 | 6 | 1 | 5/7 | 2/7; atrial fibrillation; pulmonary edema |
| Placebo | 7 | 6 | 1 | 4/7 | 4/7; atrial fibrillation; tachycardia; pacemaker insertion |
| Total | 36 | 26 | 10 | 21/36 | 16/36 |

*IABP = intra-aortic balloon pump; LVAD = left ventricular assist device; ARI = acute renal insufficiency.

loss and transfusions by treatment group are given in Table 3. The pump-prime-only dose of aprotinin and the placebo group had significantly higher blood loss ($p < 0.02$) than the highest-dosed aprotinin group. The amount of blood loss could be correlated to the aprotinin dose.

In the highest-dosed aprotinin group, the level of FgDPs (Fig. 1) significantly decreased on-pump ($p < 0.05$), rose to preoperative levels post-pump, and fell again 24 hours post-surgery. The second aprotinin-dosed group followed the same pattern, but high FgDP levels remained 24 hours post-surgery in several patients. In the lowest-dose aprotinin group (pump prime only), the high preoperative levels were even higher postoperatively, but within 24 hours of surgery, normal levels were obtained. The placebo group had very high postoperative levels which normalized within 24 hours.

The FbDPs were significantly increased postoperatively in the placebo group ($p < 0.01$) (Fig. 2). Low levels returned 24 hours after surgery, although levels were above the normal range. The two higher-dose aprotinin groups revealed only a slight postoperative elevation, whereas the lowest-dosed aprotinin group (pump prime only) had a pattern similar to the placebo group with significantly elevated levels post-surgery ($p < 0.05$).

Correlations were found between the FgDP levels and blood loss in the placebo group (0.962) and in the pump-prime-treated group (0.535), whereas there was no

**TABLE 3.**  Blood Loss and Transfusions

| Group | 24-Hr Blood Loss (ml) | Patients Transfused | | | |
|---|---|---|---|---|---|
| | | None | Platelets | RBCs | Multiple |
| High-dose aprotinin | 306 ± 53 | 2 | 0 | 8 | 1 |
| Low-dose aprotinin | 426 ± 92 | 6 | 2 | 2 | 1 |
| 2-MU pump prime | 546 ± 67* | 2 | 1 | 3 | 1 |
| Placebo | 658 ± 130* | 2 | 1 | 1 | 3 |
| Total | | 12/36 | 4/36 | 14/36 | 6/36 |

*$p < 0.02$ vs. group I.

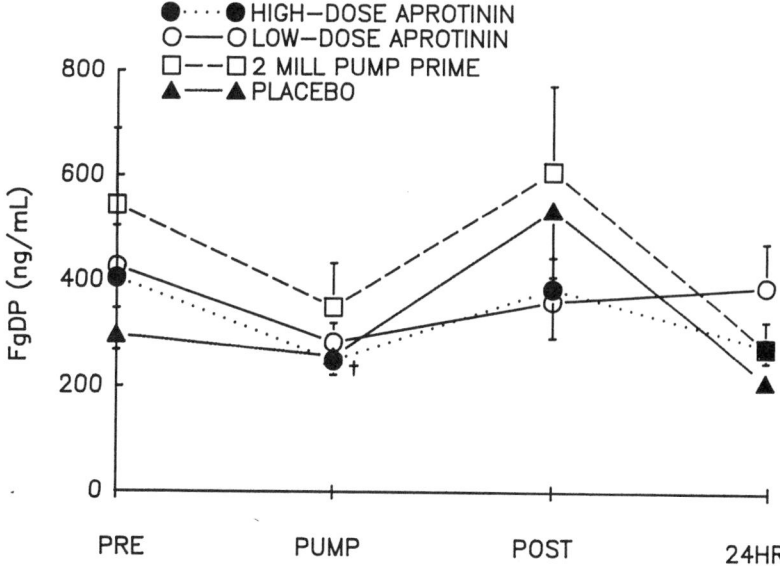

**FIGURE 1.** Fibrinogen degradation products (FgDP). Blood samples were collected from redo-CABG patients preoperatively prior to aprotinin administration after 30 minutes on-pump, immediately after administration of protamine (post-pump), and 24 hours after surgery. The mean level of FgDPs is depicted for each aprotinin/placebo treatment group. The dagger (†) indicates $p < 0.05$ versus preoperative value.

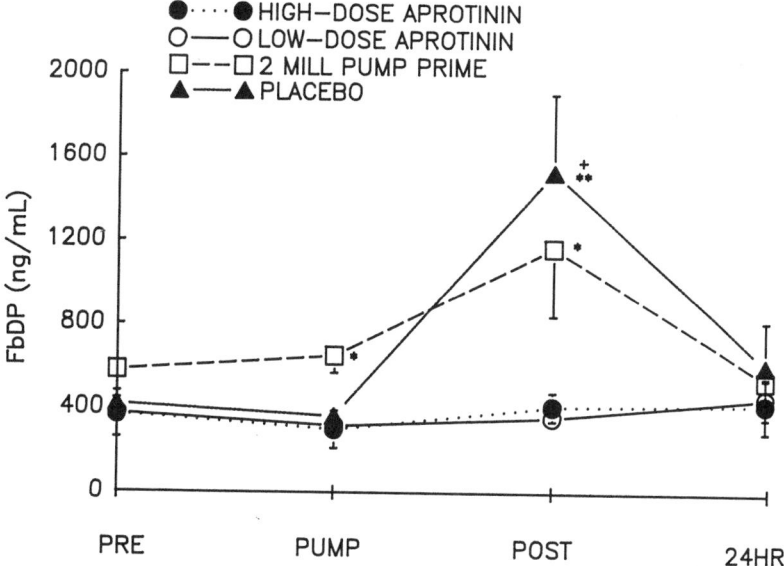

**FIGURE 2.** Fibrin degradation products (FbDP). Blood samples were collected from redo-CABG patients preoperatively prior to aprotinin administration, after 30 minutes on-pump, immediately after administration of protamine (post-pump), and 24 hours after surgery. The mean level of FbDPs is depicted for each aprotinin/placebo treatment group. The single asterisk (*) indicates $p < 0.05$ and the double asterisk (**), $p < 0.01$ versus the high-dose aprotinin value; the dagger (†) indicates $p < 0.01$ versus the preoperative value.

correlation in the two higher aprotinin-dosed groups. There was an overall correlation for all patients ($n$ = 36) between blood loss and FbDP levels (0.451). In the placebo group, a correlation between blood loss and FbDP was obtained (0.560), as well as for the pump-prime-treated group (0.442). There was no correlation between bood loss and FbDP in the two higher-dosed aprotinin groups.

Plasminogen activity levels significantly decreased on-pump ($p < 0.01$) and slowly elevated to near preoperative levels by 24 hours after surgery (Fig. 3) in all groups. The high-dose aprotinin group showed the lowest levels during surgery ($p < 0.01$).

In the three aprotinin groups, tPA levels showed a slight decrease on-pump, with an increase over preoperative levels at the postoperative blood draw (Fig. 4). These levels were near the preoperative levels 24 hours post-surgery, although these levels were higher than the normal range. In the placebo group, however, the postoperative elevation of tPA continued to increase through the next 24 hours ($p < 0.05$).

The inhibitor to tPA, PAI-1 showed a slight on-pump decrease for all groups, followed by a postoperative increase which was more marked in the placebo ($p < 0.05$) and lowest-dosed aprotinin groups (pump prime only; $p < 0.05$) (Fig. 5). At 24 hours post-surgery, a return to preoperative levels was observed only in the aprotinin groups ($p < 0.01$ high dose versus placebo).

Alpha-2 antiplasmin, a major inhibitor of plasmin, revealed elevated activity levels on-pump with all doses of aprotinin ($p < 0.01$ versus placebo) (Fig. 6). Normal activities were observed 24 hours after surgery. The placebo group showed only somewhat decreased activity on-pump, which did not normalize until 24 hours later. Because aprotinin also exhibits antiplasmin activity, the observed elevation in alpha-2 antiplasmin activity may be due to the circulating aprotinin.

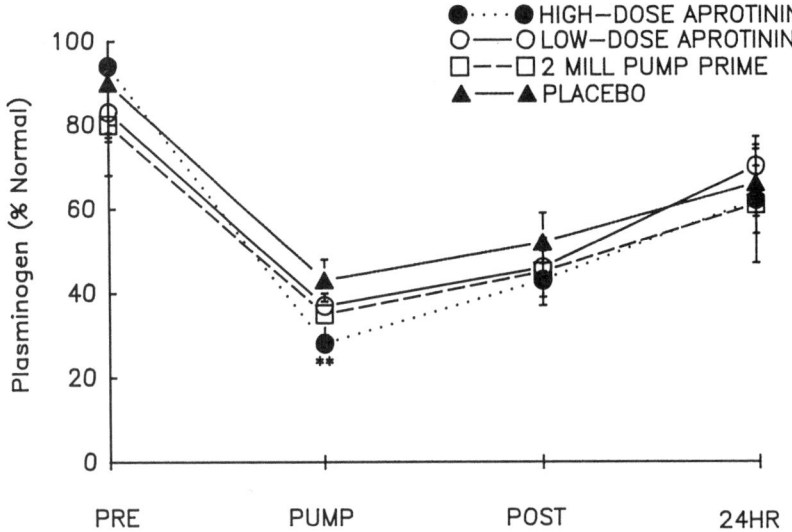

**FIGURE 3.** Plasminogen. Blood samples were collected from redo-CABG patients preoperatively prior to aprotinin administration, after 30 minutes on-pump, immediately after administration of protamine (post-pump), and 24 hours after surgery. The mean level of plasminogen is depicted for each aprotinin/placebo treatment group. The double asterisk (∗∗) indicates $p < 0.01$ versus placebo. All groups are significantly lower than the preoperative values ($p < 0.01$).

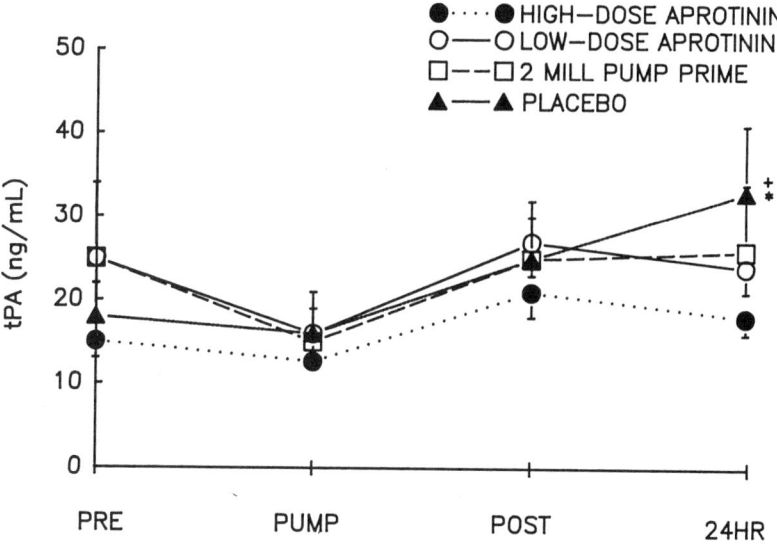

**FIGURE 4.** Tissue plasminogen activator (tPA). Blood samples were collected from redo-CABG patients preoperatively prior to aprotinin administration, after 30 minutes on-pump, immediately after administration of protamine (post-pump), and 24 hours after surgery. The mean level of tPA is depicted for each aprotinin/placebo treatment group. The asterisk (*) indicates $p < 0.05$ versus high-dose aprotinin; the dagger (†), $p < 0.05$ versus on-pump value.

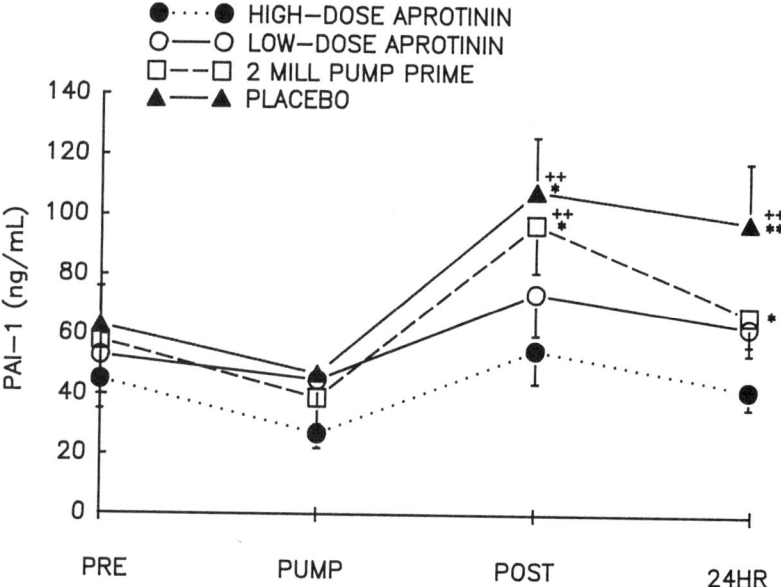

**FIGURE 5.** Plasminogen activator inhibitor (PAI-1). Blood samples were collected from redo-CABG patients preoperatively prior to aprotinin administration, after 30 minutes on-pump, immediately after administration of protamine (post-pump), and 24 hours after surgery. The mean level of PAI-1 is depicted for each aprotinin/placebo treatment group. The single asterisk (*) indicates $p < 0.05$ and the double asterisk (**), $p < 0.01$ versus high-dose aprotinin value; the double dagger (††) indicates $p < 0.01$ versus the on-pump value.

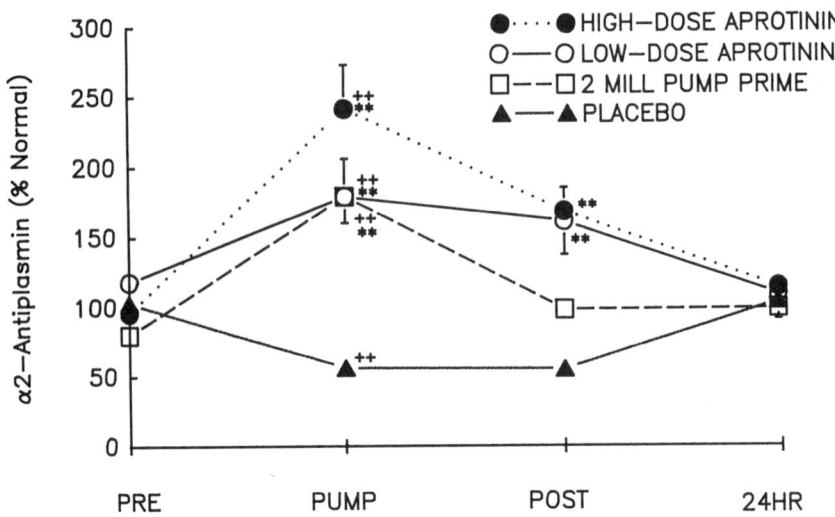

**FIGURE 6.** Alpha-2 antiplasmin. Blood samples were collected from redo-CABG patients preoperatively prior to aprotinin administration, after 30 minutes on-pump, immediately after administration of protamine (post-pump), and 24 hours after surgery. The mean level of alpha-2 antiplasmin is depicted for each aprotinin/placebo treatment group. The double asterisk (∗∗) indicates $p < 0.01$ versus the placebo value; the double dagger (††), $p < 0.01$ versus the preoperative value.

Alpha-2 macroglobulin, a slow-acting inhibitor of plasmin, revealed steadily decreasing activity in the three aprotinin groups on-pump to postoperation, maintaining low levels 24 hours later (Fig. 7). The highest-dosed aprotinin group showed the most marked postoperative decrease ($p < 0.01$). The placebo group overall revealed only a very slight decrease during surgery which lasted through 24 hours.

The actual data on each of the fibrinolytic parameters for patients in the high-dose aprotinin group compared to the placebo group are given in Table 4. A summary of the effect of the high-dose aprotinin on the fibrinolytic system during CPB is given in comparison to the non-aprotinin group in Table 5.

## Discussion

This study reveals that for patients undergoing myocardial revascularization with CPB, fibrinolysis is enhanced with surgery. The levels of tPA, the fibrinolytic activator, and the fibrinolytic inhibitor (PAI-1) are increased *with operation* in comparison with normal values. Considering the 45% hemodilution, tPA levels were more enhanced during sugery than were PAI-1 levels, and plasminogen was 57% decreased, suggesting a consumption in addition to the hemodilution. The natural inhibitors alpha-2 antiplasmin and alpha-2 macroglobulin levels revealed only minor changes with surgery. With the use of aprotinin, the fibrinolytic parameters showed only minor differences from the nonaprotinin (placebo) group *during surgery*. The exception was alpha-2 antiplasmin, which showed very elevated dose-dependent levels in all aprotinin-treated groups. This is in contrast to slightly decreased levels (hemodilution) in the placebo group. Overall, however, the increased fibrinolytic response as seen in the nonaprotinin group was attenuated with the use of

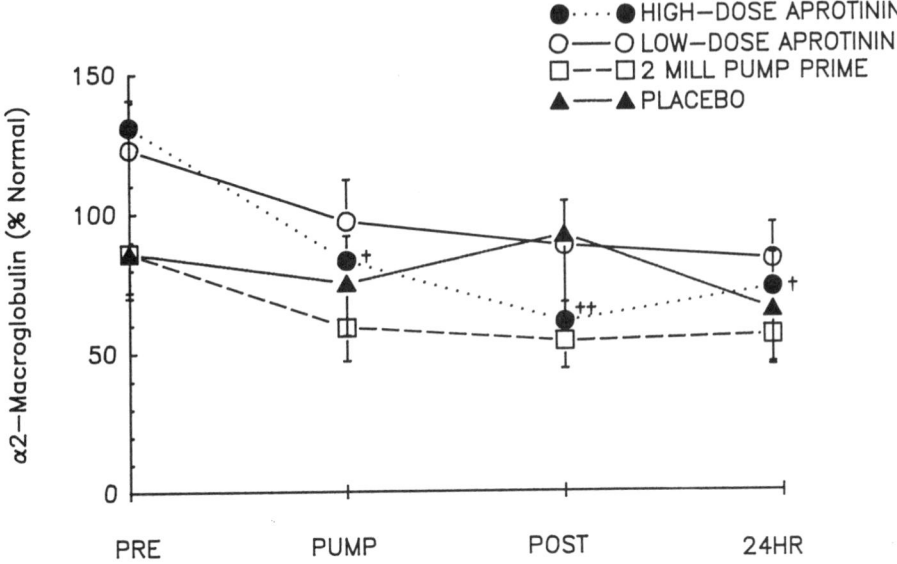

**FIGURE 7.** Alpha-2 macroglobulin. Blood samples were collected from redo-CABG patients preoperatively prior to aprotinin administration, after 30 minutes on-pump, immediately after administration of protamine (post-pump), and 24 hours after surgery. The mean level of alpha-2 macroglobulin is depicted for each aprotinin/placebo treatment group. The single dagger (†) indicates $p < 0.05$ and the double dagger (††), $p < 0.05$ versus the preoperative value.

**TABLE 4.** Fibrinolytic Values in CPB Patients with Aprotinin

| | Normal Range | | CPB Patient on Aprotinin* | CPB Patient w/o Aprotinin† |
|---|---|---|---|---|
| FgDP | 247 ± 27 ng/ml | *Pump* | 249 ± 27 | 257 ± 9 |
| | | *Postop* | 385 ± 93 | 536 ± 128 |
| | | *24 Hr* | 276 ± 29 | 211 ± 5 |
| FbDP | 232 ± 24 ng/ml | *Pump* | 300 ± 89 | 363 ± 32 |
| | | *Postop* | 411 ± 68 | 1527 ± 375 |
| | | *24 Hr* | 426 ± 131 | 607 ± 211 |
| Plasminogen | 80–120% normal | *Pump* | 28 ± 2 | 43 ± 5 |
| | | *Postop* | 43 ± 4 | 52 ± 7 |
| | | *24 Hr* | 62 ± 8 | 66 ± 8 |
| tPA | 1.5–4.5 ng/ml | *Pump* | 13 ± 6 | 16 ± 3 |
| | | *Postop* | 21 ± 3 | 25 ± 5 |
| | | *24 Hr* | 18 ± 2 | 33 ± 8 |
| PAI-1 | 4–48 ng/ml | *Pump* | 27 ± 5 | 47 ± 3 |
| | | *Postop* | 55 ± 11 | 108 ± 18 |
| | | *24 Hr* | 42 ± 6 | 98 ± 20 |
| Alpha-2 anti-plasmin | 80–120% normal | *Pump* | 241 ± 32 | 56 ± 8 |
| | | *Postop* | 168 ± 17 | 55 ± 6 |
| | | *24 Hr* | 114 ± 6 | 104 ± 13 |
| Alpha-2 macro-globulin | 80–120% normal | *Pump* | 83 ± 9 | 75 ± 19 |
| | | *Postop* | 61 ± 7 | 92 ± 29 |
| | | *24 Hr* | 73 ± 12 | 65 ± 19 |

*High-dose aprotinin group. (All data are expressed as mean ± 1 SEM.)
†Placebo group.

**TABLE 5.** Fibrinolytic System Alterations During CPB and Their Modification by Aprotinin*

| | On-Pump | | Post Pump | | 24-Hrs Post-Surgery | |
|---|---|---|---|---|---|---|
| | *CPB Patient on Aprotinin†* | *CPB Patient without Aprotinin‡* | *CPB Patient on Aprotinin†* | *CPB Patient without Aprotinin‡* | *CPB Patient on Aprotinin†* | *CPB Patient without Aprotinin‡* |
| FgDP | ↓ | sl↓↓ | NC | ↑↑ | sl↓ | sl↓ |
| FbDP | sl↓↓ | sl↓↓ | sl↑ | ↑↑ | sl↑ | ↑ |
| Plasminogen | ↓↓ | ↓↓ | ↓↓ | ↓↓ | ↓ | ↓ |
| tPA | sl↓↓ | sl↓↓ | ↑ | ↑ | sl↑ | ↑↑ |
| PAI-1 | sl↓↓ | sl↓↓ | sl↑ | ↑↑ | NC | ↑↑ |
| Alpha-2 anti-plasmin | ↑↑ | ↓ | ↑↑ | ↓ | sl↑ | NC |
| Alpha-2 macro-globulin | ↓ | sl↓↓ | ↓↓ | sl↓↓ | ↓ | sl↓↓ |

*Reference is to preoperative values. NC = no change; sl = slightly.
†High-dose aprotinin group.
‡Placebo group.

aprotinin. This was evidenced by the FbDPs and FgDPs measured on-pump, which were lowest in the high-dose aprotinin group.

After protamine was administered following CPB, there was strong evidence for enhanced fibrinolysis in the nonaprotinin group. FgDPs were increased and FbDPs were markedly increased compared to the aprotinin-treated patients. tPA and PAI-1 levels were more elevated in the nontreated patients. Alpha-2 antiplasmin was slightly decreased postoperatively, as opposed to being increased in the aprotinin patients. Alpha-2 macroglobulin steadily decreased through 24 hours postoperatively with aprotinin, perhaps indicating a consumption of the inhibitor as it bound to plasmin. The increased alpha-2 antiplasmin in the aprotinin patients may have been instrumental in controlling the enhanced fibrinolysis caused by surgery.

Twenty-four hours after surgery, most parameters returned to preoperative levels in the aprotinin groups, with the exception of alpha-2 macroglobulin which remained slightly decreased in all treated groups. Plasminogen remained low in both the aprotinin and placebo groups. FgDPs returned to normal levels 24 hours after surgery from slightly elevated preoperative levels in all groups. Interestingly, the tPA and PAI-1 levels in the non-aprotinin group, which markedly increased postoperatively, remained elevated 24 hours later, whereas the aprotinin-treated groups returned to preoperative levels, again pointing to the decreased fibrinolytic activity in the aprotinin patients.

For the fibrinolytic parameters evaluated, there was a definite dose-dependent response to aprotinin. The data of this study revealed more interindividual responses on all parameters in the two lower-dosed aprotinin-treated groups as compared to the highest dose group. Also the responses in the two lower-dosed aprotinin groups, particularly the pump-prime-group only, were relatively equal to those of the placebo group. This directly correlates with the reduced blood loss in the two higher-dosed aprotinin groups, indicating a relationship between fibrinolysis and postoperative blood loss. Because direct antifibrinolytic agents such as epsilon-aminocaproic acid reduce blood loss,[10,21] and because aprotinin clearly has an antifibrinolytic effect, at least one mechanism by which aprotinin affects blood loss is through reduction of fibrinolytic activation.

Aprotinin, being an inhibitor of plasmin, should by itself effect the functional methods of fibrinolytic parameters—in this study, the chromogenic substrate methods for plasminogen, alpha-2 antiplasmin, and alpha-2 macroglobulin. Patient data obtained using functional assays in the presence of aprotinin may not necessarily reflect true clinical conditions. This may account for the discrepancies found in the literature regarding the increase/decrease/no change of specific fibrinolytic parameters and the extent to which fibrinolysis is affected by aprotinin during surgery with CPB.[4,11,14,17,19] Moreover, attemps at pathophysiologic and mechanistic interpretations made from such data could be misleading, because false plasma levels would be demonstrated. However, the activities should still be relevant to in vivo conditions. On the other hand, blood loss, FgDP, FbDP, fibrinogen, von Willebrand factor, and platelet aggregation can be more reliably assessed, as well as immunologically assayed tPA and PAI-1 as used in this study.

We have shown a concentration-dependent decrease by aprotinin (25–200 µg/ml) on plasminogen in the assay system we used. Based on this, plasminogen was less consumed in the aprotinin patients than indicated by the test results (a false decrease is shown). This is fitting with decreased fibrinolysis. An in vitro effect by aprotinin was not observed in our alpha-2 antiplasmin or alpha-2 macroglobulin assays. However, we remain skeptical of the trueness of the values obtained in the aprotinin patient plasmas by these chromogenic assays.

We suggest that the attenuation of fibrinolysis in the aprotinin patients, as compared to the placebo-treated patients, is due to a combination of direct plasmin inhibition by aprotinin with enhanced natural inhibitor activity. The high activity of alpha-2 antiplasmin coupled with the enhanced activity of alpha-2 macroglobulin (revealed by a stronger consumption) together inhibit plasmin. In addition, tPA and PAI-1 are less affected by the trauma of surgery when aprotinin is used. The acute-phase reaction of these proteins may be blunted by the anti-inflammatory effect of aprotinin via its leukocyte-complement activity. A point of discussion is the very high PAI-1 levels in the placebo group, which should have reduced the fibrinolytic effect. Because this was not observed, we propose a mechanism whereby modulation by protein C attenuates the expected PAI-1 activity. Protein C, which inhibits PAI-1, is inhibited by aprotinin.[6] Therefore, in the aprotinin-treated groups, lowered activity levels of protein C could cause less inhibition of PAI-1 activity, allowing for decreased fibrinolytic activity.

Regarding the platelet-fibrinolysis interaction and the possible effect by aprotinin, others have reported that plasmin decreases platelet activity by internalizing the GPIb (von Willebrand factor) receptors and externalizing the GPIIb/IIIa receptors of the platelet.[5,7] The use of aprotinin during surgery inhibits the generated plasmin, thereby reducing the exposure of the platelet to plasmin.[11] We would add that the increased alpha-2 antiplasmin and PAI-1 activity act further to inhibit plasmin for an additional indirect protection. This reasoning explains an earlier study from our group whereby plasmin and aprotinin added to platelet-rich plasma in vitro did not reduce the inhibitory effect caused by plasmin.[14]

In summary, surgery with CPB produces a high degree of fibrinolysis. This is associated with high levels of tPA, which generate plasmin levels that are not compensated for by alpha-2 antiplasmin, alpha-2 macroglobulin, or PAI-1. With aprotinin at the high dose (Hammersmith regimen), fibrinolysis is significantly reduced, as affected by a lesser elevation of tPA, a dramatically higher activity level of alpha-2 antiplasmin, an enhanced activity of alpha-2 macroglobulin, and probably more active PAI-1 in comparison to the non-aprotinin-treated group. The highest dose of aprotinin in this study (630 mg) gave the most marked differences from the placebo group. The two lower doses of aprotinin (315 and 280 mg) were relatively similar in response to the placebo group. The attenuation of the fibrinolytic activation most likely also had a similar effect on platelet activation and coagulation activation by reducing the indirect effects of plasmin on these systems. The combined effects on these complex systems by the broad-spectrum inhibitor aprotinin are translated into decreased blood loss in the surgical patient.

## Acknowledgment

The authors are sincerely grateful to Harry L. Messmore, M.D., for helpful advice on this chapter and to Yelena Khenkina, M.S., for skillful technical assistance.

## References

1. Bick RL: Physiology and pathology of hemostasis during cardiac surgery. In Pifarré R (ed): Anticoagulation, Hemostasis, and Blood Preservation in Cardiovascular Surgery. Philadelphia, Hanley & Belfus, 1993, pp 23–55.
2. Bidstrup BP, Royston D, Sapsford RN, Taylor KM: Reduction in blood loss and blood use after cardiopulmonary bypass with high dose aprotinin (Trasylol). J Thorac Cardiovasc Surg 97:364–372, 1989.
3. Blakeman BP, Sullivan HJ: Surgical consideration for postoperative bleeding. In Pifarré R (ed): Anticoagulation, Hemostasis, and Blood Preservation in Cardiovascular Surgery. Philadelphia, Hanley & Belfus, 1993, pp 271–285.
4. Blauhut B, Gross C, Necek S, et al: Effects of high-dose aprotinin on blood loss, platelet function, fibrinolysis, complement, and renal function after cardiopulmonary bypass. J Thorac Cardiovasc Surg 101:958–967, 1991.
5. Cramer EM, Lu H, Caen JP, et al: Differential redistribution of platelet glycoproteins Ib and IIb-IIIa after plasmin stimulation. Blood 77:694–699, 1991.
6. España F, Estelles A, Griffin JH, et al: Aprotinin (Trasylol) is a competitive ihibitor of activated protein C. Thromb Res 56:751–756, 1989.
7. Federici AB, Berkowitz SD, Lattuada A, Mannucci PM: Degradation of von Willebrand factor in patients with acquired clinical conditions in which there is heightened proteolysis. Blood 81:720–725, 1993.
8. Fritz H, Wunderer G: Biochemistry and applications of aprotinin, the kallikrein inhibitor from bovine organs. Arzneimittelforschung 33:479–494, 1983.
9. Havel M, Teufelsbauer H, Knöbl P, et al: Effect of intraoperative aprotinin administration on postoperative bleeding in patients undergoing cardiopulmonary bypass operation. J Thorac Cardiovasc Surg 101:968–972, 1991.
10. Horrow JC, Hlavacek J, Strong MD, et al: Prophylactic tranexamic acid decreases bleeding after cardiac operations. J Thorac Cardiovasc Surg 99:70–75, 1990.
11. Huang H, Ding W, Su Z, Zhang W: Mechanism of the preserving effect of aprotinin on platelet function and its use in cardiac surgery. J Thorac Cardiovasc Surg 106:11–18, 1993.
12. John LC, Rees GM, Kovacs IB: Reduction of heparin binding to and inhibition of platelets by aprotinin. Ann Thorac Surg 55:1175–1179, 1993.
13. Levy JH, Pifarré R, Schaaf H, et al: A multicenter, double blind, placebo-controlled trial of aprotinin for reducing blood loss and the requirements for donor blood transfusion in patients undergoing repeat coronary artery bypass grafting. (In press.)
14. Louie MI, Koza MJ, Hoppensteadt D, et al: The effect of aprotinin on platelet function in cardiopulmonary bypass (CBP) patients. Thromb Haemost 69:708, 1993.
15. Loza JP, Gurewich V, Johnstone M, Pannell R: Platelet bound prekallikrein promotes pro-urokinase-induced clot lysis: A mechanism for targeting the factor XII dependent intrinsic pathway of fibrinolysis. Thromb Haemost 71:347–352, 1994.
16. Mammen EF, Koets MH, Washington BC, et al: Hemostasis changes during cardiopulmonary bypass surgery. Semin Thromb Hemost 11:281–292, 1985.
17. Marx G, Pokar H, Reuter H, et al: The effects of aprotinin on hemostatic function during cardiac surgery. J Cardiothorac Vasc Anesth 5:467–474, 1991.

18. Matzdorff AC, Green D, Cohen I, Bauer KC: Effect of recombinant aprotinin on platelet activation in patients undergoing open heart surgery. Haemostasis 23:293–300, 1993.
19. Orchard MA, Goodchild CS, Prentice CRM, et al: Aprotinin reduces cardiopulmonary bypass-induced blood loss and inhibits fibrinolysis without influencing platelets. Br J Haematol 85:533–541, 1993.
20. Pintigny D, Dachary-Prigent J: Aprotinin can inhibit the proteolytic activity of thrombin: A fluorescence and an enzymatic study. Eur J Biochem 207:89–95, 1992.
21. Taylor KM: Effect of aprotinin on blood loss and blood use after cardiopulmonary bypass. In Pifarré R (ed): Anticoagulation, Hemostasis, and Blood Preservation in Cardiovascular Surgery. Philadelphia, Hanley & Belfus, 1993, pp 129–145.
22. van den Besselaar AM, Dirven R, Bertina RM: Tissue factor-induced coagulation can be inhibited by aprotinin (Trasylol) [letter]. Thromb Haemost 69:298–299, 1993.
23. van Oeveren W, Harder MP, Roozendaal KJ, et al: Aprotinin protects platelets against the initial effect of cardiopulmonary bypass. J Thorac Cardiovasc Surg 99:788–797, 1990.
24. Wendel HP, Heller W, Galleinere MJ: Aprotinin in therapeutic doses inhibits chromogenic peptide substrate assays for protein C. Thromb Res 74:543–548, 1994.

John Francis, PhD, MRCPath

# 10
# Effects of Aprotinin on White Cells and Hemostasis

In the last decade there has been increasing resistance to the use of homologous blood transfusion for patients undergoing surgical procedures. Fears about transmissible diseases, shortages of donor blood, and even recurrence of malignant solid tumors following perioperative transfusion have stimulated the development of alternative ways of maintaining the patient's red cell volume during surgery. This has led to the development and application of predeposit autologous transfusion, autotransfusion, and pharmacologic ways of reducing perioperative bleeding.[41] The biochemical basis for the latter purpose is not well defined because the nontechnical causes of bleeding during surgery are poorly understood. Indeed, from our present understanding of the hemostatic process, such drugs might even be expected to increase bleeding or potentiate thrombosis.

## Pathogenesis of Surgical Bleeding

Excluding technical causes, why some patients bleed excessively during surgery is not known. Apart from liver transplantation and cardiopulmonary bypass surgery, relatively little work has been performed in this area. Most surgical units do not perform routine hemostatic screening preoperatively unless there is a positive personal or family history, and it is probably not economically viable to do so. Although a few previously undiagnosed congenital clotting factor deficiencies or platelet defects may present with excessive peri- and postoperative bleeding, most surgical bleeders have normal screening test results.

The postoperative behavior of coagulation factors is well established, but the perioperative changes have been less well investigated. Changes in coagulation proteins during surgery are rarely of sufficient magnitude to cause bleeding, and attention has therefore focused on the effect of surgery on the fibrinolytic system. Early studies suggested that the fibrinolytic system becomes hyperactive during major surgery,[84] although more detailed assessments were hampered by lack of appropriate laboratory methods at that time. The more recent development of techniques for measuring tissue plasminogen activator (tPA) have made it possible to demonstrate increases in fibrinolytic potential. Because tPA is normally cleared rapidly by the liver, extremely high blood levels occur during the anhepatic stage of liver transplantation and are thought to cause the severe bleeding that may accompany this procedure.[33,100] Johnson et al.[66] noted a sevenfold increase in tPA in 7 of 12 patients undergoing major abdominal surgery, whereas the other 5 individuals showed no such elevation. Because all patients had similar increases in fibrinopeptide A, coagulation was activated to the same extent. Thus, the fibrinolytic response to surgery may be very variable and might explain why only some patients bleed excessively.

A detailed study of the intraoperative changes in hemostasis in general surgery was recently reported by Kamayashi et al.[69] Activation of coagulation, as evidenced by elevation of fibrinopeptide A, occurred immediately after surgery, presumably related to the exposure of tissue factor in surgically damaged tissue. Reductions in circulating platelets, at least in gastric and liver resections, were minimal. The fibrinolytic system was markedly activated during surgery, as indicated by a pronounced rise in B-beta$_{15-42}$ fragment, a peptide cleaved from intact fibrinogen by plasmin. Comparison of the fibrinopeptide A and B-beta$_{15-42}$ levels suggested that fibrinolytic activation was greater than that of coagulation during surgical procedures.

The most extensive studies of hemostasis in surgery have been performed in patients undergoing cardiopulmonary bypass (CPB). Platelet counts fall during bypass,[96] accompanied by a marked reduction in platelet function,[86] increased bleeding times, and loss of fibrinogen receptors on the platelet membrane.[133] Preoperative use of aspirin, which interferes with platelet prostaglandin metabolism, increases blood loss in CPB.[87] Prothrombin times, activated partial thromboplastin times, and thrombin clotting times are prolonged during bypass,[5] although this cannot be attributed entirely to intravascular coagulation or hyperfibrinolysis.[88] Increased fibrinolysis is a common response to CPB,[8] increasing immediately on starting bypass and persisting throughout.[74] This fibrinolysis is due to increased tPA levels,[50,116] and increased fibrinolytic activity has been linked to the probability of bleeding.[51] Recent evidence has suggested that both complement activation and loss of platelets may be prevented by coating the bypass tubing and oxygenator with heparin.[128] This also may reduce the need for systemic heparinization, although detailed clinical studies of this approach have not yet been reported. In summary, increased fibrinolytic activity seems to be the most likely hemostatic cause of bleeding during surgery, probably due to inappropriately rapid degradation of hemostatic plugs in anastomoses and wounds. Variable impairment of platelet function interfering with primary hemostasis remains another possibility, especially in surgery associated with CPB. Potential pathways of hemostatic activation in CPB that are potential targets for aprotinin therapy are shown in Figure 1.

## Aprotinin

Aprotinin has been in clinical use for a number of years, largely as a suggested treatment for acute pancreatitis. It is a serine proteinase inhibitor obtained from bovine lung and is a relatively small molecule, having a molecular weight of 6512 and comprising 58 amino acid residues. Because of its relatively short plasma half-life, aprotinin must be given intravenously to achieve adequate blood levels, although

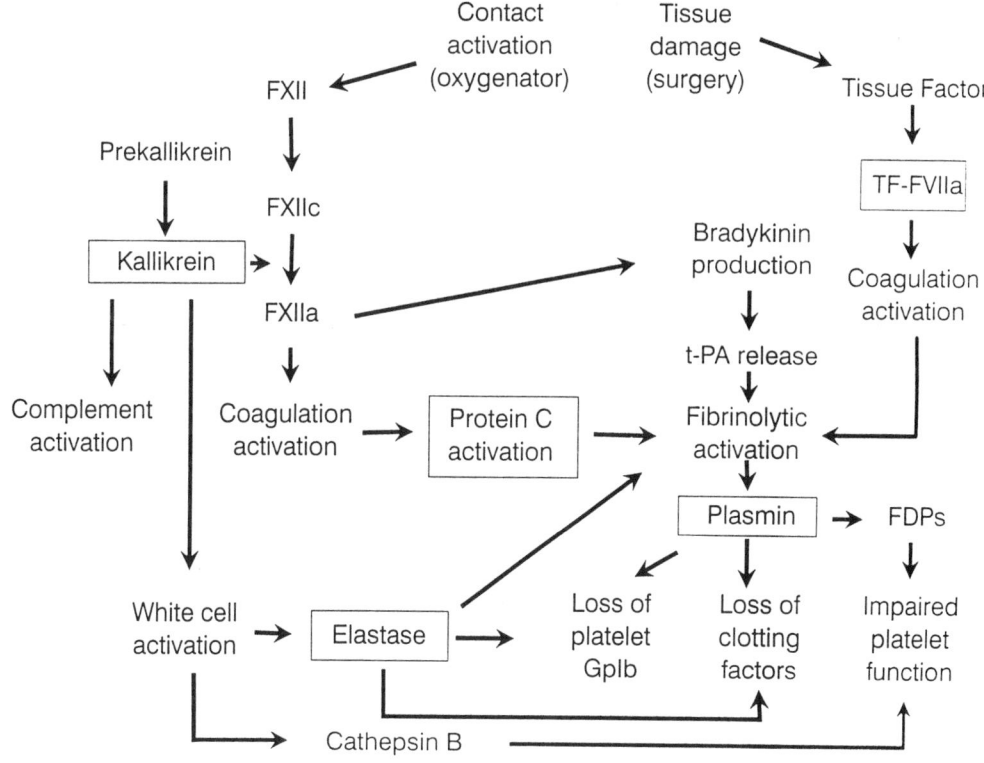

**FIGURE 1.** Potential pathways of hemostatic activation during CPB and theoretical targets *(boxed)* for the action of aprotinin.

exactly what is adequate remains controversial. It is regarded primarily as a fibrinolytic inhibitor and, for this reason, has been used to reduce blood loss in clinical situations associated with hyperfibrinolysis. These applications are given more detailed consideration elsewhere in this book and are reviewed only briefly here.

### Aprotinin in Cardiac Surgery

Aprotinin has been used in cardiac surgery for over 25 years, although its use in the high doses required to control perioperative bleeding is more recent. Early reports noted that aprotinin, given in total doses of 200,000–300,000 kallikrein-inhibiting units (KIU), had a beneficial effect on the hyperfibrinolysis associated with open-heart surgery but had little effect on blood loss.[83,120] A dose of 100,000 KIU/hr throughout surgery, however, significantly reduced the need for donor blood.[3] Further studies in Germany supported the potential for aprotinin in reducing blood loss and suggested that the effect might be dose-dependent.[52,63] More details of these early studies are given in a recent review.[104]

The use of **high-dose** aprotinin in open-heart surgery was actually designed to minimize the damaging effects of CPB on the lung. The rationale for this use was to block kallikrein and complement activation and thus reduce the inflammatory response induced by contact of the blood with the surface of the oxygenator. Because the concentration of aprotinin required to inhibit kallikrein is around 200 KIU/ml, a dose regimen designed to achieve this level was formulated. However, the most striking observation in the resultant pilot study[125] was the 50% reduction in blood loss. In fact, the target level of 200 KIU/ml was not achieved in this study, and subsequent trials therefore employed a loading dose of $2 \times 10^6$ KIU, a continuous infusion of $0.5 \times 10^6$ KIU/hr, and addition of a further $2 \times 10^6$ KIU to the pump prime.

Patients undergoing repeat open-heart surgery tend to bleed heavily, and aprotinin was especially beneficial in these cases.[105] Subsequent studies in uncomplicated open-heart surgery have confirmed the hemostatic effect of aprotinin, most studies reporting reductions in blood loss and transfusion requirements of around 40–50%.[2,11,13,30,32,40,53,55,113] Combination with autotransfusion may further reduce the need for donor blood in open-heart surgery.[2,107] Simply adding 2 MU of aprotinin to the pump prime was thought to be as effective as continuous infusion,[22] but this has not been confirmed by others.[126,127]

High-dose aprotinin resulted in an 8- to 10-fold reduction in blood loss in patients with septic endocarditis having open-heart surgery[12] and a four-fold decrease in aspirin-treated patients.[10] Thus, aprotinin may have a proportionately greater effect in patients who have the greatest blood loss. The hemostatic effect of aprotinin in aspirin-treated patients may be of considerable clinical importance, because there is some debate over whether aspirin should be discontinued before cardiac surgery, despite the increased blood loss usually encountered.[114,129] In pediatric cardiac surgery, the blood-saving effect was much less than in adults, possibly due to the more meticulous approach taken by pediatric surgeons.[15,36] However, because the time to chest closure was significantly shorter in aprotinin-treated patients[36] and postoperative bleeding seemed less,[31] aprotinin has been deemed effective in the pediatric setting. Finally, the beneficial effect of aprotinin may not be confined to the perioperative period. The drug also reduces post-CPB blood loss, even at relatively low doses,[4] although the prophylactic use of high-dose aprotinin throughout the operative period is almost certainly preferable.[9] Aprotinin has also been effective in reducing the bleeding associated with prolonged extracorporeal membrane oxygenation (ECMO).[20]

### Aprotinin in Liver Transplantation

Bleeding during liver transplantation is a major problem. Because the liver is the site of synthesis of most clotting factors and is responsible for clearing activated clotting factors from the circulation, most patients with serious liver disease have a coagulopathy. The anhepatic stage of transplantation is associated with marked hyperfibrinolysis and a bleeding diathesis.[33,100] High-dose aprotinin has significantly reduced blood loss, blood transfusion requirements, and operation time in patients undergoing orthotopic liver transplants.[23,82,90,111] Continuous-infusion aprotinin therapy appears better than repeated bolus injection in patients undergoing liver transplantation.[59]

### Aprotinin in Vascular Surgery

High-dose aprotinin was used in an open pilot study of 20 patients undergoing reconstructive surgery for aortoiliac occlusive disease.[118] Blood loss during surgery fell from a median of 1300 ml in the control group (*n* = 10) to 735 ml in aprotinin-treated patients. The median volume of transfused blood fell from 3 U to zero, and surgeons were impressed with the lack of bleeding from the wound edges and raw areas. A more extensive double-blind, placebo-controlled trial in this type of surgery has recently been completed in Southampton, England, and should be reported soon.

### Other Types of Surgery

At the time of writing, no controlled clinical trials of high-dose aprotinin have been conducted in other types of surgery. Aprotinin has been used at lower doses in neurosurgery, orthopedic surgery, and urologic surgery with varying degrees of success,[104] and it therefore seems probable that the high-dose regimen would prove reasonably effective in any type of surgery associated with significant blood loss.

A double-blind trial of aprotinin in neurosurgery (menignioma and acoustic schwannoma) is currently being conducted in Southampton, England, and will be completed before the end of 1994. We have recently described a patient who bled excessively during a craniotomy to remove a glioblastoma.[95] The patient developed the clinical and laboratory picture of acute hyperfibrinolysis and was given 30,000 KIU/kg of aprotinin intravenously, followed by 10,000 KIU/kg/hr for the next 6 hours. There was a rapid and marked improvement in the laboratory abnormalities, especially the thromboelastogram (Fig. 2), and bleeding was controlled. We have noted that many patients about to undergo surgery for removal of meningioma have laboratory evidence of hyperfibrinolysis.[94] Many of these bleed excessively during surgery, and it is therefore reasonable to assume that aprotinin, as a potent antifibrinolytic agent, may be efficacious.

## Mechanism of Action of Aprotinin

### Effects on Fibrinolysis

Aprotinin is a broad-spectrum inhibitor of serine proteinases, and many components and interactions of the hemostatic pathway are therefore potential targets of its action (Table 1). In particular, aprotinin is a potent inhibitor of plasmin, the major fibrinolytic enzyme, and kallikrein, important in the initiation of the whole-body

A

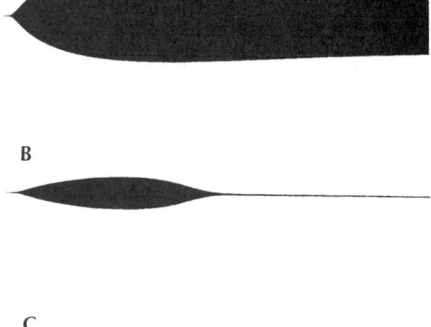

**FIGURE 2.** Effect of aprotinin on acute hyperfibrinolysis developing during neurosurgery as indicated by thromboelastography. *A*, preoperative; *B*, shortly after craniotomy during hemorrhagic crisis; *C*, 2 hours after aprotinin infusion.

B

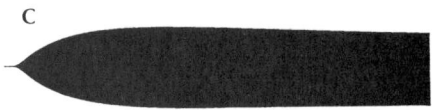

C

**TABLE 1.** Summary of Aprotinin's Reported Effects on Hemostatic Pathways

Fibrinolysis
  Inhibits plasmin directly
  Inhibits tPA release

Coagulation
  Inhibits plasma kallikrein*[†]
  Prevents loss of C1-esterase inhibitor activity by heparin[†]
  Inhibits the tissue factor–factor VIIa complex
  Binds and inhibits thrombin[‡]
  Inhibits activated protein C

Platelets
  Prevents loss of GPIb[§]
  Prevents thrombin-induced platelet aggregation
  Shortens bleeding time[§]
  Prevents impaired platelet function due to FDP
  Ameliorates drug-induced platelet function defects
  Reduces heparin binding

Endothelial cells
  Reduces platelet adherence
  Enhances von Willebrand factor synthesis
  Reduces thrombomodulin expression (?)
  Affects tissue factor expression (?)

Neutrophil function
  Inhibits in vivo neutrophil activation during surgery
  Prevents elastase release[§]
    Interfering wiht fibrinolytic activation
    Preventing degradation of coagulation factors
    Preventing platelet membrane damage

* Interfering with fibrinolytic and neutrophil activation.
† Of questionable significance for coagulation.
‡ Whether this occurs in vivo has not been demonstrated.
§ Currently controversial.

inflammatory response. However, it does not affect complement activation in CPB,[125] another central component in this process.[72] As noted earlier, hyperfibrinolysis may be an important cause of surgical bleeding, particularly in CPB and liver transplants, and this appears to be largely inhibited by aprotinin.[61,82,113] In liver transplantation, the anhepatic stage is characterized by marked shortening of the euglobulin clot lysis time and corresponding increases in tPA and cross-linked fibrin degradation products (FDP),[61] which are not observed in aprotinin-treated patients.[82] These effects are presumably related to direct inhibition of plasmin or an effect on the release of tPA[61] since aprotinin is not a a good inhibitor of tPA itself.[77] An effect on tPA release might be mediated via inhibition of kallikrein and thus bradykinin, a potent stimulator of tPA release.[61] Levels of kallikrein-like activity are lower in aprotinin-treated patients undergoing CPB, whereas kallikrein inhibition levels are much higher.[46] CPB-induced increases in plasma fibrinolytic activity are considerably greater than the increase in tPA antigen.[93] This is probably because circulating tPA is bound to PAI-1 before bypass, which then releases tPA in the absence of a corresponding increase in the inhibitor. Thus, the newly released tPA remains active in the circulation.[93] Aprotinin has no effect on tPA activity, tPA antigen, or PAI-1, and it therefore seems reasonable to assume that this agent inhibits only the formed plasmin.[83,93] Aprotinin is also an inhibitor of activated protein C,[37] which might offer an alternative explanation for its effect on fibrinolytic activation.

Even though aprotinin does not inhibit tPA directly, it markedly reduces cutaneous bleeding in rabbits,[26] dogs,[48] and rats[28] given recombinant tPA. Tranexamic acid is ineffective in this regard, although both agents reduce the incidence of cerebral bleeding in the rat model.[28] Presumably, the mechanisms of skin and cerebral bleeding due to tPA are different.

### Effects on Coagulation

Aprotinin acts as an inhibitor of the intrinsic coagulation pathway, as evidenced by a prolongation of the activated clotting time (ACT), even before the administration of heparin.[32] Aprotinin appears to act synergistically with heparin to give much longer ACTs than would normally be expected for a given heparin level[29,32,53,62,89] and has similar effects on the activated partial thromboplastin time (aPTT).[29] There is also marked variation in the sensitivity of different commercially available aPTT reagents to aprotinin, which is not related to their heparin sensitivity.[42] Thus, aprotinin seems to act as an anticoagulant yet *reduces* perioperative bleeding, an observation that seems to be at variance with our current understanding of the hemostatic mechanism. Because of this effect, it has been suggested that protamine neutralization should be based on the amount of heparin actually given and should not be calculated using the ACT.[89] Indeed, the improved hemostasis during surgery, despite the more prolonged ACT, might even obviate the need for protamine neutralization at the end of bypass.[53] This would allow retransfusion through cardiotomy suction to be continued and could thus double the volume of blood saved intraoperatively. Hunt et al.[62] have recommended that for CPB, the ACT should be run at times in excess of 750 seconds until the effects of aprotinin on postoperative thrombotic complications are accurately known. The main inhibitor of contact activation, C1-esterase inhibitor, loses some of its activity against beta-factor XIIa in the presence of heparin.[47] Aprotinin can antagonize this effect, which may add to its inhibitory activity against the contact pathway. Whether aprotinin's effect on intrinsic coagulation has any significant anticoagulant effect in vivo is debatable, as the role of contact activation of blood coagulation now seems physiologically less relevant.[18,19]

Although it has been widely assumed that intrinsic coagulation is activated through surface contact in CPB, recent data from studies using modern molecular markers have indicated that clotting activation probably occurs via the tissue factor–factor VIIa (extrinsic) pathway.[14] This is interesting in the light of studies showing that aprotinin may inhibit extrinsic coagulation through an effect on the tissue factor–factor VIIa complex.[122] Inhibition is apparently directed toward the active site of factor VIIa, but the presence of tissue factor is an absolute requirement and aprotinin does not inhibit factor Xa per se.[24] These findings may be significant in the pathogenesis of hyperfibrinolysis during CPB, which may result from clotting activation during the procedure despite the presence of high levels of heparin.[79,117] Levels of soluble tissue factor rise during CPB, and this rise was prevented by aprotinin.[71] However, as the source of plasma tissue factor has not been established, these data are difficult to interpret. Similarly, rises in plasma thrombomodulin levels during bypass can be prevented by aprotinin, without affecting the levels of proteins C and S.[16] This may reflect reduction in platelet activation and/or endothelial cell damage, a possibility that warrants further study.

The moderate anticoagulant effect of aprotinin was demonstrated by Lu et al.[79] and Orchard et al.,[93] who showed that levels of the thrombin–antithrombin III

(TAT) complex were lower following bypass than in placebo-treated individuals. However, aprotinin did not inhibit the marked rise in TAT that occurred after reversal of heparin therapy by protamine sulfate.[93] This tends to confirm the in vitro impression that a significant anticoagulant effect only occurs in the presence of heparin. In in vitro experiments, aprotinin is able to bind directly to thrombin, interfering with its ability to clot fibrinogen, cleave appropriate chromogenic substrates, and induce platelet aggregation.[97] Whether any of these activities are significant in vivo, at the doses employed, remains to be demonstrated.

In summary, the available evidence suggests that aprotinin has a moderate anticoagulant effect. Clearly this does not contribute to bleeding on the basis of clinical studies. However, it may be that lessening the degree of clotting activation, especially via the more "explosive" tissue factor pathway, helps to reduce plasmin generation by proportionally decreasing the amount of reactive fibrinolysis.

### Effects on Platelets

As detailed earlier, platelet number and function are both reduced during CPB, and this effect has been strongly implicated as a cause of bleeding during this procedure. Aprotinin has been claimed to preserve platelet-mediated hemostasis, although the mechanism of this effect is not entirely clear.[30,88,123-125,134] CPB is associated with a loss of the platelet membrane receptors involved in platelet adhesion and aggregation,[49] and this is prevented by aprotinin. The decrease in the ability of platelets to adhere is due to loss of the glycoprotein Ib receptor for von Willebrand factor.[123] Because the fibrinolytic enzyme plasmin is known to be capable of cleaving this receptor[1] and is probably inhibited by aprotinin, fibrinolytic activation was thought to offer a possible explanation for the loss of platelet function during CPB.[123]

Later work by van Oeveren et al.,[124] however, showed that the type Ib adhesive glycoproteins fell by 50% within 5 minutes of starting bypass but remained unaffected in aprotinin-treated patients. Although fibrinolysis was effectively inhibited by aprotonin, it was not apparent in controls until the end of bypass. Marked improvement of hemostasis (40% reduction in bleeding and transfusion requirements) was noted from the start of the procedure, and the authors therefore concluded that the preservation of platelet adhesive capacity was directly responsible for the reduction in blood loss. Furthermore, the loss of glycoprotein Ib occurred during the first pass of blood through the bypass circuit. The rapidity of this change, coupled with the recent demonstration that glycoprotein Ib-derived glycocalicin levels in plasma are not increased during CPB, has cast further doubt on the case for plasmin-mediated cleavage of membrane receptors.[70,78,93] In addition, earlier studies of platelet glycoprotein Ib employed gel-filtered platelets, thereby introducing the potential for an artefactual reduction in adhesive capacity through activation in vitro. When studied by whole blood flow cytometric assays which do not share this problem, no reduction in platelet membrane glycoprotein Ib was noted.[70,93] In addition, aprotinin did not ameliorate the CPB-induced reduction in ristocetin-induced platelet agglutination and collagen-induced aggregation.[93] Finally, aprotinin does not inhibit the rise in beta thromboglobulin induced by CPB, and thus it seems unlikely that plasmin plays a significant role in platelet activation under these circumstances, at least in vivo.[93] In contrast, in vitro experiments have shown that incubation of plasmin with washed platelets decreased ristocetin-induced aggregation in a dose-dependent fashion and reduced the amount of membrane glycoprotein Ib.[60] These effects were greatly lessened by pretreating the platelets with aprotinin. These authors noted similar changes during CPB, and it seems likely that the discrepancies between published studies are due to methodologic differences in testing platelet function. Interestingly, using a novel method of assessing the platelet contribution to primary hemostasis (hemostatometry) heparin was shown to significantly inhibit platelet function, an effect that could be reduced by aprotinin.[68] Aprotinin prevented binding of heparin to both activated and nonactivated platelets, suggesting that this may be a mechanism by which aprotinin preserves platelet function in CPB. Further studies of this phenomenon might be illuminating.

Edmunds and colleagues[35] recently proposed an alternative hypothesis based on the findings that plasmin exerts a direct effect on platelet aggregation and release and prolongs the bleeding time in rabbits. Platelets incubated with kallikrein also lost their ability to respond to thrombin. Thus, inhibition of plasmin and kallikrein by aprotinin could attenuate the platelet function defect and shorten bleeding times. However, Orchard and colleagues[93] showed that bleeding times were not influenced by aprotinin, being greatly prolonged ($> 30$ min) in both aprotinin and placebo-treated patients. This finding suggests that prolongation of bleeding time during CPB is mediated by factors other than plasmin, e.g., hypothermia. Plasmin is also responsible for the generation of FDP. Aprotinin reduces FDP levels during CPB, and because these fragments have significant antiplatelet activity, this may offer yet another explanation for the apparent protective effect of this drug on platelet function.[54]

Synthesis of von Willebrand factor by endothelial cells is not reduced by aprotinin[102] and may actually be increased,[56] an effect that is enhanced by prior thrombin stimulation.[56] Aprotinin reduced platelet adherence to endothelial cells and to plastic or collagen-coated tissue culture wells by a mechanism that was apparently independent of nitric oxide.[103] Whether these phenomena are important in vivo, however, remains to be demonstrated. As attractive as the "platelet preservation" theory might be, whatever the mechanism of this effect, it is not entirely sufficient to explain the ability of aprotinin to reduce blood loss. Improvements in the design of bypass equipment, including the introduction of membrane oxygenators, have reduced the damage to circulating blood platelets to the point where platelet counts are not reduced during CPB. Nevertheless, significantly bleeding may still occur and can be reduced by aprotinin.[53] Surgery other than that associated with CPB is not usually accompanied by pronounced loss of platelet function, and indeed, aprotinin has been effective in controlling bleeding in patients with severe thrombocytopenia.[44,101]

Interestingly, whereas ε-aminocaproic acid has also been shown to have beneficial effects in thrombocytopenia,[6] tranexamic acid had no effect on thrombocytopenic bleeding.[45] Aprotinin also reduces blood loss in patients having recently ingested aspirin and who are at greater risk of surgical bleeding.[10] Aspirin irreversibly interferes with platelet prostaglandin metabolism, and although this does not affect adhesion, it impairs subsequent platelet aggregation and platelet plug formation. This accounts for the increased skin bleeding times characteristic of aspirin ingestion. The observation that aprotinin can correct the excessive bleeding in patients on aspirin who subsequently undergo cardiac bypass surgery is difficult to reconcile with a platelet preservation effect since the platelets are already irreversibly compromised before surgery. Similarly, aprotinin markedly reduced bleeding time in rats treated with clopidogrel, a ticlopidine analog, in a dose-dependent manner.[57]

Presumably, intact adhesive capability is more important for surgical hemostasis than an intact aggregation response.

### Effects on White Blood Cells

Neutrophils are recruited rapidly to the site of an injury. Several components of the early inflammatory response are chemotactic for neutrophils, including platelet-derived products and fibrin fragments. The neutrophil contains many hydrolytic enzymes that can be released when the cell becomes "activated," although the best studied in relation to hemostasis is elastase.

There appear to be several triggers for the release of neutrophil elastease, but of relevance to the present discussion is that kallikrein may be responsible for some 30% of the total elastase release,[132] and thrombin may also be involved.[27] Thus, activation of coagulation at an early stage may be associated with release of elastase and other neutrophil enzymes, e.g., cathepsin G. The ability to release elastase may be increased by modest stimulation by platelets,[91] and there is evidence for complex interactions between these cell types in the pathogenesis of thrombosis and inflammation.[7,38] Plasmin directly aggregates neutrophils in a process requiring an intact active site and binding to the cell membrane via the lysine binding site of plasmin.[106] Thus, the activation of coagulation and fibrinolysis appears to be intimately involved with the activation of neutrophils and subsequent generation of elastase and other enzymes. The central roles of kallikrein and plasmin in neutrophil activation make it likely that aprotinin could inhibit these reactions, especially as it can be bound and endocytosed by these cells.[119]

The potential relevance of neutrophil activation to hemostasis lies in the fact that elastase is a potent serine protease which is known to have many effects on the coagulation and fibrinolytic systems. First, it can interfere with platelet function,[21,115] probably by proteolyzing the von Willebrand receptor glycoprotein Ib[17] and the fibrinogen receptor glycoprotein IIb/IIIa.[21,73] Second, elastase can degrade fibrinogen and most of the other coagulation factors apart from prothombin.[108] The natural inhibitors of coagulation, antithrombin III,[64] protein C,[34] protein S,[92] and tissue factor pathway inhibitor,[58] are all cleaved by elastase, and in the case of ATIII, this inactivation is promoted by heparin.[67,110] Interestingly, elastase may cleave prekallikrein to kallikrein,[109] which may represent a positive feedback mechanism for further elastase release.

Elastase removes the kringle$_{1-4}$ structure from plasminogen, yielding the so-called "mini-plasminogen."[81] Des-kringle$_{1-4}$ plasminogen is more readily activated by tPA and urokinase-type plasminogen activator (uPA) than the native molecule and does not require cofactors for its activation by tPA.[81] In addition, elastase cleaves alpha-2 antiplasmin and plasminogen activator inhibitor (PAI).[81] The net effect of these activities is to enhance fibrinolysis. Indeed, elastase is regarded as an alternative pathway of fibrinolytic activation.[80,81,98,99] Because plasmin generation is probably very important in the pathogenesis of surgical bleeding, neutrophil elastase may also be implicated.

Neutrophils become activated during surgical procedures.[25,121] Activation in vivo results in a failure to respond to exogenous stimuli in vitro.[75] Thus, the cells demonstrate reduced chemotaxis, bacterial killing, and oxidative metabolism. We have recently shown that bipolar shape formation (a test of locomotor capacity), chemotaxis, and nitroblue tetrazolium reduction (a measure of superoxide generation) all became abnormal during major vascular surgery.[43,76] However, all three tests remained normal in patients receiving high-dose aprotinin.[43,76] The reason for these findings in aprotinin-treated patients was not studied directly but may reflect inhibition of kallikrein and plasmin, since as discussed, both of these may activate neutrophils. Because the cells were not activated in vivo, they remained able to respond to exogenous stimuli in vitro, showing normal locomotor capacity, chemotaxis, and oxidative burst.

In our study of major vascular surgery, elastase release was not measured. However, elastase may be released during surgical procedures, and this is certainly true of CPB both in vivo[39,125] and in vitro.[112,130] Elastase release may be inhibited by aprotinin,[125,131] although others have not found this to be the case.[85] In some studies at least, patients treated with aprotinin have had lower plasma levels of elastase,[125] which may be related to the protective effect that this agent appears to have on neutrophils during surgery. As noted earlier, neutrophils can be activated by kallikrein,[35] and this pathway can thus presumably be blocked by aprotinin.[131] In addition, kallikrein inhibition retards the activation of factor XII, which, in turn, reduces the formation of factors XIIa and XIIf. Both the latter fragment and plasmin directly activate C1, the first component of the complement pathway, which can facilitate neutrophil activation and elastase release. Thus, aprotinin has an inhibitory effect on at least three pathways of neutrophil activation.

It should be noted that interactions between activated neutrophils and primary hemostasis are probably *local* events, and as such, it would be difficult to provide *systemic* evidence of these phenomena. However, it is not inconceivable that prevention or reduction of local neutrophil activation and subsequent elastase-mediated degradation of primary platelet plugs might contribute to the beneficial effect of aprotinin on primary hemostasis. Further studies in this interesting area are certainly justified.

## Conclusions

A number of different pharmacologic approaches to the reduction of surgical bleeding have been tried. Of the agents used, aprotinin has given the most impressive results and the body of experience, especially in cardiac surgery, is greatest with this drug. Despite considerable research, however, the mode of action of aprotinin in securing hemostasis remains unknown. Recent research has revealed a number of pathways by which aprotinin may reduce bleeding, especially during CPB. However, these studies have certainly not provided the whole answer, and it is tempting to speculate that aprotinin acts by inhibiting the function of an as yet unidentified enzyme (or enzymes), probably involved in primary hemostasis. Alternatively, a known enzyme, possibly in the fibrinolytic system, may act in a manner that remains to be completely elucidated. Interestingly, the fact that a drug that inhibits bleeding does not also seem to potentiate thrombosis challenges many current concepts of hemostasis. Further research in this fascinating area may shed new light on the hemostatic mechanism.

## References

1. Adelman B, Michelson AD, Loscalzo J, et al: Plasmin effect on platelet glycoprotein IB–von Willebrand factor interaction. Blood 65:32–40, 1985.
2. Alajmo F, Calamai G, Perna AM, et al: High-dose aprotinin: Hemostatic effects in open heart operations. Ann Thorac Surg 48:536–539, 1989.

3. Ambrus JL, Schimert G, Lajos TZ, et al: Effect of antifibrinolytic agents and estrogens on blood loss and blood coagulation factors during open heart surgery. J Med 2:65–81, 1971.
4. Angelini GD, Cooper GJ, Lamarra M, Bryan AJ: Unorthodox use of aprotinin to control life-threatening bleeding after cardiopulmonary bypass. Lancet 335:799–800, 1990.
5. Bachmann F, McKenna R, Cole ER, Najafi H: The hemostatic mechanism after open-heart surgery: I. Studies on plasma coagulation factors and fibrinolysis in 512 patients after extracorporeal circulation. J Thorac Cardiovasc Surg 70:76–85, 1975.
6. Bartholomew JR, Salgia R, Bell WR: Control of bleeding in patients with immune and non-immune thrombocytopenia with aminocaproic acid. Arch Intern Med 149:1959–1961, 1989.
7. Bazzoni G, Dejana E, Delmaschio A: Platelet–neutrophil interactions: Possible relevance in the pathogenesis of thrombosis and inflammation. Haematologica 76:491–499, 1991.
8. Bentall HH, Allwork SP: Fibrinolysis and bleeding in open-heart surgery. Lancet 1:4–8, 1968.
9. Bidstrup B: Aprotinin for bleeding after cardiopulmonary bypass [letter]. Lancet 335:1535–1536, 1990.
10. Bidstrup BP, Royston D, McGuiness C, Sapsford RN: Aprotinin in aspirin-pretreated patients. Perfusion 5(Suppl):77–81, 1990.
11. Bidstrup BP, Royston D, Sapsford RN, Taylor KM: Reduction in blood loss and blood use after cardiopulmonary bypass with high-dose aprotinin (Trasylol). J Thorac Cardiovasc Surg 97:364–372, 1989.
12. Bidstrup BP, Royston D, Taylor KM, Sapsford RN: Effect of aprotinin on need for blood transfusion in patients with septic endocarditis having open-heart surgery [letter]. Lancet i:366–367, 1988.
13. Blauhut B, Gross C, Necek S, et al: Effects of high-dose aprotinin on blood loss, platelet function, fibrinolysis, complement, and renal function after cardiopulmonary bypass. J Thorac Cardiovasc Surg 101:958–967, 1991.
14. Boisclair MD, Philippou H, Lane DA: Thrombogenic mechanisms in the human: Fresh insights obtained by immunodiagnostic studies of coagulation markers. Blood Coag Fibrinol 4:1007–1021, 1993.
15. Boldt J, Knothe C, Zickmann B, et al: Aprotinin in pediatric cardiac operations—Platelet function, blood loss, and use of homologous blood. Ann Thorac Surg 55:1460–1466, 1993.
16. Boldt J, Zickmann B, Schindler E, et al: Influence of aprotinin on the thrombomodulin/protein C system in pediatric cardiac operations. J Thorac Cardiovasc Surg 107:1215–1221, 1994.
17. Brower MS, Levin RI, Garry K: Human neutrophil elastase modulates platelet function by limited proteolysis of membrane glycoproteins. J Clin Invest 75:657–666, 1985.
18. Broze GJ: Tissue factor pathway inhibitor and the revised hypothesis of blood coagulation. Trend Cardiovasc Med 2:72–77, 1992.
19. Broze GJ, Gailani D: The role of factor XI in coagulation. Thromb Haemost 70:72–74, 1993.
20. Brunet F, Mira JP, Belghith M, et al: Effects of aprotinin on hemorrhagic complications in ARDS patients during prolonged extracorporeal $CO_2$ removal. Intensive Care Med 18:364–367, 1992.
21. Bykowska K, Pawlowska Z, Clernlewski C, et al: Different effects of human neutrophil elastase on platelet glycoproteins IIb and IIIa of resting and stimulated platelets. Thromb Haemost 64:69–73, 1990.
22. Carrel T, Bauer E, Laske A, et al: Low-dose aprotinin for reduction of blood loss after cardiopulmonary bypass. Lancet 337:673, 1991.
23. Cauchie P, Pradier O, Dejonckheers M, et al: DIC, fibrinolysis and aprotinin treatment during orthotopic liver transplantation (OLT) [abstract]. Thromb Haemost 65:1089, 1991.
24. Chabbat J, Porte P, Tellier M, Steinbuch M: Aprotinin is a competitive inhibitor of the factor-VIIa–tissue factor complex. Thromb Res 71:205–215, 1993.
25. Christou NV, Tellado JM: In vitro polymorphonuclear neutrophil function in surgical patients does not correlate with anergy but with 'activating' processes such as sepsis or trauma. Surgery 106:718–724, 1989.
26. Clozel JP, Banken L, Roux S: Aprotinin: An antidote for recombinant tissue-type plasminogen activator (rt-PA) active in vivo. J Am Coll Cardiol 16:507–510, 1990.
27. Cohen WM, Wu HF, Featherstone GL, et al: Linkage between blood coagulation and inflammation—Stimulation of neutrophil tissue kallikrein by thrombin. Biochem Biophys Res Commun 176:315–320, 1991.
28. De Bono DP, Pringle S, Underwood I: Differential effects of aprotinin and tranexamic acid on cerebral bleeding and cutaneous bleeding time during rt-PA infusion. Thromb Res 61:159–163, 1991.

29. de Smet AA, Joen MC, van Oeveren W, et al: Increased coagulation during cardiopulmonary bypass by aprotinin. J Thorac Cardiovasc Surg 100:520–527, 1990.
30. Dietrich W, Barankay A, Dilthey G, et al: Reduction of homologous blood requirement in cardiac surgery by intraoperative aprotinin application—Clinical experience in 152 cardiac surgical patients. Thorac Cardiovasc Surg 37:92–98, 1989.
31. Dietrich W, Mossinger H, Spannagl M, et al: Hemostatic activation during cardiopulmonary bypass with different aprotinin dosages in pediatric patients having cardiac operations. J Thorac Cardiovasc Surg 105:712–720, 1993.
32. Dietrich W, Spannagl M, Jochum M, et al: Influence of high-dose aprotinin treatment on blood loss and coagulation patterns in patients undergoing myocardial revascularization. Anesthesiol 73:1119–1126, 1990.
33. Dzik WH, Arkin CF, Jenkins RL, Stump DC: Fibrinolysis during liver transplantation in humans: Role of tissue-type plasminogen activator. Blood 71:1090–1095, 1988.
34. Eckle I, Seitz R, Egbring R, et al: Protein-C degradation in vitro by neutrophil elastase. Biol Chem Hoppe Seyler 372:1007–1013, 1991.
35. Edmunds LH, Niewiarowski S, Colman RW: Aprotinin. J Thorac Cardiovasc Surg 101:1103–1104, 1991.
36. Elliot MJ, Allen A: Aprotinin in paediatric cardiac surgery. Perfusion 5(Suppl):73–76, 1990.
37. Espana F, Estelles A, Griffin JH, et al: Aprotinin (Trasylol) is a competitive inhibitor of activated protein C. Thromb Res 56:751–756, 1989.
38. Faint RW: Platelet neutrophil interactions—Their significance. Blood Rev 6:83–91, 1992.
39. Faymonville ME, Pincemail J, Duchateau J, et al: Myeloperoxidase and elastase as markers of leukocyte activation during cardiopulmonary bypass in humans. J Thorac Cardiovasc Surg 102:309–317, 1991.
40. Fraedrich G, Weber C, Bernard C, et al: Reduction of blood transfusion requirement in open heart surgery by administration of high doses of aprotinin—preliminary results. Thorac Cardiovasc Surg 37:89–91, 1989.
41. Francis JL: The use of drugs to reduce blood loss during surgery. Hematol Rev Commun 7:85–99, 1992.
42. Francis JL, Howard C: The effect of aprotinin on the response of the activated partial thromboplastin time (APTT) to heparin. Blood Coag Fibrinol 4:35–40, 1993.
43. Francis JL, Thompson JF, Lord RA, et al: Effects of aprotinin on haemostasis and neutrophil function in vascular surgery. In Samama CM (ed): Hemostasis and Thrombosis in Cardiovascular Surgery. Oxford, Arnette Blackwell, 1993, pp 97–110.
44. Frater RW: Aprotinin and open heart operations [letter]. Ann Thorac Surg 49:851–852, 1990.
45. Fricke W, Alling D, Kimball J, et al: Lack of efficacy of tranexamic acid in thrombocytopenic bleeding. Transfusion 31:345–348, 1991.
46. Fuhrer G, Gallimore M, Hoffmeister HE, Heller W: Aprotinin in cardiopulmonary bypass: Effects on the plasma kallikrein system and blood loss [abstract]. Fibrinolysis 4(Suppl 3):62, 1990.
47. Fuhrer G, Gallimore MJ, Heller W, Hoffmeister HE: Aprotinin in cardiopulmonary bypass: Effects on the Hageman factor (FXII)–kallikrein system and blood loss. Blood Coag Fibrinol 3:99–104, 1992.
48. Garabedian HD, Gold HK, Leinbach RC, et al: Bleeding time prolongation and bleeding during infusion of recombinant tissue-type plasminogen activator in dogs: Potentiation by aspirin and reversal with aprotinin. J Am Coll Cardiol 17:1213–1222, 1991.
49. George JN, Pickett EB, Saucerman S, et al: Platelet surface glycoproteins: Studies on resting and activated platelets and platelet membrane microparticles in normal subjects, and observations in patients during adult respiratory distress syndrome and cardiac surgery. J Clin Invest 78:340–348, 1986.
50. Giuliani R, Szwarcer E, Aquino EM, Palumbo G: Fibrin-dependent fibrinolytic activity during extracorporeal circulation. Thromb Res 61:369–373, 1991.
51. Gram J, Janetzko T, Jespersen J, Buhn HD: Enhanced effective fibrinolysis following the neutralization of heparin in open heart surgery increases the risk of post-surgical bleeding. Thromb Haemost 63:241–245, 1990.
52. Hack G, Kirchoff PG, Popov-Cenic S, et al: Aprotinin bei operationen am offen herzen. Med Welt 34:726–731, 1983.
53. Harder MP, Eijsman L, Roozendaal KJ, et al: Aprotinin reduces intraoperative and postoperative blood loss in membrane oxygenator cardiopulmonary bypass. Ann Thorac Surg 51:936–941, 1991.

54. Hauert J, Parise P, Callegari P, et al: Modification of haemostatic parameters during cardiopulmonary bypass (CPB): Effect of aprotinin [abstract]. Thromb Haemost 65:1029, 1991.

55. Havel M, Teufelsbauer H, Knobl P, et al: Effect of intraoperative aprotinin administration on postoperative bleeding in patients undergoing cardiopulmonary bypass operation. J Thorac Cardiovasc Surg 101:968–972, 1991.

56. Havel MP, Griesmacher A, Weigel G, et al: Aprotinin increases release of von Willebrand factor in cultured human umbilical vein endothelial cells. Surgery 112:573–577, 1992.

57. Herbert JM, Bernat A, Maffrand JP: Aprotinin reduces clopidogrel-induced prolongation of the bleeding time in the rat. Thromb Res 71:433–441, 1993.

58. Higuchi DA, Wun TC, Likert KM, Broze GJ: The effect of a luekocyte elastase on tissue factor pathway inhibitor. Blood 79:1712–1719, 1992.

59. Himmelreich G, Muser M, Slama K, et al: Hemostatic chnages in orthotopic liver transplantation (OLT) as well as postoperative albumin synthesis are influenced by different intraoperative aprotinin applications [abstract]. Thromb Haemost 65:1089, 1991.

60. Huang HM, Ding WX, Su ZK, Shang WZ: Mechanism of the preserving effect of aprotinin on platelet function and its use in cardiac surgery. J Thorac Cardiovasc Surg 106:11–18, 1993.

61. Hunt BJ, Cottam S, Segal H, et al: Inhibition by aprotinin of tPA-mediated fibrinolysis during orthotopic liver transplantation. Lancet 336:381, 1990.

62. Hunt BJ, Segal H, Yacoub M: Monitoring heparin by the activated clotting time when aprotinin is used during cardiopulmonary bypass [abstract]. Thromb Haemost 65:1025, 1991.

63. Huth C, Hoffmeister HE: Einsatz von proteinasen-inhibitoren waehrend der extrakorporalen zirkulation-wirkungsverbesserung durch optimierung der dosis in einer klinischen studie. In Dudziak R, Kirchoff PG, Reuter HG, Schumann F (eds): Proteolyse und Proteinasen-inhibition in der Hertz- und Geffaschirurgie. Stuttgart, Schattauer, 1985, pp 243–253.

64. Jochum M, Lander S, Heimburger N, Fritz H: Effect of human granulocytic elastase on isolated human antithrombin III. Hoppe Seylers Z Physiol Chem 362:103–112, 1981.

65. John LCH, Rees GM, Kovacs IB: Reduction of heparin binding to and inhibition of platelets by aprotinin. Ann Thorac Surg 55:1175–1179, 1993.

66. Johnson EJ, Hariman H, Hampton KK, et al: Fibrinolysis during major abdominal surgery. Fibrinolysis 4:147–151, 1990.

67. Jordan RE, Kilpatrick J, Nelson RM: Heparin promotes the inactivation of antithrombin by neutrophil elastase. Science 237:777–779, 1987.

68. Kalter RD, Saul CM, Wetstein L, et al: Cardiopulmonary bypass: Associated hemostatic abnormalities. J Thorac Cardiovasc Surg 77:427–435, 1979.

69. Kamayashi J, Sakon M, Yokota M, et al: Activation of coagulation and fibrinolysis during surgery analyzed by molecular markers. Thromb Res 60:157–167, 1990.

70. Kestin AS, Valeri CR, Khuri SF, et al: The platelet function defect of cardiopulmonary bypass. Blood 82:107–117, 1993.

71. Kim T, Hoppensteadt D, Moran S, et al: The effects of aprotinin treatment during CABG on TFPI, tissue factor and other hemostatic parameters. Thromb Haemost 69:1290, 1993.

72. Kirklin JK, Westaby S, Blackstone JW, et al: Complement and the damaging effects of cardiopulmonary bypass. J Thorac Cardiovasc Surg 86:845–857, 1983.

73. Kornecki E, Ehrlich VH, De Mars DD, Lenox RH: Exposure of fibrinogen receptors in human platelets by surface proteolysis with elastase. J Clin Invest 77:750–756, 1986.

74. Kucuk O, Kwaan HC, Frederickson J, et al: Increased fibrinolytic activity in patients undergoing cardiopulmonary bypass operation. Am J Hematol 23:223–229, 1986.

75. Lord RA: Assessment of neutrophil function: An introduction. Med Lab Sci 46:347–356, 1989.

76. Lord RA, Roath OS, Thompson JF, et al: Effect of aprotinin on neutrophil function after major vascular surgery. Br J Surg 79:517–521, 1992.

77. Lotterberg R, Sjak-Shie N, Fazlebas AT, Roberts RM: Aprotinin inhibits urokinase but not tissue type plasminogen activator. Thromb Res 49:549–556, 1988.

78. Lu H, Commin PL, Soria J, et al: Haemostasis in patients undergoing cardiopulmonary bypass: The effect of aprotinin [abstract]. Thromb Haemost 65:1027, 1991.

79. Lu H, Soria C, Commin PL, et al: Hemostasis in patients undergoing extracorporeal circulation: The effect of aprotinin (Trasylol). Thromb Haemost 66:633–637, 1991.

80. Machovich R, Owen WG: An elastase-dependent pathway of plasminogen activation. Biochemistry 28:4517–4522, 1989.

81. Machovich R, Owen WG: The elastase-mediated pathway of fibrinolysis. Blood Coag Fibrinol 1:79–90, 1990.

82. Mallett SV, Cox D, Burroughs AK, Rolles K: Aprotinin and reduction of blood loss and transfusion requirements in orthotopic liver transplantation [letter]. Lancet 336:886–887, 1990.

83. Mammen EF: Neutral protease inhibitors in extracorporeal circulation. Ann NY Acad Sci 146:754–762, 1968.

84. Mansfield AO: Alterations in fibrinolysis associated with surgery and venous thrombosis. Br J Surg 59:754–757, 1972.

85. Marx G, Pokar H, Reuter A, et al: The effects of aprotinin on hemostatic function during cardiac surgery. J Cardiothorac Vasc Anesth 5:467–474, 1991.

86. McKenna R, Bachmann F, Whittaker B, et al: The hemostatic mechanism after open-heart surgery: II. Frequency of abnormal platelet function during and after extracorporeal circulation. J Thorac Cardiovasc Surg 70:298–308, 1975.

87. Michelson EL, Morganroth J, Torosian M, MacVaugh H: Relation of preoperative use of aspirin to increased mediastinal blood loss after coronary artery bypass graft surgery. J Thorac Cardiovasc Surg 76:694–697, 1978.

88. Nagaoka H, Innami R, Murayama F, et al: Effects of aprotinin on prostaglandin metabolism and platelet function in open herat surgery. J Cardiovasc Surg 32:31–37, 1991.

89. Najman D, Walenga JM, Hoppensteadt D, et al: The effects of aprotinin on anticoagulant monitoring: Implications in cardiovascular surgery [abstract]. Thromb Haemost 65:1336, 1991.

90. Neuhaus P, Bechstein WO, Lefebre O, et al: Effect of aprotinin on intraoperative bleeding and fibrinolysis in liver transplantation. Lancet 2:924–925, 1989.

91. Nicolini FA, Wilson AC, Mehta P, Mehta JL: Comparative platelet inhibitory effects of human neutrophils and lymphocytes. J Lab Clin Med 116:147–152, 1990.

92. Oates AM, Salem HH: The binding and regulation of protein-S by neutrophils. Blood Coag Fibrinol 2:601–607, 1991.

93. Orchard MA, Goodchild CS, Prentice CRM, et al: Aprotinin reduces cardiopulmonary bypass-induced blood loss and inhibits fibrinolysis without influencing platelets. Br J Haematol 85:533–541, 1993.

94. Palmer JD, Francis DA, Francis JL, Roath OS: Plasmin-related systems and meningiomas [abstract]. Clin Hemorheol 13:5424, 1993.

95. Palmer JD, Francis DA, Roath OS, et al: Hyperfibrinolysis during intracranial surgery: Effect of high dose aprotinin. J Neurol Neurosurg Psychiatry 1994 (in press).

96. Pike OM, Marquiss JE, Weiner RS, Brechenridge AT: A study of platelet counts duing cardiopulmonary bypass. Transfusion 12:119–122, 1972.

97. Pintigny D, Dachary-Prigent J: Aprotinin can inhibit the proteolytic activity of thrombin: A fluorescence and an enzymatic study. Eur J Biochem 207:89–95, 1992.

98. Plow E: The major fibrinolytic proteases of human leukocytes. Biochim Biophys Acta 630:47–56, 1980.

99. Plow EF: Leukocyte elastase release during blood coagulation: A potential mechanism for activation of the alternative fibrinolytic pathway. J Clin Invest 69:564–572, 1982.

100. Porte RJ, Bontempo FA, Knot EAR, et al: Systemic effects of tissue plasminogen activator-associated fibrinolysis and its relation to thrombin generation in orthotopic liver transplantation. Transplantation 47:978–984, 1989.

101. Roath OS, Majer RV, Smith AG: The use of aprotinin in thrombocytopenic patients: A preliminary evaluation. Blood Coag Fibrinol 1:235–239, 1990.

102. Royston BD, Royston D, Coade SB, et al: Aprotinin does not inhibit the release of PG12 or vWF from cultured human endothelial cells. Thromb Haemost 67:172–175, 1992.

103. Royston BD, Royston D, Pearson JD: Aprotinin inhibits platelet adhesion to endothelial cells. Blood Coag Fibrinol 3:737–742, 1992.

104. Royston D: The serine antiprotease aprotinin (Trasylol): A novel approach to reducing postoperative bleeding. Blood Coag Fibrinol 1:55–69, 1990.

105. Royston D, Bidstrup BP, Taylor KM, Sapsford RN: Effect of aprotinin on need for blood transfusion after repeat open-heart surgery. Lancet ii:1289–1291, 1987.

106. Ryan TJ, Lai L, Malik AB: Plasmin generation induces neutrophil aggregation: Dependence on the catalytic and lysine binding sites. J Cell Physiol 151:255–261, 1992.

107. Santoli E, Scrofani R, Santoli C: How should the risk of bank blood transfusion in open heart operations be minimized? [letter]. Ann Thorac Surg 50:1021–1022, 1990.

108. Schmidt W, Egbring R, Havemann K: Effect of elastase-like and chymotrypsin-like neutral proteases from human granulocytes on isolated clotting factors. Thromb Res 6:315–326, 1975.

109. Shibuya Y, Tanaka H, Nishino N, et al: Activation of human plasma prekallikrein by *Pseudomonas aeruginosa* elastase in vitro. Biochim Biiophys Acta 1097:23–27, 1991.
110. Sie P, Dupouy D, Dol F, Boneu B: Inactivation of heparin cofactor II by polymorphonuclear leukocytes. Thromb Res 47:657–664, 1987.
111. Smith O, Hazlehurst G, Brozovic B, et al: Impact of aprotinin on blood transfusion requirements in liver transplantation. Transfusion Med 3:97–102, 1993.
112. Stahl RF, Fisher CA, Kucich U, et al: Effects of simulated extracorporeal circulation on human leukocyte elastase release, superoxide generation, and procoagulant activity. J Thorac Cardiovasc Surg 101:230–239, 1991.
113. Szecsi J, Betonyi E, Redai I, et al: Effect of acute aprotinin (Gordox) therapy on hemostasis in heart surgery patients, with special reference to hyperfibrinolysis. Orv Hetil 131:2809–2814, 1990.
114. Taggart DP, Siddiqui MAA, Wheatley DJ: Aspirin and blood loss. Ann Thorac Surg 51:693–694, 1991.
115. Taki M, Miura T, Inagaki M, et al: Influence of granulocyte elastase-like proteinase (ELP) on platelet functions. Thromb Res 41:837–846, 1986.
116. Tanaka K, Tanabe H, Morimoto T, et al: Increased fibrinolytic activity caused by cardiopulmonary bypass and ventricular assist device [abstract]. Fibrinolysis 4(Suppl 3):61, 1990.
117. Teufelsbauer H, Proidl S, Havel M, Vukovich T: Early activation of hemostasis during cardiopulmonary bypass: Evidence for thrombin mediated hyperfibrinolysis. Thromb Haemost 68:250–252, 1992.
118. Thompson JF, Roath OS, Francis JL, et al: Aprotinin in vascular surgery. Lancet 335:911, 1990.
119. Thomson AW, Pugh-Humphreys RGP, Tweedie DJ, Horne CHW: Effects of the antiprotease Trasylol® on peripheral blood leucocytes. Experientia 34:528–530, 1978.
120. Tice DA, Worth MH, Clauss RH, Reed GH: The inhibition by Trasylol of fibrinolytic activity associated with cardiovascular operations. Surg Gynecol Obstet 119:71–74, 1964.
121. Utoh J, Yamamoto T, Utsunomiya T, et al: Effect of surgery on neutrophil functions, superoxide and leukotriene production. Br J Surg 75:682–685, 1988.
122. van den Besselaar AMHP, Dirven R, Bertina RM: Tissue factor-induced coagulation can be inhibited by aprotinin. Thromb Haemost 69:298–299, 1993.
123. van Oeveren W, Eijsman L, Roozendaal KJ, Wildevuur CRH: Platelet preservation by aprotinin during cardiopulmonary bypass. Lancet ii:644, 1988.
124. van Oeveren W, Harder MP, Roozendaal KJ, et al: Aprotinin protects platelets against the initial effect of cardiopulmonary bypass. J Thorac Cardiovasc Surg 99:788–797, 1990.
125. van Oeveren W, Jansen NJG, Bidstrup BP, et al: Effects of aprotinin on hemostatic mechanisms during cardiopulmonary bypass. Ann Thorac Surg 44:640–645, 1987.
126. Vandenvelde C, Bergmann P, Dubois-Primo J, et al: Clinical and biological effects of preoperative aprotinin in cardiopulmonary bypass (CPB) surgery [abstract]. Thromb Haemost 65:1026, 1991.
127. Vandenvelde C, Fondu P, Duboisprimo J: Low-dose aprotinin for reduction of blood loss after cardiopulmonary bypass. Lancet 337:1157–1158, 1991.
128. Videm V, Mollnes TE, Garred P, Svennevig JL: Biocompatibility of extracorporeal circulation: In vitro comparison of heparin-coated and uncoated oxygenator circuits. J Thorac Cardiovasc Surg 101:654–660, 1991.
129. Violaris AG, Angelini GD: Aspirin and blood loss. Ann Thorac Surg 51:693, 1991.
130. Wachtfogel YT, Kucich U, Hack CE, et al: Aprotinin inhibits the contact, neutrophil, and platelect activation systems during simulated extracorporeal perfusion. J Thorac Cardiovasc Surg 106:1–10, 1993.
131. Wachtfogel YT, Kucich U, Hack CE, et al: Aprotinin inhibits the contact, neutrophil, and platelet activation systems during simulated extracorporeal perfusion. Thromb Haemost 69:778, 1993.
132. Wachtfogel YT, Kucich U, James HL, et al: Human plasma kallikrein releases neutrophil elastase during blood coagulation. J Clin Invest 72:1672–1677, 1983.
133. Wenger RK, Lukasiewicz H, Mikuta BS, et al: Loss of platelet fibrinogen receptors during clinical cardiopulmonary bypass. J Thorac Cardiovasc Surg 97:235–239, 1989.
134. Wildevuur CRH, Eijsman L, Roozendaal KJ, et al: Platelet preservation during cardiopulmonary bypass with aprotinin. Eur J Cardiothorac Surg 3:533–538, 1989.

Jawed Fareed, PhD
Walter Jeske, BS
Debra Hoppensteadt, MS, MT(ASCP)
Jeanine M. Walenga, PhD
Roque Pifarré, MD

# 11

# Drug Interactions with Aprotinin

Aprotinin, a wide-spectrum serine protease inhibitor, was first isolated from mammalian lungs and is now also produced by recombinant technology.[37] Aprotinin is a polypeptide with a molecular weight of 6.2 kDa; minor variations in the molecular weight of various molecular forms have been noted. The N terminus of this 58-amino acid protein contains the Arg-Pro-Asp sequence, which is believed to be involved in producing its antiprotease effects. The C terminus of aprotinin contains the Ala-Gly-Gly sequence.

Aprotinin interacts with various endogenous proteins, but its most important effect is to antagonize serine proteases, such as factor XIIa, kallikrein, plasmin, protein Ca, and several thrombolytic enzymes (Table 1). Thus, aprotinin can be used as a potent inhibitor in clinical states that generate abnormally high amounts of these enzymes and thus result in varying degrees of hemodynamic and bleeding complications.[26,35]

Aprotinin also modulates cellular responses, producing varying degrees of cytoprotective effects[22,26] (Table 2). Most of these responses are due to the inhibition of proteolytic enzymes that modulate cellular activation.[26,37] However, because aprotinin contains six arginine residues, it also may act as a nitric oxide donor. Thus drugs capable of nitric oxide generation may exhibit an additive or synergistic response to aprotinin. Aprotinin inhibits many of the granulocytic enzymes of leukocyte and macrophage origin and may be able to stabilize the cellular integrity of endothelial cells by inhibiting various enzymes involved in the necrotic process. Although its actions on fibroblasts are currently unknown, aprotinin produces various modulatory actions on platelets and smooth muscle cells.

Aprotinin also may be capable of interacting with various endogenous serine protease inhibitors (serpins) (Table 3). One of its basic actions on these serpins is protective. Because aprotinin inhibits various proteolytic enzymes, it may protect against the digestion of protease inhibitors, which in turn may potentiate the physiologic function of the inhibitors. With the exception of antithrombin III and

**TABLE 1.** Enzymes Inhibited by Aprotinin

| Enzyme | Degree of Inhibition | Physiologic Consequences |
|---|---|---|
| Plasma kallikrein | 4+ | Inhibition of coagulation and kinin generation |
| Glandular kallikrein | 4+ | Inhibition of kinin generation |
| Factor XIIa | 3+ | Inhibition of coagulation, fibrinolysis, and clotting process |
| Tissue factor/factor VIIa | 1+ | Inhibition of clotting process |
| Plasmin | 3+ | Inhibition of thrombolysis |
| Plasminogen activator | 1–3+ | Inhibition of thrombolysis |
| Protein Ca | 1+ | Hemostatic restoration, inhibition of thrombolysis |
| C1-esterase | 2+ | Anti-inflammatory action |
| Neutrophil elastase | 1+ | Anti-inflammatory action |
| Cathepsins | ± | Cellular modulation |

heparin cofactor II, the inhibitory spectrum of many protease inhibitors is similar to that of aprotinin. Thus, aprotinin may improve the inhibition of various enzymes, producing either additive or potentiating effects.

It is clear that aprotinin has multiple sites of action, both plasmatic and cellular. Furthermore, it is capable of various endogenous interactions. Thus its use with other drugs may result in significant interactions. Although data are limited, several recent studies have addressed the interaction of aprotinin with other drugs, and additional studies are currently under way.[2,3,16,17,25]

## Experimental and Clinical Studies

Several experimental studies have examined the interactions of aprotinin with drugs and biologically active proteins, but data from clinical studies are limited.[14,19,23] Table 4 summarizes the possible interactions of aprotinin with anticoagulant and antithrombotic drugs.

Heparin is capable of releasing tissue factor pathway inhibitor (TFPI) from the vascular system.[1] TFPI is an endogenous, polyfunctional inhibitor of proteases; one of its domains, which structurally resembles aprotinin, may be capable of inhibiting elastase and cathepsins. Thus, aprotinin may potentiate the action of released TFPI. Although several studies have demonstrated the release of TFPI during heparinization, no interaction with aprotinin has yet been reported.

**TABLE 2.** Modulation of Cellular Responses by Aprotinin

| Cells | Modulation |
|---|---|
| Polymorphonuclear leukocytes | Inhibition of granulocytic enzymes; cytostabilization |
| Macrophages | Inhibition of tissue factor and granulocytic enzymes |
| Endothelial cells | Inhibition of tPA; cytostabilization |
| Fibroblasts | Unknown |
| Smooth muscle cells | Modulation of contractile actions (mediated by NO?) |
| Platelets | Cytoprotection; inhibition of endopeptidases; probable NO-mediated regulation |

tPA = tissue-type plasminogen activator; NO = nitric oxide.

**TABLE 3.** Interactions of Aprotinin with Serpins

| Serpin | Interaction |
| --- | --- |
| Antithrombin III | Not known |
| Heparin cofactor II | Not known |
| Plasminogen activator inhibitor | Additive |
| Alpha-2 antiplasmin | Synergistic |
| Alpha-2 macroglobulin | Additive |
| Alpha-1 antitrypsin | Additive |
| C1-esterase inhibitor | Additive |
| Tissue factor pathway inhibitor | Synergistic |

Laurel and coworkers described the effect of aprotinin on the activation of Hageman factor.[21] Because Hageman factor is strongly activated during contact activation and may initiate the clotting, kallikrein, and fibrinolytic processes, its inhibition is a major mechanism by which aprotinin mediates its action during cardiopulmonary bypass (CPB) surgery. In a strongly anticoagulated environment, as during heparinization, the clotting process is completely inhibited. Thus the primary actions of aprotinin are directed to the inhibition of the plasmin and kallikrein formed during contact activation. The initial inhibition of factor XIIa is therefore important in the control of bleeding.

Azougagh and coworkers reported the effect of aprotinin on heparin and heparin neutralization by protamine.[3] In the experimental setting, aprotinin inhibits the clotting process in vitro and the prolongation of bleeding time in vivo but does not alter the protamine neutralization profile in vivo. A clinical study validating these observations is not yet available.

**TABLE 4.** Interactions of Aprotinin with Anticoagulant, Antithrombotic, and Thrombolytic Drugs

| Drug | Possible Mechanism | Consequence |
| --- | --- | --- |
| Heparin-related agents | Inhibition of prophylactic action; release of TFPI | Control of bleeding; augmented cytoprotection |
| Antiplatelet drugs | Cytoprotection; prevention of consumption | |
| Endothelial lining modulators | Unknown | |
| Viscosity modulators | Unknown | |
| Thrombolytic agents | Inhibition of thrombolysis | Antagonism of thrombolytic effects |
| Recombinant hirudin | None | |
| Direct antithrombin peptides | Augmentation | Increased effects |
| Protein Ca | Inhibition of thrombolytic pathway | Antagonism |
| Antithrombin III and heparin cofactor II | Unknown | |
| TFPI | Augmentation of protease inhibitory effects | Synergism |

TFPI = tissue factor pathway inhibitor

Najman and coworkers reported the first clinical evidence that aprotinin produces a significant effect on the anticoagulant action of heparin, as measured by conventional methods.[25] An augmented increase in the activated clotting time (ACT) in the presence of aprotinin led the investigators to suggest the possibility of underheparinization in aprotinin-treated patients. Thus, later reports of isolated adverse effects in aprotinin-treated patients may be due to an underdosing of heparin because of a falsely elevated ACT. The same study provided evidence that aprotinin also inhibits the platelet aggregation response in normal, healthy volunteers, whereas heparinized patients undergoing CPB surgery showed no deficits. Based on these data, the investigators concluded that the effect of aprotinin on the hemostatic system and its interaction with heparin must be considered to optimize safety and efficacy during CPB surgery. A more valid method of determining absolute levels of heparin and total anticoagulant potential may be useful in optimizing heparin use during bypass surgery.[12,18,25]

Aprotinin produces several effects on platelets and protects them from consumption during CPB surgery. The effects of aprotinin on various endothelial-modulating drugs and viscosity facilitators are not yet known. To varying degrees aprotinin inhibits fibrinolytic agents—one of the main mechanisms of its hemostatic effect. Futhermore, it also protects platelets from the digestive action of plasmin and related enzymes. However, aprotinin is a potent inhibitor of the fibrinolytic process and should be used with caution in the management of patients treated with fibrinolytic agents. On the other hand, aprotinin can be used to reverse the effect of the fibrinolytic agent if desired.

Although aprotinin does not modulate the antithrombotic actions of recombinant hirudin, it may augment the action of the new nonspecific inhibitors of proteases, such as efegatran and argatroban. Aprotinin has been reported to inhibit protein Ca and can be used as an antidote for the antagonism of this protease.[32] No information has been reported about the interaction of aprotinin with antithrombin III and heparin cofactor II.

Because of the structural and functional homology, it is speculated that aprotinin may augment the action of TFPI as well as inhibit its degradation. Aprotinin has been reported to inhibit the tissue factor–factor VIIa complex,[9] which is a primary target of the inhibitory action of TFPI. At high plasma levels (3–5 U/ml) heparin is capable of releasing large amounts of TFPI; simultaneous administration of aprotinin may augment this effect.

Table 5 lists anticoagulants and their potential interactions with aprotinin. Currently several newer anticoagulants, such as recombinant hirudin, hirulog, and synthetic peptide inhibitors (e.g., efegatran and argatroban), are under development for use during CPB surgery. Although the interactions of heparin and aprotinin with these agents are under investigation, no in vitro or in vivo study is yet available. Because peptides such as argatroban and efegatran are also mild inhibitors of

**TABLE 5.** Interactions of Aprotinin with Anticoagulant Drugs

| Drug | Interaction |
| --- | --- |
| Heparin | Variable |
| Hirudin | None |
| Hirulog | None |
| Synthetic peptides (efegatran, argatroban) | Augmentation of antithrombotic actions |

plasmin and other fibrinolytic enzymes, they may augment the inhibitory actions of aprotinin in the fibrinolytic system. Therefore, for optimal development of aprotinin, such interactions should be taken into account.

A large number of patients requiring CPB surgery are pretreated with antiplatelet drugs such as aspirin. In addition, they also may take various other drugs, such as calcium channel blockers, antiarrythmics, or antihypertensive drugs (e.g., angiotensin-converting enzyme inhibitors). Most patients treated with antiplatelet agents present with preexisting hemostatic compromise. However, other cardiovascular drugs have no significant effects on the hemostatic process at therapeutic dosages. Because the mechanisms of action of antiplatelet drugs vary widely, they may exhibit complex interactions with aprotinin. It has been suggested that aprotinin stabilizes the membrane glycoproteins and inhibits generation of cytosolic proteases during CPB. Thus, aprotinin produces a protective effect on platelets. Table 6 lists the potential interactions of aprotinin with antiplatelet drugs. The bleeding effect of aspirin may be neutralized by aprotinin, but additional data are needed to validate various assumptions. Aprotinin is expected to augment the cytoprotective effects of dipyridamole, but experimental data are not available to support this hypothesis. The simultaneous use of aprotinin and the newly developed monoclonal antibodies to glycoprotein (GP) IIb/IIIa, synthetic antiplatelet agents, and omega-3 fatty acids may result in synergistic interactions that lead to clinical compromise and thus should be investigated carefully.

Table 7 presents a list of potential mechanisms by which aprotinin may interact with antiplatelet and platelet-restoring agents and thus protect platelets from consumption. Considerable investigative work has been carried out on this subject. Aprotinin inhibits the binding of heparin to platelet surfaces, antagonizes the plasmin-mediated digestion of platelet glycoproteins, and inhibits proteases involved in the digestion of platelet cytosolic proteins. All of these mechanisms protect the functional and structural integrity of platelets and other cells.[30] Thus, when aprotinin is administered with other thrombocytoprotective drugs such as dipyridamole or defibrotide, a stronger hemostatic result may be observed. Because the mechanisms of different antiplatelet drugs vary widely, they interact with aprotinin at multiple sites. Overall, aprotinin antagonizes the bleeding promoted by aspirin and certain GP IIb/IIIa inhibitors.

The initial development of aprotinin was based on its potent inhibition of various proteases. Disorders such as pancreatitis and uncontrolled activation of proteases were considered to be the main clinical indications for its use.[37] Because of the factor XIIa mediation of the fibrinolytic process, which is activated during CPB surgery, and because of the feedback amplification of the kallikrein-mediated augmentation of factor XII, aprotinin may inhibit the fibrinolytic process at multiple sites, including the following:

**TABLE 6.**  Interactions of Aprotinin with Antiplatelet Drugs

| Antiplatelet Agent | Interaction |
|---|---|
| Aspirin | Antagonism |
| Dipyridamole | Synergism of cytoprotective effects |
| Monoclonal antibodies to glycoprotein IIb/IIIa | Unknown |
| Omega-3 fatty acids | Unknown |
| Peptides and proteins | Variable |

**TABLE 7.**   Potential Mechanisms by which Aprotinin May Interact with Antiplatelet and Platelet-restoring Agents

| Mechanism | Clinical Outcome |
| --- | --- |
| Inhibition of heparin binding to platelet surface | Restoration of normal function of platelets |
| Inhibition of plasmin-mediated digestion of membrane glycoproteins | Protection of the functional integrity of platelet glycoprotein complexes (IIb/IIIa and Ib) |
| Inhibition of proteases involved in digesting platelet cytosolic proteins | Regulatory role of granular peptides is protected |

1. Inhibition of the contact activation process
2. Inhibition of the factor XIIa-mediated activation of prekallikrein to kallikrein
3. Inhibition of the feedback amplification of factor XIIa generation by kallikrein
4. Inhibition of kallikrein
5. Inhibition of plasmin
6. Inhibition of factor XIIa and kallikrein-mediated plasmin activation

Table 8 lists various thrombolytic agents and their potential interaction with aprotinin. All of these fibrinolytic agents are inhibited by aprotinin to varying degrees. In several initial studies aprotinin has been used as an antidote for bleeding complications induced by thrombolytic agents. Whereas aprotinin produces a mild effect on the protease activation step, it strongly inhibits the generation of plasmin. Futhermore, it also inhibits the plasmin-mediated effects on both plasmatic proteins and platelets, as listed below:

1. Direct inhibition of plasmin
2. Plasmin-mediated formation of Lys-plasminogen
3. Plasmin-mediated digestion of factor VII (VIIa)
4. Plasmin-mediated digestion of platelet glycoproteins
5. Other proteolytic functions of plasmin

Several reports have described the use of aprotinin in the control of bleeding associated with hemostatic agents,[10,13,15] and experimental models have shown its antagonistic effect on various thrombolytic agents.[13,16] Schneider et al. demonstrated that aprotinin antagonizes the interaction between aspirin and tissue-type plasminogen activator (tPA), which results in bleeding.[28] Thrombolytic therapy with the uncontrolled use of antiplatelet agents is often associated with bleeding. Because the patients are heavily heparinized, excessive production of plasmin leads to

**TABLE 8.**   Interactions of Aprotinin with Thrombolytic Agents

| Agent | Interaction |
| --- | --- |
| Streptokinase | Antagonism |
| Urokinase | Antagonism |
| Tissue-type plasminogen activator | Antagonism |
| Prourokinase | Antagonism |
| Ancrod | Unknown |

impairment of the hemostatic system at various sites. Garabedian and coworkers demonstrated that aprotinin is highly effective in controlling hemorrhage in dogs.[13]

A systematic comparison of aprotinin with epsilon aminocaproic acid (EACA) has not been made. Such a study should be carried out to confirm the efficacy of aprotinin in neutralizing thrombolytic agents. The interaction of aprotinin with thrombolytic agents may become important in cases of failed thrombolysis when the patient is taken for emergency CPB surgery. In such cases, the levels of aprotinin should be taken into account for optimizing the use of heparin and additional aprotinin.

Table 9 lists the modulatory action of aprotinin on heparin-mediated plasmatic and cellular effects. Information about this mediation is limited. However, significant clinical consequences in terms of both efficacy and safety can be projected. Combined inhibition of the factor VIIa–tissue factor complex results in decreased platelet consumption, because both agents are capable of producing this effect. Aprotinin inhibits activation of factor XIIa and in heparinized patients inhibits only the fibrinolytic and kallikrein/kinin systems. Aprotinin also reduces the binding of heparin to platelet membranes[20] and restores their functional and structural integrity. Heparin releases endogenous tPA, whereas aprotinin effects its inhibition. This also may result in restoration of hemostasis. One of the most interesting mediating effects on the function of heparin is the release of TFPI, a tri-Kunitz domain protease inhibitor. The third Kunitz domain of TFPI has a structure similar to that of aprotinin (Fig. 1). This domain is also known to inhibit enzymes such as elastase. Because heparin significantly increases the circulating level of TFPI, administration of aprotinin may lead to synergistic inhibition of both the tissue factor–factor VIIa complex and elastase.

The structures of the transmembrane procoagulant tissue factor and TFPI are compared in Figure 2. Massive amounts of tissue factor are generated in bypass surgery. In addition to triggering activation of the clotting processes, tissue factor, through receptor-mediated mechanisms, also activates macrophages, fibroblasts, and other cellular components, leading to the generation of various cytokines and autocoids. Both aprotinin and endogenously released TFPI are capable of inhibiting these activation processes. Thus, some of the beneficial effects are attributable to aprotinin- and heparin-mediated release of TFPI. This may not be the case when site-directed thrombin inhibitors, such as hirudin and hirulog, are used as anticoagulants for CPB surgery.

**TABLE 9.** Aprotinin Modulation of Heparin-mediated Plasmatic and Cellular Effects

| Effect | Clinical Outcome |
| --- | --- |
| Inhibition of factor VIIa–tissue factor complex | Decreased activation of tissue factor-mediated mechanisms |
| Inhibition of factor XIIa activation | Control of factor XIIa-mediated protease processes |
| Reduction of heparin binding to platelet membranes | Platelet function modulation |
| Inhibition of heparin-mediated release of tissue-type plasminogen activator | Control of thrombolysis-mediated bleeding |
| Enhanced inhibition of the tissue factor–factor VIIa complex | Control of tissue factor–factor VIIa-mediated cellular release and plasmatic activation processes resulting in decreased thrombotic processes |

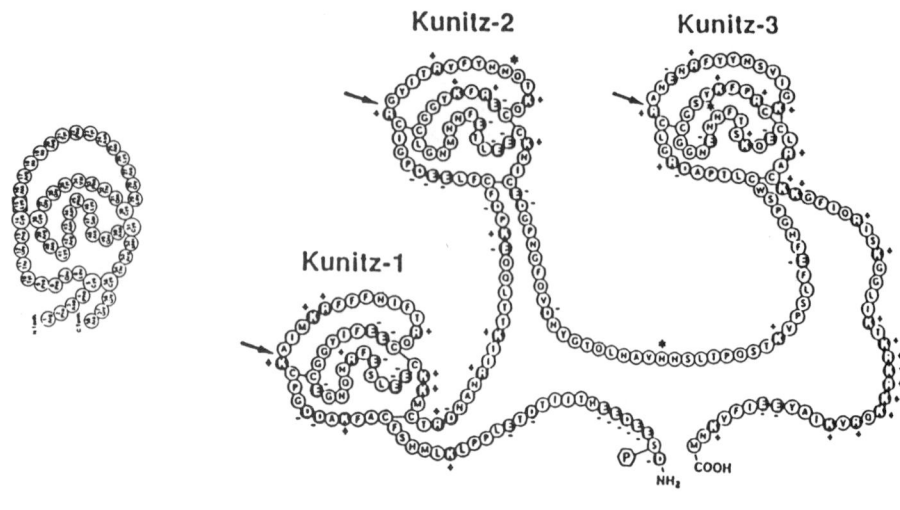

**Kunitz-2**   **Kunitz-3**

**Kunitz-1**

Aprotinin                Tissue Factor Pathway Inhibitor

**FIGURE 1.** Comparison of the structures of aprotinin and tissue factor pathway inhibitor (TFPI). Both are classified as Kunitz-type inhibitors. Aprotinin is a broad-spectrum protease inhibitor, whereas TFPI inhibits factor Xa, tissue factor–factor VIIa complex, and elastase. The tissue factor–factor VIIa complex and elastase inhibitory actions of aprotinin and TFPI may be mutually synergistic.

Table 10 summarizes data about the release of TFPI during CPB surgery. Heparinization causes the release of a massive amount of TFPI. Protamine results in the neutralization of heparin and reuptake of TFPI at various vascular sites. The effect of aprotinin on this reuptake is not yet known.

Striking similarities between aprotinin and the newly developed recombinant hirudin are also evident (Fig. 3). Recombinant hirudin, a potent, highly specific thrombin inhibitor, is currently under development for use in interventional cardiovascular procedures.[36] Despite the structural similarities between the two proteins, no data are available on their interaction; carefully designed studies are crucial. More recently, several recombinant aprotinin homologs with different inhibitory specificities have been developed.[8] Because these homologs may have a stronger potential for interactions with hirudin, optimal pharmacologic development requires systematic studies. It also has been suggested that aprotinin may be coupled to hirudin and hirudin-related peptides. The pharmacologic properties of such hybrids should be carefully investigated.

## Additional Considerations

Aprotinin has been used for several years to protect biologically active proteins from proteolytic digestion. Drugs currently prepared through recombinant technology that are protein in nature are preserved with aprotinin. Multiple dosing of such drugs may provide sizeable amounts of aprotinin in the circulation, but to a large degree this is inconsequential. Large amounts of aprotinin, however, may inhibit certain proteases, with both positive and negative outcomes.

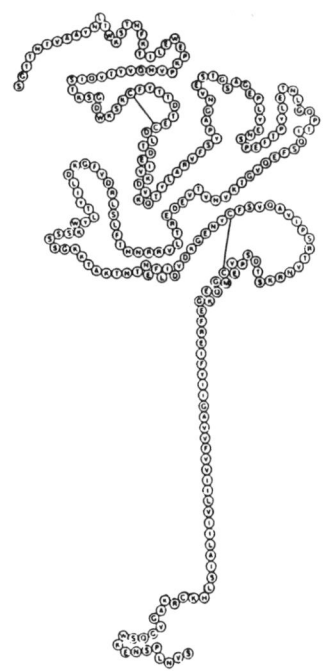

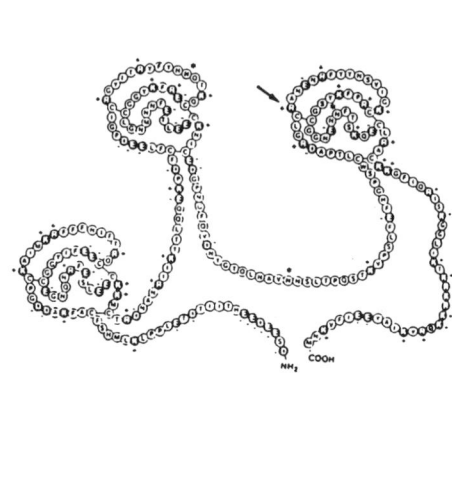

Tissue Factor      Tissue Factor Pathway Inhibitor

**FIGURE 2.** Comparison of the primary structure of tissue factor with tissue factor pathway inhibitor (TFPI). Tissue factor is a transmembrane protein with both plasmatic and tissue-factor receptor activation properties. TFPI selectively inhibits tissue factor and its mediated responses. Thus, in addition to controlling coagulation activation, this inhibition is also involved in the control of inflammatory responses.

The actions of various pharmacologically active agents, including recombinant erythropoietin, factor VIII, plasma products, desmopressin (DDAVP), and angiotensin-converting enzyme inhibitors, can be modulated by aprotinin (Table 11). Morimoto et al.[23] demonstrated that aprotinin and other enzyme inhibitors potentiate the nasal absorption of vasopressin and its analog, DDAVP, possibly by protecting these peptides from digestion in the nasal cavity. Thus, aprotinin also protects endogenously several of the peptide mediators and growth factors. In another study, aprotinin was shown to protect insulin degradation in the ileum by inhibiting various proteolytic enzymes at the site.[24] Such localized delivery of various peptides to sites with preexisting protease inhibitors may have obvious beneficial effects.

**TABLE 10.** Tissue Factor Pathway Inhibitor Release during Cardiovascular Bypass Surgery

| Group | Tissue Factor Pathway Inhibitor (ng/ml)* |
|---|---|
| Baseline | $110 \pm 20$ |
| After heparinization | $630 \pm 68$ |
| After protamine neutralization | $190 \pm 26$ |

* All results represent the mean $\pm$ 1 SD of 10 individual cases. TFPI antigen was measured.

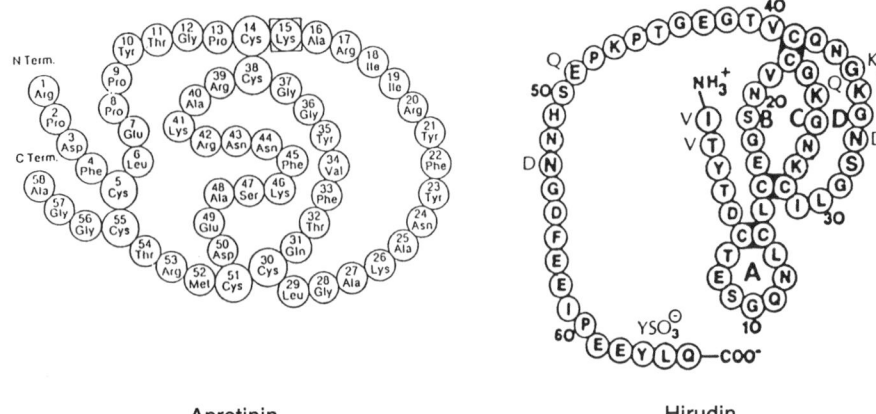

|  |  |
|---|---|
| Aprotinin | Hirudin |

**FIGURE 3.** Comparison of the primary structures of aprotinin and hirudin. Both proteins have similar molecular weights. Both are now produced by recombinant technology. Aprotinin is a broad-spectrum inhibitor, whereas hirudin is monospecific.

Plasma proteins for biologic use, such as protein Ca, factor concentrates, and blood products (e.g., platelets and granulocytes), also can be protected by the addition of aprotinin to the buffers used for their preparation and isolation.[22,32]

## Summary

It is clear that aprotinin is a polyfunctional agent. The data about its interactions with heparin, thrombolytics, and platelets are convincing. Overall, these interactions favor the use of aprotinin. Beneficial outcomes include restoration of hemostatic function, reduction of fibrinolytic activation, and inhibition of tissue factor-mediated pathways (with anti-inflammatory effects). Despite these protective effects, aprotinin has been associated with adverse outcome such as stroke; in addition, incorrect dosage calculation for aprotinin and other drugs (e.g., heparin) may result in adverse outcomes due to mutually synergistic effects.[4–7,11,33–35] High-dose aprotinin has been reported to produce renal dysfunction and intravascular coagulation, leading to hypothermic circulatory arrest.[27] Some patients required reoperations; those who died exhibited multiple pathologic symptoms in the

**TABLE 11.** Interactions of Aprotinin with Various Drugs

| Drug | Interaction |
|---|---|
| Biologically active peptides (growth factors, erythropoietin) | Protection against proteolytic degradation (both endogenous and exogenous) |
| Desmopressin | On-site protection of the molecular integrity of platelet membrane |
| Insulin | Site-specific protection; enhanced bioavailability |
| Angiotensin-converting enzyme inhibitors | Protection |
| Bradykinin antagonists | Synergism |
| Blood products | Protection of functional properties |

vascular system. Whether this effect was due to drug interaction or another manifestation remains unknown. Severe anaphylactic shock due to repeated application of aprotinin following intrathoracic aortic replacement also has been reported.[29] In two patients severe anaphylactic shock required cardiopulmonary resuscitation.[31] A nonoptimized dosage of aprotinin may result in either thrombotic or bleeding complications, which probably are due to interactions with endogenous modulators or drugs administered for various purposes. Aprotinin remains a drug of high therapeutic index and leads to an adverse outcome only in the presence of predisposing factors or drugs capable of interaction.

# References

1. Abildgaard U, Sandset PM, Lindahl AK: Tissue factor pathway inhibitor. In Poller L (ed): Recent Advances in Blood Coagulation, 6th ed. Edinburgh, Churchill Livingstone, 1993, pp 105–124.
2. Alston TA, D'Ambra MN: Aprotinin does not neutralize heparin [letter]. Ann Thorac Surg 57:516, 1994.
3. Azougagh Oualane F, Toulemonde F, Doutremepuich F, Doutremepuich C: Effects of aprotinin on heparin activities and heparin neutralization with protamine. Thromb Res 68:185–193, 1992.
4. Baubillier E, Cherqui D, Dominique C, et al: A fatal thrombotic complication during liver transplantation after aprotinin administration. Transplantation 57:1664–1666, 1994.
5. Bayo M, Ferrandiz M, Casas JI, et al: Allergic reaction following the administration of aprotinin in mitral valve replacement [letter]. Revista Espanola de Anestesiologia y Reanimacion. 41:123–124, 1994.
6. Blauhut B, Lundsgaard-Hansen P: Reply to invited letter concerning: Aprotinin [letter]. J Thorac Cardiovasc Surg 103:386–387, 1992.
7. Bohrer H, Fleischer F, Lang J, Vahl C: Early formation of thrombi on pulmonary artery catheters in cardiac surgical patients receiving high-dose aprotinin. J Cardiothorac Anesth 4:222–225, 1990.
8. Brinkmann T, Schnierer S, Tschesche H: Recombinant aprotinin homologue with new inhibitory specificity for cathepsin G. Eur J Biochem 202:95–99, 1991.
9. Chabbat J, Porte P, Tellier M, Steinbuch M: Aprotinin is a competitive inhibitor of the factor VIIa–tissue factor complex. Thromb Res 71:205–215, 1993.
10. Clozel JP, Banken L, Roux S: Aprotinin: An antidote for recombinant tissue-type plasminogen activator (rt-PA) active in vivo. J Am Coll Cardiol 16:507–510, 1990.
11. Cottineau C, Moreau X, Drouet M, et al: Anaphylactic shock during the use of high doses of aprotinin in cardiac surgery. Ann Fr Anesth Reanim 12:590–593, 1993.
12. Farooqi N, DeHert S, Vlaeminck R, et al: Effects of low doses of aprotinin on clotting times activated with celite and kaolin. Acta Anaesthesiol Belg 44(3):87–92, 1993.
13. Garabedian HD, Gold HK, Leinbach RC, et al: Bleeding time prolongation and bleeding during infusion of recombinant tissue-type plasminogen activator in dogs: Potentiation by aspirin and reversal with aprotinin. J Am Coll Cardiol 17:1213–1222, 1991.
14. Gersbach P, Lammle B, Schupbach P, et al: Major coagulation disorders when using aprotinin—observations on a case. Thorac Cardiovasc Surg 39(4):196–198, 1991.
15. Girolami A: Inhibition by aprotinin [letter]. J Lab Clin Med 122:757, 1993.
16. Herbert JM, Bernat A, Maffrand JP: Aprotinin reduces clopidogrel-induced prolongation of the bleeding time in the rat. Thromb Res 71:433–441, 1993.
17. Hunt BJ, Murkin JM: Heparin resistance after aprotinin [letter]. Lancet 341:126, 1993.
18. Hunt BJ, Segal HC, Yacoub M: Guidelines for monitoring heparin by the activated clotting time when aprotinin is used during cardiopulmonary bypass [letter]. J Thorac Cardiovasc Surg 104:211–212, 1992.
19. Hunt BJ, Cottam S, Segal H, et al: Inhibition by aprotinin of tPA-mediated fibrinolysis during orthotopic liver transplantation [letter]. Lancet 336:381, 1990.
20. John LC, Rees GM, Kovacs IB: Reduction of heparin binding to and inhibition of platelets by aprotinin. Ann Thorac Surg 55:1175–1179, 1993.
21. Laurel MT, Ratnoff OD, Everson B: Inhibition of the activation of Hageman factor (factor XII) by aprotinin (Trasylol). J Lab Clin Med 119:580–585, 1992.

22. Mazoyer E, Boizard-Boval B, Pidard D, et al: Platelet membrane glycoproteins and platelet functions during storage in the presence of a proteinase inhibitor. Thromb Res 62(3):165–175, 1991.
23. Morimoto K, Yamaguchi H, Iwakura Y, et al: Effects of proteolytic enzyme inhibitors on the nasal absorption of vasopressin and an analogue. Pharm Res 8:1175–1179, 1991.
24. Morishita M, Morishita L, Takayama K, et al: Site-dependent effect of aprotinin, sodium caprate, Na2EDTA and sodium glycocholate on intestinal absorption of insulin. Biol Pharm Bull 16:68–72, 1993.
25. Najman DM, Walenga JM, Fareed J, Pifarré R: Effects of aprotinin on anticoagulant monitoring: Implications in cardiovascular surgery. Ann Thorac Surg 55:662–666, 1993.
26. Royston BD, Royston D, Pearson JD: Aprotinin inhibits platelet adhesion to endothelial cells. Blood Coagul Fibrinol 3:737–742, 1992.
27. Saffitz JE, Stahl DJ, Sundt TM, et al: Disseminated intravascular coagulation after administration of aprotinin in combination with deep hypothermic circulatory arrest. Am J Cardiol 72:1080–1082, 1993.
28. Schneider J: Interactions of saruplase with acetylsalicylic acid, heparin, glyceryl trinitrate, tranexamic acid and aprotinin in a rabbit pulmonary thrombosis model. Arzneimittelforsch 40:1180–1184, 1990.
29. Schulze K, Graeter T, Schaps D, Hausen B: Severe anaphylactic shock due to repeated application of aprotinin in patients following intrathoracic aortic replacement. Eur J Cardiothorac Surg 7:495–496, 1993.
30. Sunamori M, Sultan I, Suzuki A: Effect of aprotinin to improve myocardial viability in myocardial preservation followed by reperfusion. Ann Thorac Surg 52:971–978, 1991.
31. Sundt TM III, Kouchoukos NT, Saffitz JE, et al: Renal dysfunction and intravascular coagulation with aprotinin and hypothermic circulatory arrest. Ann Thorac Surg 55:1418–1424, 1993.
32. Taby O, Chabbat J, Steinbuch M: Inhibition of activated protein C by aprotinin and the use of the insolubilized inhibitor for its purification. Thromb Res 59:27–35, 1990.
33. Umbrain V, Christiaens F, Camu F: Intraoperative coronary thrombosis: Can aprotinin and protamine be incriminated? J Cardiothorac Vasc Anesth 8:198–201, 1994.
34. van den Besselaar AM, Dirven R, Bertina RM: Tissue factor-induced coagulation can be inhibited by aprotinin (Trasylol) [leter]. Thromb Haemost 69:298–299, 1993.
35. van Oeveren V, van Oeveren B, Wildevuur CR: Anticoagulation policy during use of aprotinin in cardiopulmonary bypass [letter]. J Thorac Cardiovasc Surg 104:210–211, 1992.
36. Walenga JM, Koza J, Soon BS, et al: Evaluation of CGP 39393 as the anticoagulant in cardiopulmonary bypass operation in a dog model. Ann Thorac Surg 1994 (in press).
37. Westaby S: Aprotinin in perspective. Ann Thorac Surg 55:1033–1041, 1993.

Ch.R.H. Wildevuur, MD, PhD
L. Eijsman, MD, PhD
H.C. Hemker, MD, PhD

# 12

# Aprotinin and Hemostasis in Cardiopulmonary Bypass

Impaired hemostasis has been associated with cardiopulmonary bypass (CPB) from its very beginning, contributing significantly to the morbidity and mortality related to cardiac surgery. During the past 40 years, however, technically improved CPB circuits strongly diminished these problems of hemostasis. Nevertheless, impaired hemostasis has not yet been eliminated entirely. This is demonstrated by a more recent achievement, proving that blood loss can be reduced to about half in routine cardiac surgery by using the protease inhibitor aprotinin.

The use of CPB causes massive contact-phase and complement activation as the blood interacts with the nonphysiological surfaces of the CPB circuit. Contact-phase activation starts the cascade of the kinin-generating system, the intrinsic coagulation pathway, and the fibrinolytic system. As massive activation of the **intrinsic** coagulation pathway leads to systemic thrombin generation, patients undergoing CPB have to be heparinized to prevent disseminated intravascular clotting. Heparinization also makes retransfusion of pericardially shed blood possible, which, by contact with tissue, has additionally been activated via the **extrinsic** coagulation pathway. So far, no systematic attempts have been made to inhibit the activation of the kinin-generating and fibrinolytic pathways or the complement system. As specific assays to determine the effect of blood activation during CPB on the different pathways are now available, insight into systemic blood activation, particularly into the major factors leading to impaired hemostasis and the effects of aprotinin during CPB, has increased.

## Hemostatic Mechanisms at the Bleeding Sites during Surgery

Upon incision and thus the cutting of blood vessels, platelets immediately adhere onto the de-endothelialized vascular wall structures, such as collagen fibers, basement membranes, and microfibrils. This prompt reaction is caused by various accessible glycoprotein receptors on platelets for von Willebrand factor (vWF), collagen, and laminin. For instance, glycoprotein (GP) Ib receptors on the platelet membrane bind to collagen fibrils via tissue-bound vWF.

At the same time, tissue factor activates the extrinsic coagulation pathway, which generates thrombin. Thrombin binds readily to the platelets by a specific thrombin receptor. This binding induces further platelet activation, such as a conformational change of the GPIIb-IIIa receptor and a "flip-flop" reaction of the platelet membrane. In this activation process, the cyclo-oxygenase pathway is involved. This process is, therefore, inhibited by aspirin. The conformational change of the GPIIb-IIIa complex transforms it into the main fibrinogen receptor. It thus enables platelet–platelet interaction, which leads to platelet aggregation.

The "flip-flop" reaction involves the transportation of negatively charged phospholipids from the inner side of the phospholipid bilayer to the outer layer of the platelet membrane, thus exposing a negatively charged, procoagulant phospholipid surface. This amplifies thrombin formation by providing the appropriate phospholipid surface for cofactors (factor Va and factor VIIIa) that cause a strong, positive feedback activation of the coagulation factors (factors IXa and Xa). Thus, thrombin sparks thrombin generation explosively.

The activation of platelets is also followed by a change in the shape of platelets (i.e., pseudopod formation) and microvesicle shedding, which enlarges the procoagulant surfaces, contributing to the explosive increase of thrombin generation. Thrombin also induces a release of the platelets' granule contents, which play a role in local hemostatis. Adenosine diphosphate (ADP), released from the dense bodies, stimulates platelet aggregation, whereas serotonin, released from the granules, causes local vasoconstriction.

Thrombin that is generated within the platelet plug, polymerizes fibrinogen into fibrin, which leads to the formation of a more solid, hemostatic plug. At the site of an arterial lesion, local thrombin generation should be explosive. If not, thrombin would be washed-out by the fast blood flow. However, explosive thrombin generation should only lead to local hemostatic plug formation, not to disseminated intravascular coagulation. Therefore, the positive feedback activation of cofactors (factors Va and VIIIa) should be counteracted by activation of negative feedback systems. This is effectuated by tissue factor plasma inactivator (TFPI) and antithrombin III but particularly by the protein C and protein S systems. The protein C system is activated by the binding of thrombin to the receptor thrombomodulin on the surface of endothelial cells. During this process, thrombin loses its procoagulant properties. In conjunction with protein S and the phospholipid platelet membrane, activated protein C inactivates Va and VIIIa into Vi and VIIIi, thereby ending further prothrombin conversion.

When thrombin is generated systemically, the level of activated protein C increases before any change in the level of factor V, fibrinogen, or platelets can be observed. This regulation of protein C seems to play a pivotal role in preventing disseminated intravascular coagulation.

In addition, by neutralizing the inhibitor of the tissue-type plasminogen activator (PAI), activated protein C stimulates fibrinolysis. Fibrinolysis, i.e., the splitting of polymerized fibrin strands, is caused by the proteolytic enzyme plasmin. Plasmin arises from plasminogen, a process that is induced by plasminogen activators such as tissue-type plasminogen activator (tPA). The release of tPA from endothelial cells is stimulated by various factors that also activate clotting. Although tPA by itself is a poor plasminogen activator, counteracted in plasma by plasminogen-activator inhibitors like PAI-1, its activity increases hundredfold in the presence of fibrin. This explains why tPA is primarily effective in hemostatic plugs.

When tPA is present, fibrin monomers on the platelet surface accelerate local plasminogen activation to form plasmin, which internalizes the GPIb receptors on platelets.[2] This might help to prevent circulating platelets from continuing to adhere and participate in the initial, local hemostatic process. In addition to splitting fibrin, plasmin cleaves fibrinogen and the GPIb receptors.

All these features of plasmin dynamically balance the hemostatic plug formation induced by thrombin. Local hemostatic plug formation is further controlled by intact endothelial cells. These produce heparan sulfate, which enhances the inhibiting effect of downstream antithrombin III on thrombin. Stimulated by thrombin, the intact endothelial cells also release prostacyclin ($PGI_2$), a potent inhibitor of platelet activation that stops the positive feedback activation of thrombin by platelets.

The above-described, classical picture of hemostasis at the site of vascular damage has been extended by the more recent demonstration of the profound effects of shear-stress on the processes leading to thrombus formation.[20] At surgical bleeding sites (predominantly vasoconstricted capillaries and arterioles), flowing blood is exposed to high shear-forces. These shear-forces induce the release of the intracellular multimeric vWF of platelets, which immediately binds to the GPIb receptors on the platelets' surface. This binding causes the transmembrane calcium channels to open, leading to an influx of calcium into the platelets. This calcium influx activates processes that lead to a functional change of GPIIb-IIIa, enabling its binding to vWF.

The repeating subunit structure of these large multimers of vWF offers an array of interaction sites, making multivalent binding to the GPIIb-IIIa receptors on the platelet membrane possible, thereby increasing the number of contact points and the affinity (strength) of interaction.[5] As a result, the overall force, linking platelets to the surface or to one another or to both, is increased. This then effectively opposes the shear-stress that flowing blood exerts on the platelet plug formation. In contrast to thrombin-induced platelet aggregation, shear-induced platelet aggregation is independent of the cyclo-oxygenase pathway[17] and, therefore, not inhibited by aspirin.

When platelets in flowing blood are not activated and shear-forces are low, platelets can adhere to and spread on a surface in case the GPIb platelet receptors "recognize" immobilized vWF. In addition, GPIIb-IIIa receptors can bind to fibrinogen, and cohesion with other platelets can proceed. These processes can occur even when platelets are inhibited by aspirin. However, when GPIb binds to immobilized vWF or soluble vWF (at higher shear-rates), or when thrombin binds to thrombin receptors independent of shear-forces, platelets do become activated. Both strong platelet adherence and platelet aggregation to oppose high shear-forces are particularly effectuated by activated GPIIb-IIIa receptors binding to multimeric vWF.

It is clear that the local circumstances at the site of vascular damage determine effective hemostatic plug formation, which primarily depends on platelet adhesion and aggregation. It is important to realize that two platelet mechanisms contribute to hemostasis: the ligand- (thrombin)-induced platelet activation and the shear-induced platelet activation. The first depends on the cyclo-oxygenase pathway; the second does not.

## Factors Affecting Hemostasis in Cardiopulmonary Bypass

Increasing numbers of patients presenting for coronary artery bypass grafting are treated with **aspirin**. Therefore, hemostasis may already be impaired before surgery, as described in the preceeding discussion. In this regard, a prophylactic dose of 100 mg of aspirin does not seem to affect hemostasis additionally in CPB, whereas a higher dose of 325 mg does.[22,25]

Another anticoagulant that might affect the hemostatic function of platelets is **heparin**, which is routinely used to prevent clotting in the CPB circuit. In about one-third of patients undergoing CPB, heparin interferes with the binding of vWF to GPIb platelet receptors, thereby affecting platelet adhesion.[11] **Hemodilution** of about 50%, due to the clear prime of the circuit, affects hemostasis, probably to a small extent.

As mentioned earlier, the use of CPB leads to **massive contact-phase and complement activation**, as blood interacts with the nonphysiological surfaces of the CPB circuit. This leads to activation of the **intrinsic** pathway of the coagulation and fibrinolytic systems and subsequent thrombin and plasmin generation (Fig. 1). Thrombin and plasmin are agonists with a high affinity for binding to the platelet surface, thereby affecting the GPIb receptor (Fig. 2) and, thus, the platelet's hemostatic function.[1]

Moreover, at various points of the CPB circuit, high shear-forces are generated, which activate platelets to adhere strongly to thrombogenic surfaces and aggregate. This reduces the number of circulating platelets. In addition, high shear-forces damage erythrocytes, resulting in release of adenosine diphosphate (ADP). ADP is an additional strong agonist for platelet aggregation and further affects the hemostatic capacity of platelets.

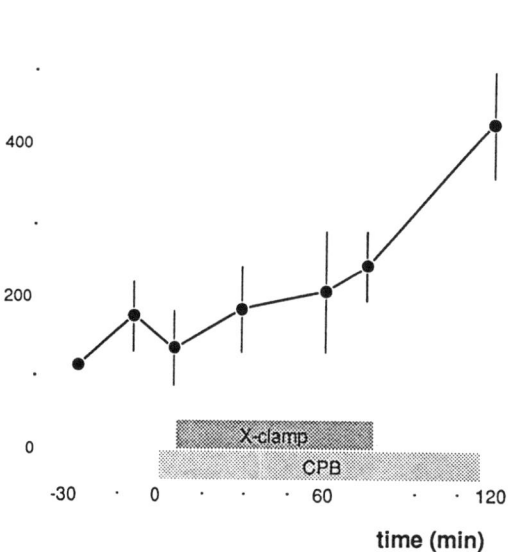

Bβ 15-42 (%)

**FIGURE 1.** B-beta$_{15-42}$, a specific marker for disseminated intravascular coagulation (systemic thrombin generation), expressed as a percentage of initial values, increased continuously during CPB.

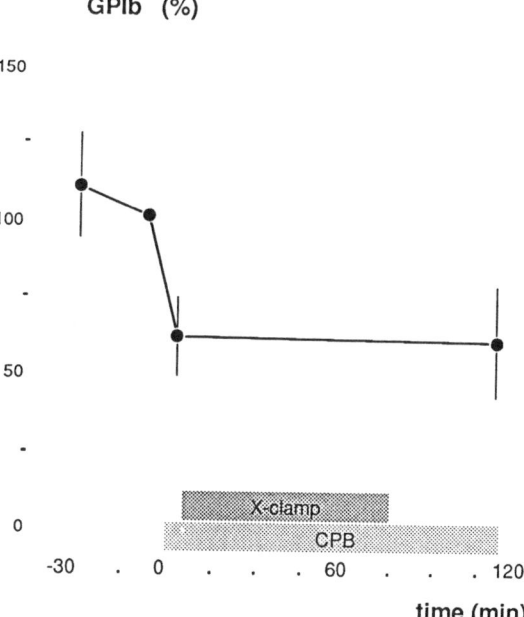

**GPIb (%)**

**FIGURE 2.** Platelet glycoprotein receptor Ib (GPIb), expressed as a percentage of pre-CPB values, decreased by 40% at the onset of CPB.

time (min)

Another source of blood activation that affects hemostasis during CPB is the translocation of **endotoxin** from the gut into the circulation.[8,10] This process is likely to be associated with the disturbed microcirculation of the gut mucosa during CPB. Under normal circumstances, the gut mucosa acts as an active barrier to prevent translocation of endotoxin. Endotoxin causes contact activation, stimulates monocytes and macrophages to produce cytokines, and strongly activates endothelial cells to release tPA, all of which interfere with the mechanisms involved in hemostasis.

Systemic blood activation is also caused by the **recirculation of pericardially shed blood** via cardiotomy suction. This blood has been in extensive contact with tissue, which particularly leads to activation of the extrinsic pathways of coagulation and fibrinolysis.[23]

A contributing factor that induces systemic blood activation is the **reperfusion** of heart and lungs after CPB.[7] This is due to the fact that tPA, released following ischemic damage of endothelial cells in these organs during aortic cross clamping, enters the blood circulation, subsequently stimulating fibrinolysis. The administration of **protamine** to neutralize heparin when ending CPB is also known to affect platelet hemostatic function.[29]

The above factors make it clear that platelet hemostatic function and capacity are affected and fibrinolysis is activated **during** CPB due to multiple factors. These factors together cause impaired hemostasis **after** CPB. Of importance also is that the enzymatic activity of antiproteases, physiologically counteracting the activation of the described plasmatic systems, becomes inhibited by **hypothermia**, routinely employed during CPB.

The reproducible, substantial improvements in hemostasis during and after CPB achieved by administering the antiprotease aprotinin points to a broad protective effect of aprotinin on the mechanisms of hemostasis induced by the multiple factors mentioned. It has been demonstrated that aprotinin prevents the interaction of heparin with vWF, eliminating the interference of heparin with platelet hemostatic function.[12] In addition, aprotinin in synergism with heparin strongly inhibits the activation of the **intrinsic** coagulation pathway (Fig. 3) that is due to contact activation by blood-material interaction and/or endotoxin translocation.[3] Moreover, aprotinin is an effective inhibitor of plasmin. Effective inhibition of thrombin and plasmin by aprotinin leads to preservation of platelet GPIb receptors (Fig. 4).[6,27,28,32] This importantly contributes to maintain hemostasis (Fig. 5). The strong inhibition of fibrinolysis enhances this effect even more.[16]

The mechanism by which protamine affects platelet function is unclear, and studies on the effect of aprotinin in this regard are needed. Interestingly, improved hemostasis by aprotinin administration can also be achieved in patients using prophylactic aspirin (Figs. 6 and 7).[22,25] An explanation of this effect is that shear-induced platelet reactivity, which is independent of the cyclo-oxygenase pathway, could be preserved by aprotinin. This emphasizes the essential role of this mechanism in platelet plug formation at multiple bleeding sites during surgery.[20]

Shear-induced platelet reactivity can be measured by doing a Thrombostat test.[13] This is an in vitro bleeding test, perfusing whole blood through an artificial arteriole (ID 190 $\mu$m) under constant pressure (40 mm Hg). This generates a shear-stress of 128 dyn/cm$^2$, which can be compared with the value estimated at the surgical bleeding site. By the induced shear-stress, platelets are activated and stick to the collagen filter at the end of the capillary, thus forming a platelet hemostatic plug. It is important to add ADP onto the filter to prevent an abnormally prolonged test result being obtained in patients treated with aspirin.[14] The binding of released platelet–vWF induced by ADP seems to play a dominant role in platelet plug formation by this specific shear-rate, which is not affected by aspirin.[17]

Although the results of the in vivo bleeding test correlate with the in vitro bleeding test,[13] the in vivo test is more sensitive for detecting the various factors influencing hemostasis.[19] For example, the clotting system and the cyclo-oxygenase pathway tend to affect the in vivo test.[19,30] Furthermore, CPB influences the in vivo

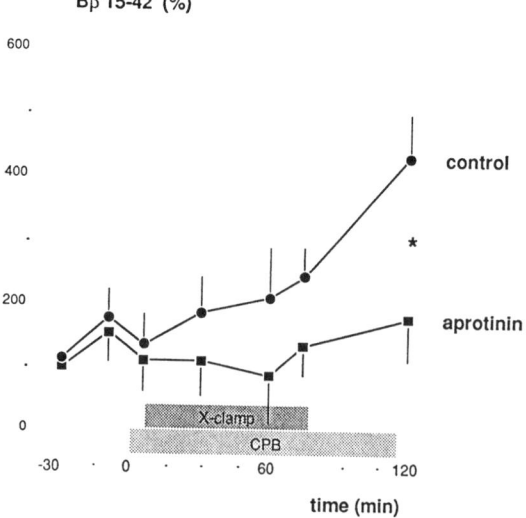

**FIGURE 3.** Generation of the B-beta$_{15-42}$ fragment, the molecular marker for disseminated intravascular coagulation, was completely inhibited by aprotinin administration (6 million KIU).

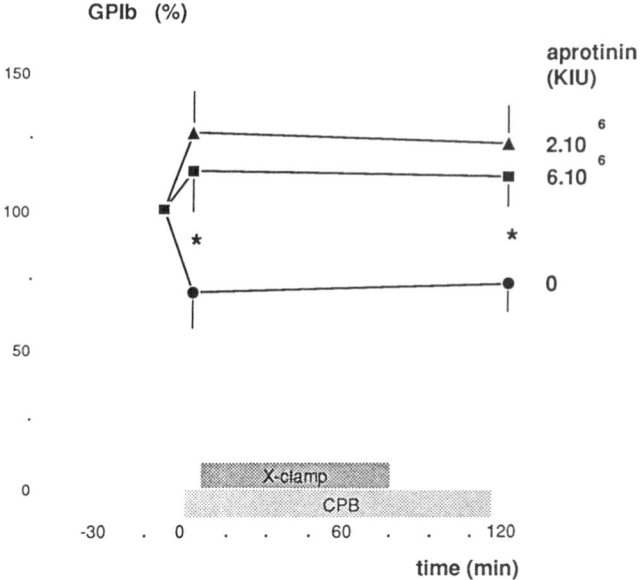

**FIGURE 4.** Platelet glycoprotein receptor IB (GPIb) changes during CPB, expressed as a percentage of pre-CPB values in aprotinin-treated patients given only 2 million KIU in the pump prime or combined with an additional bolus of 2 million KIU given at induction of anesthesia and a continuous infusion of 2 million KIU until protamine administration (total, 6 million KIU) or placebo. GPIb receptors remained preserved with aprotinin independent of the dose during CPB.

test, depending on various factors, e.g., skin temperature, vasotonic medication, and blood pressure.[26] Therefore, the in vitro test during CPB is more specifically useful for monitoring the shear-induced pathway of platelets, which seems to play a major role in hemostasis, particularly in aspirin-treated patients.

In a recent study, we demonstrated the alteration in hemostasis induced by the shear-induced platelet activation during CPB in aspirin-treated and non-aspirin-treated patients. Before CPB, the bleeding volume during the Thrombostat test was equal for both groups. Systemic heparinization influenced these test results only

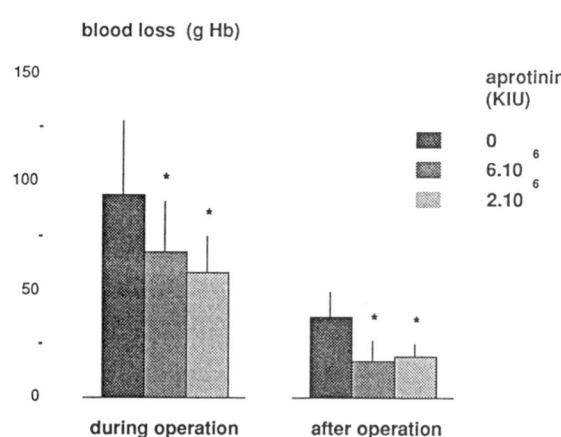

**FIGURE 5.** Blood loss, expressed in grams of hemoglobin content (g Hb), during and after operation in patients treated with 6 million KIU and 2 million KIU of aprotinin, was equally reduced and significantly ($*p < 0.05$) lower than in patients receiving placebo.

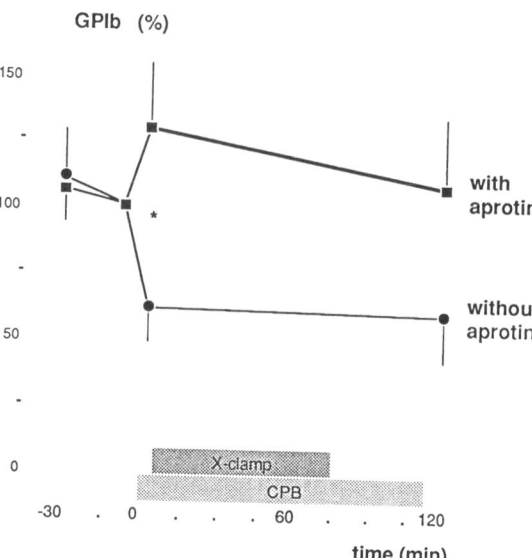

**FIGURE 6.** Platelet glycoprotein receptor (GPIb) was significantly (*$p < 0.05$) reduced at the onset or CPB in non-aprotinin-treated patients independent of aspirin pretreatment. Aprotinin administration (2 million KIU in the pump prime), both in patients with or without aspirin pretreatment, preserved platelet GPIb receptors during CPB.

slightly, which signals that the effect of the clotting system is only minor.[24] After starting CPB, bleeding volume in both groups increased abruptly. This indicates that the hemostatic capacity of platelets rapidly and strongly diminishes. During CPB, however, the hemostatic capacity of the platelets was significantly more affected in the aspirin-treated patients than in the non-aspirin-treated patients.

The reported, initial decrease of platelet membrane glycoprotein antigens (GPIb) during CPB[27,32] might partly reflect the loss of the hemostatic capacity of platelets during the Thrombostat test. In both groups, the shear-induced platelet aggregation recovered partly after CPB, but the hemostatic capacity of the platelets remained significantly more affected in aspirin-treated patients than in placebo-treated patients. This higher vulnerability of aspirin-treated patients for impaired hemostasis induced by CPB, however, can be modified by aprotinin administration.[22,25]

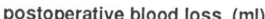

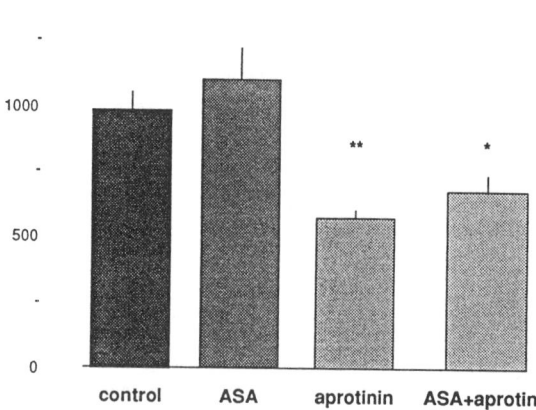

**FIGURE 7.** Postoperative blood loss during 24 hours after operation. Aprotinin significantly decreased blood loss in aspirin-treated and non-aspirin-treated patients (*$p < 0.05$ comparing aspirin-treated patients with aspirin/aprotinin-treated patients; **$p < 0.05$ comparing non-treated patients and aprotinin-treated patients).

It is interesting that the dose of aspirin seems to cause a different shear-induced reactivity of platelets in vitro,[18] which might also be reflected in the clinical CPB situation. Although the mechanism is still unclear, it underlines the broad protective effect of aprotinin. This might also explain the reproducibility of the hemostatic effect of aprotinin in various centers, independent of the differences in the various circumstances that can influence hemostasis.

On the other hand, the broad and potent action of a natural protease inhibitor like aprotinin might also have unwanted side effects. Because of its inhibitory effect on fibrinolysis and the natural anticoagulant protein C system, aprotinin causes a shift in favor of thrombosis. This aprotinin-induced imbalance is likely rebalanced by systemic heparinization during CPB. However, when aprotinin administration is started at the induction of anaesthesia, i.e., before heparin is given, or when aprotinin is still active after protamine has neutralized heparin, the antifibrinolytic properties may tend to work in favor of thrombin (fibrin) formation.

Particularly during coronary artery bypass grafting, there is a risk of thrombosis in the vein grafts, as these grafts are mostly de-endothelialized after implantation, thus forming an ideal activation site for platelet adherence. Moreover, reports of disseminated intravascular clotting after deep hypothermia and circulatory arrest in patients treated with aprotinin[31] demonstrate the danger of uncontrolled inhibition of the protein C system under these circumstances, despite systemic heparinization. The rationale is therefore to limit aprotinin administration to the period of systemic heparinization and to moderate hypothermia.

Several reports[21,28] have shown that 2 million KIU of aprotinin added to the pump prime has an effect on hemostasis that is comparable to that for the initially proposed dose scheme of 6 million KIU (which also covers the period before and after heparinization).[28] However, the 6-million-KIU dose has an inhibitory effect on the balance of natural anticoagulation, which is present before and after systemic heparinization. Although a dose of 2 million KIU of aprotinin, to be added to the pump prime only, is therefore theoretically safer than the 6-million-KIU dose, this low dose might not protect sufficiently against all the mentioned factors that have the potential to affect hemostasis during CPB.

Shortly after the aorta cross-clamp is released, a sharp rise in tPA and fibrinolytic activity was observed.[4] One has to realize that these effects can be caused by multiple coinciding factors: recirculation of heart and lungs, increase of cardiotomy suction, and end of hypothermia. As these factors might vary from center to center, a variable protective effect of just 2 million KIU of aprotinin in the prime can be expected. Although this might lower the high reproducibility rate and effectiveness of the 6-million-KIU dose scheme, it could prevent the potential side effects of aprotinin and it certainly reduces the costs.

With all this in mind, it is important to realize that efforts to improve hemostasis during CPB are primarily aimed at reducing or, if possible, eliminating the need for blood products because of their inherent risks. To achieve this goal, several cardiac centers have instituted a strict blood salvage protocol, which includes postoperative retransfusion of preoperatively donated autologous blood. Also in this situation, a low dose of aprotinin should be considered, because it can contribute substantially to reducing the use of blood products.[21] On the other hand, when postoperative retransfusion of preoperatively donated autologous blood leads to the preservation of a substantial number of platelets that do not endure the negative effects of blood activation caused by CPB, the protective effect of 2 million KIU of aprotinin on circulating platelets might not be so impressive anymore.

However, potentiating effects are seen when heparin-coated circuits, the use of which reduces complement activation,[9] are primed with 2 million KIU of aprotinin.

In a recent study,[15] none of the separate variables, i.e., neither heparin coating nor aprotinin, improved hemostasis, but their combination did. Another observation in this study was that the inflammatory reaction, which determines length of stay in the intensive care unit, was also significantly milder following the combined use of heparin coating and aprotinin.

The gradually expanding knowledge of the mechanisms affecting blood activation during CPB indicates that for CPB techniques, multiple improvements are still required. In regard to the use of drugs such as aprotinin, it is essential to find the optimal dose and to avoid potential side effects. Finally, all other measures that reduce blood activation and limit the use of blood products should also be taken when employing CPB.

## References

1. Adelman B, Michelson AD, Loscalzo J, et al: Plasmin effect on platelet glycoprotein IB–von Willebrand factor interactions. Blood 65:32–40, 1985.
2. Cramer EM, Lu H, Caen JP, et al: Differential redistribution of platelet glycoproteins Ib and IIb-IIIa after plasmin stimulation. Blood 77:694–699, 1991.
3. De Smet AAEA, Chan Njoek Joen M, van Oeveren W, et al: Increased anticoagulation during cardiopulmonary bypass by aprotinin. J Thorac Cardiovasc Surg 100:520–527, 1990.
4. Eijsman L: Cardiopulmonary Bypass and Hemostasis. Groningen, University Press, 1992.
5. Federici AB, Bader R, Pagarius S, et al: Binding of von Willebrand factor (vWF) to glycoproteins (GP) Ib and IIb-IIIa complex: Affinity is related to multimeric size. Br J Haematol 73:93–99, 1989.
6. Huang H, Ding W, Su Z, Zhang W: Mechanisms of the preserving effect of aprotinin on platelet function and its use in cardiac surgery. J Thorac Cardiovasc Surg 106:11–18, 1993.
7. Jansen NJG, van Oeveren W, van den Broek L, et al: Inhibition of the reperfusion phenomena in cardiopulmonary bypass by dexamethasone. J Thorac Cardiovasc Surg 102:515–525, 1991.
8. Jansen NJG, van Oeveren W, Gu YJ, et al: Endotoxin release and tumor necrosis factor formation during cardiopulmonary bypass. Ann Thorac Surg 55:744–748, 1992.
9. Jansen PGM, te Velthuis H, Huybregts MAJM, et al: Reduced complement activation and improved postoperative course after cardiopulmonary bypass with heparin-coated circuits. J Thorac Cardiovasc Surg (submitted).
10. Jansen PGM, te Velthuis H, Oudemans-van Straaten H, et al: Perfusion-related factors of endotoxin release during cardiopulmonary bypass. Eur J Cardiothorac Surg 8:125–129, 1994.
11. John LCH, Rees GM, Kovacs IB: Inhibition of platelet function by heparin. J Thorac Cardiovasc Surg 105:816–822, 1993.
12. John LCH, Rees GM, Kovacs IB: Reduction of heparin binding to and inhibition of platelets by aprotinin. Ann Thorac Surg 55:1175–1179, 1993.
13. Kratzer MAA, Born GVR: Simulation of primary hemostasis in vitro. Haemostasis 15:357–362, 1985.
14. Kretschmer V, Schikor B, Sohngen D, Dietrich G: In vitro bleeding test: A simple method for the detection of aspirin effects on platelet function. Thromb Res 56:593–602, 1989.
15. Loisance D, Jansen PGM, Lebesnerais P, Wildevuur ChRH: Synergistic effect of heparin-coated circuits with aprotinin prime for cardiac surgery on blood loss, blood use and intensive care stay. J Thorac Cardiovasc Surg (submitted).
16. Lu H, Soria C, Ommin PL, et al: Hemostasis in patients undergoing extracorporeal circulation: The effect of aprotinin (Trasylol). Thromb Haemost 66:633–637, 1991.
17. Moake JL, Turner NA, Stathopoulos NA, et al: Shear-induced platelet aggregation can be mediated by vWF released from platelets as well as by exogenous large or unusually large vWF multimers, required adenosine diphosphate, and is resistant to aspirin. Blood 71:1366–1374, 1988.
18. Ratnatunga CP, Edmondson SF, Rees GM, Kovacs IB: High-dose aspirin inhibits shear-induced platelet reaction involving thrombin generation. Circulation 85:1077–1082, 1982.

19. Rodgers RPC, Levin J: A critical reappraisal of the bleeding time. Semin Thromb Hemost 16:1–20, 1990.
20. Ruggeri M: Mechanisms of shear-induced platelet adhesion and aggregation. Thromb Haemost 70:119–123, 1993.
21. Schönberger JPAM, Everts PAM, Husam Ercan EKP, et al: Low-dose aprotinin in internal mammary bypass operations contributes to important blood saving. Ann Thorac Surg 54:1172–1177, 1992.
22. Tabuchi N, Gallandat Huet RCG, Sturk A, Wildevuur ChRH: Aprotinin preserves hemostasis in aspirin-treated patients undergoing cardiopulmonary bypass. Ann Thorac Surg (in press).
23. Tachubi N, de Haan J, Boonstra PW, van Oeveren W: Activation of fibrinolysis in the pericardial cavity during cardiopulmonary bypass. J Thorac Cardiovasc Surg 106:823–833, 1993.
24. Tabuchi N, de Haan J, van Oeveren W: Rapid recovery of platelet function after cardiopulmonary bypass. Blood 82:2930–2931, 1993.
25. Tabuchi N, van Oeveren W, Eijsman L, et al: Preserved hemostasis during the combined use of aprotinin and aspirin in CABG operations. In Friedel N, Hetzler R, Royston D (eds): Blood Use in Cardiac Surgery. Darmstadt, Steinkopff Verlag, 1991, pp 245–251.
26. Valeri CR, Khabbaz K, Khuri SF, et al: Effect of skin temperature on platelet function in patients undergoing extracorporeal bypass. J Thorac Cardiovasc Surg 104:108–116, 1992.
27. Van Oeveren W, Eijsman L, Roozendaal KJ, Wildevuur ChRH: Platelet preservation by aprotinin during cardiopulmonary bypass. Lancet 1586:644, 1988.
28. Van Oeveren W, Harder MP, Roozendaal KJ, et al: Aprotinin protects platelets against the initial effect of cardiopulmonary bypass. J Thorac Cardiovasc Surg 99:788–797, 1990.
29. Velders AJ, van den Dungen JJAM, Westerhof NJW, Wildevuur ChRH: Platelet damage by protamine administration: Protection by reducing protamine or by prostacyclin ($PGI_2$) treatment. Artif Organs 3:318, 1979.
30. Weiss HJ, Lages B: Studies of thromboxane B2, platelet factor 4, and fibrinopeptide A in bleeding-time blood of patients deficient in von Willebrand factor, platelet glycoprotein Ib and IIb-IIIa, and storage granules. Blood 82:481–490, 1993.
31. Westaby B, Forni A, Dunning J, et al: Aprotinin and bleeding in profoundly hypothermic perfusion. Eur J Cardiothorac Surg 8:87–91, 1994.
32. Wildevuur ChRH, Eijsman L, Roozendaal KJ, et al: Platelet preservation during cardiopulmonary bypass with aprotinin. Eur J Cardiothorac Surg 3:533–538, 1990.

Roque Pifarré, MD
Maher Istanbouli, CCP
Jamal Sinno, CCP
Jodi Cava, CCP

# 13

# Monitoring of Anticoagulation during Cardiopulmonary Bypass in Patients Treated with Aprotinin

Cardiopulmonary bypass (CPB) became possible only because anticoagulation with heparin was available. Systemic anticoagulation is required to prevent coagulation of the blood when it comes in contact with the foreign surfaces of the heart-lung machine. Heparin is used for this purpose because it inhibits thrombin, thus preventing the creation of fibrin.

The complexity of hemostatic control during CPB requires careful consideration. A clear understanding is necessary of the variables associated with the therapeutic use of heparin, its neutralization with protamine, and the individual nature of these responses. The protocol for anticoagulation during CPB has varied greatly from institution to institution. In 1975, Bull et al.[5] made an important contribution by showing the differences in, and variability of, the anticoagulation response. These authors recommended routine monitoring of anticoagulation during CPB with the activated coagulation time (ACT).[4] This method eliminates the uncertainty during CPB, one of the major factors in excessive postoperative blood loss.[1] Monitoring heparin concentration directly has been advocated by others.[14,21]

The large surface of the extracorporeal circulation apparatus results in a massive thrombotic stimulus, leading to the activation of factor XII. The end result of this contact activation is the production of a systemic inflammatory response. Activation of factor XII initiates a series of cascades involving the coagulation system, plasmin fibrinolysis, kallikrein, and complement activation.[15] Aprotinin is being used in many clinical situations to improve hemostasis in patients undergoing CPB.[2] It inhibits kallikrein, plasmin, trypsin, and chymotrypsin and affects receptors on platelet membranes.[25] The decrease in blood loss in CPB operations with use of aprotinin has been attributed to preservation of the adhesive capacity of platelets.[11]

Monitoring of anticoagulation during CPB is most important. The importance of ascertaining the proper dose of heparin during CPB cannot be overemphasized. The amount of heparin given must be carefully calculated. Too high a dose can lead to bleeding, whereas too low a dose can lead to clotting. This is even more important when aprotinin is being used. The celite ACT does not display its normal sensitivity and linearity in patients treated with aprotinin. Instead, the celite ACT is abnormally prolonged. Awareness of this prolongation is critical to maintain the proper concentration of heparin in the blood and, therefore, adequate anticoagulation.

## Heparin Administration Protocol

The heparin dose, when aprotinin is not used, is calculated at the Loyola University Medical Center as a total dose of 200 U (2 mg) per kg of body weight. During CPB, the ACT is maintained above 400 s. Several doses of 2000–3000 U of heparin are added to the oxygenator, if needed, to maintain the ACT above the level of 400 s.

The heparin is administered directly into the right atrium of the heart by the surgeon before cannulating the aorta and right atrium for CPB. This method of administration accomplishes two objectives: (1) it ensures that the heparin has entered the central circulation, and (2) it ensures the full dose of heparin has been administered. Heparin administered in a peripheral line may not reach the central circulation, with possible catastrophic results.

Other teams use an initial dose of 300–400 U/kg of body weight. They may also add 10,000–20,000 U of heparin in the priming fluid used for the extracorporeal circuit. During bypass, heparin is added at a rate of 50–100 U/kg/hr. Monitoring anticoagulation with the ACT and the heparin analyzer (Hepcon, Medtronic Hemotec, Englewood, CO) has convinced us that the lower dosage is safe and the higher dose unnecessary. We believe that the more heparin you use, the more postoperative bleeding you will face. Our findings[1,21] agree with those of Metz and Keats.[17]

In a multicenter, double-blind, placebo-controlled trial of aprotinin for reducing blood loss in patients undergoing repeat coronary artery bypass grafting, it was recommended that prior to cannulation of the heart, a heparin loading dose of at least 350 U/kg be administered to the patient. Additional heparin was administered to maintain the heparin concentration at 2.7 U/ml during CPB using a heparin/protamine titration performed with the Hepcon heparin monitoring system[16] (Table 1).

## Monitoring of Anticoagulation

No practical test of heparin-induced anticoagulant effect was available until the ACT was introduced by Hattersley in 1966.[10] Bull et al.[4,5] in 1975 produced two classic papers, pointing out the need for heparin and protamine dosing protocols using the ACT. Their publication became the turning point for heparin management during CPB, marking the transition from an empirical heparin dosing to a structured approach using the ACT.

**TABLE 1.**  Control of Anticoagulation During Aprotinin Use

| | |
|---|---|
| Heparin loading dose | 350 U/kg |
| Add heparin to maintain heparin concentration (Hepcon) at | 2.7 U/ml |
| ACT (celite) | > 750 s |
| ACT (kaolin) | > 500 s |

At present, the laboratory tests for heparin monitoring fall into two categories: clotting time and measurements of blood heparin concentration.

## Aprotinin and the Celite ACT Test

Giving aprotinin (at high dose and half-dose) has been shown to reduce perioperative and postoperative blood loss and the need for blood transfusion in cardiac patients.[2,3,16,23] The hemostatic benefits of aprotinin are attributed to its antifibrinolytic property, its capacity to preserve platelet function, and its inhibition of the activation of the intrinsic coagulation system.[8,11,18,25]

It has become apparent that aprotinin prolongs the ACT measured with celite in patients whose blood has been anticoagulated with heparin.[7,25] In most institutions, the ACT (celite) is used intraoperatively during CPB to monitor anticoagulation with heparin. The normal value of ACT in a control population is $107 \pm 13$ s.[10] Heparin administration results in a linear prolongation of the celite ACT up to values $> 600$ s, at which point the ACT no longer performs in a linear fashion.

Adequate anticoagulation with heparin during CPB is achieved if the ACT is maintained at $\geq 400$ s,[30] although it has been questioned whether this level is valid when aprotinin is administered. In 1990, de Smet et al.[7] reported a synergistic prolongation of the ACT in patients undergoing CPB with aprotinin. However, in 1990, based on in vitro studies indicating that aprotinin affects the extrinsic clotting system and the protein C system, Van Oeveren and associates[25] advised against changing heparinization regimes and cautioned that the ACT should not be used to monitor heparinization in aprotinin-treated patients in CPB. In 1992, Hunt and associates[12,13] also warned against changes in heparinization protocols, but they suggested that an ACT of $> 750$ s should be maintained to compensate. Wang and associates[28] showed that prolongation of the ACT in heparinized, aprotinin-treated patients undergoing CPB was present when celite was used as the surface activator. However, they did not find this ACT-prolonging effect when kaolin was used as an activator. In a randomized study, the same authors[27] concluded that the increased ACTs of blood anticoagulated with heparin during CPB in aprotinin-treated patients are likely due to the use of celite as the surface activator rather than to aprotinin-enhanced anticoagulation of heparin. The ACTs measured with kaolin activator are insensitive to the presence of aprotinin and remain comparable to the ACTs in the control group.

A clinical study by Cosgrove et al.[6] used the celite-ACT $> 400$ s as a minimum level of anticoagulation. This trial showed a possible increase in thrombotic complications after patients undergoing repeat coronary artery bypass were treated with aprotinin, raising the question of whether aprotinin could be prothrombotic. The results of a multicenter randomized study by Levy et al.[16] showed no such complications. It was concluded that the complications reported by Cosgrove and associates[6] might have resulted from inadequate heparinization due to the belief that aprotinin decreased the heparin requirements.

In a study done at our own institution,[19] we concluded that the so-called anticoagulant effect of aprotinin as determined by the celite-ACT is not heparin-like, and aprotinin does not affect thrombin formation and the coagulation cascade as heparin does. It is therefore not appropriate to assume that the increased ACT (celite) in aprotinin-treated patients undergoing CPB warrants reduced heparinization as suggested by some investigators.[7] We believe that such reduced heparinization would, in fact, lead to reduced anticoagulation and possible adverse thrombotic events.

### Aprotinin and the Kaolin ACT Test

The kaolin ACT has been shown to be less affected by the administration of aprotinin. Kaolin is similar to celite in the sense that it activates the intrinsic coagulation pathway via factor XII, known as the contact factor. Kaolin appears to be a better contact activator than celite because it functions efficiently in the presence of aprotinin, probably due to its different surface structure. Kaolin is made of hydrated aluminum silicate, whereas celite is made of a diatomaceous earth. According to Wendel et al.,[29] the factor XII levels were more reduced with kaolin than celite, and this difference was more pronounced in the presence of aprotinin.

These two systems to measure ACTs are very different. The Medtronic Hemotec uses kaolin activator. It uses 0.4 ml of whole blood injected into each of two plastic cartridges, and then a mechanical plunger that moves in and out of these blood samples. The initial plunger movement mixes the whole blood with kaolin activator, and the plunger continues to rise and fall until clot forms. The absence of plunger fall is detected photo-optically, stops the timer, and determines the ACT.

The Hemochron machine (International Technidyne Corp., Edison, NJ) uses a magnet inside prewarmed glass specimen tubes that hold the diatomaceous earth activator (celite). Once the blood is inside the tube, the tube rotates inside the machine. As the blood clots, it displaces the magnet and the switch is activated. The ACT is the time it takes to displace the magnet a given distance.

Wang et al.,[27] as well as Wendel and associates,[29] have suggested the use of the kaolin ACT for monitoring of heparin-induced anticoagulation in patients treated with aprotinin therapy. Taylor[24] has recommended that levels of at least 750–800 s should be maintained during CPB when high-dose aprotinin therapy is being used and anticoagulation is monitored with the celite ACT.

### Heparin/Protamine Titration and Aprotinin

In a recent multicenter randomized study,[16] the level of heparin anticoagulation in the presence of aprotinin was monitored using the Hepcon heparin-monitoring system and heparin/protamine titration (HPT) (Table 1). In the HPT, the concentration of heparin is calculated on the basis of a known concentration of protamine. The titration is performed in a six-channel cartridge. Each channel contains a different level of protamine sulfate and an equal amount of dilute thromboplastin, into which is injected 0.2 ml of fresh whole blood. At the initiation of the test, the reagents are mixed with the blood sample, activating blood coagulation; the protamine in each channel neutralizes a specific amount of heparin. The first channel to clot is the channel in which the amount of protamine most closely neutralizes all of the heparin in the blood without an excess of either agent. The end point of the test is the detection of clot formation, as measured by the rate of fall of the plunger mechanism in each cartridge channel. The plunger assembly falls rapidly through an unclotted sample, but the fibrin web formed during clotting impedes the rate of descent. The rate of fall is detected by a photo-optical system located in the activator assembly of the instrument. With HPT, a target heparin concentration (e.g., 2–4 U/ml) can be used to guide heparin dosing.

It must be taken into account, however, that monitoring the heparin concentration via HPT reflects only the amount of heparin circulating in the patient and does not depict heparin response. Using HPT to monitor heparin concentration will not identify cases of heparin resistance. Those cases, instead, will be identified with the ACT. Another important clinical distinction is that the circulating heparin level, provided by the HPT system, reflects total circulating heparin, not functional circulating heparin. Protamine has an affinity for all heparin, whether it is functional (bound to antithrombin III) or not. Therefore, the circulating heparin levels do not accurately reflect the functional circulating heparin levels.

Monitoring anticoagulation during CPB has been controversial. Gravlee et al.[9] stated that heparin dosing during CPB cannot be guided by monitoring heparin concentrations. Wang et al.[27] reported that the heparin concentration determined by HPT failed to match the heparin dose in 43% of the measurements. It has been our practice to use the celite-ACT and measurement of the heparin concentration simultaneously in all our cases, and we are satisfied with the results.[22]

## High-Dose Thrombin Time and Aprotinin

The thrombin time is considered to be the most effective, sensitive, and specific test for monitoring heparin at low levels. Instead of measuring the intrinsic coagulation pathway (contact activation of factor XII) with ACT, the thrombin time measures the final step in the coagulation cascade: It measures the conversion of fibrinogen into fibrin in the presence of thrombin. It has not been practical, however, to use the conventional thrombin time for monitoring heparin during CPB due to the high concentration of heparin in these patients, compared with the low concentration of thrombin reagents employed.

The modification introduced by Hemochron (Hemochron HiTT, International Technidyne Corp.) is intended for the purpose of monitoring high levels of heparin anticoagulation. The high-dose thrombin time (HiTT) test employs a specific concentration of thrombin such that high levels of heparin may be monitored. The high concentration of thrombin provides a heparin-specific assay unaffected by minor decreases in fibrinogen or the accumulation of fibrinogen degradation products (DPTs). The specificity for heparin provides a high correlation between the HiTT value and the circulating heparin level following a bolus dose. The HiTT test provides a measure of the heparin response and the functional circulating heparin level in a single test. The reason is that the thrombin reagent in the HiTT is neutralized only by the heparin/antithrombin III complex and not free-floating heparin.

The HiTT assay is used in a manner similar to the ACT for monitoring heparin. The patient is infused with heparin as required to maintain the desired target range. The advantages of the HiTT assay are that it is a heparin-specific assay and is not affected by hypothermia or hemodilution, and more important, it is not influenced by concomitant aprotinin. The disadvantages most frequently mentioned are that it requires meticulous technique for sample collection and assay procedure. Precise volume transfer and specimen mixing are required for accurate test results.

## Summary

Monitoring of anticoagulation during CPB when aprotinin is used is of paramount importance. The proper level of anticoagulation must be maintained. Failure to do so can result in serious complications, such as graft thrombosis, stroke, and acute myocardial infarction.

In the multicenter, double-blind, placebo-controlled trial of aprotinin, the heparin loading dose was 350 U/kg. During CPB, heparin was added to maintain the heparin concentration at 2.7 U/ml. The ACT (celite) was also used and maintained above 750 s. When the kaolin ACT is used, it should be maintained above 500 s (Table 1). When this approach was used, there was no difference in the incidence of stroke, graft thrombosis, acute myocardial infarction, and renal failure between the aprotinin groups and the placebo group.

## References

1. Babka R, Colby C, El-Etr A, Pifarre R: Monitoring of intraoperative heparinization and blood loss following cardiopulmonary bypass surgery. J Thorac Cardiovasc Surg 73:700–783, 1977.
2. Bidstrup BP, Royston D, Sapsford RN, Taylor KM: Reduction in blood loss and blood use after cardiopulmonary bypass with high dose aprotinin (Trasylol). J Thorac Cardiovasc Surg 97:364–372, 1989.
3. Bidstrup BP, Royston D, Taylor KM, Sapsford RN: Effect of aprotinin on need for blood transfusion in patients with septic endocarditis having open heart surgery. Lancet 1:366–367, 1988.
4. Bull BS, Huse WM, Brauer FS, Korpeman RA: Heparin therapy during extracorporeal circulation: II. The use of a dose-response curve to individualize heparin and protamine dosage. J Thorac Cardiovasc Surg 69:685–689, 1975.
5. Bull RS, Korpeman RA, Huse WM, Briggs BD: Heparin therapy during extracorporeal circulation: I. Problems inherent in existing heparin protocols. J Thorac Cardiovasc Surg 69:674–684, 1975.
6. Cosgrove DM III, Heric B, Lytle BW, et al: Aprotinin therapy for reoperative myocardial revascularization: A placebo control study. Ann Thorac Surg 54:1031–1038, 1992.
7. de Smet AAEA, Joen MCN, Van Oeveren W, et al: Increased anticoagulation during cardiopulmonary bypass by aprotinin. J Thorac Cardiovasc Surg 100:520–527, 1990.
8. Dietrich W, Spannagl M, Jochum M, et al: Influence of high dose aprotinin treatment on blood loss and coagulation patterns in patients undergoing myocardial revascularization. Anesthesiology 93:1119–1126, 1990.
9. Gravlee GP, Hadston WS, Rothberger HK, et al: Heparin dosing and monitoring for cardiopulmonary bypass: A comparison of techniques with measurements of subclinical plasma coagulation. J Thorac Cardiovasc Surg 99:518–527, 1990.
10. Hattersley PG: Activated coagulation time of whole blood. JAMA 196:150, 436, 4401, 1966.
11. Havel M, Tenfelsbauer H, Knobl P, et al: Effect of intraoperative aprotinin administration on postoperative bleeding in patients undergoing cardiopulmonary bypass operation. J Thorac Cardiovasc Surg 1010:968–972, 1991.
12. Hunt BJ, Segal H, Yacoub M: Aprotinin and heparin monitoring during cardiopulmonary bypass. Circulation 86(suppl II):II-410–II-412, 1992.
13. Hunt BJ, Segal HC, Yacoub M: Guidelines for monitoring heparin by the activated clotting time when aprotinin is used during cardiopulmonary bypass. J Thorac Cardiovasc Surg 104:211–212, 1992.
14. Jobes DR, Schwartz AJ, Ellison N, et al: Monitoring heparin anticoagulation and its neutralization. Ann Thorac Surg 31:161–166, 1981.
15. Kirklin JK, Westaby S, Blackstone EH, et al: Complement and damaging effects of cardiopulmonary bypass. J Thorac Cardiovasc Surg 96:845–857, 1983.
16. Levy JH, Pifarre R, Schaaf H, et al: A multicenter, double blind, placebo-controlled trial of aprotinin for reducing blood loss and the requirements for donor blood transfusion in patients undergoing repeat coronary artery bypass grafting. (In press.)
17. Metz S, Keats AS: Low activated coagulation time during cardiopulmonary bypass does not increase postoperative bleeding. Ann Thorac Surg 49:440–444, 1990.
18. Nagaoka H, Innamic R, Murayama F, et al: Effects of aprotinin on prostaglandin metabolism and platelet function in open heart surgery. J Cardiovasc Surg 32:31–37, 1991.
19. Najman DM, Walenga JM, Fareed J, Pifarre R: Effects of aprotinin on anticoagulants monitoring: Implications in cardiovascular surgery. Ann Thorac Surg 55:662–666, 1993.

20. Penner JA: Experience with a thrombin clotting time assay for measuring heparin activity. Am J Clin Pathol 61:645, 1974.
21. Pifarre R, Babka R, Sullivan HJ, et al: Management of postoperative heparin rebound following cardiopulmonary bypass. J Thorac Cardiovasc Surg 81:378–381, 1981.
22. Pifarre R, Sullivan H, Montoya A, et al: Management of blood loss and heparin rebound following cardiopulmonary bypass. Semin Thromb Hemost 15:173–177, 1989.
23. Royston D, Bistrup BP, Taylor KM, Sapsford NN: Effect of aprotinin on need for blood transfusions after repeat open-heart surgery. Lancet ii:1289–1291, 1987.
24. Taylor KM: Perioperative approaches to coagulation defects. Ann Thorac Surg 56:578–582, 1993.
25. Van Oeveren W, Harder MP, Roozendaal KJ, et al: Aprotinin protects platelets against the initial effect of cardiopulmonary bypass. J Thorac Cardiovasc Surg 99:788–797, 1990.
26. Wang JS, Lin CY, Karp RB: Do we have a way to measure the adequacy of heparinization during cardiopulmonary bypass? Anesth Analg 74:51–53, 1992.
27. Wang JS, Lin CY, Hung WT, Karp RB: Monitoring of heparin-induced anticoagulation with kaolin-activated clotting time in cardiac surgical patients treated with aprotinin. Anesthesiology 77:1080–1084, 1992.
28. Wang JS, Lin CY, Hung WT, et al: In vitro effects of aprotinin on activated clotting time measured with different activators. J Thorac Cardiovasc Surg 104:1135–1140, 1992.
29. Wendel HP, Heller W, Gallimore MJ, et al: The prolonged activated clotting time (ACT) with aprotinin depends on the type of activator used for measurement. Blood Coag Fibrinol 4:41–45, 1993.
30. Young JH, Kleker CT, Doty OS: Adequate anticoagulation during cardiopulmonary bypass determined by activated clotting time and the appearance of fibrin monomer. Ann Thorac Surg 26:231–240, 1978.

Michael N. D'Ambra, MD
Theodore Alston, MD, PhD

# 14

## Is Kaolin the Ideal Way to Monitor Anticoagulation with Heparin in Aprotinin-treated Patients?

Studies in Europe and the United States have documented the efficiency and safety of aprotinin in reducing postoperative bleeding and homologous blood transfusion in patients undergoing cardiopulmonary bypass (CPB).[2,7,10] However, confusion resulted when it was discovered that the activated clotting time (ACT), the standard method for monitoring the adequacy of heparin anticoagulation during CPB, was prolonged in the presence of aprotinin. It was erroneously suggested that aprotinin provided additional anticoagulation effects and that heparin doses therefore could be maintained or reduced.[1,4]

### Kaolin vs. Celite Activators

The thesis that aprotinin allows the use of lower heparin doses was subsequently rejected.[8] To compensate for the variability in ACT when aprotinin is used, the recommendation was made that the ACT should be maintained not at the usual standard of 400 seconds but at 750 seconds[5] or not used at all.[12] Subsequent investigation demonstrated that the effect of aprotinin on the ACT depends on the type of activator used in measuring the ACT. When celite is used as an activator, ACT is prolonged with the combined use of aprotinin and heparin compared with heparin alone. The use of kaolin as the activator under the same circumstances results in no prolongation.[13,14] Confusion in ACT interpretation may lead to inadequate heparinization while the patient is on CPB. In addition, the problems of protamine overdose and heparin resistance may be compounded.[6]

Wang and associates[13,14] recommend that heparin anticoagulation in patients treated with aprotinin should be evaluated with the kaolin-ACT (K-ACT). They compared celite-ACTs (C-ACTs) and K-ACTs of heparin-anticoagulated blood with and without aprotinin. They used a Hemochron system (International Technidyne, Edison, NJ) for both C-ACTs and K-ACTs. A Hepcon/HMS system (Medtronic HemoTec, Englewood, CO) was used to measure both the heparin concentration

## ACT's: Hepcon(HR), Kaolin(K), Celite(C)
## Aprotinin (A) and Control (C) Groups

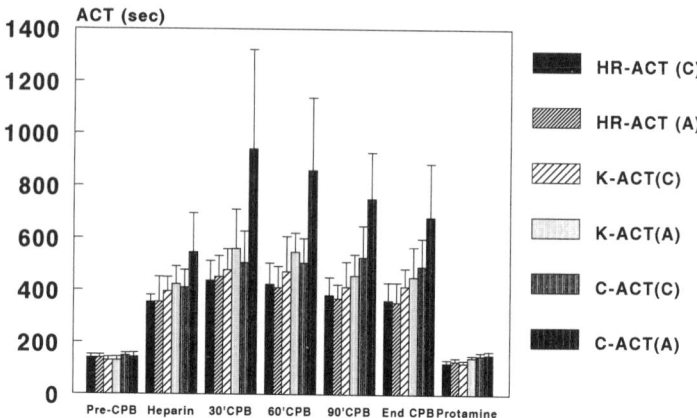

**FIGURE 1.** ACTs at various times, as measured with C-ACT, K-ACT, and the Hepcon/HMS system (HR-ACT) in the aprotinin (A) and control (C) groups. In the patients who received both heparin and aprotinin, C-ACTs were significantly longer than K-ACTs and HR-ACTs. In the group that had aprotinin alone (no heparin treatment), there was no significant difference among the C-ACTs, K-ACTs, or HR-ACTs. (From Wang J-S, Lin C-Y, Hung W-T, Karp RB: Monitoring of heparin-induced anticoagulation with kaolin-activated clotting time in cardiac surgical patients treated with aprotinin. Anesthesiology 77:1080–1084, 1992, with permission.)

and the high-range ACT (HR-ACT); the Hepcon/HMS system uses kaolin as a surface activator.

Patients were divided into four groups: (1) those who received both heparin and aprotinin, (2) those who received heparin alone, (3) those who received aprotinin alone, and (4) those who received neither. In the patients who received both heparin and aprotinin, C-ACTs were significantly longer than K-ACTs and HR-ACTs. In the group that received aprotinin alone, C-ACTs, K-ACTs, and HR-ACTs showed no significant difference. These results confirm that the C-ACT, but not the K-ACT, is affected only when both aprotinin and heparin are used. Figure 1 and Table 1 illustrate the changes in all ACTs in both aprotinin-treated and control patients.[14]

**TABLE 1.** Comparison of Activated Clotting Times with Different Activators

| | Activated Clotting Time (sec) | | | |
|---|---|---|---|---|
| | Heparin | | No Heparin | |
| | Aprotinin | Control | Aprotinin | Control |
| HR-ACT (kaolin) | 406 | 423 | 135 | 132 |
| K-ACT | 502 | 465 | 127 | 127 |
| C-ACT | 784 | 496 | 143 | 140 |

From Wang J-S, Lin C-Y, Hung W-T, Karp RB: Monitoring of heparin-induced anticoagulation with kaolin-activated clotting time in cardiac surgical patients treated with aprotinin. Anesthesiology 77:1080–1084, 1992, with permission.

None of the K-ACTs showed significant variability, whether performed by the Hemochron or Hepcon/HMS systems. K-ACTs and HR-ACTs remained at comparable levels in all four groups of patients throughout CPB (Table 1, Fig. 1). The C-ACTs showed no significant variation in the control groups that were not treated with aprotinin, whether or not heparin was used (Fig. 1, Table 1).

The average HR-ACTs were consistently lower than K-ACTs and C-ACTs during anticoagulation and CPB in both the aprotinin-treated and control groups (Table 1), possibly because the method of evaluation and dose of kaolin are different in the Hepcon /HMS and Hemochron systems. This finding could be problematic, because a lower ACT requires a higher dose of heparin and thus a higher dose of protamine, both of which are associated with increased postoperative blood loss.[3]

## Adsorption of Aprotinin by Kaolin

We investigated the possible etiology of the insensitivity of kaolin-ACT to aprotinin. Aprotinin was added to human serum at an initial concentration of 200 KIU/ml, an average clinical value. The aprotinin-containing serum was incubated for 1 minute with increasing quantities of either kaolin or celite and then assayed for residual aprotinin. For reference, at an hematocrit value of 40%, the whole-blood ACT test has 10 mg of clay for each ml of plasma. Figure 2 shows that above 6 mg/ml of clay, all of the aprotinin is removed by kaolin within 60 seconds, whereas most of the aprotinin is not removed by celite at clay concentrations as high as 20 mg/ml.

Thus kaolin powder adsorbs aprotinin onto its surface and so removes the drug from solution in plasma. Under the usual conditions of the ACT, the kaolin can remove 99% of the aprotinin in < 1.0 minute from blood containing a plasma level of 200 KIU/ml. Therefore, a K-ACT with aprotinin is essentially the same as a C-ACT without aprotinin. This finding does not explain the mechanism of the effect of aprotinin on C-ACTs, but its inhibition of the contact activator is assumed to play a role.

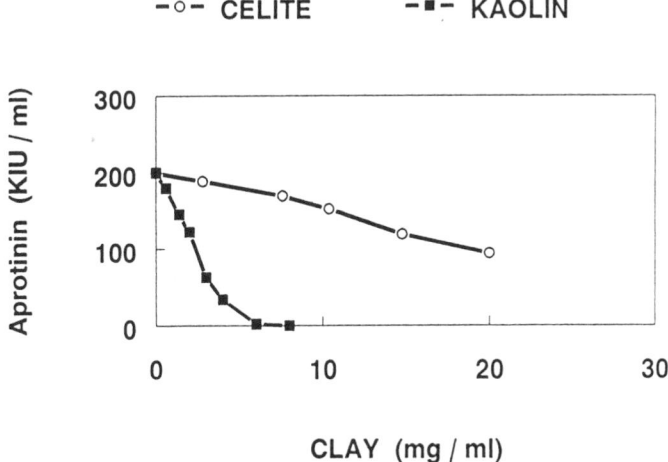

**FIGURE 2.** Serum aprotinin levels after 60 seconds for increasing concentrations of either kaolin (o) or celite (■) clay coagulation activators. Note that within 60 seconds an ACT obtained with 7.5 mg/ml or greater of kaolin clay is completely free of aprotinin in solution.

### Effect of High Doses of Aprotinin on Kaolin-Activated Clotting Time

At very high doses of aprotinin, the K-ACT may not be reliable. Levels above 600 KIU/ml can be attained by rapid bolusing of a 2 million KIU aprotinin loading dose in a normal-sized patient. Because the blood sample used to confirm heparinization is usually drawn after aprotinin dosing, the serum level of aprotinin in the sample depends on how recently and how rapidly the aprotinin was administered. The target serum level of aprotinin with the high-dose (Hammersmith) regimen is approximately 200 KIU/ml. According to International Technidyne Corporation, manufacturer of the Hemochron ACT system, the K-ACT is less affected by low-to-moderate levels of aprotinin (80–180 KIU/ml but becomes less precise as the dose of aprotinin reaches 180 to 500 KIU/ml.[9] As the aprotinin level rises above 180–200 KIU/ml, the kaolin in the tube becomes oversaturated with aprotinin; thus free aprotinin prolongs the ACT, as it does with the C-ACT. Therefore, if the K-ACT is used, the loading dose of aprotinin (2,000,000 KIU) should not be given as a bolus but rather as a short infusion over 20–30 minutes. Thus the loading dose can be administered without causing excessively high serum levels that skew the ACT.

## Current Heparin Management Protocols

Van Oeveren and associates[12] advise against using the ACT for guidance in heparin anticoagulation when aprotinin is administered. Hunt and coworkers[5] and Royston[11] recommend that an ACT of more than 750 seconds rather than the normally accepted ACT of 400–480 seconds should be the goal for CPB patients treated with aprotinin. They do not, however, specify whether C-ACT or K-ACT should be used.[5,11,12] Although Wang and associates[14] found that C-ACTs reached levels of more than 750 seconds in patients receiving both aprotinin and heparin, they recommend use of the K-ACT to monitor heparinization during CPB.

Many centers use the K-ACT routinely in patients undergoing CPB with and without aprotinin as adjunct treatment. The Cardiac Anesthesia Group at Massachusetts General Hospital routinely used the K-ACT with a fixed-dose heparin regimen for the past 4 years (unpublished data). The protocol is as follows:

1. Aprotinin test dose: 1 ml (1.4 mg or 10,000 KIU).
2. Loading dose of aprotinin: 200 ml (280 mg or 2,000,000 KIU), given over 20–30 minutes.
3. Bolus of heparin: 300 U/kg (400 U/kg with heparin infusion), followed by 100 U/kg/hr.
4. K-ACT is performed to confirm heparinization (> 400 seconds) but not to titrate heparin. If K-ACT is less than 400 seconds, an additional 100 U/kg of heparin is given and K-ACT is repeated.
5. Constant infusion of aprotinin: 50 ml/hr (70 mg/hr or 500,000 KIU/hr).

If circulatory arrest is required, infusion of aprotinin is stopped and heparin (100 U/kg) is given immediately before arrest.

## Conclusion

The clinician has a number of choices for monitoring heparin in the patient who receives aprotinin. The choice depends on local preferences, availability of equipment, and surgical routines. No method is ideal, but evidence suggests that K-ACT avoids the confounding in vitro effects of aprotinin on the evaluation of heparinization. Thus the same method of monitoring can be used in aprotinin-treated as well as routine patients. If C-ACT is used, aprotinin must not be thought of as a heparin-sparing agent in vivo.

## References

1. de Smet AAEA, Joen MCN, van Oeveren W, et al: Increased anticoagulation during cardiopulmonary bypass by aprotinin. J Thorac Cardiovasc Surg 100:520–527, 1990.
2. Dietrich W, Barankay A, Hahnel C, Richter JA: High-dose aprotinin in cardiac surgery: Three years' experience in 1,784 patients. J Cardiothorac Vasc Anesth 6:324–327, 1992.
3. Gravlee GP, Haddon WS, Rothberger HK, et al: Heparin dosing and monitoring for cardiopulmonary bypass. A comparison of techniques with measurement of subclinical plasma coagulation. J Thorac Cardiovasc Surg 99:518–527, 1990.
4. Harder MP, Eijsman L, Roozendall KJ, et al: Aprotinin reduces intraoperative and postoperative blood loss in membrane oxygenator cardiopulmonary bypass. Ann Thorac Surg 51:936–941, 1991.
5. Hunt BJ, Segal H, Yacoub M: Aprotinin and heparin monitoring during cardiopulmonary bypass. Circulation 86(Suppl II):II-410–II-412, 1992.
6. Hunt BJ, Murkin JM: Heparin resistance after aprotinin [letter]. Lancet 341:126, 1993.
7. Lemmer JH Jr, Stanford W, Bonney SL, et al: Aprotinin for coronary bypass operations: Efficacy, safety, and influence on early saphenous vein graft patency. A multicenter, randomized, double-blind, placebo-controlled study. J Thorac Cardiovasc Surg 107:543–553, 1994.
8. Najman DM, Walenga JM, Fareed J, Pifarré R: Effects of aprotinin on anticoagulant monitoring: Implications in cardiovascular surgery. Ann Thorac Surg 55:662–666, 1993.
9. Package Insert for ACT by HEMOCHRON, Edison, NJ: International Technidyne Corporation.
10. Royston D, Bidstrup BP, Taylor KM, Sapsford RN: Effect of aprotinin on need for blood transfusion after repeat open-heart surgery. Lancet ii:1289–1291, 1987.
11. Royston D: High-dose aprotinin therapy: A review of the first five years' experience. J Cardiothorac Vasc Anesth 6:76–100, 1992.
12. van Oeveren W, van Oeveren B, Wildevuur CRH: Anticoagulation policy during use of aprotinin in cardiopulmonary bypass [letter]. J Thorac Cardiovasc Surg 104:210–211, 1992.
13. Wang J-S, Lin C-Y, Hung W-T, et al: In vitro effects of aprotinin on activated clotting time measured with different activators. J Thorac Cardiovasc Surg 104:1135–1140, 1992.
14. Wang J-S, Lin C-Y, Hung W-T, Karp RB: Monitoring of heparin-induced anticoagulation with kaolin-activated clotting time in cardiac surgical patients treated with aprotinin. Anesthesiology 77:1080–1084, 1992.

Ulana Leskiw, MD
Jerrold H. Levy, MD

# 15

# Antigenicity of Protamine and Aprotinin in Cardiac Surgery

Any foreign polypeptide has the potential to elicit an allergic response. As early as 1967, anaphylactic shock was reported in a patient who received aprotinin for the treatment of pancreatitis.[13] The spectrum of hypersensitivity reactions reported in association with aprotinin administration ranges from urticaria and hypotension to frank cardiovascular collapse and death.[2,9,13,30] Aprotinin bears many similarities to protamine, a drug whose allergic potential has been extensively investigated. This chapter discusses general aspects of anaphylactic and anaphylactoid reactions, reviews the literature regarding hypersensitivity reactions to aprotinin, and provides recommendations for the use of this drug.

## Anaphylactic and Anaphylactoid Reactions

Anaphylaxis may be defined as "an immediate-onset allergic reaction produced by the immunologically mediated release of physiologically active substances from mast cells and basophils."[19] Clinical manifestations of anaphylactic reactions may include any combination of the following signs and symptoms: erythema, pruritus, urticaria, angioedema, upper airway obstruction/laryngeal edema, bronchospasm, nausea, vomiting, diarrhea, hypotension, vascular collapse, and death.[19] The term *anaphylaxis* was introduced in 1902, when Richet and Portier,[25] who were attempting to immunize dogs to sea anemone toxin, found that the second sublethal injection of toxin produced a profound hypersensitivity reaction with shock and death. Rather than conferring immunity, the first sublethal dose had sensitized the dogs to the antigen, and thus they coined the word *ana* (against) *phylaxis* (protection).

Classic **anaphylactic reactions** are type I, or immediate hypersensitivity, immunologic reactions. These reactions are IgE-mediated and require previous exposure of the patient to an antigen. Patient exposure to the foreign substance results in the production of antigen-specific IgE antibodies that are bound to the surfaces of mast cells and basophils.[19] Upon rechallenge of the patient, the antigen bridges two adjacent IgE molecules on the cell surface, initiating cellular activation and resulting in the release of a number of mediators which contribute to the inflammatory process.[19] Among the mediators released are histamine, tryptase, acid hydrolases, chemotactic factors, arachidonic acid metabolites (leukotrienes and prostaglandins), and platelet-activating factor. In addition, eosinophils and neutrophils are recruited by chemotactic factors to the site of the reaction and may participate in it.[19]

Immunogenicity refers to the ability of a molecule to act as an antigen to stimulate the immune response. The specificity of this response to produce unique antibodies against a particular molecule is another important characteristic. Molecular size and degree of foreignness to the recipient are two factors that influence the immunogenicity and specificity of a molecule.[19] In order to initiate an anaphylactic reaction, an antigen must be polyvalent, i.e., capable of binding two or more adjacent IgE molecules. Large molecules, such as proteins, are generally able to stimulate an immune response on their own, whereas small molecules are only able to initiate a response if they first bind to host proteins. Among the substances known to produce anaphylaxis via classical IgE-mediated mechanisms are penicillin, protamine, foreign proteins, and muscle relaxants.[19] Clinical tests that may be used to detect specific IgE antibodies include skin tests and radioallergosorbent tests (RASTs).

In contrast to the classic IgE-mediated anaphylactic reactions, similar syndromes may be precipitated by non–IgE-mediated mechanisms. These **anaphylactoid reactions**, or pseudoallergic reactions as they have been called, cannot be clinically distinguished from true anaphylaxis.[19] They are IgE-independent and rely on the nonimmunologic release of mediators.[19] Among the agents that have the potential to produce these IgE-independent reactions are complement anaphylatoxins (C3a and C5a) and certain compounds capable of causing direct mast cell degranulation. The complement anaphylatoxins C3a and C5a are generated by activation of the complement cascade. This activation may occur via one of two pathways. In the classic pathway, IgG or IgM binds to the antigen, forming immune complexes which then activate the cascade. In the alternative pathway, certain substances can activate the complement cascade nonimmunologically. Once generated, the anaphylatoxins can cause the release of mediators from mast cells and basophils.[19] In addition to anaphylatoxin-mediated reactions, some substances are capable of causing histamine release by direct mast cell degranulation. Examples of compounds that are known to produce anaphylactoid reactions by this mechanism are ionic radiocontrast media, opiates, muscle relaxants, and vancomycin.[19]

## Aprotinin

Aprotinin is a small-molecular-weight polypeptide that is isolated from bovine lung tissue. It is a basic protein with a molecular weight of approximately 6,500. Over the years, the available preparations of aprotinin have become better purified, and the typically administered dose of drug has increased. As a foreign protein, aprotinin should be able to stimulate an immune response on its own, without the need for hapten formation or prior binding to host proteins. It is interesting that aprotinin bears a number of similarities to protamine, a drug that has been well studied with respect to associated hypersensitivity reactions and their possible mechanisms. Protamine is also a basic polypeptide isolated from a foreign (fish) source, and it has a similar molecular weight of approximately 5,000. Because of these similarities, information gained about the antigenicity of protamine may provide some important perspectives on the allergic potential of aprotinin as well.

## Experience with Protamine

Protamine is not a highly immunogenic substance, perhaps because of similarity to human histone proteins. One patient group that has been found to be at greater risk for adverse reactions to protamine are diabetics taking neutral protamine Hagedorn (NPH) insulin. NPH insulin contains 0.35–0.4 mg of protamine/100 units of insulin. In a prospective study of 1,551 patients receiving protamine for neutralization of heparin during cardiac surgery, Levy et al.[22] reported that the incidence of adverse reactions was 2% (1/50) in patients taking NPH insulin and 0.06% (1/1,501) in all other patients. Similar numbers were reported in their subsequent retrospective review of an additional 3,245 patients receiving protamine during cardiac surgery. In that series, 0.6% (1/160) of NPH insulin-dependent diabetics and 0.06% (2/3,085) of the other patients exhibited adverse reactions.[21] Patients with fish allergy or prior vasectomy were originally thought to be at increased risk as well, but prospective evaluation did not reveal a greater incidence of allergic reactions in these groups.[21] It has also been suggested that prior patient exposure to protamine may increase the risk of an allergic reaction. However, considering the generally low incidence of protamine reactions and the large number of patients who receive the drug during cardiac surgery, vascular surgery, and cardiac catheterization, it seems unlikely that a single intravenous dose results in significant sensitization.

Three mechanisms have been postulated to account for the adverse reactions that occur after protamine administration: direct mast cell degranulation and histamine release, activation of complement, and antibody-mediated responses. The first mechanism, direct mast cell degranulation, was initially supported by animal studies which suggested that protamine could cause direct release of histamine.[28] However, the most recent evidence indicates that this is probably not a significant mechanism of human protamine reactions. Studies from human mast cells have not demonstrated significant histamine release with clinically relevant concentrations of protamine.[20,27] Direct activation of complement by protamine-heparin complexes has been shown to occur.[4,15] Again, however, this seems unlikely to be the mechanism responsible for most protamine reactions, because protamine activation of complement occurs with some frequency without ill effect, whereas the actual incidence of protamine reactions is low.

IgE- and possibly IgG-mediated mechanisms are most likely responsible for the hypersensitivity reactions that occur in association with protamine administration. In a case-control study, Weiss et al.[33] evaluated 27 patients who had suffered acute reactions to intravenous protamine and 43 patients who had received the drug without ill effect. The patients were grouped into protamine-insulin-dependent diabetics and patients who had never been exposed to protamine. A RAST was used to determine antiprotamine IgE antibody levels. The authors found that 9 of 13 patients who had manifested reactions and had been taking protamine insulin had antiprotamine IgE antibodies. These antibodies were not detected in any of the patients in the other groups. In patients who had previously received protamine insulin, the presence of antiprotamine IgE antibodies was a significant risk factor for acute protamine reactions, with a relative risk of 95. In the same group, the presence of antiprotamine IgG was also a risk factor with a relative risk of 38.

## Case Reports and Estimated Incidence of Hypersensitivity Reactions to Aprotinin

Over the 30 years since aprotinin's introduction into foreign markets, a number of reports of hypersensitivity reactions to the drug have been published (Table 1). Most of the early reports came from studies investigating aprotinin's efficacy in the treatment of pancreatitis. Hansson and Lenninger[13] described a study patient who developed hypotension, dyspnea, and urticaria in association with aprotinin administration, but was rapidly resuscitated with epinephrine, theophylline, and hydrocortisone. In another series, Baden et al.[2] described a patient who, immediately after aprotinin infusion, developed urticaria and a weak pulse and progressed to cardiac arrest. Despite all attempts, he was unable to be resuscitated.[2] Bauer et al.[3] reported a patient who developed dyspnea, loss of consciousness, wheezing, hypotension, and bradycardia immediately after aprotinin infusion but was resuscitated with epinephrine and sodium bicarbonate. Of note, two of these three patients has been previously exposed to the drug. Less severe reactions reported in association with aprotinin included urticaria[13] and hypotension.[2]

Further reports of anaphylactic-type reactions followed.[17,18,26] The case described by Proud and Chamberlain[26] illustrates some of the difficulties encountered in determining the etiology of an adverse drug reaction. The patient suffered a rash that was initially attributed to ampicillin and later attributed to endotoxemia. Unfortunately, a repeat dosage of aprotinin caused a hypotensive episode that resulted in severe brain damage. More recent case reports of anaphylactic-type reactions have involved patients who received aprotinin during cardiothoracic or aortic surgery.[5,8,30,34] Of the five patients described in these last four reports, four had previously received aprotinin.

The actual incidence of hypersensitivity reactions occurring in association with aprotinin therapy appears to be relatively low. A retrospective review published in 1966 reported that among 2,373 cases of aprotinin administration in the literature, 2 cases of shocklike reaction had occurred, an incidence of 0.08%.[7] Freeman et al.[12] performed a small retrospective review to determine the overall incidence of hypersensitivity reactions to aprotinin in their patients. During 136 courses of aprotinin therapy, they observed 1 case of hypotension with bronchospasm and tachycardia and 1 case of urticaria, for an incidence of anaphylactic/anaphylactoid reactions of 0.74% (1/136) and an incidence of minor allergic reactions of 0.74% (1/136). Fraedrich et al.[11] observed 2 anaphylactic reactions in 350 patients receiving aprotinin, for an incidence of 0.57%. In one study of 538 patients who received aprotinin for the treatment of pancreatitis, 4 patients (0.74%) developed a rash which necessitated discontinuation of therapy.[24] Dietrich et al.,[9] in a large study of patients receiving aprotinin during cardiac surgery, reported 3 episodes of hypotension in 902 patients, for an incidence of minor hypersensitivity reactions of 0.33%.

The above-mentioned surveys do not specify what percentage of their study patients had been previously exposed to aprotinin. However, at least 8 of 13 cases reported in the preceding paragraph occurred in patients with prior exposure to the drug. Clearly, the incidence of adverse reactions may depend on whether or not the patients had received aprotinin in the past. Recognizing that prior treatment with this foreign polypeptide may result in sensitization of the patient and, therefore, a greater risk of hypersensitivity reactions, Freeman et al.[12] conducted a controlled study to determine the incidence of adverse effects after reexposure to the drug. In a study of 15 patients who received multiple doses of aprotinin, the authors performed ocular sensitivity tests prior to repeat dosing, with the intention of halting therapy in patients who developed positive sensitivity tests. (Dilute solutions of aprotinin were used to perform the tests, and the development of acute conjunctivitis constituted sensitization.) No conjunctival reactions were seen and none of the patients developed allergic reactions during subsequent treatment with aprotinin. The authors concluded that the drug could safely be used repeatedly provided that prior sensitivity testing was done.*

Notwithstanding the lack of allergic reactions noted in this small study, it is clear from Table 2 that a significant number of patients who experienced hypersensitivity reactions after aprotinin had been previously exposed to the drug. Furthermore, the percentage of patients so treated may be underestimated in our table, because some of the studies and case reports do not specify whether or not the patient previously received the drug. Individuals may have been exposed to aprotinin during treatment for pancreatitis, during cardiac surgery, or upon treatment with certain biological glues that incorporate aprotinin. In contrast to the study by Freeman, Schulze at al.[30] reported an incidence of suspected anaphylactic reactions of 5.8% (5/86 patients) in patients with repeat exposure to aprotinin; however, no mention was made of immunologic testing to validate the etiology of the reactions.

Estimated incidences of hypersensitivity reactions to aprotinin, derived from the number of adverse reactions reported and the number of patients presumed to have been treated with the drug, have been provided by Miles, Inc. (Table 3). In an analysis of adverse drug effects observed in patients treated with aprotinin in Germany up until 1966, the estimated incidence of side effects was 0.1%. This figure was derived by multiplying the number of reported cases by two (to allow for under-reporting) and dividing by the number of patients estimated to have been treated with the drug. Based on similar assumptions, the incidence of anaphylaxis in patients treated with aprotinin in Germany from 1980–1982 was estimated to be 0.007%. Similarly, data from Japan for the period form 1967–1982 yielded an estimated incidence of adverse reactions of 0.018%. In Japan, the incidence of adverse reactions upon first exposure to the drug was estimated to be between 0.009–0.17%, somewhat less than the incidence of 0.023–1.13% estimated for cases of repeat exposure.

Further data from pharmaceutical studies are provided in Table 4 (Trasylol package insert, 1994). During exposure for the first time in the United States, there were no cases of anaphylaxis noted among 398 and 299 patients in controlled and open studies, respectively. There are only small numbers of patients in the United States who have received aprotinin for a repeat exposure, and only 1 patient has been reported to have anaphylaxis on reexposure. In foreign studies of patients without prior exposure to the drug, the incidence of anaphylaxis in controlled and open studies was, respectively, 0.35% (7/1,996 patients) and 0.16% (3/1,873

---

* The usefulness of the ocular sensitivity test as a screen for patient sensitization is questionable. At least one report describes an anaphylactic-type reaction after repeat aprotinin administration in a patient with a negative ocular sensitivity test.[17]

**TABLE 1.** Hypersensitivity Reactions Reported in Association with Aprotinin Administration

| Study (Year) | No. of Patients | Dose of Aprotinin (if specified) | Description of Reaction | Prior Exposure to Aprotinin | Comments |
|---|---|---|---|---|---|
| Hansson, 1967[13] | 2 | — | Urticaria | Yes, in 1 of 2 patients | — |
| | 1 | — | Hypotension, dyspnea, urticaria → resuscitated | Yes | — |
| Nodine, 1968[24] | 4 | — | Rash | Unspecified | — |
| Baden, 1969[2] | 2 | — | Hypotension | Unspecified | — |
| | 1 | 100,000 U | Urticarial rash → weak pulse → cardiac arrest → unable to be resuscitated | Yes (2 mos prior) | — |
| Bauer, 1971[3] | 1 | 300,000 KIU | Agitation, dyspnea, cyanosis → loss of consciousness, wheezing, hypotension, bradycardia → resuscitated | No | — |
| Levy, 1974[18] | 1 | ~1,700 U | Chest pain → loss of consciousness, hypotension, tachycardia → resuscitated | Unspecified | — |
| Proud, 1976[26] | 1 | Initially, ~1,700 KIU | Rash, hypotension | Yes (2 wks prior) | — |
| | | Later, only 30 s of a slow infusion of 200,000 KIU | Rash, hypotension → cardiorespiratory arrest → severe irreversible brain damage | | |
| Freeman, 1983[12] | 1 | — | Tachycardia, hypotension, bronchospasm → resuscitated | No | — |
| | 1 | — | Urticarial rash | Yes | — |
| La Ferla, 1984[17] | 1 | 500,000 KIU | Cardiac arrest → resuscitated | Yes | Reaction occurred despite negative ocular sensitivity testing |

| Study | No. | Dose | Reaction | Prior Exposure | Comments |
|---|---|---|---|---|---|
| Yanagihara, 1985[35] | 18 | — | Shock, urticaria, erythema, fever, vomiting | Yes in 7/18; no in 8/18; unknown in 3/18 | Subsequently 10/18 patients had positive RAST |
| Schuler, 1987[29] | 1 | 250,000 KIU | Urticaria, bronchospasm, shock → resuscitated | Yes, twice | Subsequently, skin testing and RAST were positive |
| Bohrer, 1990[5] | 1 | 625,000 KIU | Hypotension, flushing → resuscitated | Unspecified | Patient was a 3.4-yr-old, 12-kg boy |
| Wuthrich, 1992[34] | 1 | — | Flushing, bronchospasm, hypotension → resuscitated | Yes (2 mos prior) | Subsequent RAST testing of serum samples:<br>• Sample taken 1 mo before reexposure: RAST Class II positive<br>• Samples taken 8 days and 3 mos after reaction: RAST Class I positive |
| Dietrich, 1992[9] | 3 | — | Mild circulatory depression → prompt response to vasopressor therapy | Yes | — |
| Schulze, 1993[30] | 1 | 2 million KIU | Erythema → hypotension, bradycardia → cardiac arrest → resuscitated | Yes (5 mos prior) | — |
| | 1 | 750,000 KIU | Erythema → hypotension, tachycardia → cardiac arrest → resuscitated | Yes (2 mos prior) | — |
| Dewachter, 1993[8] | 1 | — | Hypotension, tachycardia, flushing → resuscitated | Yes (2 mos prior) | Subsequent radioimmunoassay and skin tests were positive |

**TABLE 2.** Reported Incidence of Hypersensitivity Reactions due to Aprotinin

| Source (Year) | Incidence of Anaphylactic/ Anaphylactoid Reactions | Incidence of Minor Allergic Reactions |
|---|---|---|
| Overall incidences | | |
| Bumm, 1966[4] | 0.08% (2/2373) | — |
| Hansson, 1967[13] | 1.03% (1/97 patients) | 2.06% (2/97 patients) |
| Nodine, 1968[24] | 0 (0/538 patients) | 0.74% (4/538 patients) |
| Baden, 1969[2] | 4.17% (1/24 patients) | 8.33% (2/24 patients) |
| Bauer, 1971[3] | 1.92% (1/52 patients) | — |
| Freeman, 1983[12] | 0.74% (1/136 courses) | 0.74% (1/136 courses) |
| Fraedrich, 1991[11] | 0.57% (2/350 patients) | — |
| Dietrich, 1992[9] | 0 (0/902 patients) | 0.33% (3/902) |
| Incidences in patients with prior exposure to aprotinin | | |
| Freeman, 1983[12] | 0 (0/15 patients)* | — |
| Schulze, 1993[30] | 5.81% (5/86 patients) | — |

\* Patients were pretested with ocular sensitivy tests.

patients). In studies of foreign marketing, the incidence of anaphylaxis was 0.0036% (5/140,000 patients) in patients without prior treatment with aprotinin. For patients with prior exposure to the drug, foreign marketing studies revealed an incidence of anaphylaxis of 0.19% (13/7,000), approximately 50 times greater than for patients without prior exposure.

## Immunologic Tests and Possible Mechanisms of Hypersensitivity Reactions Associated with Aprotinin

To investigate the possibility that an antibody-mediated mechanism was responsible for at least some of the hypersensitivity reactions to aprotinin, Yanagihara and Shida[35] tested for specific IgE and IgG antibodies in serum from 18 patients with pancreatitis who developed allergic or anaphylactic-type reactions after receiving the drug. The reactions included fever, rash, urticaria, erythema, vomiting, and shock. Of the 18 patients, 7 had been previously treated with aprotinin, 8 received aprotinin for the first time, and 3 had an unknown history of previous aprotinin exposure. Serum samples were obtained within 1 week of the reaction, again at 2–4 weeks after the reaction, and finally at 8 weeks after the reaction. Serum was tested for specific anti-aprotinin IgE antibody by RAST and for specific anti-aprotinin IgG antibody by agar gel diffusion and/or passive cutaneous anaphylaxis in guinea pigs. Overall, 10 of the 18 patients (55.6%) showed a positive RAST in at least one sample. Of the 7 patients who had been previously treated with aprotinin, 71.4% (5/7) had positive RAST; of the 8 patients who received aprotinin for the first

**TABLE 3.** Estimated Incidence of Hypersensitivity Reactions to Aprotinin*

| | Estimated Incidence of Reactions |
|---|---|
| Germany to 1966 | Adverse effects 0.1% |
| Germany 1980–1982 | Anaphylaxis 0.007% |
| Japan 1967–1982 | Adverse effects 0.018% |

\* Based on cases reported to the manufacturer and number of patients believed to have been treated with the drug. Data provided by Miles, Inc.

**TABLE 4.** Incidence of Anaphylactic Reactions to Aprotinin*

|  | No Prior Trasylol Exposure | Prior Trasylol Exposure |
|---|---|---|
| U.S. controlled studies | 0/398 | 0/0 |
| U.S. open studies | 0/299 | 1/6 |
| Foreign controlled studies | 7/1996 = 0.35% | 0/0 |
| Foreign open studies | 3/1873 = 0.16% | (1) |
| Foreign marketing | 8/140,000 = 0.0036% | 13/7000 = 0.19% |

* Data from Trasylol package insert, 1994.

time, 37.5% (3/8) had positive RAST; and of the 3 patients with an unknown history of exposure, 66.7% (2/3) had positive RAST. Of 2 patients with a history of drug allergy (to pyrazolone-derived drugs), 1 had a positive RAST and the other had a negative RAST. Anti-aprotinin IgG antibody, however, was not detected in any of the 13 patients who were tested for it.

The investigators also studied 44 patients who had received aprotinin without adverse effects. Of these 44 patients, 42 received aprotinin therapy for the first time and 2 had an unknown history of exposure to the drug. Serum samples were collected before aprotinin administration, immediately after drug infusion, at 2 weeks after infusion, and finally at 8 weeks after infusion. Following treatment with aprotinin, 31.8% (14/44) of the patients had positive RAST. Of note, the mean total dose of aprotinin administered was greater in the group of patients with positive RAST than in those with negative RAST ($336.6 \pm 76.6 \times 10^4$ KIU vs. $64.5 \pm 18.5 \times 10^4$ KIU). Furthermore, most of the patients with positive RAST had received aprotinin for several days, whereas most of those with negative RAST had received only a single dose. Agar gel diffusion did not detect anti-aprotinin IgG antibody in any of the 44 patients. Finally, the authors tested 9 healthy volunteers and 8 atopic patients with bronchial asthma. Both skin tests (using dilute solutions of aprotinin, i.e., $10^4$ g/ml or 7.143 KIU/ml) and RASTs for anti-aprotinin IgE antibody were performed. All of the skin tests and RASTs were negative.

Other investigators have documented, by means of positive skin tests and RASTs, the presence of specific anti-aprotinin IgE antibodies in patients who suffered hypersensitivity reactions to the drug. Schuler et al.[29] described a 25-year-old man who, upon the third administration of aprotinin, developed urticaria, bronchospasm, and shock. Subsequent RAST and skin testing with dilute aprotinin were both positive. Wuthrich et al.[34] reported the case of a 3-year-old boy who developed an anaphylactic-type syndrome upon repeat dose of aprotinin 2 months after initial treatment. Three serum samples were analyzed by RAST: a sample that had been drawn 1 month before the second surgery and frozen, a sample drawn 8 days after the incident, and a sample drawn 3 months after the incident. The RAST results were, respectively: 3.4 U/ml (class II, positive), 0.6 U/ml (class I, weakly positive), and 0.4 U/ml (class I, weakly positive).[34] Dewachter et al.[8] studied a patient who developed a hypersensitivity reaction after her second exposure to aprotinin. Radioimmunoassay performed on a serum sample drawn on the day of the incident confirmed the presence of anti-aprotinin IgE antibodies; skin tests (both prick tests and intradermal test at $10^{-1}$) performed 6 weeks later were positive.

Anti-aprotinin IgG and IgM antibodies have also been documented in patients treated with the drug. Dietrich et al.[10] reported that two of their patients who showed signs of allergic reactions were subsequently found to have anti-aprotinin IgG and IgM antibodies. Fraedrich et al.[11] stated that 30% of their patients who received aprotinin had developed specific anti-aprotinin IgG antibodies when tested at least 6 months later, while 40% of the patients had developed specific anti-aprotinin IgM antibodies. These data are in contrast to the results of Yanagihara and Shida,[35] who did not detect anti-aprotinin IgG in any of their patients.

These results clearly indicate that aprotinin has the potential to induce specific anti-aprotinin IgE antibodies in some patients. Thus, an IgE-mediated mechanism may be postulated for some of the hypersensitivity reactions. However, the presence of IgE antibody does not prove definitively that aprotinin is acting as an antigen rather than eliciting an anaphylactoid reaction by one of the other mechanisms described earlier. Establishment of the relative risk of immunospecific IgE antibodies for clinically manifest allergic reactions requires the evaluation of treated controls.[32] Of interest, in one of the case reports in which a positive RAST was documented[34] and in five of the patients with a positive RAST in Yanagihara and Shida's study,[35] the RAST index, and therefore anti-aprotinin IgE levels, declined over time. A similar phenomenon has been documented in patients with immediate hypersensitivity to penicillin.[16]

Obviously, many questions remain. The roles of IgG and IgM antibodies are unclear. In addition, a number of the reported hypersensitivity reactions occurred upon first exposure to the drug. Several mechanisms may be postulated to account for these reactions which occurred upon initial treatment. First, the patient may have become sensitized during an unrecognized exposure to aprotinin in the past. However, such a mechanism could not explain all cases. Cross-sensitization to bovine proteins may be a second possible mechanism. Siegel and Werner[31] reported a patient who had an allergic reaction to aprotinin and later developed allergies to beef, milk, and other bovine products. Again, such cross-sensitization is unlikely to account for more than a few cases, at most. Finally, the most likely mechanism for the reactions that occurred upon initial exposure is that aprotinin was administered concomitantly with other drugs capable of producing hypersensitivity reactions. Anaphylaxis upon first exposure to aprotinin noted in early reports may also have been due to preservatives or even to original preparations that were less purified.

## Clinical Implications

The consequences of anaphylactic and anaphylactoid reactions can be devastating, particularly in patients with limited cardiovascular reserve. Unfortunately, the patients who derive the greatest benefit from the use of aprotinin are frequently also the patients with the poorest cardiac function—patients undergoing reoperations, valve replacement, heart transplantation, or surgery for congenital heart disease. These patients are least able to tolerate even the slightest hemodynamic compromise. Moreover, not only do the anaphylaxis-associated hypotension and arrhythmias pose grave risks, but histamine itself may act as a coronary vasoconstrictor and systemic vasodilator.[19] There are data to suggest that patients with cardiovascular disease may be particularly susceptible to the coronary artery-constricting effects of histamine.[19] Furthermore, most patients receive aprotinin sometime after the induction of general anesthesia. Among patients who suffer anaphylaxis while under general anesthesia, circulatory collapse is the most common manifestation.[19]

As discussed in the preceding sections of this chapter, it appears that the group of patients at greatest risk of suffering a hypersensitivity reaction are those who have been previously treated with aprotinin. In Europe, individuals may have received aprotinin for a wide variety of indications, including treatment of pancreatitis, prophylaxis of pancreatitis in upper abdominal surgery, treatment of shock, and prophylaxis of hemorrhage (especially in cardiac surgery). In addition, aprotinin has been used as a component of certain biological glues. In the United States, the drug was used in trials for the treatment and prophylaxis of pancreatitis and prophylaxis of hemorrhage. It has recently been approved for use in cardiac surgery. However, as noted earlier, hypersensitivity reactions to aprotinin may also occur in patients who have not previously received the drug, most likely due to occult or unknown exposure. Therefore, we recommend that all patients receive a test dose of 1 ml of the drug approximately 10 minutes prior to the full loading dose. For patients who are known to have received aprotinin in the past, particular caution is necessary. Anaphylactic reactions are dose-independent and may occur even after the administration of a small 1-ml test dose. Therefore, in this group of patients, we recommend some form of testing for sensitization even prior to the test dose.

As noted earlier, both immediate-type (wheal and flare) skin testing and RASTs detect specific IgE antibodies. For most drug allergies, skin testing is the more readily available and has been widely used. Some experts, in fact, believe that immediate-type skin testing is the most useful test for IgE antibody for the majority of drugs, because it carries the greatest likelihood of positive results.[1] Skin testing does carry a small risk of anaphylaxis and, therefore, should be performed by a trained individual with full resuscitation equipment available.[19] RAST obviously does not involve any risk of anaphylaxis, but it is not as readily available and there is no evidence that the results are more reliable than those obtained by skin testing. Of note, both skin-test-positive/RAST-negative and skin-test-negative/RAST-positive patients with anaphylactic reactions have been identified.[23]

Two types of skin tests that have been well described are the prick-puncture test (in which the test solution is placed on the arm and introduced into the epidermis by a small needle) and the intradermal test (in which the solution is injected directly into the dermis).[6] The prick-puncture test is less sensitive but more specific than the intradermal test, possibly because it introduces fewer molecules of the drug. In general, the intradermal test should not be performed unless preceded by a negative prick-puncture test. For the prick-puncture test, a small drop of test solution is placed on the volar surface of the forearm. A 25- or 26-gauge needle is passed through the drop and introduced into the epidermis at a low angle with the bevel facing up. The needle tip is lifted upward slightly, elevating the epidermis. The needle tip is withdrawn, and 1 minute later, the test solution is wiped away. A wheal $> 3$ mm in diameter is likely to represent clinical allergy.

Any time a skin test is performed, both negative and positive control tests should be done as well. The negative control test consists of the diluent used to prepare the test solution (dermographic patients will exhibit a positive reaction with the negative control). Positive controls are placed to ensure that the patient is not poorly responsive to histamine or immunosuppressed. For the prick-puncture test, morphine base in a concentration of 1 mg/ml may be used as a positive control. It is important to note that certain medications, notably antihistamines, tricyclic antidepressants, phenothiazines, and some sympathomimetics, may inhibit or decrease a positive reaction. Corticosteroids may exert an effect on the response as well. It has been recommended that high doses of glucocorticoids be reduced prior to skin testing, whereas low doses (i.e., $< 15$ mg of prednisolone/day) be continued.[6]

It is unknown whether pretreatment with antihistamines and corticosteroids offers any measure of protection to patients at risk for hypersensitivity reactions to aprotinin. Prednisone and diphenhydramine have been shown to reduce the incidence of adverse reactions in patients who have a history of reactions to radiocontrast media.[14] Most contrast dye reactions are believed to be due to mast cell degranulation and not true immune responses. Whether the beneficial effects of pretreatment would apply in cases of aprotinin hypersensitivity is unstudied.

For patients who are to be exposed to aprotinin again for a subsequent cardiac surgical procedure, a plan should be available for urgent institution of cardiopulmonary bypass should circulatory collapse occur. This is of particular importance in patients undergoing reoperations. The patients in this category are most likely to receive aprotinin, but they obviously have difficult access for aortic and right atrial cannulation. In these cases, therefore, thought should be given to cannulation, or at least exposure, of the femoral vessels or aorta prior to administration of the drug. It is also probably prudent in these cases to avoid adding aprotinin to the pump prime until the full intravenous loading dose has been given without ill effect. The risk versus benefit of aprotinin should be considered. Although routine administration involves loading the patient with aprotinin prior to skin incision, the ability to rapidly institute cardiopulmonary bypass should be available for known second-time aprotinin exposure.

In cases where a hypersensitivity reaction to aprotinin is believed to have occurred, it is important to attempt to establish aprotinin definitively as the offending agent. As mentioned previously, many drugs which are administered intraoperatively, often in close temporal association with aprotinin, are known to produce hypersensitivity reactions. Common culprits include antibiotics, muscle relaxants, and latex. Therefore, for patients who have manifested symptoms of a hypersensitivity reaction after aprotinin, subsequent immunologic testing seems prudent.

## Conclusion

Although aprotinin has a long history of safe administration, hypersensitivity reactions to the drug do occur. Based on an analysis of the currently available literature, the incidence of anaphylactic reactions to aprotinin may be estimated at < 0.5%. Patients who have been previously treated with the drug appear to be at increased risk for adverse reactions. The mechanism of aprotinin hypersensitivity reactions remains incompletely elucidated. However, evaluation of patients who have suffered anaphylactic reactions to aprotinin has revealed, in some cases, the presence of specific anti-aprotinin IgE antibodies, whether demonstrated by immediate-type skin testing or RAST. Thus, it appears that an IgE-mediated mechanism may account for a significant number of aprotinin hypersensitivity reactions. Whether other non–IgE-mediated mechanisms such as IgG antibodies, complement activation, or direct histamine release are also of clinical importance in the pathogenesis of these reactions is as yet unclear.

In view of the potential for hypersensitivity reactions to aprotinin, all patients should receive a test dose of 1 ml prior to administration of the full loading dose. Although no data are currently available evaluating the role of allergy testing for subsequent exposure, patients with known (or strongly suspected) previous exposure to the drug should probably undergo some form of testing for sensitization prior to administration of even the test dose. Particular care should be exercised in patients undergoing reoperation who may have difficult access for cannulation for cardiopulmonary bypass. Further studies are needed to delineate more clearly the mechanisms of hypersensitivity reactions to aprotinin and to establish quantitatively the usefulness of immediate-type skin testing and RAST as screening and diagnostic tools in this area.

# References

1. Adkinson NF: Tests for immunological drug reactions. In Rose NR, Friedman H, Fahey JL (eds): Manual of Clinical Laboratory Immunology, 3rd ed. Washington, DC, American Society for Microbiology, 1986, pp 692–697.
2. Baden H, Jordal K, Lund F, Zachariae F: Prophylactic and curative action of Trasylol in pancreatitis: A double-blind trial. Scand J Gastroenterol 4:291–295, 1969.
3. Bauer J, Futterman S, Dreiling DA: Anaphylactic shock secondary to initial Trasylol administration. Am J Gastroenterol 56:542–544, 1971.
4. Best N, Sinosich MJ, Teisner B, et al: Complement activation during cardiopulmonary bypass by heparin-protamine interaction. Br J Anaesth 56:339–343, 1984.
5. Bohrer H, Bach A, Fleischer F, Lang J: Adverse haemodynamic effects of high-dose aprotinin in a paediatric cardiac surgical patient. Anaesthesia 45:853–854, 1990.
6. Bousquet J, Michel F-B: In vivo methods for study of allergy: Skin tests, techniques, and interpretation. In Middleton E, Reed CE, Ellis EF, et al (eds): Allergy: Principles and Practice, 4th ed. St. Louis, Mosby, 1993, pp 573–588.
7. Bumm HW, Hindermann J, Durr W, Dressler S: Die seltene Beobachtung von Unvertraglichkeit serscheinungen gegenuber dem Fermentinaktivator praparat Trasylol. Zentralbl Chir 91:1029, 1966.
8. Dewachter P, Mouton C, Masson C, et al: Anaphylactic reaction to aprotinin during cardiac surgery. Anaesthesia 48:1110–1111, 1993.
9. Dietrich W, Barankay A, Hahnel C, Richter JA: High-dose aprotinin in cardiac surgery: Three years' experience in 1784 patients. J Cardiothorac Vasc Anesthesiol 6:324–327, 1992.
10. Dietrich W, Hahnel C, Richter JA: Routine application of high-dose aprotinin in open-heart surgery: A study on 1784 patients. Anesthesiology 73:A146, 1990.
11. Fraedrich G, Neukamm K, Schneider T, et al: Safety and risk/benefit assessment of aprotinin in primary CABG. In Freidel N, Hetzer R, Royston D (eds): Blood Use in Cardiac Surgery. New York, Springer-Verlag, 1991, pp 221–231.
12. Freeman JG, Turner GA, Venables CW, Latner AL: Serial use of aprotinin and incidence of allergic reactions. Curr Med Res Opin 8:559–561, 1983.
13. Hansson K, Lenninger S: Proteinase inhibitors in acute pancreatitis. Eur J Surg Suppl 378:103–109, 1967.
14. Kelly JF, Patterson R, Lieberman P, et al: Radiographic contrast media studies in high-risk patients. J Allergy Clin Immunol 62:181–184, 1978.
15. Kirklin JK, Chenoweth DE, Naftel DC, et al: Effects of protamine administration after cardiopulmonary bypass on complement, blood elements, and the hemodynamic state. Ann Thorac Surg 41:193–199, 1986.
16. Kraft D, Roth A, Mischer P, et al: Specific and total serum IgE measurements in the diagnosis of penicillin allergy: A long-term follow-up study. Clin Allergy 7:21–28, 1977.
17. LaFerla GA, Murray WR: Anaphylactic reaction to aprotinin despite negative ocular sensitivity tests. BMJ 289:1176–1177, 1984.
18. Levy AH: Unusual reaction to Trasylol. Can Med Assoc J 111:1304, 1974.
19. Levy JH: Anaphylactic Reactions in Anesthesia and Intensive Care, 2nd ed. Boston, Butterworth-Heinemann, 1992.
20. Levy JH, Faraj BA, Zaidan JR, Camp VML: Effects of protamine on histamine release from human lung. Agents Actions 28:70–72, 1989.
21. Levy JH, Schweiger IM, Zaidan JR, et al: Evaluation of patients at risk for protamine reactions. J Thorac Cardiovasc Surg 98:200–204, 1989.
22. Levy JH, Zaidan JR, Faraj BA: Prospective evaluation of risk of protamine reactions in patients with NPH insulin-dependent diabetes. Anesth Analg 65:739–742, 1986.
23. Marquardt DL, Wassermann SI: Anaphylaxis. In Middleton E, Reed CE, Ellis EF, et al (eds): Allergy: Principles and Practice, 4th ed. St. Louis, Mosby, 1993, pp 1525–1536.

24. Nodine JH, Greberman M: Proteinase inhibitors in human pancreatitis: Digital computer analysis of clinical research data. Ann NY Acad Sci 146:564–578, 1968.
25. Portier MM, Richet C: D l'action anaphylactique de certains venins. CR Soc Biol 54:170–172, 1902.
26. Proud G, Chamberlain J: Anaphylactic reaction to aprotinin. Lancet 2:48–49, 1976.
27. Sauder RA, Hirschman CA: Protamine-induced histamine release in human skin mast cells. Anesthesiology 73:165–167, 1990.
28. Schnitzler S, Renner H, Pfuller U: Histamine release from rat mast cells induced by protamine sulfate and polyethylene imine. Agents Actions 11:73–74, 1981.
29. Schuler TM, Frosch PJ, Arza D, Wahl R: Anaphylaktische Reaktion auf Aprotinin. Munch Med Wochenschr 129:816–817, 1987.
30. Schulze K, Graeter T, Schaps D, Hausen B: Severe anaphylactic shock due to repeated application of aprotinin in patients following intrathoracic aortic replacement. Eur J Cardiothorac Surg 7:495–496, 1993.
31. Siegel VM, Werner M: Allergische Pankreititis bei einer Sensibilisierung gegen den Kallikrein Trypsin Inaktivator. Dtsch Med Wochenschr 90:1712–1716, 1965.
32. Weiss ME, Adkinson NF, Hirschman CA: Evaluation of allergic drug reactions in the perioperative period. Anesthesiology 71:483–486, 1989.
33. Weiss ME, Nyhan D, Peng Z, et al: Association of protamine IgE and IgG antibodies with life-threatening reactions to intravenous protamine. N Engl J Med 320:886–892, 1989.
34. Wuthrich B, Schmid P, Schmid ER, et al: IgE-mediated anaphylactic reaction to aprotinin during anaesthesia. Lancet 340:173–174, 1992.
35. Yanagihara Y, Shida T: Immunological studies on patients who received aprotinin therapy. Arerugi 34:899–904, 1985.

## Harry L. Messmore, Jr., MD

# 16

# Potential Medical Indications for Aprotinin

Aprotinin is a basic proteinase inhibitor with specificity for the serine proteases trypsin, glandular and plasma kallikrein, plasmin, activated protein C, and thrombin.[8,37] It is purified from bovine tissues (pancreas, salivary gland, lung), and its chemical structure (58 amino acids) and molecular weight (6,512 daltons) have been determined. It is inactive when taken orally but is fully active when given intravenously. Aprotinin has a half-life of about 2 hours and is not excreted in the urine. It is well tolerated, with few side effects or allergic reactions reported on initial or subsequent use.

The most potent and clinically apparent pharmacologic effect of aprotinin is antifibrinolysis exerted through the inhibition of plasmin. Aprotinin has a weak anticoagulant effect in vitro through the inhibition of kallikrein and thrombin, but these effects are not significant in vivo. Because of its inhibition of plasmin and kallikrein, aprotinin's primary in vivo effects are antifibrinolytic and anti-inflammatory. Secondary effects via these same mechanisms may result in prohemostatic properties that account for its ability to promote hemostasis via impairment of prourokinase activity and preservation of von Willebrand factor activity in fibrinolytic states.[8,35]

Because of these properties, aprotinin may prove to be clinically useful in treating some clinical disorders in which it has not yet been fully evaluated. These include bleeding disorders involving hemorrhage from mucosal surfaces, from angiodysplasia and malignant neoplasms, during treatment with extracorporeal circuits (other than cardiopulmonary bypass), in central nervous system bleeds, following thrombolytic therapy, in sepsis with shock, and in trauma with shock and adult respiratory distress syndrome. It may also prove useful in treatment of hemangiomatosis and acquired alpha-2-antiplasmin deficiency and in patients with severe liver disease who have mucosal bleeding or who are undergoing liver transplantation or major surgery. Treatment of primary hemorrhagic disorders such as hemophilia, von Willebrand's disease, and alpha-2-plasmin inhibitor deficiency may at times benefit from the antifibrinolytic properties of this drug.

**TABLE 1.** Medical Indications for Aprotinin*

| |
|---|
| Acute pancreatitis |
| Abnormal bleeding |
|   Surgical |
|   Mechanical trauma |
|   Aneurysm |
|   Ruptured intracranial aneurysm |
|   Post-thrombolytic therapy |
|   Traumatic hemorrhagic shock |
|   Obstetric-gynecologic |
|   Liver transplantation (orthotopic) |

* Based on preliminary evidence showing benefit when the drug was given.

Even severe cases of thrombocytopenic states may benefit until more definitive treatment is available.

Aprotinin has a number of surgical indications which are reviewed in other chapters in this volume. It is less clear if aprotinin has potential medical indications, and these are the subject of this review. Table 1 lists the medical disorders in which there is a rationale for using aprotinin and in which preliminary evidence shows benefit when the drug was given. Table 2 lists those disorders that have not as yet been treated with aprotinin but for which there is an excellent rationale for using this drug. In some instances, these disorders have been successfully treated with antifibrinolytic drugs of the synthetic type. In other instances, the effect of aprotinin would be due to its anti-inflammatory, antikallikrein, or antiprotease properties other than antifibrinolytic. These medical indications and theoretical medical uses are discussed in the following sections.

## Medical Indications for Aprotinin

### Pancreatitis

Pancreatitis is associated with local and systemic effects due to the release of digestive enzymes (amylase, lipase, trypsin, chymotrypsin) that incite a severe inflammatory reaction. Local hemorrhage and circulatory collapse can occur in some patients. Because aprotinin inhibits trypsin as well as tissue- and plasma-generated kallikrein, it would be expected to have value in this disorder. Despite

**TABLE 2.** Potential Medical Indications for Aprotinin

| |
|---|
| Mucosal hemorrhage not responding to usual modes of therapy (oral, esophageal, gastric, intestinal) |
| Hemophilic disorders and von Willebrand's disease (mild bleeding, dental procedures, joint hemorrhage, mucosal bleeding, circulatory inhibitors of coagulation factors) |
| Vascular disorders (giant hemangioma [via induction of thrombosis], hemorrhagic telangiectasia) |
| Refractory thrombocytopenia with hemorrhage |
| Shock, traumatic and septic |
| Malignant neoplasms (via modulation of metastases, thermoradiotherapy of head and neck neoplasms) |
| Severe corneal injuries |
| Platelet preservation in the blood bank |
| Fibrin glue, neurosurgical uses |

this rationale, there is no good clinical evidence for its efficacy in terms of reduced mortality.[35]

### Abnormal Bleeding

Excessive plasmin activity, either local or systemic, rarely causes bleeding in the absence of a break in the vascular system. For that reason, bleeding with excessive fibrinolysis is clinically important in surgical settings, particularly with cardiopulmonary bypass surgery.[4,12,26] Aprotinin has been shown to be highly effective in such cases, as a number of chapters in this book attest. It is reasonable to expect that certain other surgical settings might also be associated with hyperfibrinolysis.

When there is excessive bleeding, and usual measures to stop it are not effective, it would be appropriate to consider local or, more rarely, systemic fibrinolysis. Local fibrinolysis may be difficult to detect by laboratory testing, but the finding of fibrin or fibrin degradation products (D-dimer, fibrin, or fibrinogen split products) in the blood should support any suspicion of local fibrinolysis.[36] Decrease in plasminogen, alpha-2-antiplasmin, or fibrinogen levels in the absence of overt disseminated intravascular coagulation (decrease in antithrombin III) would strongly suggest systemic fibrinolysis, which is rare except in systemic thrombolytic therapy.[25,27,29,30,34,36] Aprotinin may reduce bleeding caused by antiplatelet drugs, which may be important in surgical patients receiving such drugs (clodipogrel-ticlopidine).[16] It also blocks the antiplatelet effects of heparin.[18]

A broad understanding of the risks and potential benefit of antifibrinolytic therapy with aprotinin is needed to make a clinical judgment in such cases. However, if all reasonable therapeutic approaches have been tried, and the hemorrhage is life-threatening or may result in severe disability, an empiric approach may be warranted.[34] The hazard of aprotinin therapy is likely to be less than the hazard of blood products. It is uncertain whether the use of two empiric treatments simultaneously, such as desmopressin acetate (DDAVP) and aprotinin, would be safe. If excessive local fibrinolysis is present, the local level of von Willebrand factor may be low due to lysis by plasmin.[9,10] The use of aprotinin may permit the local level of von Willebrand factor to rise and promote platelet adhesion. The administration of DDAVP may not compensate for the local fibrinolysis.

Because there are very few studies to support this concept, except in surgery for prostatic carcinoma where local fibrinolysis due to urokinase has been fully established as a cause, more studies are urgently needed.[21,25] Aprotinin, in combination with synthetic antifibrinolytic drugs, has been successfully used to stop bleeding during and following prostate surgery.[35] It is of interest that aprotinin is not excreted in the urine, and that the urokinase in the urine continues to convert plasminogen to plasmin and lysis of clots in the bladder may still occur.[35] It is highly probable that kallikrein on the surface of platelets in the clots is inhibited by aprotinin. This interrupts the natural pathway of the activation of prourokinase in the tissues by platelet kallikrein, resulting in decreased local fibrinolysis.[20]

Although it would be a relative contraindication to administer short-term aprotinin to a patient with deep vein thrombosis (a common occurrence in trauma and major surgical patients), the benefit of using it may well outweigh the risk, except in overt disseminated intravascular coagulation where its use would be clearly contraindicated.

Mechanical trauma resulting in tissue injury, fractures, hemorrhage, shock, and adult respiratory distress syndrome has been studied for the effects of aprotinin on mortality rate and respiratory insufficiency. Patients receiving aprotinin benefited as compared with placebo-treated controls, but not more than a group receiving heparin.[35] Treatment of ruptured intracranial aneurysm with aprotinin to prevent rebleeding has been carried out in combination with a synthetic antifibrinolytic drug (tranexamic acid). It has been postulated that the post-hemorrhagic vasospasm would be lessened by aprotinin because of its effects on the kallikrein-kinin system.[35]

It is important to be able to block the effects of plasminogen activators such as streptokinase and urokinase, because they may result in serious and life-threatening hemorrhage by destroying preformed hemostatic plugs. Studies in animals demonstrated that the fibrinolytic (thrombolytic) activity and resultant bleeding from wounds can be stopped by aprotinin.[7,13] It is reasonable to treat bleeding associated with thrombolytic therapy with aprotinin only if other measures have been exhausted and the bleeding is threatening to be fatal or seriously disabling, because human trials for this purpose have not yet been done.[15] When given after thrombolytic therapy for acute myocardial infarction, aprotinin could cause abrupt reocclusion of the coronary vessel and result in death. The same is true for thrombolytic therapy for other arterial thrombotic problems, such as cerebral or femoral arterial thrombosis.

Obstetric and gynecologic hemorrhage have been treated with aprotinin in the past. Surprisingly, aprotinin was efficacious when given for abruptio placenta and disseminated intravascular coagulation. It is questionable whether these good results can be confirmed by a randomized prospective trial.[35] It has been found to be beneficial when used to decrease menorrhagia in women with an intrauterine device (IUD). It may prove to be useful when incorporated into these devices.[35]

Aprotinin has been studied extensively in liver transplantation, where the incidence of serious hemorrhage is quite high, as is the use of blood products to treat the coagulopathy in these patients. A major factor has been excessive fibrinolysis, which is the reason aprotinin has been studied.[1,2,27,36] The results have been variable, and further studies are needed to define its role as a prophylactic or therapeutic agent in this setting.

## Potential Medical Indications for Aprotinin

In the unusual circumstance of circulating inhibitor to factor VIII, where factor VIII is not effective for treatment of serious hemorrhage, trials of aprotinin might be unwarranted. This could be studied in hemophilic dog or pig models. In hereditary alpha-2-antiplasmin deficiency, aprotinin should be a valuable drug to control serious hemorrhage.[24]

Certain vascular disorders might be effectively treated with aprotinin. The first is giant hemangioma, which may be very disabling, disfiguring, and painful. Attempts at control or eradication by radiation therapy with or without corticosteroids (Kasabach-Merritt syndrome in children) have not been successful in older children and adults. The use of antifibrinolytic drugs plus infusions of cryoprecipitate to raise the fibrinogen and factor VIII–von Willebrand factor levels has occasionally been effective.[31] It is possible that aprotinin, alone or in combination with epsilon aminocaproic acid (EACA), would be as effective as the combination of EACA and cryoprecipitate. One might then avoid the hazard of a blood product.

Hereditary hemorrhagic telangiectasia is a disorder of small vessels that may cause localized mucosal, pulmonary, or central nervous system hemorrhage. Local fibrinolytic activity has been demonstrated in these vascular lesions,[19] and treatment with synthetic inhibitors has proven to be successful in stopping the bleeding in some cases, although a prospective study has never been done.[19,29] Aprotinin could be applied or sprayed topically on the nasal mucosa, which would be quite useful because severe chronic epistaxis with iron deficiency anemia is such a problem for these patients. There may be a role for aprotinin in severe thrombocytopenic states with bleeding. It may be as effective as EACA for this indication, and in certain circumstances in which parenteral treatment is necessary, it could be the drug of choice. One study has demonstrated its effectiveness for this indication.[14] One theoretical advantage over EACA is that aprotinin does not impair platelet function.[17,22]

It seems paradoxical that aprotinin would be useful in septic shock, and certainly its use in humans for this purpose should be limited to experimental protocols. A study reported in 1989 involving 20 critically ill patients showed a benefit over controls in terms of pulmonary function and platelet counts, but there was no difference in mortality.[28] An interesting animal study of pigs in septic shock due to live *Escherichia coli* infusion given aprotinin or sham (Ringer's solution) showed an advantage with aprotinin in terms of consumption coagulopathy and cardiopulmonary hemodynamics.[33] A study of endotoxemia in goats showed that aprotinin failed to alter the pathophysiology of cardiopulmonary impairment.[38]

Traumatic shock has benefited from aprotinin therapy in several studies. As was pointed out in one review, the inhibitory effect on plasmin does not seem to have a deleterious effect on disseminated intravascular coagulation in these patients.[35] Malignant neoplasms that secrete plasminogen activators or activate the fibrinolytic system indirectly may cause serious hemorrhage. Classically, this may occur on a systemic basis with depletion of fibrinogen as well as with dissolution of fibrin. Acute promyelocytic leukemia and prostatic carcinoma are well known for this, and aprotinin could, in some circumstances, be a useful therapy.[30] Malignant melanoma and hepatoma or cholangiocarcinomas may exhibit intense local fibrinolysis with hemorrhage. This is particularly notable on the surface of the liver or around metastases to the brain (author's experience). Aprotinin could be of palliative use in these circumstances.

Aprotinin has been used experimentally in animals and humans to alter the behavior of metastasizing tumors or to enhance the benefit of thermoradiotherapy.[11,21,23] Because some tumors appear to be able to metastasize by lysing fibrin that is binding the cells together and others are able to implant as metastatic sites by forming fibrin, it is not possible to predict what harm or benefit may come from giving aprotinin without clinical human studies. Some neoplasms in animal models are favorably influenced by aprotinin.[11,21]

A study in an experimental model has shown benefit from aprotinin in the treatment of severe corneal injury. The study showed that high plasmin activity occurs early in the course of the injury. Invasion of inflammatory cells into the corneal stroma is inhibited by the use of aprotinin, accelerating the healing phase.[6]

The use of aprotinin along with thrombin inhibitors and antiplatelet clumping agents in stored platelet concentrates has been shown to permit storage of platelets for up to 15 days at room temperature with retention of viability. Whether these platelets will circulate for a reasonable length of time is as yet unknown.[3]

It has been shown that fibrin glue that incorporates aprotinin into the formulation is useful as a hemostatic agent, particularly in brain surgery.[35]

A final proposed use of aprotinin that might have clinical use is the protection of ischemic myocardium. This has been shown to be feasible in acute myocardial infarction in humans, but the study was done before the widespread use of thrombolytic therapy.[5] Aprotinin would be contraindicated in patients receiving thrombolytic drugs because it would counteract their effects.[10] It may, however, be useful in preserving myocardium during prolonged hypothermic cardioplegia followed by reperfusion.[32]

## Summary

Aprotinin is a very useful drug that has potential for a number of new indications as basic and clinical research continues. Its ability to reverse the prolonged bleeding time associated with thrombolytic therapy suggests that it could be very useful in a number of acquired and hereditary bleeding disorders for which there is relatively ineffective therapy currently available or for which available therapy is associated with short-term or long-term risks (blood products).

## References

1. Azad SC, Kratzer MAA, Groh J, et al: Intraoperative and postoperative re-evaluation of hemostasis in orthotopic liver transplantation. Semin Thromb Hemost 19:233–241, 1993.
2. Beckstein WO, Riess H, Blumhardt G, et al: Aprotinin in orthotopic liver transplantation. Semin Thromb Hemost 19:262–267, 1993.
3. Bode AP, Miller DT: The use of thrombin inhibitors and aprotinin in the preservation of platelets stored for transfusion. J Lab Clin Med 113:753–758, 1989.
4. Brunet E, Mira JP, Belghith M, et al: Effects of aprotinin on hemorrhagic complications in ARDS patients during prolonged extracorporeal $CO_2$ removal. Intens Care 18:364–367, 1992.
5. Cecna-Seldner FA, Villarreal J: Effect of the kallikrein inhibitor aprotinin in myocardial ischemia and necrosis in man. Angiology 31:488–496, 1980.
6. Cejkova J, Lojda Z, Dropcova S, Kadlecova D: The histochemical pattern of mechanically or chemically injured rabbit cornea after aprotinin treatment: Relationships with the plasmin concentration of the tear fluid. Histochem J 25:438–445, 1993.
7. Clozel JP, Banken L, Roux S: Aprotinin: An antidote for recombinant tissue-type plasminogen activator (rt PA) active in vivo. J Am Coll Cardiol 16:507–510, 1990.
8. Dubber AHC, McNichol GP, Uttley D, Douglas AS: In vitro and in vivo studies with Trasylol, an anticoagulant and a fibrinolytic inhibitor. Br J Haematol 14:31–49, 1968.
9. Federici AB, Berkowitz SD, Lattuada A, Mannucci PM: Degradation of von Willebrand factor in patients with acquired clinical conditions in which there is heightened proteolysis. Blood 81:720–725, 1993.
10. Federici A, Berkowitz S, Zimmerman T, Mannucci PM: Proteolysis of von Willebrand factor after thrombolytic therapy in patients with acute myocardial infarction. Blood 79:38–44, 1992.
11. Gabor M: The role of hemostasis and fibrinolysis in the metastatic spread of cancer. Semin Thromb Hemost 10:61–70, 1984.
12. Gallimore MJ, Heller W, Fuhrer G, et al: Contact activation, heparins and cardiopulmonary bypass. Thromb Haemost 69:92–93, 1993.
13. Garabedian H, Gold H, Leinbach R, et al: Bleeding time prolongation and bleeding during infusion of recombinant tissue-type plasminogen activator in dogs: Potentiation by aspirin and reversal with aprotinin. J Am Coll Cardiol 17:1213–1222, 1991.
14. Gardner FH, Helmer RE: Aminocaproic acid: Use in control of hemorrhage in patients with amegakaryocytic thrombocytopenia. JAMA 243:35–37, 1980.
15. Gimple LW, Gold HK, Leinbach RC, et al: Correlation between template bleeding times and spontaneous bleeding during treatment of acute myocardial infarction with recombinant tissue-type plasminogen activator. Circulation 80:581–588, 1989.
16. Herbert JM, Bernat A, Maffrand JP: Aprotinin reduces clopidogrel-induced prolongation of the bleeding time in the rat. Thromb Res 71:433–441, 1993.

17. Jensen R, Ens G: DDAVP, EACA and other pharmacologic agents used to maintain hemostatic integrity. Clin Hemost Rev 5:1, 1991.
18. John LCH, Rees GM, Kovacs IB: Reduction of heparin binding to and inhibition of platelets by aprotinin. Ann Thorac Surg 55:1175–1179, 1993.
19. Kwaan HC, Silverman S: Fibrinolytic activity in lesions of hereditary hemorrhagic telangiectasia. Arch Dermatol 107:571–573, 1973.
20. Loza JP, Gurewich P, Johnstine M, Pannell R: Platelet-bound prekallikrein promotes pro-urokinase induced clot lysis: A mechanism for targeting the factor XII dependent intrinsic pathway of fibrinolysis. Thromb Haemost 71:347–352, 1994.
21. Markus G: The role of hemostasis and fibrinolysis in the metastatic spread of cancer. Semin Thromb Hemost 10:61–70, 1984.
22. Matzdorff AC, Green D, Cohen I, Bauer KD: Effect of recombinant aprotinin in platelet activation in patients undergoing open heart surgery. Haemostasis 23:293–300, 1993.
23. Mikhalkin IA, Iashvili ZG, Bykov VL: Thermoradiotherapy combined with a proteolysis inhibitor (Contrical) in the treatment of head and neck cancer. Oncology 50:344–347, 1993.
24. Miles LA, Plow EF, Donnelly KJ, et al: A bleeding disorder due to deficiency of $\alpha_2$-antiplasmin. Blood 59:1246–1251, 1982.
25. Okajima K, Kohno I, Soe G, et al: Direct evidence for systemic fibrinogenolysis in patients with $\alpha_2$ plasmin inhibitor deficiency. Am J Hematol 45:16–24, 1994.
26. Orchard MA, Goodchild CS, Prentice CRM, et al: Aprotinin reduces cardiopulmonary bypass-induced blood loss and inhibits fibrinolysis without influencing platelets. Br J Haematol 85:533–541, 1993.
27. Paramo JA, Rocha E: Hemostasis in advanced liver disease. Semin Thromb Hemost 19:184–188, 1993.
28. Putterman C: Aprotinin therapy in septic shock [letter]. Acta Chir Scand 155:367, 1989.
29. Saba HI, Morelli GA, Longrino LA: Treatment of bleeding in hereditary hemorrhage telangiectasia with aminocaproic acid. N Engl J Med 330:1789–1790, 1994.
30. Schwartz BS, Williams EC, Conlou M, Mosher DF: Epsilon-aminocaproic acid in the treatment of patients with acute promyelocytic leukemia and acquired $\alpha_2$-plasmin inhibitor deficiency. Ann Intern Med 105:873–877, 1986.
31. Stahl RL, Henderson JM, Hooks MH, et al: The therapy of Kasabach-Merritt syndrome with cryoprecipitate plus intra-arterial thrombin and aminocaproic acid. Am J Hematol 36:272–274, 1991.
32. Sunamori M, Sulton I, Suzuki A: Effect of aprotinin to improve myocardial viability in myocardial preservation followed by reperfusion. Ann Thorac Surg 52:971–978, 1991.
33. Svartholm E, Haglund U, Ljungberg J, Hedner V: Influence of aprotinin, a protease inhibitor, on porcine *E. coli* shock. Acta Chir Scand 155:7–13, 1989.
34. Valentin S, Williamson P, Sutton D: Reduction of acute hemorrhage with aprotinin. Anaesthesia 48:405–406, 1993.
35. Vertraete M: Clinical application of inhibitors of fibrinolysis. Drugs 29:236–261, 1985.
36. Welte M, Groh J, Azad S, et al: Effect of aprotinin in coagulation parameters in liver transplantation. Semin Thromb Hemost 19:297–299, 1993.
37. Wendel HP, Heller W, Gallimore MJ: Aprotinin in therapeutic doses inhibits chromogenic peptide substrate assays for protein C. Thromb Res 74:543–548, 1994.
38. Winn R, Gleisner J, Maunder R, et al: Lung permeability and hemodynamics during endotoxemia: Effect of aprotinin. J Surg Res 41:620–626, 1986.

**W. Dietrich, MD**
**H. Mössinger, MD**

# 17

# The Use of Aprotinin in Pediatric Cardiopulmonary Bypass

Pediatric cardiac surgery is an ongoing challenge not only for the surgeon but also for the anesthesiologist. The types of operation vary substantially, and even a familiar diagnosis often requires a total different approach. Physiology differs considerably in children and adults, and the anesthesiologist often has to deal with an immature physiologic system. An important aspect of pediatric physiology for cardiac surgery is the effect of the hemostatic derangement due to cardiopulmonary bypass (CPB) on bleeding tendency. CPB in infants and neonates differs in several aspects from CPB in adult patients: the degree of hemodilution and blood exchange is greater, the temperature variations are more pronounced and the artificial surface of the bypass circuit, which may induce blood damage, is much larger in relation to the body surface area. Consequently, the impact of CPB on hemostasis and all other cascade systems of the body is more distinct than in adult patients.

Many of the surgical procedures for congenital malformations are more complex than those performed in adults, and many reoperations, including preliminary palliations, are necessary. Apart from surgically induced bleeding, the major cause of blood loss is an acquired coagulopathy. Impaired platelet function, due either to the mechanical effect of CPB or to the influence of hemostatic activation on platelets during CPB, is the main cause of postoperative bleeding.[23,44] Four important alterations affect the coagulation system in infants undergoing CPB:

1. Maturational differences in the hemostatic system of infants younger than 6 months are significant. Plasma concentrations of the vitamin K-dependent factors (II, VII, IX, X) protein C and protein S, and of the four factors of the contact system (Hageman factor [factor XII], prekallikrein, high-molecular-weight kininogen, and factor XI)[1] are lower in healthy, full-term neonates, probably because of the decreased rate of hepatic synthesis. On the other hand, platelet count, fibrinogen concentration, and the activity of other coagulation factors are comparable in neonates and adults, although in neonates certain elements may exist in a dysfunctional form.[22] Within the first half year of life the coagulation system matures and becomes similar to that of adults. The immature coagulation system does not lead to increased

bleeding tendency in healthy infants, probably because the balance between activators and inhibitors is maintained. But generation of thrombin and subsequent formation of fibrin are delayed when the hemostatic system becomes activated.

2. Cyanotic children demonstrate an impaired hemostatic system, which is related directly to the degree of polycythemia. Low platelet count and abnormal function, hypofibrinogenemia and decreased concentrations of factors V, VII, and VIII, and increased fibrinolysis are often seen in such patients.[13] In addition, some of them are taking hemostatically active medication.

3. The hemodilution caused by CPB in children is extreme compared with that in adults. The priming volume may surpass 2–3 times the estimated blood volume. Concentrations of coagulation factors have been shown to decrease by 50% and platelet count by 70% in neonates, despite blood priming of the oxygenator.[22]

4. Cardiac operations are regularly performed in deep hypothermia or circulatory arrest, which may further impair platelet function.[30,40] Yet the effect of low temperatures on the hemostatic system, with or without circulatory arrest, remains unclear.

Cardiac surgery in infants is associated with a substantial inflammatory response to CPB as measured by enhanced complement activation.[24] Greeley et al.[16] demonstrated a significant increase in release of thromboxane during CPB in infants, probably as a result of platelet activation. Despite conflicting data from other studies,[13] these results are consistent with the concept that inflammatory response to CPB is more pronounced in infants. Because complement activation is linked to the activation of other cascade systems, it is conceivable that hemostatic activation, which results in impaired hemostasis and increased bleeding tendency, plays a major role in pediatric cardiac surgery. The hemostatic alteration induced by CPB seems to be of a more global nature in infants than in adults.

## Pharmacologic Methods to Reduce Bleeding

In adults, many attempts have been made to reduce bleeding after CPB by pharmacologic intervention. Desmopressin acetate (DDAVP) was introduced enthusiastically into cardiac surgery;[34] the prostacyclin analogue iloprost[21] was used with only moderate effect on blood loss but considerable impact on peripheral resistance; and the antifibrinolytics epsilon-aminocaproic acid (EACA) and tranexamic acid are reported to decrease postoperative blood loss significantly.[20] The most impressive results, however, were obtained recently with the use of high-dose aprotinin, a proteinase inhibitor derived from bovine lung tissue. Aprotinin has antifibrinolytic properties in lower concentrations and in higher concentrations also acts as a kallikrein inhibitor, therefore attenuating the contact activation of the hemostatic system.[14] The literature confirming the efficacy of aprotinin continues to expand. Many studies[1,2,6,9,26,33,38] have demonstrated convincingly that it reduces the intra- and postoperative blood loss in adults undergoing cardiac surgery by 40–50%.

Information about pharmacologic intervention to reduce bleeding in pediatric cardiac surgery is limited. McClure and Izsak[27] studied the effect of EACA and found a reduction in blood loss from 62 to 35 ml/kg in children with cyanotic heart disease, whereas in acyanotic children the reduction (29 to 26 ml/kg) was not significant. In 1989 Seear et al.[35] investigated the effect of DDAVP on postoperative blood loss after cardiac operations in children. They studied 60 patients with a mean age of 46 and 64 months and a body weight of 15 and 20 kg, respectively. All patients underwent surgery for congenital heart disease. The difference in total postoperative blood loss in the desmopressin-treated children (40 ± 33 ml/kg) and the placebo group (31 ± 38 ml/kg) was not significant. In addition, no significant difference was found in hemostatic parameters. The authors concluded that DDAVP provided no hemostatic advantage in children undergoing cardiac operations.

At the beginning of the 1980s, the first experience with aprotinin in cardiac surgery in neonates and infants was reported. Popov-Cenic and Urban[31] found that aprotinin significantly reduced postoperative blood loss by more than 50% (51.8 to 22.4 ml/kg/24 hr) after open-heart surgery. The dosage regimen, however, varied from that applied in other studies. Aprotinin therapy was begun 1 or 2 days before surgery and continued until the first postoperative day. The total dose of aprotinin given in the operating room was approximately 100,000–200,000 KIU/kg. This treatment, however, was not introduced as a routine procedure in pediatric surgery.

Elliott and Allen[12] published preliminary results of aprotinin therapy in pediatric cardiac patients. The dosage, based on body surface area, was $2 \times 1.7 \times 10^6$ KIU/m² plus a continuous dose of $4 \times 10^5$ KIU/m². Thus, the total dosage was approximately $1–2 \times 10^6$ KIU per patient. They found a statistically significant reduction in chest closure time, which was particularly evident in patients with anatomic correction of transposition of the great arteries (42 ± 9 min in the aprotinin group vs. 138 ± 75 min in the historical control group). Blood loss and transfusion requirement showed no significant difference.

Müller et al.[29] reported the results of cardiac surgery, including long bypass procedures and deep hypothermia with circulatory arrest, in 205 children who weighed 2–36 kg. They administered $2 \times 3.5–5 \times 10^4$ KIU/kg of aprotinin and an additional dose of $2–3 \times 10^4$ KIU/kg/hr. Patients were compared with a historical control group (n = 100). Blood loss was significantly reduced (154 ± 184 vs. 210 ± 195 ml), as was the requirement for homologous blood. Patients treated with aprotinin required 25 ± 71 ml of whole blood and 42 ± 86 ml of packed red cells vs. 88 ± 146 ml of whole blood and 42 ± 86 ml of packed red cells in the control group. Herynkopf et al.[19a] administered 50,000 KIU of aprotinin in a double-blind, placebo-controlled study of 30 children up to 11 years. Blood loss reduction was about 30% (12.1 vs 17.7 ml/kg) but not significant in this small sample. Sixty-four percent of aprotinin-treated patients and only 25% of the controls did not need any homologous blood products postoperatively (p < 0.03). The number of donors was also significantly lower in the aprotinin group (1.07 vs 2.75) but this difference might have been enhanced by a transfusion policy using more whole blood in the aprotinin group in contrast to packed cells and fresh frozen plasma in the control group.

Because of the encouraging results of the use of aprotinin in adult cardiac patients within the last few years, a study of the role of aprotinin in pediatric cardiac surgery was considered worthwhile. The study is described in detail below.

## Aprotinin Study in Pediatric Cardiac Patients

We investigated the effect of high-dose aprotinin in a prospective, randomized study that used different dosages in 60 patients (body weight < 10 kg) undergoing open-heart surgery for various congenital heart lesions.[8] Patients with an expected bypass time longer than 120 minutes were excluded from the protocol. Assignment to one of three groups, each containing 20 patients, was random. Patients in the low-dose group (group L) received a bolus of 15,000 KIU/kg of aprotinin after induction of anesthesia and an additional bolus of 15,000 KIU/kg into the pump of the heart-lung machine. In the high-dose group (group H) the dosage of aprotinin was doubled: 30,000 KIU/kg after induction of anesthesia and 30,000 KIU/kg in the pump prime. Patients without aprotinin treatment served as controls.

Standard anesthetic techniques with fentanyl and flunitrazepam were used in all cases. All patients were anticoagulated with 375 U/kg mucosa heparin before CPB. The extracorporeal circuit consisted of a bubble oxygenator and nonocclusive roller pumps. The oxygenator was primed in all patients with 500 ml of homologous blood; 5,000 units of heparin were added to the pump prime. Patients underwent surgery either in deep hypothermic circulatory arrest (DHCA) at a rectal temperature of 20°C or in hypothermia with a rectal temperature of 26°C and a flow rate of 2.4 to 1.2/L/min/m². After completion of CPB, residual heparin was antagonized by protamine chloride (ratio 1:1.5).

Blood samples were drawn at the following times: (1) after induction of anesthesia but before infusion of aprotinin; (2) 5 minutes after onset of CPB; (3) 30 minutes after onset of CPB or, in patients undergoing DHCA, 15 minutes after the end of circulatory arrest; (4) at the end of CPB; and (5) at the end of the operation. From these samples the split products of the crosslinked fibrin were measured by two independent immunoassays, based on monoclonal antibodies to D-dimers. Degradation products of fibrinogen (FgDP), total degradation products, the complex of thrombin with antithrombin III (TAT), $F_{1+2}$ prothrombin fragments, and elastase in complex with a $\alpha_1$-protease inhibitor (PMN elastase) were determined by sandwich enzyme-linked immunosorbent assays (ELISAs) using polyclonal and monoclonal antibodies. The concentration of fibrin monomers was measured by an immunoassay with monoclonal antibodies directed against the N-terminal of a chain of human fibrin.

Spontaneous fibrinolytic activation in the native samples and in their euglobulin fraction was estimated by use of plasminogen-containing human fibrin plates.[41] Any development of a lysis area, regardless of size, was considered to be an indication of plasminogen activator(s) in the sample. For global coagulation tests, routinely applied clotting methods were used. Blood loss via the chest tubes was measured in the intensive care unit 6, 12, and 24 hours postoperatively. Plasma concentrations of aprotinin were quantified by a competitive ELISA, according to Müller-Esterl et al.[30] Heparin levels were measured by chromogenic substrate methods. Heparin anticoagulation was controlled by the activated clotting time (ACT), using a celite activator (Hemochron 400). Nonparametric tests were used for data analysis.

The results of the study are presented in more detail elsewhere.[8] The mean age of the patients was 211 ± 189 days in the control group compared with 263 ± 189 days (group L) and 349 ± 305 days (group H). The mean body weights were 5.5 ± 1.8 kg (control group), 6.2 ± 1.9 kg (group L), and 6.3 ± 2.5 kg (group H). Fourteen patients in the control group, 13 in group L, and 10 in group H underwent DHCA. Specific diagnoses are summarized in Table 1.

Our investigation corroborates the results of recent studies[1,2,17,19] of the use of high-dose aprotinin in adult patients undergoing cardiac surgery. We found a dose-dependent attenuation of the deleterious effect of CPB on hemostatic activation as well as a reduction of bleeding tendency in pediatric patients treated with aprotinin compared with the untreated control group.

As expected, plasma concentrations of aprotinin 30 minutes after onset of CPB were significantly higher (99 ± 25 KIU/ml) in group H than in group L (73 ± 30 KIU/ml) but did not reach levels found in adults when corresponding doses of aprotinin are used. The parameters of fibrinolysis were reduced on a dose-dependent basis. All split products of fibrinogen or fibrin were significantly lower in the two

**TABLE 1.** Diagnoses of Pediatric Patients

|  | Control | Low | High | Total |
|---|---|---|---|---|
| Tetralogy of Fallot | 1 | 2 | 0 | 3 |
| Transposition of the great arteries | 5 | 3 | 3 | 11 |
| Tricuspid atresia | 0 | 2 | 0 | 2 |
| Complete atrioventricular septal defect | 1 | 5 | 5 | 11 |
| Ventricular septal defect | 6 | 1 | 8 | 15 |
| Miscellaneous | 7 | 7 | 4 | 18 |
| Total | 20 | 20 | 20 | 60 |

aprotinin groups compared with the control group; the lowest concentrations were measured in group H. There was only a tendency toward reduction in clotting activation in the aprotinin groups. The concentration of fibrin monomere was significantly lower in the aprotinin groups than in the control group at the end of surgery, but TAT-complexes and $F_{1+2}$ fragments were unaffected.

The ACT was longer than 1,000 seconds in all groups during CPB. None of the patients required additional heparin to increase the ACT. Plasma concentrations of heparin 30 minutes after onset of CPB were $3.1 \pm 0.5$ U/ml. The blood loss was $9.4 \pm 5.3$ ml/kg in the control group, $8.7 \pm 6.3$ ml/kg in group L, and $5.6 \pm 1.8$ ml/kg in group H 6 hours postoperatively ($p < 0.05$). The total blood loss before removal of the chest tube showed no significant differences among the groups. No differences were found in the requirement of homologous blood. Two units of fresh whole blood were used for all patients during and after operation, including the pump prime. Thus, the donor exposure was the same in all groups.

## Aprotinin Dosage in Pediatric Cardiac Surgery

The main difference between the results of aprotinin studies in pediatric and adult patients[9] was the fact that no difference in clotting inhibition was noticeable. On the other hand, plasma concentrations of aprotinin were very low and did not reach the target concentration of 200 KIU/ml. The low plasma levels of aprotinin in the first study, suspected to be ineffective in suppressing coagulation activity, were the starting point of a complementary study[28] (Table 2), which added a fourth group of patients who received very high dosages of aprotinin (30,000 KIU/kg before induction of anesthesia, usually with 500,000 KIU added to the prime volume, regardless of body weight which was $< 10$ kg in most patients). This regimen was based on estimation of the dilution effect of the prime volume, which is relatively invariable (between 500 and 700 ml) for pediatric patients. Values of 400 KIU/ml in the fourth

**TABLE 2.** Dosages of Aprotinin

|  | n | Start of Operation (KIU/kg) | Pump Prime (KIU/kg) |
|---|---|---|---|
| Controls | 22 | 0 | 0 |
| Low dose | 33 | 15,000 | 15,000 |
| Medium dose | 27 | 30,000 | 30,000 |
| High dose | 14 | 30,000 | 60,000 (total minimum-500,000 KIU) |

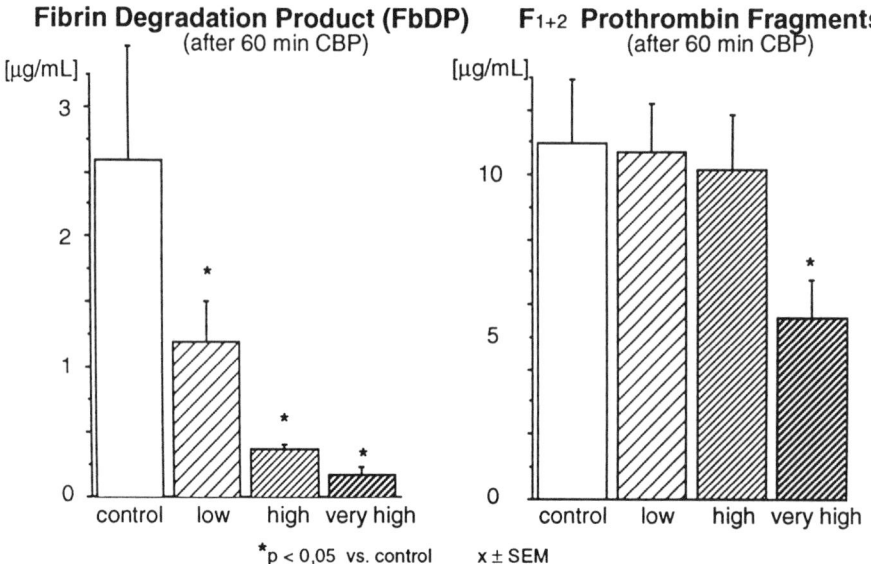

**FIGURE 1.** Attenuation of fibrinolysis (illustrated by fibrin degradation products) is dose-dependent and noticeable even with low dosages of aprotinin, whereas a suppression of clotting activity is reached only with a very high dosage (demonstrated by $F_{1+2}$ prothrombin fragments).

group surpassed by far the kallikrein-inhibiting level of aprotinin (200 KIU/ml). The TAT complex and $F_{1+2}$ fragments, indicators for clotting activation, were significantly reduced compared with the other three groups (Fig. 1). Fibrin and fibrinogen split products were further attenuated, demonstrating once more the strongly dose-related effect on the suppression of fibrinolysis. Blood loss and blood requirement, however, were not reduced compared with the other groups.

## Blood Loss and Aprotinin Therapy

In the above studies blood loss for 6 hours postoperatively was significantly reduced in the two high-dose aprotinin groups, but no convincing reduction was achieved after 24 hours, even in the highest-dose group. Furthermore, the reduction was negligible in clinical terms. Homologous blood requirement—calculated in units instead of milliliters—did not differ among the groups. Although measurements usually are made in milliliters, clinical importance is achieved only with a reduction in units, i.e., number of donor exposures.

Differing success in preventing blood loss may be explained also by divergent losses in untreated patients. We measured a 24-hour blood loss of 17 ml/kg compared with 31 ml/kg,[35] 52 ml/kg,[37] 65 and 29 ml/kg,[27] 38 ml/kg,[12] and 16.5 ml/kg.[29] Because hemorrhage and tamponade are poorly tolerated in infants, surgical hemostasis should be more meticulous (note the 4 times longer-lasting chest closure time for arterial switch operations in the Great Ormand Street series[12]). As stated, patients with an expected CPB time longer than 120 minutes were excluded from our protocol, because we were convinced that the bleeding tendency in long-lasting operations was reduced by aprotinin. Such patients benefit most from aprotinin treatment and were not excluded in other studies.

Despite irrefutable evidence that aprotinin reduces bleeding tendency and blood loss in adults, the results in pediatric patients are conflicting. Boldt et al.[4] studied the influence of two different dosages of aprotinin on blood loss and platelet function in pediatric cardiac patients up to a weight of 20 kg. The authors used a dosage of 20,000 KIU/kg after induction and 20,000 KIU/kg to the pump prime in one group and 35,000 KIU/kg (bolus) and 35,000 KIU/kg (prime) plus a continuous infusion of 10,000 KIU/kg/hr, respectively. Patients were compared with an untreated control group. The total dosage of aprotinin was $256 \times 10^6$ KIU and 475,000 KIU, respectively. The authors found no significant differences in platelet function among the groups. In addition, blood loss and homologous blood requirement did not differ significantly.

The same investigators studied the influence of aprotinin on the thrombomodulin/protein C systems. They investigated 30 children undergoing operation for congenital heart disease with a body weight of $10 \pm 7$ kg and $12 \pm 9$ kg and a mean age of about 3 years. Patients with reoperations were excluded from the protocol. The aprotinin-treated group (dosage: 30,000 KIU/kg [bolus], 30,000 KIU/kg [pump prime], and 30,000 KIU/kg every hour during CPB) was compared with a control group. The plasma concentration of thrombomodulin was reduced in the aprotinin-treated group. However, the interpretation of this finding remains unclear, and further studies are warranted to elucidate the influence of aprotinin on endothelial-derived coagulation. Again, the study demonstrated no reduction in bleeding tendency or homologous blood requirement due to aprotinin.

To date, the database of information about the use of aprotinin in pediatric cardiac surgery is not strong. Table 3 summarizes the results of aprotinin treatment in pediatric cardiac surgery. Some evidence suggests that the dosages of aprotinin used in pediatric studies lead to a lower plasma concentration compared with adult dosages and, therefore, may be too low. The influence on bleeding tendency may be less pronounced than in adult patients and not of clinical relevance. However, clinical evidence suggests that pediatric patients undergoing repeat cardiac operations or with expected long pump times will benefit from aprotinin therapy. Further studies are needed to evaluate the role of aprotinin treatment in pediatric cardiac surgery.

## Side Effects of Aprotinin

What are the disadvantages of aprotinin therapy? As a heterologous protein, aprotinin has antigenic properties and carries the risk of allergic and anaphylactic reactions, as described in adults.[7] In addition to one case report of an allergic reaction to aprotinin in a pediatric cardiac patient,[3] we observed two rather severe events in our experience, which now includes more than 1800 applications in children. Both were reoperative patients, and both had received aprotinin at the first operation. After aprotinin was discontinued and circulation was stabilized with high doses of vasopressors, the operation continued.

The risk of allergic reaction will increase in the future, because with widespread use the chance of reexposure to aprotinin will expand. Hence aprotinin should be given only to the monitored patient in the operating room and only after the administration of a test dose. If previous contact to aprotinin is known or suspected, prophylactic administration of antihistamines and corticosteroids is highly recommended. We strongly recommend the use of a test dose and the start of aprotinin infusion when the surgeon is ready to initiate CPB—i.e., at the time of aortic cannulation.

**TABLE 3.**  Studies with Aprotinin in Pediatric Cardiac Surgery

| | n | Max Weight (kg) | Mean Weight (kg) | Dosage | | | 24-hr Blood loss | | Remarks |
|---|---|---|---|---|---|---|---|---|---|
| | | | | Bolus (KIU/kg) | CPB (KIU/kg) | Additional Dosage (KIU/kg/h) | Aprotinin (ml/kg) | Control (ml/kg) | |
| Popov and Cenic (Bonn, 1982) | 150 | 12 | 4,8 | 45,000 | 300,000/ prime | 300,000/h 45,000 post-operatively | 22.4 | 51.8 | Continued application 2 days pre- and 1 day post-operatively |
| Elliot and Allen (London, 1990) | 12 | Neonates | 3.4 ± 0.7 | Approximately 100,000 (240 mg/m²) | Approximately 100,000 (240 mg/m²) | 0 | 39 ± 39 | 43 ± 5 | Only switch operations |
| Müller (Hannover, 1992) | 205 | 36 | 12.7 ± 7.1 | 35–50,000 | 35–50,000 | 20–30,000 | 12.1 ± 14.4 | 16.5 ± 15.3 | |
| Boldt (Gießen, 1993) | 42 | 20 | 13.2 ± 7.6 | 20,000 35,000 | 20,000 35,000 | 20,000 10,000 ? | 28 ± 10 27 ± 10 | 28 ± 7 | |
| Dietrich and Mössinger (München, 1993) | 60 | 10 | 6.0 ± 2.1 | 15,000 30,000 | 15,000 30,000 | 0 0 | 15.2 ± 9.7 11.3 ± 4.6 | 16.6 ± 8.7 | CPB > 2 hr excluded |
| Mössinger and Dietrich (München, 1993) | 96 | 25 | 6.7 ± 4.2 | 30,000 | 500,000/ prime | 0 | 17.6 ± 10.8 | 17.1 ± 8.9 | |
| Boldt (Gießen, 1994) | 30 | Children | 10.9 ± 7.5 | 30,000 | 30,000 | 30,000 | 19.2 ± 9.2 | 18.2 ± 10.1 | |
| Herynkopf (Porto Alegro, 1994) | 30 | 36 | 16.5 | 20,000 | 20,000 | 10,000 | 12.1 | 17.7 | |

Two retrospective reports[36,42] have assessed the influence of deep hypothermic circulatory arrest (DHCA) and aprotinin on renal function and coagulation in adult patients. It was speculated that the combination of no blood flow and low temperature may lead to activation of the coagulation system with disastrous consequences. Surgery for congenital heart disease is often performed in deep hypothermia or DHCA. We demonstrated[10] that low temperatures lead to increased activation of the hemostatic system. In our study 60% of patients underwent surgery with DHCA. The coagulation profile was better in aprotinin-treated patients than in the control group, and no signs of hypercoagulability were evident postoperatively. During the last 5 years at our institution DHCA with aprotinin was used in about 500 children, and we detected none of the harmful consequences described by Sundt et al.[36] in adult patients. Thus, our experience indicates that deep hypothermia does not constitute a contraindication for the use of aprotinin, at least in pediatric patients.

## Mode of Aprotinin Action

During CPB the hemostatic system is activated by the contact of blood with the artificial surfaces of the heart-lung machine. Contact activation (Hageman factor [factor XII], prekallikrein, high-molecular-weight kininogen, and factor XI) has no role in in-vivo coagulation.[15] Nevertheless, during CPB, which is a highly artificial system, contact activation seems to play an important role, leading to the generation of thrombin and finally to formation of fibrin. Fibrinolysis also is activated during this process. The contact activation with the conversion of prekallikrein to kallikrein launches the activation of the cascade systems, including the intrinsic pathway of coagulation, fibrinolysis, the classic complement pathway, and the kinin-kininogen system. Neutrophil activation takes place at the same time. Heparin inhibits only one component of the contact activation system, the formation of fibrin. Because thrombin already bound to fibrin is less inhibitable by heparin,[40] fibrin formation and polymerization take place despite heparin treatment during CPB.[11]

In lower concentrations, aprotinin inhibits fibrinolysis. In higher dosages, as used in adult cardiac surgery since 1987, it also inhibits kallikrein.[39] The inhibition of kallikrein results in an inhibition of the contact phase of coagulation. The contribution of contact activation to clinically significant activation of hemostasis, however, remains controversial. Thrombin generation, an indicator of reduced clotting activation, was decreased in adults.[9] We demonstrated that high-dose aprotinin attenuates not only fibrinolytic activity but also the generation of thrombin. Thus, aprotinin has anticoagulatory properties.[32] Because thrombin is a very powerful platelet activator,[43] a reduction in its generation ultimately leads to diminished stimulation of platelets. Improved preservation of platelet function has been described in patients treated with aprotinin.[25] This improvement is not an effect of direct aprotinin action on platelets but rather an indirect effect caused by decreased generation of thrombin and/or plasmin.

The present pediatric study shows that aprotinin attenuates fibrinolytic activation on a dose-dependent basis, as indicated by a reduction in fibrin split products. The aprotinin dose was calculated in accordance with the dosage used in adults. Pediatric patients are treated with a total dosage of $6-7 \times 10^6$ KIU, corresponding to $7-10 \times 10^4$ KIU/kg. In contrast to adult studies, decreased formation of thrombin, as indicated by reduced formation of TAT complex or $F_{1+2}$, was not found with pediatric dosages, possibly because of the relatively low plasma concentrations of aprotinin (peak levels in the range of 100 compared with 200 KIU/ml in adults), which were not able to inhibit kallikrein activation.

Such low concentrations are the consequence of greater dilution of aprotinin in the prime volume. Accordingly, in a subsequent study[28] we raised plasma concentrations by adding a fixed dosage of $5 \times 10^5$ KIU to the pump prime. TAT complex and $F_{1+2}$ fragments remained significantly lower with this dosage, thus supporting the hypothesis that clotting activation is suppressed with plasma concentrations of aprotinin exceeding 200 KIU/ml (in fact, the mean peak plasma level was 400 KIU/ml). A very high dosage of aprotinin[28] produces not only the dose-dependent effect on fibrinolysis but also decreases clotting activation, as assessed by formation of $F_{1+2}$ (see Fig. 1).

Information about platelet activation as the main source of bleeding[18] in pediatric patients is limited. It is not known whether other or additional mechanisms play a role in hemostatic activation compared with adults. Further studies are essential to elucidate the mode of hemostatic derangement in pediatric patients undergoing cardiac surgery.

Based on our results, we recommend the following dosage regimen in pediatric cardiac surgery:

30,000 KIU/kg as a bolus, with 60,000 KIU/kg added to the pump prime
(minimum: 500,000 KIU/patient)

This regimen takes into account the more pronounced hemodilution in pediatric patients. If much lower priming volumes of the oxygenators are feasible, an alternative dosage of 1,000 KIU/ml prime volume seems to be a practical solution.

Should aprotinin be given to all pediatric cardiac patients on a routine basis? In terms of bleeding tendency, the indication is questionable. But the routine use of aprotinin may maintain a more physiologic hemostatic state, with less activation of the hemostatic system. Little is known about the general consequences of activation of the cascade systems. Attenuation of this process with the use of aprotinin may lead to a better outcome. Our clinical experience in about 1800 children also supports the routine use of aprotinin in all pediatric cardiac operations. Long-lasting procedures and reoperations seem to be even more susceptible to its beneficial effects.

## Conclusion

Neonates and infants undergoing cardiac surgery have a higher risk of hemostatic derangement, with the possible consequence of increased postoperative bleeding, than adult patients. Reports in the literature about the extent of bleeding in pediatric patients vary substantially, possibly because of different techniques of surgical hemostasis. Priming of the heart-lung machine with blood and/or fresh frozen plasma may mask hemostatic defects induced by the immature coagulation system of neonates.

Studies in adults treated with aprotinin during the last 5 years consistently reported a reduction in bleeding tendency. The present studies demonstrate a similar reduction in pediatric patients. Even if aprotinin is not as effective in terms of reduced bleeding and blood conservation in infants as in adults, its use attenuates hemostatic activation during CPB. Maintenance of a more physiologic balance in the hemostatic system provides the rationale for the routine use of aprotinin in pediatric patients. Undoubtedly, however, aprotinin seems to be indicated in reoperations and all complex and long-lasting procedures. The optimal dosage remains in doubt. Taking into account the vast range in weight and blood volume of pediatric patients as well as the required priming volume of different types of oxygenators, a variable regimen is desirable but perhaps impractical. In pediatric patients we recommend a total dosage of aprotinin between 100,000 and 150,000 KIU/kg, depending on body weight and dilution.

## References

1. Bidstrup BP, Royston D, Sapsfort RN, Taylor KM: Reduction in blood loss and blood use after cardiopulmonary bypass with high dose aprotinin (Trasylol). J Thorac Cardiovasc Surg 97:364–372, 1989.
2. Blauhut B, Gross C, Necek S, et al: Effects of high-dose aprotinin on blood loss, platelet function, fibrinolysis, complement, and renal function after cardiopulmonary bypass. J Thorac Cardiovasc Surg 101:958–967, 1991.
3. Böhrer H, Bach A, Fleischer F, Lang J: Adverse haemodynamic effects of high-dose aprotinin in a pediatric cardiac surgical patient. Anaesthesia 45:853–854, 1990.
4. Boldt J, Knothe C, Zickmann B, et al: Comparison of two aprotinin dose regimes in pediatric cardiac surgery: Influence on platelet function and blood loss. J Thorac Cardiovasc Surg 105:705–711, 1993.
5. Boldt J, Zickmann B, Schindler E, et al: Influence of aprotinin on the thrombomodulin protein C system in pediatric cardiac operations. J Thorac Cardiovasc Surg 107:1215–1221, 1994.
6. Cosgrove DM, Heric B, Lytle BW, et al: Aprotinin therapy for reoperative myocardial revascularization: A placebo-controlled study. Ann Thorac Surg 54:1031–1038, 1992.
7. Dietrich W, Barankay A, Hahnel C, Richter JA: High-dose aprotinin in cardiac surgery: Three years' experience in 1,784 patients. J Cardiothorac Vasc Anesth 6:324–327, 1992.
8. Dietrich W, Mössinger H, Spannagl M, et al: Hemostatic activation during cardiopulmonary bypass with different aprotinin dosages in pediatric patients having cardiac operations. J Thorac Cardiovasc Surg 105:712–720, 1993.
9. Dietrich W, Spannagl M, Jochum M, et al: Influence of high-dose aprotinin treatment on blood loss and coagulation pattern in patients undergoing myocardial revascularization. Anesthesiology 73:1119–1126, 1990.
10. Dietrich W, Spannagl M, Mössinger HJ, Richter JA: Fibrin formation during CPB with and without circulatory arrest in operations of congenital heart diseases. Anesthesiology 75:A76, 1991.
11. Dietrich W, Spannagl M, Schramm W, et al: The influence of preoperative anticoagulation on heparin response during cardiopulmonary bypass. J Thorac Cardiovasc Surg 102:505–514, 1991.
12. Elliott M, Allen A: Aprotinin in pediatric cardiac surgery. Perfusion 5:73–76, 1990.
13. Fleming W, Sarafian L, Leschen M, et al: Serum concentrations of prostacyclin and thromboxane in children before, during, and after cardiopulmonary bypass. J Thorac Cardiovasc Surg 92:73–78, 1986.
14. Fritz H, Wunderer G: Biochemistry and applications of aprotinin, the kallikrein inhibitor from bovine organs. Arzneim Forsch/Drug Res 33:479–494, 1983.
15. Furie B, Furie BC: Molecular and cellular biology of blood coagulation. N Engl J Med 326:800–806, 1992.
16. Greeley W, Bushman G, Kong D, et al: Effects of cardiopulmonary bypass on eicanoid metabolism during pediatric cardiovascular surgery. J Thorac Cardiovasc Surg 95:842–849, 1988.
17. Harder MP, Eijsman L, Roozendaal KJ, et al: Aprotinin reduces intraoperative and postoperative blood loss in membrane oxygenator cardiopulmonary bypass. Ann Thorac Surg 51:936–941, 1991.
18. Harker LA: Bleeding after cardiopulmonary bypass. N Engl J Med 314:446–448, 1986.
19. Havel M, Teufelsbauer H, Knobl P, et al: Effect of intraoperative aprotinin administration on postoperative bleeding in patients undergoing cardiopulmonary bypass operation. J Thorac Cardiovasc Surg 101:968–972, 1991.

19a. Herynkopf F: Aprotinin in children undergoing correction of congenital heart defects. J Thorac Cardiovasc Surg 103:517–527, 1992.

20. Horrow JC, Hlavacek J, Strong MD, et al: Prophylactic tranexamic acid decreases bleeding after cardiac operations. J Thorac Cardiovasc Surg 99:70–74, 1990.

21. Kappa JR, Horn D, NcIntosh CL, et al: Iloprost (ZK 36374), a new prostacyclin analogue, permits open cardiac operation in patients with heparin-induced thrombocytopenia. Surg Forum 36:285–286, 1985.

22. Kern FH, Morana NJ, Sears JJ, Hickey PR: Coagulation defects in neonates during cardiopulmonary bypass. Ann Thorac Surg 54:541–546, 1992.

23. Kestin A, Valeri C, Khuri S, et al: The platelet function defect of cardiopulmonary bypass. Blood 82:107–117, 1993.

24. Kirklin JK, Westaby S, Blackstone EH, et al: Complement and the damaging effects of cardiopulmonary bypass. J Thorac Cardiovasc Surg 86:845–857, 1983.

25. Lavee J, Savion N, Smolinsky A, et al: Platelet protection by aprotinin in cardiopulmonary bypass: Electron microscopic study. Ann Thorac Surg 53:477–481, 1992.

26. Lu H, Soria C, Commin PL, et al: Hemostasis in patients undergoing extracorporeal circulation: The effect of aprotinin (Trasylol). Thromb Haemost 66:633–637, 1991.

27. McClure P, Izsak J: The use of epsilon-aminocaproic acid to reduce bleeding during cardiac bypass in children with congenital heart disease. Anesthesiology 40:604, 1974.

28. Mössinger H, Dietrich W, Spannagl M, et al: High-dose aprotinin reduces not only fibrinolytic, but also clotting activation in pediatric cardiac surgery. Proceedings of the 15th SCA Meeting, 1993, p 249.

29. Müller H, Alken A, Ziemer G, et al: Aprotinin in pediatric cardiopulmonary bypass surgery. J Cardiothorac Vasc Anesth 6:100, 1992.

30. Müller-Esterl W, Oettl A, Truscheit E, Fritz H: Monitoring of aprotinin plasma levels by an enzyme-linked immunosorbent assay (ELISA). Fresenius Z Anal Chem 317:718, 1984.

31. Popov-Cenic S, Urban AE, Noë G: Studies on the cause of bleeding during and after surgery with a heart-lung machine in children with cyanotic and acyanotic congenital cardiac defects and their prophylactic treatment. In McConn R (ed): The Role of Chemical Mediators in the Pathophysiology of Acute Illness and Injury. New York, Raven Press, 1982, pp 229–242.

32. Quereshi A, Lamont J, Burke P, et al: Aprotinin: The ideal anti-coagulant? Eur J Vasc Surg 6:317–320, 1992.

33. Royston D, Taylor KM, Bidstrup BP, Sapsford RN: Effect of aprotinin on need for blood transfusion after repeat open-heart surgery. Lancet ii:1289–1291, 1987.

34. Salzman EW, Weinstein MJ, Weintraub RM, et al: Treatment with desmopressin acetate to reduce blood loss after cardiac surgery. A double-blind randomized trial. N Engl J Med 314:1402–1406, 1986.

35. Seear MD, Wadsworth LD, Rogers PC, et al: The effect of desmopressin acetate (DDAVP) on postoperative blood loss after cardiac operations in children. J Thorac Cardiovasc Surg 98:217–219, 1989.

36. Sundt TM, Kouchoukos NT, Saffitz JE, et al: Renal dysfunction and intravascular coagulation with aprotinin and hypothermic circulatory arrest. Ann Thorac Surg 55:1418–1424, 1993.

37. Urban AE, Brecher AM, Popov-Cenic S: Blutungen nach intrakardialen operativen Eingriffen im Säuglingsalter: Klinische Relevanz und perioperative Therapie. In Dudziak R, Kirchoff PG, Reuter HD, Schumann F (eds): Proteolyse und Proteinaseninhibition in Herz- und Gefäß-chirurgie. Stuttgart, Schattauer, 1985, pp 273–278.

38. van Oeveren W, Jansen NJG, Bidstrup BP, et al: Effects of aprotinin on hemostatic mechanisms during cardiopulmonary bypass. Ann Thorac Surg 44:640–645, 1987.

39. Verstraete M: Clinical application of inhibitors of fibrinolysis. Drugs 29:236–261, 1985.

40. Weitz JL, Hudoba M, Massel D, et al: Clot-bound thrombin is protected from inhibition by heparin-antithrombin III is susceptible to inactivation by antithrombin III-independent inhibitors. J Clin Invest 86:385–391, 1990.

41. Wendt P, Fritsch A, Schulz F, et al: Proteinases and inhibitors in plasma and peritoneal exudate in acute pancreatitis. Hepatogastroenterol 31:277–281, 1984.

42. Westaby S, Forni A, Dunning J, et al: Aprotinin and bleeding in profoundly hypothermic perfusion. Eur J Cardiothorac Surg 8:82–86, 1994.

43. Winters K, Santoro S, Miletich J, Eisenberg P: Relative importance of thrombin compared with plasmin-mediated platelet activation in response to plasminogen activation with streptokinase. Circulation 84:1552–1560, 1991.

44. Woodman R, Harker L: Bleeding complications associated with cardiopulmonary bypass. Blood 76:1680, 1990.

**Ben Bidstrup, FRACS, FRCSEd**

# 18

## Pretreatment with Aprotinin and Aspirin

Because aspirin is widely used in the treatment of cardiac disease, many patients presenting for open-heart surgery have been exposed to it within 7–10 days. Bleeding problems associated with recent aspirin exposure increase costs related to time spent in intensive care and hospital as well as use of blood products. Studies in the United States and Europe demonstrate that aprotinin reduces bleeding and use of blood products by 50% in both non–aspirin-treated and aspirin-treated patients. Other drugs have been investigated less widely, without the consistent effect of high-dose aprotinin.

To use currently available blood conservation strategies cost effectively, patients at high risk of bleeding must be identified preoperatively. Current pathology testing does not facilitate application of risk stratification to predict the potential for excessive postoperative bleeding. Stratification is done by identifying groups according to other characteristics, such as previous surgery, presence of preexisting problems, and exposure to drugs, especially aspirin. Aspirin irreversibly acetylates prostaglandin G/H synthase, resulting in a permanent inability to produce thromboxane $A_2$, another prostaglandin derivative. Aspirin is effective rapidly and permanently. Platelets are unable to resynthesize new proteins because of their anuclear nature.[15] The effect of low doses of aspirin ($<100$ mg/day) is cumulative. Platelet turnover requires 8–10 days, leading to slow recovery after cessation of therapy. Aspirin is efficacious in the prevention of complications related to cardiovascular disease. In particular, morbid events related to unstable angina, subendocardial myocardial infarction, and recent myocardial infarction are reduced.[7,11,13,18] Effects on primary prevention of cardiac events have been less apparent. In postoperative cardiac surgical patients the use of aspirin improves saphenous vein graft patency.[10]

For the above reasons, many patients who undergo cardiac surgery, especially coronary artery bypass grafting, have been exposed to aspirin. Clinical aspects of aspirin exposure are related to platelet dysfunction, including increased skin bleeding time, as demonstrated by Ferraris et al.[8] shortly after a single dose of aspirin. Their study showed an increase in postoperative bleeding at 12 hours from $916 \pm 482$ ml to 1513 ± 978 ml as well as the following increases in use of blood products; packed red cells, 1.8 to 4.4 units; platelets, 0.2 to 1.3; and packs and fresh frozen plasma, 0.78 to 3.6 units. Patients with bleeding times that exceeded 9 minutes were excluded because the authors considered such patients to be at considerably increased risk of postoperative bleeding, although few data support this conclusion.

As a part of the Veterans' Administration trial assessing changes in patency of aortocoronary bypass graft (ACBG), patients in several groups received aspirin preoperatively. Patients receiving aspirin 12 hours before surgery showed an increase in postoperative bleeding and in use of homologous blood products. In addition, the rate of reoperation increased from 1.7% to 6.6%.[19]

Bashein et al.[1] demonstrated that aspirin exposure was associated not only with an increase in blood usage (9.5 vs. 3.0 units) but also with a significant increase in morbidity, which resulted in longer intensive care (4.7 vs. 2.1 days) and hospital stays (10.9 vs. 7.0 days). They demonstrated a 1.82 times greater risk of reoperation for bleeding in patients exposed to aspirin within 7 days of surgery. In the current medicoeconomic climate this can have a major impact; the authors estimated that costs for aspirin-pretreated patients increased from $9400 to $14,000. In a prospective review, Taggart et al.[20] evaluated the effect of continued use of low-dose aspirin in 202 patients. They found increased use of blood products and increased frequency of reoperation but no prolongation of hospital stay (mean = 8 days). The mean stay needs to be compared with the North American average, which often is less than 6 days. No significant relationship was found with the actual dose of aspirin (75, 150, and 300 mg/day). Cobbe supported the continued use of aspirin (and streptokinase) in an editorial in the *British Medical Journal*, based on the results of the GISSI studies. Holden responded that the continued concomitant use of aspirin was associated with significant morbidity, and Gay argued not only that aspirin should be discontinued but also that blood banks should provide fresh whole blood rather than fractionated blood products for patients with open-heart surgery. This raises the issue of alternatives to reduce the donor exposure of such patients.[9] Several groups have reported an incidence of excessive bleeding in the range of 20%. One group requires the use of large quantities of blood components (6–10 platelet packs, 4 units of fresh frozen plasma, 2–4 units of cryoprecipitate and packed red cells). Such requirements may expose patients to approximately 18 donors. Furthermore, the cost of blood products may exceed $2,000, depending on costs related to repeated cross-matching.

Although the hemostatic defect associated with aspirin is believed to be related to the irreversible acetylation of cycloxygenase, little work has been done to determine the effect during cardiopulmonary bypass. The Geissen group examined the effect of preoperative aspirin on the usual parameters of blood loss as well as on other markers of platelet function. Aggregometry was performed with several agonists (adenosine diphosphate, 1.0 $\mu$mol/L, 2.0 $\mu$mol/L; collagen; and adrenalin). Postoperative blood loss was significantly higher in the ACBG group exposed to aspirin 5–7 days preoperatively compared with the control group undergoing aortic valve replacement (AVR), which was exposed to neither aspirin nor other anticoagulants. Aggregation parameters showed marked reductions in all tested variables in the ACBG vs. AVR groups, despite no significant preoperative differences. Other explanations for such differences are possible, given that the procedures differ in many ways.[5]

Various policies have been adopted to deal with the increased bleeding tendency due to preoperative exposure to aspirin. Many centers defer surgery until the effect of aspirin has worn off (usually 8–10 days). This policy may place the unstable patient at increased risk of cardiac events before surgery. In many cases, surgery is undertaken, and aspirin-associated morbidity is accepted. Aprotinin (Trasylol, Bayer AG, Leverkusen, Germany) has been shown in many clinical studies to be highly efficacious in reducing postoperative bleeding. However, because many of the early studies excluded the previous use of aspirin,[3,16,21] it seemed reasonable to assess the effect in patients who remained on aspirin therapy.

A reasonable body of evidence now shows the efficacy of aprotinin in aspirin-treated patients. In a placebo-controlled, double-blind study, Murkin and colleagues randomized patients exposed to aspirin within 48 hours of surgery to receive the high-dose regimen of aprotinin[3] or an equivalent volume of placebo. One important difference was that the infusion was continued until the patient was admitted to intensive care. The 57 patients included 45 undergoing coronary bypass surgery (42 with internal mammary artery [IMA] grafts), 5 undergoing ACBG plus valve procedure, and 2 undergoing valve procedure alone. Both groups were similar in demography, distribution of procedure, and aspirin therapy. The aprotinin-treated patients had significantly lower blood loss intraoperatively, postoperatively, and in total. As a result, the proportion of patients receiving packed red cells during the hospital stay was significantly lower. The use of IMA grafts was a significant predictor of higher intraoperative blood loss, but this trend was reversed with aprotinin. The overall duration of operation and time in intensive care and hospital were shorter in the aprotinin-treated patients. The incidence of adverse events, especially those which may be related to ischemic events or graft thrombosis, were examined postoperatively. Perioperative myocardial infarction was reported in 1 aprotinin-treated patient and 3 placebo-treated patients. Central nervous system events occurred in 1 and 4 patients in each group, respectively.[14] The authors considered that the difference may indicate a protective effect of serine protease inhibitors on cerebral damage during cardiopulmonary bypass.

In the multicenter study reported by Lemmer and associates, patients were stratified according to aspirin exposure. In patients who had received aspirin, the effect of aprotinin was still evident.[12] Schönberger retrospectively reviewed the effect of low-dose aspirin and low-dose aprotinin in 75 patients, of whom 25 had received low dose aspirin without aprotinin, 25 had received both aspirin and aprotinin, and 25 had received neither. The blood requirements tended to be higher in patients treated with aspirin than in the control group. However, blood loss was significantly decreased in patients exposed to aprotinin as well as aspirin.[17]

In an open pilot study Bidstrup and coauthors examined the effect of aprotinin and aspirin usage in 44 nonrandomized patients. They reported a greater than 50% reduction in postoperative blood loss and significant reductions in need for blood products.[4] Based on these data, a randomized, placebo-controlled study was carried out in 60 patients, all of whom had continued to take aspirin until less than 24 hours before surgery. The study found a 50% reduction in postoperative hemoglobin loss (Table 1), a similar reduction in postoperative blood loss, and a greater proportion

**TABLE 1.** Reduction of Hemoglobin Loss, Chest Drainage, and Exposure to Red Cells

|  | Hemoglobin Loss | Chest Drainage (6 hrs) | No Donor Blood (%) |
| --- | --- | --- | --- |
| Aprotinin | 11.41 (7.86) | 194.8 (100.8) | 23.3 |
| Placebo | 36.01 (31.3) | 504.3 (309.3) | 56.7 |
| Significance | $p < 0.001$ | $p < 0.001$ | $p = 0.008$ |

**TABLE 2.**  Distribution of Adverse Effects between the Two Groups*

|  | Aprotinin | Placebo |
|---|---|---|
| Atrial fibrillation/flutter | 7 | 11 |
| Wound infection | 2 | 2 |
| Perioperative myocardial infarction | 2 | 2 |
| Neurologic disturbance | 1 | 1 |
| Pneumothorax | 1 | 0 |
| Resternotomy | 1 | 1 |

*There were no statistically significant differences between the two groups.

of patients who did not receive homologous blood products. The incidence of adverse events was equally distributed between the two groups; the most common was atrial fibrillation. Changes in renal function were not significant. The incidence of perioperative myocardial infarction was also equally distributed between the two groups (Table 2) (Bidstrup, unpublished data).

A study involving 41 centers in the United Kingdom examined the use of aprotinin in 671 high-risk patients. Many of the patients admitted to the study had been exposed to aspirin. Overall blood use was 2 units/patient (median). Adverse events, including 1 graft occlusion, were reported in only 3% of patients.[2]

The use of the antifibrinolytic agents epsilon aminocaproic acid and tranexamic acid has not been specifically reported in this subgroup of patients. Desmopressin has had varying results in reducing postoperative bleeding. Dilthey and coworkers in Munich examined the effect of desmopressin in 40 patients who had continued to use aspirin to within 5 days of surgery. The authors found no significant change in postoperative bleeding but reported a reduction in packed red cell transfusion.[6]

Economic and medical pressures in patients undergoing coronary bypass surgery now dictate that both delay in surgery and a prolonged hospital stay are unacceptable. In aspirin-treated patients, these factors may be inversely related. One approach is to include as part of the blood conservation strategy pharmacologic interventions that reliably reduce the risks associated with aspirin exposure. Numerous prospective clinical trials as well as a large-scale prospective review demonstrate that aprotinin is highly efficacious in this area. The risk/benefit ratio in this subgroup of patients seems extremely favorable, and the possible effect of aprotinin on graft patency can be reversed with continued exposure to aspirin.

# References

1. Bashein G, Nessly ML, Rice AL, et al: Preoperative aspirin therapy and reoperation for bleeding after coronary artery bypass surgery. Arch Intern Med 151:89–93, 1991.
2. Bidstrup BP, Harrison J, Royston D, et al: Aprotinin therapy in cardiac operations: A report on use in 41 cardiac centers in the United Kingdom. Ann Thorac Surg 55:971–976, 1993.
3. Bidstrup BP, Royston D, Sapsford RN, Taylor KM: Reduction in blood loss and blood use after cardiopulmonary bypass with high dose aprotinin (Trasylol). J Thorac Cardiovasc Surg 97:364–372, 1989.
4. Bidstrup BP, Royston D, McGuiness C, Sapsford RN: Aprotinin in aspirin-pretreated patients. Perfusion 5:77–81, 1990.
5. Boldt J, Knothe C, Zickmann B, et al: The effects of preoperative aspirin therapy on platelet function in cardiac surgery. Eur J Cardiothorac Surg 6:598–602, 1992.
6. Dilthey G, Dietrich W, Spannagl M, Richter JA: Influence of desmopressin acetate on homologous blood requirements in cardiac surgical patients pretreated with aspirin. J Cardiothorac Vasc Anesth 7:425–430, 1993.

7. Elwood P, Sweetnam P: Aspirin and secondary mortality after myocardial infarction. Lancet 2:1313–1315, 1979.
8. Ferraris VA, Ferraris SP, Lough FC, Berry WR: Preoperative aspirin ingestion increases operative blood loss after coronary artery bypass grafting. Ann Thorac Surg 45:71–74, 1988.
9. Gay WJ: Aspirin, blood loss, and transfusion [editorial comment]. Ann Thorac Surg 50:345–345, 1990.
10. Goldman S, Copeland J, Moritz T, et al: Starting aspirin therapy after operation: Effects on early graft patency. Circulation 84:520–526, 1991.
11. Juul MS, Edvardsson N, Jahnmatz B, et al: Double-blind trial of aspirin in primary prevention of myocardial infarction in patients with stable chronic angina pectoris. Lancet 340:1421–1425, 1992.
12. Lemmer J Jr, Stanford W, Bonney SL, et al: Aprotinin for coronary bypass operations: Efficacy, safety, and influence on early saphenous vein graft patency. A multicenter, randomized, double-blind, placebo-controlled study. J Thorac Cardiovasc Surg 107:543–551; discussion, 551–553, 1994.
13. Lewis H, Davis J, Archibald D, et al: Protective effects of aspirin against acute myocardial infarction and death in men with unstable angina: Results of a Veterans Administration Cooperative Study. N Engl J Med 309:396–403, 1983.
14. Murkin JM, Lux J, Shannon NA, et al: Aprotinin significantly decreases bleeding and transfusion requirments in patients receiving aspirin and undergoing cardiac operations. J Thorac Cardiovasc Surg 107:554–561, 1994.
15. Patrono C: Aspirin as an antiplatelet drug. N Engl J Med 330:1287–1294, 1994.
16. Royston D, Bidstrup BP, Taylor KM, Sapsford RN: Aprotinin decreases the need for postoperative blood transfusions in patients having open heart surgery. Bibl Cardiol 73–82, 1988.
17. Schönberger JP, Bredee JJ, van-Oeveren W, et al: Preoperative therapy of low-dose aspirin in internal mammary artery bypass operations with and without low-dose aprotinin. J Thorac Cardiovasc Surg 106:262–267, 1993.
18. Second International Study of Infarct Survival (ISIS 2) Collaborative Group: Randomized trial of intravenous streptokinase, oral aspirin, both or neither among 17,187 cases of suspected acute myocardial infarction: ISIS-2. Lancet 2:349–360, 1988.
19. Sethi GK, Copeland JG, Goldman S, et al: Implications of preoperative administration of aspirin in patients undergoing coronary artery bypass grafting. Department of Veterans Affairs Cooperative Study on Antiplatelet Therapy. J Am Coll Cardiol 15:15–20, 1990.
20. Taggart DP, Siddiqui A, Wheatley DJ: Low-dose preoperative aspirin therapy, postoperative blood loss, and transfusion requirements. Ann Thorac Surg 50:425–428, 1990.
21. van Oeveren W, Janssen N, Bidstrup BP, et al: Effects of aprotinin on haemostatic mechanisms in cardiopulmonary bypass. Ann Thorac Surg 44:640–645, 1987.

**Manuel Concha, MD**
**Ignacio Muñoz, MD**

# 19

## Experience with Low-Dose Aprotinin

With the advent of cardiac surgery using extracorporeal circulation (ECC), there has been great concern over perioperative and immediate postoperative bleeding and the ensuing high degree of morbidity and mortality, especially in patients at high risk of hemorrhage. These high-risk patients include those who have previously undergone one or more sternotomies, patients with severe sepsis or serious clotting disorders, and those who are receiving perioperative treatment with anticoagulants or fibrinolytic agents. In such patients, the risk of mortality and the occurrence of complications attributable to bleeding is very high, and numerous attempts have been made by researchers worldwide to alleviate this problem.

One of the most important advances in cardiac surgery has been the discovery in 1987 by Royston et al.[1] of the hemostatic effects of aprotinin, a serine protease inhibitor, in the course of experiments aimed at reducing inflammation in various organs and systems during ECC,[2-6] a concept previously developed by Kirklin et al.[7] After a number of trials using a drug whose mechanism of action was relatively unknown, an aprotinin dose regimen was calculated. This regimen was based on attaining a concentration of roughly 200 KIU/ml of plasma. In in vitro tests, this amount proved sufficient to totally inhibit kallikrein, the primary mediator of the cascade of inflammatory phenomena responsible for, among other things, the hemostatic disorders taking place during and after extracorporeal surgery.

The standard, or Hammersmith, dosage[8] of aprotinin was thus established and has since been employed in numerous randomized tests with large numbers of patients in Europe and the United States.[9-19] All these tests have shown the drug to be highly effective, achieving a mean reduction in postoperative blood loss of around 50%, together with considerable reduction in autologous blood transfusion requirements and the appreciable morbidity this entails[20,21] Aprotinin also reduces bleeding-related complications, particularly in hemostatic reoperation, which has been shown to involve a high risk of mortality and complications.[22]

Although the mechanism of action of aprotinin has yet to be fully identified, a number of tests have highlighted its ability to conserve platelet function and reduce the fibrinolysis triggered by the passage of blood across endothelium-free surfaces, and the consequent cascade of inflammatory phenomena.[23-35] The complication rate in these tests was extremely low, and a high-dose regimen has since been established and employed in most surgical centers.

## Aprotinin at Lower Dosage

It should be noted that the commonly used dose regimen conceals a number of gray areas. Firstly, it is an absolutely empirical dosage, based on phenomena observed in vitro and subsequently validated in clinical trials; these phenomena, however, are part of a complex biological mechanism which is currently largely unknown. Secondly, the Hammersmith dosage fails to take into consideration factors such as weight and body surface area; the dosage actually administered may vary widely as a function of these factors, although clinical trials suggest that body surface area may not be of crucial importance.[18]

The kinetics of aprotinin remain partially unknown, because no direct relationship has been established between the dose employed and the plasma levels achieved, nor between plasma levels and the criteria for clinical efficacy. These criteria are, in any case, difficult to establish.

The high cost of aprotinin has led some authors to test lower dosage protocols, with a view both to cutting costs and to reducing further the very low rate of complications and side effects attributed to aprotinin.[20,36-42,74-76] Moreover, in order to be validated, dose regimens for aprotinin, or indeed any other drug intended to prevent bleeding complications, must prove effective in terms of the criteria laid down by Royston et al.[75] They must, therefore, afford a reduction in postoperative bleeding and in homologous blood requirements comparable to the reductions obtained using the regimens commonly employed to date.

Schonberger et al.[40] studied a group of 100 consecutive patients undergoing coronary revascularization. These patients received a pump prime dose of $2 \times 10^6$ KIU of aprotinin as the sole measure to combat postoperative bleeding. Patients undergoing a single mammary bypass showed postoperative bleeding of 684 ml, as compared to 1,237 ml in patients not receiving aprotinin ($p < 0.01$). The difference, though still statistically significant, was less marked in patients undergoing bilateral mammary bypass. Of the control group, 8% of patients underwent reoperation due to bleeding, compared with none from the aprotinin group. Hemoderivative requirements were 0.5 in the experimental group, as against 2.05 in the control group, and 78% of aprotinin-treated patients required no hematologic drugs compared to 45% in the control group.

Kawasujii et al.[37] made a randomized study of 27 patients undergoing cardiac revascularization surgery. Half of these patients received a pump prime dose of 30,000 KIU aprotinin/kg followed by maintenance infusion of 7,500 KIU/kg/hour of operation. Postoperative blood loss was 803 ml/patient in the aprotinin group versus 1,277 ml/patient in the control group ($p < 0.05$). Similar results were reported by van Oeveren et al.,[29,43] Carrel et al.,[39] Covino et al.,[38] and Schomberger et al.[40] In all these studies, reductions were seen in postoperative bleeding and the need for hematologic drugs on a par with those obtained using the dosage described by Royston.

The protection of platelet function by aprotinin at this dose regimen was studied by Lavee et al.,[44] who showed via electron microscopy that there were important differences in platelet aggregation capacity in patients treated with a low dosage of aprotinin after cardiopulmonary bypass (CPB) compared to untreated patients. Kawasujii et al.[37] described the effects of low-dose aprotinin on platelet action and on various aspects of hemostasis. The results of both studies showed major advantages of the use of low-dose aprotinin with respect to the preservation of platelet function, prevention of fibrinolysis, and several aspects of hemostasis. These advantages are comparable with those described by several authors reporting on the Hammersmith dosage of aprotinin.[23–25,29–35]

There is a strong indication in all the above results that lower doses of aprotinin may be just as effective as those initially recommended. These findings call for studies of larger patient groups treated at this dosage.

Carrel et al.[39] carried out a randomized study of four patient groups receiving no aprotinin, a low pump prime dose, a low intravenous dose at the start of operation, and the Hammersmith dosage. Treatment was highly effective in the reduction of postoperative bleeding and of homologous blood requirements in the group receiving the low pump prime dose, equivalent to results for the group treated with high dosages. This would suggest that, just as other authors have reported for low dosages,[29] the benefits of lower-dose aprotinin seem to be due to the preservation of platelet adhesiveness, avoiding the activation of platelets when blood comes into contact with the surface of the oxygenator and the ECC tubing lines at the beginning of CPB; this may be witnessed by a 50% reduction in the initial value of glycoprotein Ib during the first few minutes of ECC, an unmistakable sign of platelet activation, and gives rise to marked reduction in hemostatic capacity. For this reason, it is important when using lower-dose aprotinin, that the drug be inside the ECC circuit at the very start of CPB in order to counteract the adverse events taking place there on beginning the operation. The observation that identical doses administered intravenously lacked efficacy appear to support this theory.[39]

## Experience at Reina Sofia Hospital

Our experience began in October 1990. From March 1991 to December 1993, a study was made of 663 consecutive adult patients undergoing operation at this center. Various types of operation were performed with ECC, always using one single dose of $2 \times 10^6$ KIU of aprotinin as the pump prime dose to prevent hemorrhagic complications. Various parameters for this group were compared with those of another group of 762 consecutive patients undergoing operation at the same center between May 1988 and February 1991. The latter group received no aprotinin and thus served as a control.

Groups were similar in age, functional class, pathologic distribution, and percentage of patients at high risk of postoperative bleeding. Protocols for anesthesia, ECC, myocardial protection, surgical techniques, and postoperative care were those commonly used and similar for both patient groups. The characteristics of the patients are listed in Table 1.

## Protocol

A single dose comprising 200 ml of solution containing 280 mg ($2 \times 10^6$) of aprotinin (Trasylol, Bayer AG, Leverkusen, Germany) was administered. Patients received initial anticoagulation treatment with 3 mg heparin/kg before cannulation

**TABLE 1.** Patient Characteristics

|  | Aprotinin | Control | Total |
|---|---|---|---|
| CABG | 208 | 307 | 515 |
| Valvular | 368 | 405 | 773 |
| Heart transplantation | 101 | 50 | 151 |
| Total | 663 | 762 | 1425 |

CABG = coronary artery bypass graft.

for CPB. Activated coagulation time (ACT) was taken every 20–30 minutes (Hemochron, International Technidyne Corp., Edison, NY). ACT was maintained at > 800 s during ECC, with more heparin being added as required. When the cannulas were removed, heparin was neutralized by protamine sulfate at 1 mg/mg heparin. Drainage tubes were placed in the pericardial cavity and pleural spaces as required, and continuous suction was applied to the thoracic cavity.

## Intraoperative Anticoagulation Monitoring

The ACT of all patients was periodically monitored during ECC and kept > 800 s to ensure a safety margin, allowing for the lengthening of the ACT produced exclusively by aprotinin in the presence of heparin, as described by other authors for high doses of aprotinin.[18,45-50] This lengthening of the ACT is an artifact of the measuring method produced by aprotinin on the presence of heparin[33] and should neither be interpreted as an anticoagulant effect of aprotinin nor indicate the possibility of using lower doses of heparin—which may produce thrombotic events (see below).

## Postoperative Blood Loss

Mean postoperative bleeding at 18 hours postoperation was $470 \pm 336$ ml in the aprotinin group and $873 \pm 741$ ml in the control group over the entire series of patients ($p < 0.001$), reaching a reduction of 46.1% in postoperative drain loss, comparable with that reported by several authors for the Hammersmith dosage.[10-18] Reduction in bleeding was just as significant in the total group of patients, in coronary revascularization, and in valve and heart transplant operations (Fig. 1).

## Reoperation due to Bleeding

The need for early reoperation on a patient because of excessive bleeding is an important factor in an unfavorable prognosis, as it is usually associated with major hemodynamic disorders, huge homologous blood requirements, possible cardiac tamponade, frequent need for emergency operations under unfavorable hemodynamic conditions, thorax openings in the intensive care unit, occasional need for renewed ECC to control bleeding, and the occasional intervention by staff not completely familiar with cardiac surgery. Moreover, patients requiring hemostatic exploration because of excessive blood loss or due to the risk or presence of cardiac tamponade are frequently those at highest risk before operation; these patients have various associated factors of bleeding risk such as previous cardiac surgery, sepsis, and coagulopathy. They are often patients in a precarious clinical situation

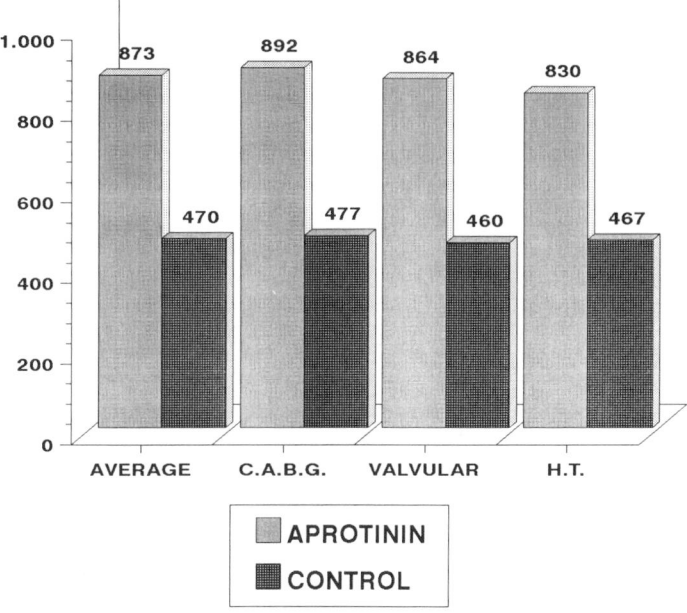

**FIGURE 1.** Postoperative bleeding (expressed in ml at 18 hours postoperatively) in the total group of patients. CABG = coronary artery bypass graft; HT = heart transplantation.

or who have undergone complicated or high-risk surgery. For all the foregoing reasons, reoperation due to bleeding carries with it a special risk of complications and a high peri- and postoperative mortality rate.

At the Cleveland Clinic,[22] a study was made of a series of 1,500 consecutive patients undergoing coronary reoperation. The authors concluded that excessive postoperative bleeding specifically requiring hemostatic reoperation was the greatest source of mortality and of early and late morbidity in the postoperative phase of these patients, with an incidence of reoperation of 7%. For all the above reasons, we believe that the incidence of reoperation is an important prognostic factor in cardiac surgery, and that its reduction could be adopted as an important criterion to be used along with the classic criteria when describing the efficacy of commonly used hemostatic agents, especially aprotinin.

In our series of patients, there was no reoperation due to bleeding in the group of patients treated with aprotinin and 10 reoperations in the control group: 4 of these were in transplanted patients, 3 in heart surgery, and 3 in valve surgery patients (Table 2). Patients undergoing reoperation generally received extensive transfusion and had long, complicated postoperative periods. In our experience, few reoperations due to blood loss revealed a specific site of bleeding, and the removal of clots and the extraction of hematomas was usually sufficient to stop bleeding.

## Patients with a High Risk of Bleeding

In our experience and as generally reported, subgroups of patients may be identified in whom a greater number of hemorrhagic complications can be expected, e.g., those having previous ECC surgery, active infective endocarditis, preoperative disorders of coagulation parameters, previous prolonged ECC, and heart transplantation.

**TABLE 2.** Reoperations for Bleeding

|  | Aprotinin Group | Control Group | % |
|---|---|---|---|
| CABG | 0 | 3 | 0.97 |
| Valvular | 0 | 3 | 0.7 |
| Heart transplantation | 0 | 4 | 8 |
| Total | 0 | 10 | 1.38 |

These are the patients with higher rates of morbidity and mortality owing to hemorrhagic complications and are thus those who would theoretically benefit most from treatments aimed at reducing bleeding.

### Previous ECC Surgery

It was for this patient group that the high-dose regimen of aprotinin was first established.[1] In almost every one of these patients, there is a history of one or more sternotomies and serious adhesions of the cardiac structures, and thus they run a greater risk of increased bleeding.[18] Very serious hemorrhagic accidents may occur in the operating theater,[51] and there is a particular danger of an increase in diffuse bleeding during the postoperative phase, which could lead to serious complications in these patients.[19,22]

In our experience, 14.5% of the entire series of patients required reoperation: 16.4% in the aprotinin group and 12.8% in the control group. Postoperative blood loss during the first 18 hours was $578 \pm 376$ ml for the aprotinin group and $1,104 \pm 856$ ml for the control group, thus exhibiting a 47.6% reduction in postoperative hemorrhage ($p < 0.001$). This efficacy in hemorrhage reduction is comparable to that reported by other authors using high doses,[19,20] though lower than the figures presented by Royston et al. in their first description of high doses in a limited series of 11 patients.

### Active Endocarditis

This group includes a subgroup of patients at high risk of bleeding due to several factors. Firstly, the widespread sepsis affecting these patients produces grave coagulopathy, as well as hepatic damage leading to a deficit in prothrombin and other coagulation factors. Patients often have a history of one or more previous operations for prosthetic endocarditis, which in itself constitutes an important risk factor. These operations are usually laborious and complicated and so involve prolonged periods of CPB (which itself is an important factor in the risk of bleeding). These patients are therefore at high risk of hemorrhage and its secondary morbidity and death.[18,46,52]

In the patient series studied at our center, there were 43 confirmed or highly suspected cases of active endocarditis. Postoperative blood loss at 18 hours was $514 \pm 305$ ml in the aprotinin group and $1,041 \pm 801$ ml in the control group ($p < 0.001$), for a reduction of 50.6% in the group treated with aprotinin. These results are in line with those reported for the Hammersmith dosage.[19,52]

### Preoperative Coagulopathy

This group includes patients having preoperative prothrombin activity measured at $< 50\%$ and/or a platelet count $< 100,000/dl$. The majority of these patients were being maintained on oral dicumarol anticoagulants because either they were fitted with mechanical prostheses or they had a high risk of thromboembolic disease; they underwent emergency operation, leaving no time to standardize coagulation. Others were patients on the waiting list for heart transplantation and had associated bleeding risk factors. Others were patients on prolonged heparin treatment for various reasons, which could cause thrombocytopenia through peripheral capture of platelets, heparin-induced antibody creation, or other means.[53] Deliberately excluded from this group were coronary revascularization patients with uninterrupted treatment with aggregation-inhibitors; these patients were treated as a group apart, owing to the complications involved.

There were 252 patients having these characteristics, 16.8% of the total. Median blood loss at 18 hours postoperatively was 586 ± 305 ml for the aprotinin-treated group and 1,267 ± 801 ml for the control group, giving a reduction of 69.5% in postoperative blood loss ($p < 0.001$).

### Prolonged ECC

Since the introduction of ECC, its effects on hemostasis have been noted, mainly in the reduction of the total number of platelets through their destruction or capture at hepatic and peripheral levels.[26-28] Additionally, the continual aspiration of blood has proved to be a leading factor in the decrease in the number of platelets after ECC, particularly if there is intense suction.[53]

More important than the reduction in the number of platelets is the loss of functionality these platelets suffer, mainly as a result of their activation as they touch the sides of the artificial, endothelium-free surfaces during CPB, as previously described. This platelet dysfunction may or may not be reversible, and in most cases, recovery depends on other factors such as the duration of ECC. Changes to other coagulation factors have also been noted at different moments during ECC.[27] Kirklin et al.[54] described inflammatory reaction of the entire body secondary to CPB. Resulting from this are the above-mentioned changes to the number of platelets and their capacity for adhesion and aggregation, as well as activation of the complement and the kallikrein-bradykinin system—the inflammation mediator in different organs and systems—plus the depletion of several factors of the intrinsic coagulation system and activation of fibrinolysis. Many, if not all, of these events increase linearly with the duration of CPB, and so prolonged ECC times should be considered as a hemorrhage risk factor in the immediate postoperative period. It is worth repeating that prolonged perfusion usually goes hand-in-hand with other associated hemorrhage risk factors, so these patients will have a substantial morbidity and death rate secondary to blood loss.

In the experience of the authors, there were 220 patients with an ECC time > 120 minutes, which we considered to be the limit of prolonged ECC. Postoperative blood loss in the group treated with aprotinin was 471 ± 305 ml, compared to 1,033 ± 798 ml for the control group ($p < 0.001$), giving as 54.4% reduction in bleeding in the aprotinin group.

### Cardiac Transplantation

Patients undergoing cardiac transplantation greatly benefit from the reduction of bleeding achieved using aprotinin. They often have previous cardiac surgery, are on the waiting list for transplantation and receiving oral anticoagulation, and frequently have hepatic congestion through right insufficiency and thus display coagulopathy.

Operations often have a prolonged ECC time, especially in reoperations. Additionally, certain drugs are employed perioperatively, such as the antithymocyte (ATC) globulin, which may cause hypoprothrombinemia and a tendency to bleed. Also, as they are immunodepressed patients, they benefit from receiving fewer transfusions in view of the risk of infectious diseases, especially cytomegalovirus.[18]

In Reina Sofia Hospital, 161 orthotopic cardiac transplantations were performed, of which 25.4% were reoperations with previous ECC, 51.5% were anticoagulated using dicumarol with a prothrombin activity of < 50% at operation, and 31.6% had ECC times > 120 minutes. Postoperative blood loss was 467 ± 349 ml for the aprotinin group and 930 ± 714 ml for the control ($p < 0.001$). There were also fewer complications in the aprotinin-treated group, and 4 patients required reoperation in the control group versus none of the aprotinin group. Reduction in blood loss was 47.9%.

### Aspirin-treated Patients

This specific group of coronary revascularization patients prior to operation had been receiving aspirin as a platelet aggregation inhibitor. Aspirin has the property of reducing the death rate for coronary ischemia by 10% to 15% and the rate of myocardial infarction by 30%,[56,57] so it is advisable to continue aggregation inhibition up until the moment of operation as a prophylaxis against ischemic events. Moreover, studies show that the use of aggregation-inhibiting drugs during the preoperative and perioperative period increases the early permeability of vein bypasses,[57,58] thus decreasing early and late morbidity and death. On the other hand, the inhibition of cyclo-oxygenase produced by aspirin is not immediately reversible, and if the drug is not suspended 7–10 days before operation, it lengthens the bleeding time and produces an appreciable increase in perioperative and postoperative blood loss, as reported by various authors.[59,60]

The use of high doses of aprotinin has proved effective in decreasing blood loss in patients who had not discontinued taking aspirin, either because of emergency operation or because they preferred the benefits of the treatment despite the risks involved (roughly 40% of patients). Marked reductions were seen in complications in hemorrhage and in homologous blood.[61,62]

Tabuchi et al.[63] reported major benefits when using lower doses of aprotinin (2 × 10⁶ KIU as the pump prime dose) in patients treated with aspirin right up to operation; they achieved a reduction in blood loss from 1,096 ± 121 ml down to 672 ± 65 ml in a randomized study of 40 patients. In the present study there were 102 patients whose previous aspirin treatment was either not suspended at all or was not suspended with enough time before operation (19.8% of coronary surgery). Median blood loss at 18 hours postoperation was 451 ± 316 ml for the group treated with our aprotinin protocol as compared to 1,027 ± 806 ml for the control group ($p < 0.001$). Blood loss was reduced by 56%, confirming the efficacy of the treatment in this high-risk subgroup.

### Patients Having Previous Thrombolysis

In this section are included those patients who had received an intravenous thrombolysis regimen for acute myocardial infarction (streptokinase, urokinase, or plasminogen activator) and who, for various reasons, required coronary revascularization within 24 hours of completing treatment, or those patients who in the course of a failed angioplasty or complications in the hemodynamic laboratory received intracoronary thrombolysis using the above agents and who then underwent operation within 24 hours. In this study, there were 34 such patients. The aprotinin-treated group had a median blood loss of 840 ± 639 ml compared to 1,870 ± 1,143 ml for the control group ($p < 0.01$). These results agree with those of other authors using high doses and prove the effectiveness of the drug in a large subgroup of patients with a high risk of hemorrhage occurring during surgical intervention. Blood loss was reduced by 55%. The differences in postoperative blood loss in all high-risk patients are shown in Figure 2.

## Hemorrhage Risk Score

Until now, we have dealt with proving the effectiveness of treatment with the aprotinin regimen which we followed in our series of patients and in various subgroups of these patients who were considered to be at high risk, explaining the reasons for this in each case. Nevertheless, since the start of our experience with aprotinin, we have believed that not all of those patients categorized as high risk had the same degree of risk of postoperative bleeding, because, as we have argued previously, there are patients in whom several of these risk factors may overlap simultaneously and, in such cases, the possibility of hemorrhagic complications

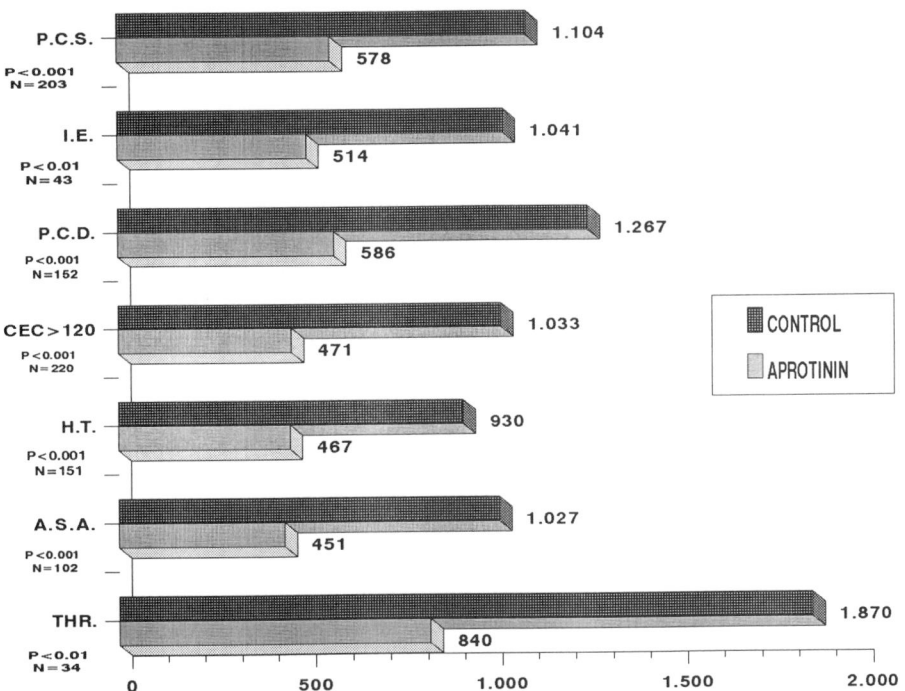

**FIGURE 2.** Postoperative bleeding (expressed in ml at 18 hours postoperatively) in high-risk patients. PCS = previous cardiac surgery (extracorporeal); IE = infective endocarditis (active); PCD = preoperative coagulation disorders; ECC > 120 = extracorporeal circulation time longer than 120 min; HT = heart transplantation. ASA = previous treatment with aspirin not discontinued (CABG patients); THR = surgery in the first 24 hours after thrombolysis (CABG patients).

would obviously increase. In the same way, we have concerns as to whether in this group of patients (whom we could consider to have a risk of bleeding which rises with the number of risk factors involved), treatment using our aprotinin regimen would be as effective as that observed in patients with isolated risk factors, or if the benefit obtained perhaps might decrease or increase. This point seemed particularly worthy of investigation, because proportionately more and more patients undergoing operation are falling into this category. Thus every patient in our series was assigned one point for each of the blood-loss risk factors mentioned (previous ECC, previous coagulopathy, ECC time > 120 min, active endocarditis, and cardiac transplantation). Patients were then grouped by their score of 0–5 for hemorrhagic risk, postoperative blood loss was studied for each group, and comparison was made between patients receiving aprotinin and controls. The group of coronary patients receiving continued preoperative aspirin treatment was included in the preoperative coagulopathy group.

There were 600 patients with a zero score for blood loss, 42% of the total series; these patients could be categorized as having a low risk of hemorrhagic complications, and perhaps the use of special methods to avoid bleeding might be argued against when reduced prevalence of hemorrhage and economic questions are taken into account. Postoperative blood loss was $441 \pm 348$ ml for the aprotinin-treated group and $705 \pm 519$ ml for the controls ($p < 0.001$). Reduction due to aprotinin was 37.4%, notably less than in other patients, but still appreciable. However, as discussed later, this type of patient is not exempt from hemorrhagic complications.

A score of 1 was recorded in 492 patients (34.5% of the total). Postoperative blood loss was $475 \pm 246$ ml for the aprotinin group and $1,105 \pm 769$ ml for the control ($p < 0.001$), so reduction in blood loss was 57%, clearly much greater than in the low-risk patients. There were 226 patients with 2 associated risk factors, representing 15.8% of the total. Postoperative blood loss $530 \pm 368$ ml for the aprotinin group and $1,270 \pm 904$ ml for the control ($p < 0.001$), and thus a reduction of 58.2%. In 104 patients with a score of 3, 7.29% of the total, there was postoperative blood loss of $634 \pm 369$ ml for the aprotinin group and $1,530 \pm 987$ ml for the control ($p < 1.001$), a reduction of 59.6%. Finally, 16 patients scored 4— there was no score of 5. Here, median blood loss was $655 \pm 443$ ml for the aprotinin group and $2,288 \pm 768$ ml for the controls, a reduction of 71.3% ($p < 0.01$). These results are shown in Table 3 and in Figure 3.

It is clear that postoperative bleeding increases linearly with risk score, becoming strikingly excessive in high-score groups not receiving aprotinin (Fig. 4), with significant differences between them. However, when aprotinin was used

**TABLE 3.**   Postoperative Bleeding in Relation to the Risk Score

| Score | Patients | Aprotinin Group (ml blood loss) | Control Group (ml blood loss) | p-Value | Bleeding Reduction |
|---|---|---|---|---|---|
| Average | 1425 | $470 \pm 336$ | $873 \pm 741$ | $< 0.001$ | 46.1% |
| 0 | 600 | $441 \pm 348$ | $705 \pm 519$ | $< 0.001$ | 37.4% |
| 1 | 492 | $475 \pm 246$ | $1105 \pm 769$ | $< 0.001$ | 57.0% |
| 2 | 226 | $530 \pm 368$ | $1270 \pm 904$ | $< 0.01$ | 58.2% |
| 3 | 104 | $634 \pm 369$ | $1530 \pm 987$ | $< 0.001$ | 59.6% |
| 4 | 16 | $655 \pm 443$ | $2288 \pm 768$ | $< 0.01$ | 71.3% |

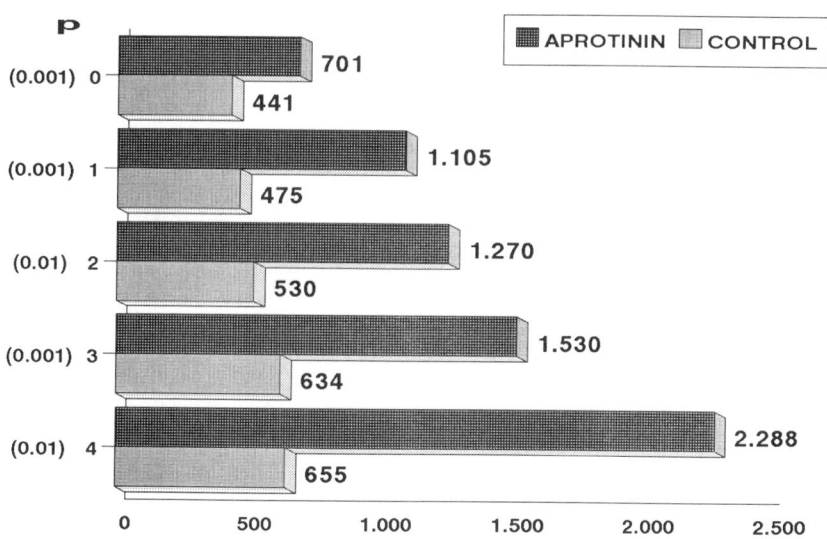

**FIGURE 3.** Postoperative bleeding (expressed in ml at 18 hours postoperatively) in relation to the hemorrhage risk score.

(Fig. 5), these differences, although still present, were much more discrete. A pattern is revealed in which aprotinin treatment, although useful in all patient groups and at all degrees of blood loss risk, is particularly useful in patients with a high risk of hemorrhage and is more beneficial the greater the degree of risk of postoperative bleeding.

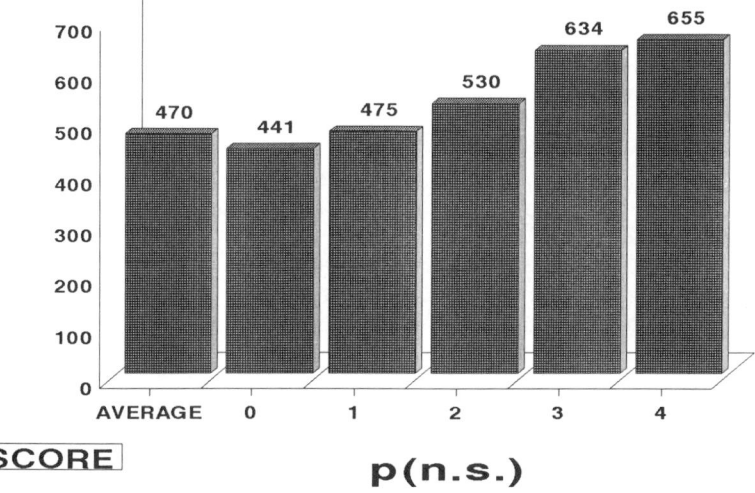

**FIGURE 4.** Postoperative bleeding in relation to the hemorrhage risk score in patients treated with low-dose aprotinin.

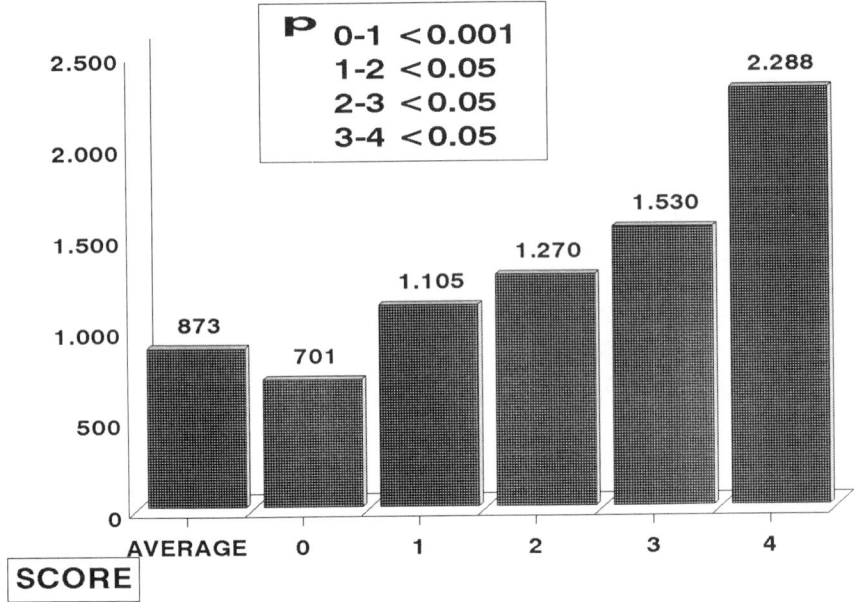

**FIGURE 5.** Postoperative bleeding in relation to the hemorrhage risk score in control group patients.

## Hemorrhagic Events

Until now, we have concentrated on showing the effectiveness of low-dose aprotinin treatment in terms of significant decreases in postoperative bleeding in the entire patient population and in subgroups of patients. With an aim to further illustrate the value of the treatment and the regimen used by our group and other researchers, we use the term "hemorrhagic event" to represent the appearance of any of the following hemorrhagic complications, which we judged to have a high rate of morbidity and death:

- Excessive bleeding in the operating theater which greatly holds up closure, due to the need for hemostatic exploration.
- Reoperation due to excessive bleeding from the intensive care unit in the first 24 hours postoperation.
- Postoperative bleeding of $> 1,500$ ml in the first 18 hours.
- Need for the transfusion of $> 5$ U of homologous whole blood or red cell concentrate.

Obviously, a patient would commonly suffer several associated hemorrhagic events, as these associate readily. All patients in the series who had at least one of these events were investigated to establish a criterion for the effectiveness of our aprotinin regimen.

The entire group of patients receiving aprotinin had a total of 18 hemorrhagic events compared to 80 in the control ($p < 0.001$), a decrease of 77.5% attributable to the use of aprotinin. Grouped by pathology, the differences were just as substantial and significant (Table 4). There were 0.02 events/patient in the aprotinin group compared to 0.1 in the control.

Interestingly, as the hemorrhagic risk score rose, there were proportionately more hemorrhagic events. Hence, in patients with a zero score, there were 8 and

**TABLE 4.** Hemorrhagic Events

| | Aprotinin Group | Control Group | Events/Patient (Aprotinin/Control) | Reduction* | p-Value |
|---|---|---|---|---|---|
| Total group | 18 | 80 | 0.02/0.1 | 77.5 | < 0.001 |
| CABG | 7 | 28 | 0.03/0.09 | 75 | < 0.05 |
| Valvular | 9 | 42 | 0.02/0.1 | 78.5 | < 0.05 |
| Heart transplantation | 2 | 10 | 0.01/0.2 | 80 | < 0.05 |
| Score 0 | 8 | 16 | 0.003/0.006 | 50 | <0.001 |
| Score 1 | 2 | 22 | 0.008/0.08 | 90.9 | < 0.001 |
| Score 2 | 6 | 19 | 0.04/0.23 | 68.4 | < 0.001 |
| Score 3 | 1 | 15 | 0.01/0.3 | 93.3 | < 0.001 |
| Score 4 | 1 | 8 | 0.1/0.88 | 87.5 | ns |

*RED = reduction in hemorrhagic event by aprotinin.

16 hemorrhagic events in aprotinin and control patients, respectively, with 0.003 and 0.006 events/patient, a decrease of 50%. For a score of 1, there were 2 and 22 events, respectively ($p < 0.001$), with 0.008 and 0.08 events/patient, a decrease of 90.9%. In patients scoring 2, there were 6 and 19 hemorrhagic events ($p < 0.001$), with 0.04 and 2.23 events/patient, a decrease of 68.4%. Patients scoring 3 had 1 and 15 hemorrhagic events, respectively ($p < 0.0019$), with 0.01 and 0.3 events/patient, a reduction of 93.3% in the aprotinin-treated group. Finally, in the few patients scoring 4, there were 1 and 8 hemorrhagic events, respectively, a decrease of 87.5% in hemorrhagic events (Table 5).

It can be clearly seen that treatment with low-dose aprotinin is effective in all patients, and its benefits increase proportionally as the patient accumulates associated hemorrhagic risk factors. It should be noted that the patients with the highest scores have an extremely high rate of morbidity and death attributable to hemorrhage, and so the benefits of using aprotinin treatment, as seen from the present figures for the above-described regimen, may play an important role in avoiding serious complications.

## Aprotinin and Platelet Count

As has been discussed elsewhere in this review, most researchers now agree that the action of aprotinin does not affect the total number of platelets to any greater extent than occurs in the actual CPB[24–26,29–35,43,44,53,54,66]; its action lies in the

**TABLE 5.** Complications

| | Aprotinin Group | Control Group | p-Value |
|---|---|---|---|
| Perioperative myocardial infarction | 19(9.6%) | 27(8.8%) | ns |
| Stroke | 20(2.1%) | 18(3.1%) | ns |
| Stroke with permanent sequelae | 4(0.45%) | 5(0.78%) | ns |
| Renal failure | 47(7.3%) | 51(5.7%) | ns |
| Dialysis | 10(1.5%) | 8(1.04%) | ns |
| Allergic reactions | 0 | 0 | ns |

preservation of platelet adhesiveness and their capacity for aggregation, achieved by preventing their activation at the start of ECC. Nevertheless, we studied the reduction in platelet numbers post-ECC. There was a loss of 40.7% in aprotinin-treated patients compared with 40.5% in the controls. These results are practically identical and serve to confirm current opinion. Other parameters studied such as activated partial thromboplastin time, prothrombin activity, fibrinogen, and Quick's test revealed no significant differences between aprotinin-treated and untreated patients.

## Thrombotic Phenomena

Because aprotinin treatment at the various dosages described produces a marked reduction in both postoperative bleeding and all kinds of hemorrhagic events, and because its detailed mechanism of action remains largely unknown, it is worth considering—from a purely theoretical viewpoint—that the drug might produce a state of hypercoagulability and thus give rise to thrombotic phenomena, especially in high-risk patients. Some authors[67,68] have described increased thrombus formation in the central catheters during extracorporeal surgery performed on aprotinin-treated patients, which may support this theory.

### Myocardial Infarction

Recently, in a randomized study of 169 patients undergoing reoperation for coronary surgery at Cleveland Clinic, Cosgrove et al.[20] reported an increased incidence of perioperative infarction (as measured by electrocardiographic criteria) and an alarming incidence (50%) of thrombosis in venous grafts in patients treated with various aprotinin regimens. These results have not, however, been confirmed by other workers who have studied this topic. Jegarden et al.,[69] in a series of 52 patients undergoing operation for arterial coronary revascularization, reported 99% permeability and an extremely low rate of perioperative acute myocardial infarction. Bidstrup et al.,[70] using magnetic resonance imaging, studied permeability in 269 venous bypasses and concluded that there were no differences in permeability between aprotinin-treated and untreated patients. Numerous studies have reported similar findings.[71,72] As Cosgrove et al. commented in the discussion of their results, and as we have also remarked elsewhere, the root of the problem may lie in the maintenance of ACT at 400 s in the Cleveland Clinic study; thus, the lengthening of this parameter by aprotinin was not taken into account, and the patients may have received insufficient anticoagulation.

Moreover, the group in question was undoubtedly at high risk of perioperative infarction. The same methodology is used at Reina Sofia Hospital, where the ECG of patients is serially studied and the criterion for acute myocardial infarction is set by the appearance of a new Q wave in an ECG taken at 48 hours. We had an acute myocardial infarction index of 9.6% for the aprotinin group and 8.8% for the control ($p$ = not significant). Subsequently, 100 consecutive patients received myocardial revascularization while treated with our aprotinin protocol; within 72 hours postoperation, all of these patients were submitted to a technetium pyrophosphate radioisotope study to detect perioperative acute myocardial infarction. The detected incidence was 5.5%.

The above results lead us to conclude that aprotinin, at the dosage employed in our studies, does not create any special risk of acute myocardial infarction in the perioperative period, and this despite the fact that our center has a patient profile which indicates that coronary revascularization entails a considerable risk of ischemic events.

### Strokes

Another acknowledged complication of extracorporeal surgery is the occurrence of cerebrovascular accidents,[73,74] particularly in patients having widespread arteriopathy, as often presented by coronary cases and in elderly patients. This incidence could theoretically increase due to the use of aprotinin, although authors studying this point[75,76] have found no significant differences when using aprotinin.

In the present study, we examined all patients developing any kind of neurologic signs during the immediate postoperative period. Each patient was subjected to computed tomography (CT) as soon as their condition permitted. Patients with cerebral hemorrhage or those having a pathology that would explain their clinical state were excluded. Only those who had clearly suffered ischemic accidents were included. A total of 38 patients (2.6%) presented with ischemic cerebrovascular accidents taking place during the perioperative period and visualized by CT. Of these, 29 progressed favorably, and on discharge, their neurologic disorders had cleared up, either spontaneously or after short periods of rehabilitation (76.3% of the cerebrovascular accidents). The remaining 9 patients still suffered chronic sequelae on discharge or died as a result of the ischemic accident.

There was no difference in the incidence of strokes (self-limited cerebrovascular accident) or of serious strokes (chronic sequelae or death) in aprotinin-treated and untreated patients; there was a 2.1% total incidence of ischemic cerebrovascular accident, 1.6% recovery from cerebrovascular accident on discharge, and 0.45% chronic sequelae for the aprotinin group, as against 3.1%, 2.3%, and 0.78%, respectively, for the control group ($p$ = not significant).

## Renal Insufficiency

Some authors have suggested the possibility of a nephrotoxic effect of high-dose aprotinin or have described it under fixed circumstances,[20,77-81] whereas others have discovered no important effects on renal function.[19,43,66] In the present study, patients were categorized as having renal dysfunction when they displayed normal creatine levels before operation and had levels > 1.5 mg/dl immediately after operation, or if they showed an increase of 0.5 mg/dl compared to preoperative levels. A patient was categorized as having grave renal insufficiency when a technique such as hemodialysis, peritoneal dialysis, or hemofiltration was deemed necessary.

A total of 98 patients had some kind of renal insufficiency (6.5%), and 18 of these were classed as grave (1.2%). No significant differences were found between aprotinin-treated patients and the control group (7.3% renal insufficiency and 1.5% grave renal insufficiency in the aprotinin group versus 5.7% and 1.04%, respectively, in the controls; $p$ = not significant).

## Allergic Reactions

Despite the heterologous (bovine) origin of the protein and the ensuing possibility of various types and degrees of allergic reaction, the actual incidence of such reactions was extremely low, < 1%. Some authors have described anaphylactic reactions[82-87] for which previous exposure to the drug would theoretically have been necessary. For this reason Royston et al.[18] advise that administration of the first dose be gradual, testing with 1 ml of aprotinin.

In the present study, no significant allergic reactions were observed. There was no incidence of hemodynamic deterioration when aprotinin was introduced into the circulatory flow, nor was there evidence of bronchial spasm, serious cutaneous rash, or other, despite the absence of prior tests with the drug. We do, nevertheless, view such testing as advisable.

In our series of patients there were, moreover, 20 patients who had to undergo short-term reoperation due to various causes. They had been treated with aprotinin in the foregoing operation and were thus re-exposed to the drug, thereby incurring a high risk of anaphylaxis. No major allergic reactions were observed in these patients.

## Conclusions

Based on the above results, the firm opinion of the authors is that a regimen of $2 \times 10^6$ KIU of aprotinin is highly effective in the prevention of hemorrhagic complications in patients undergoing operation involving ECC. The effectiveness of this dose is comparable to that of higher doses and may thus minimize undesirable effects and reduce costs.

If this aprotinin regimen is used, the authors believe it crucial to administer the drug as the pump prime dose, so that its effect will be immediate when blood first makes contact with the surfaces of the ECC line; otherwise, the efficacy of the drug may decrease or even disappear altogether. Therein may lie the explanation for the similarity in effectiveness between low and high doses of aprotinin, since both regimens have the same pump prime dosage, and that may be the most efficacious part of the Hammersmith dose in the prevention of bleeding. The empirical nature of the dose and the mystery which still surrounds the pharmakinetics of the drug and its detailed mechanism of action mean that this will remain as a reasonable doubt, for future research to resolve.

As this chapter has shown, this treatment regimen is effective for all kinds of patients, even for those categorized as low risk, who as we have seen are not totally exempt from hemorrhagic events. The relatively low cost of this dosage, its proven efficacy, and the almost complete absence of undesirable side effects mean that it may be used in large series of patients, which will probably result in any remaining doubts being clarified.

Particular emphasis is placed on the usefulness of the drug with the stated protocol when administered to patients categorized as at high risk of bleeding. We firmly believe that enormous benefits may be obtained. The results indicate that this treatment should be much more extensive than it is at present.

A large number of patients had multiple factors indicating risk of bleeding, with the ensuing high risk of secondary complications. We consider that the usefulness of low-dose aprotinin has been clearly demonstrated, and its relative usefulness is likely to increase when there is a higher risk of hemorrhagic complications.

The possibility of hemorrhagic events in patients with a high risk score must be regarded as unacceptable; these events probably constitute one of the main causes of morbidity and death, so any means at our disposal should be employed to minimize this possibility. Aprotinin could undoubtedly play an important role in such cases.

The rate of complications at our center attributable to aprotinin has been practically nil, similar to that of most authors. There is no basis at this moment for claims that aprotinin, especially at low dosage, may produce hypercoagulability, thrombosis, renal insufficiency, or clinically significant allergic reactions, although the reactions referred to in the literature do bear further investigation.

This chapter has attempted to provide an overview of the usefulness of low-dose aprotinin in cardiac surgery. Hopefully, the inclusion of an exhaustive study of a large series of patients further contributes to the review. Likewise, to evaluate the efficacy of the drug, wider criteria than those previously employed have been used, i.e., theoretical discussion of the effectiveness of low dosage, systemized study of all subgroups of patients considered to be at high risk, and selective investigation of all patient groups in whom the possibility of hemorrhagic complications increased with the association of different risk factors.

## Perspectives

Future research should throw more light on the lesser-known aspects of aprotinin and its safety in use. It would appear, however, that there is no question of the drug's safety; moreover, the undeniable beneficial effects far outweigh any risks involved. The optimum regimen for aprotinin dosage and the method of administration most suited to the minimum efficacy dose must be determined.

This year at our center, we are beginning a randomized study using three different aprotinin regimens in the pump prime dose. All three may be described as low-dose regimens and will furthermore be determined according to the weight and body surface area of the patient. The results of this study will add to our knowledge of this drug when administered at low dosage.

A more detailed knowledge of the effects and mechanism of action of aprotinin, along with its ideal regimen for administration, will certainly be paramount to minimizing the serious consequences of the hemorrhagic complications that have arisen since the very beginnming of cardiac surgery.

## References

1. Royston D, Bidstrup BP, Taylor KM, Sapsford RN: Effect of aprotinin on the need for blood transfusion after repeat open heart surgery. Lancet 2:1289–1291, 1987.
2. Royston D, Minty BD, Wallwork J, et al: The effect of surgery with cardiopulmonary bypass on alveolar-capillary barrier function in man. Ann Thorac Surg 40:133–142, 1985.
3. Royston D, Braude S, Nolop DB, Hughes JMB: 113m-Indium protein flux does not reflect degree or outcome in respiratory failure. Am Rev Respir Dis 139:A380, 1989.
4. Royston D, Fleming JS, Desai JB, et al: Increased peroxide product generation associated with open heart surgery: Evidence for free radical generation. J Thorac Cardiovasc Surg 91:759–766, 1986.
5. Blauth C, Arnold J, Schulemberg W, et al: Cerebral microembolism during cardiopulmonary bypass: Retinal microvascular studies in vivo with fluorescein angiography. J Thorac Cardiovasc Surg 95:668–676, 1988.
6. Royston D: Blood cell activation in cardiopulmonary bypass. Semin Thorac Cardiovsc Surg 2:341–357, 1990.
7. Kirklin JK, Westaby S, Blackstone EH, et al: Complement and the damaging effects of cardiopulmonary bypass. J Thorac Cardiovasc Surg 86:845–852, 1983.

8. Fritz R, Wunderer G, Jochum M: Biochemie und anwendung des kallicreininhibitors aprotinin. Drug Res 33:479–494, 1983.

9. Royston D: The serine antiprotease aprotinin (Trasylol): A novel approach to reducing postoperative bleeding. Blood Coag Fibrinol 1:55–69, 1990.

10. Harder MP, Eijsman L, Roozendaal KJ, et al: Aprotinin reduces intraoperative and postoperative blood loss in membrane oxygenator cardiopulmonary bypass. Ann Thorac Surg 51:936–941, 1991.

11. Alajmo F, Calamai G, Perna A, et al: High dose aprotinin: Hemostatic effect in open heart operations. Ann Thorac Surg 48:536–539, 1989.

12. Dietrich W, Barankay A, Dilthey G, et al: Reduction of homologous blood requirement in cardiac surgery by intraoperative aprotinin application: Clinical experience in 152 cardiac surgical patients. Thorac Cardiovasc Surg 37:92–98, 1989.

13. Fraedrich G, Weber C, Bernard C, et al: Reduction of blood transfusion requirement in open heart surgery by administration of high doses of aprotinin: Preliminary results. Thorac Cardiovasc Surg 37:89–91, 1989.

14. Dietrich W, Spannagl M, Jochum M, et al: Influence of high dose aprotinin treatment on blood loss and coagulation patterns in patients undergoing myocardial revascularization. Anesthesiology 73:1119–1126, 1990.

15. Havel M, Teufelsbauer H, Knobl P, et al: Effect of intraoperative aprotinin administration on postoperative bleeding in patients undergoing cardiopulmonary bypass operation. J Thorac Cardiovasc Surg 101:968–972, 1991.

16. Bidstrup BP, Royston D, Sapsford RN, Taylor KM: Reduction in blood loss use after cardiopulmonary bypass with high dose aprotinin (Trasylol). J Thorac Cardiovasc Surg 97:364–372, 1989.

17. Royston D: Aprotinin in open heart surgery. Perfusion 5(Suppl):63–72, 1990.

18. Royston D: High dose aprotinin therapy: A review of the first five years experience. J Cardiothorac Vasc Anesth 6:76–100, 1992.

19. Bidstrup B, Harrison J, Royston D, et al: Aprotinin therapy in cardiac operations: A report on use in 41 cardiac centers in the United Kingdom. Ann Thorac Surg 55:971–976, 1993.

20. Cosgrove DM, Heric B, Lytle DW, et al: Aprotinin therapy for reoperative myocardial revascularization: A placebo controlled study. Ann Thorac Surg 54:1031–1038, 1992.

21. Bove JR: Transfusion associated hepatitis and AIDS: What is the risk? N Engl J Med 317:242–245, 1987.

22. Little BW, Loop FD, Cosgrove DM, et al: Fifteen hundred coronary reoperations: Results and determinant of early and late survival. J Thorac Cardiovasc Surg 93:847–859, 1987.

23. Taylor KM: Perioperative approaches to coagulation defects. Ann Thorac Surg 56:S78–S82, 1993.

24. Emerson TE: Pharmacology of aprotinin and efficacy during cardiopulmonary bypass. Cardiovasc Drug Rev 7:127–140, 1989.

25. Westaby S: Aprotinin in perspective. Ann Thorac Surg 55:1033–1041, 1993.

26. Mohr R, Golan M, Martinowitz U, et al: Effect of cardiac operation on platelet. J Thorac Cardiovasc Surg 92:434–441, 1986.

27. Mammen EF, Koet MH, Washington BC, et al: Hemostatic changes during cardiopulmonary bypass surgery. Semin Thromb Hemost 11:281–292, 1985.

28. Bick RL: Hemostasis defect associated with cardiac surgery, prosthetic devices, and other extracorporeal circuits. Semin Thromb Hemost 11:249–280, 1987.

29. Van Oeveren W, Harder MP, Roozendaal KS, et al: Aprotinin protects platelets against the initial effect of cardiopulmonary bypass. J Thorac Cardiovasc Surg 99:788–797, 1990.

30. Wachtfogel Y, Kucich U, Hach E, et al: Aprotinin inhibits the contact, neutrophil, and platelet activation systems during simulated extracorporeal perfusion. J Thorac Cardiovasc Surg 106:1–10, 1993.

31. Joachim B, Knothe C, Bernbried Z, et al: Platelet function in cardiac surgery: Influence of temperature and aprotinin. Ann Thorac Surg 55:652–658, 1993.

32. John L, Rees G, Kovacs I: Reduction of heparin binding to an inhibition of platelet by aprotinin. Ann Thorac Surg 55:1175–1179, 1993.

33. Huang H, Ding W, Su Z, Zhang W: Mechanism of the preserving effect of aprotinin on platelet function and its use in cardiac surgery. J Thorac Cardiovasc Surg 106:11–18, 1993.

34. Van Oeveren W, Eijsman L, Roozendaal KJ, et al: Platelet preservation by aprotinin during cardiopulmonary bypass. Lancet 2:644, 1988.

35. Gardaz JP, Hauert J, Chassot PG, et al: Modification of hemostatic parameters during cardiopulmonary bypass: Effects of high dose aprotinin. Anesthesiology 74(A):991, 1991.

36. Taylor KM: Effect of aprotinin on blood loss and blood use after cardiopulmonary bypass. In Pifarré R (ed): Anticoagulation, Hemostasis, and Blood Preservation in Cardiovascular Surgery. Philadelphia, Hanley & Belfus, 1993.
37. Kawasuji M, Ueyama K, Sakakibara N, et al: Effect of low dose aprotinin on coagulation and fibrinolysis in cardiopulmonary bypass. Ann Thorac Surg 55:1205–1209, 1993.
38. Covino E, Iorio D, Marino L, et al: Low dose aprotinin as blood saver in open heart surgery. Eur J Cardiothorac Surg 5:414–418, 1991.
39. Carrel T, Bauer E, Laske A, et al: Low dose aprotinin also allows reduction of blood loss after cardiopulmonary bypass. Lancet 337:673, 1991.
40. Schonberger J, Everts P, Erean H, et al: Low dose aprotinin in internal mammary artery bypass operation contributes to important blood saving. Ann Thorac Surg 54:1172–1176, 1992.
41. Concha M, Montero A, Arizon JM, et al: Trasplante cardíaco ortotópico: Estudio de la morbimortalidad precoz: Experiencia del Hospital Reina Sofia (Córdoba). Rev Esp Cardiol 46:93–100, 1993.
42. Concha M, Anguita M: Trasplante Cardíaco: Experiencia Hospital Universitario Reina Sofia. Córdoba (1986–1991). Córdoba, Servicio de Publicaciones Universidad de Córdoba, 1992, p 28.
43. Van Oeveren W, Jansen NJ, Bidstrup BP, et al: Effects of aprotinin on haemostatic mechanism during cardiopulmonary bypass. Ann Thorac Surg 44:640–645, 1987.
44. Lavee J, Savion N, Smolinsky A, et al: Platelet protection by aprotinin in cardiopulmonary bypass: Electron microscopic study. Ann Thorac Surg 53:477–481, 1992.
45. Royston D, Bidstrup BP, Sapsford RN, Taylor KM: Reduced blood loss after open heart surgery with aprotinin is associated with an increase in the activated clotting time (ACT). J Cardiothorac Anesth 3:80, 1989.
46. Najman D, Walenga J, Fareed J, Pifarre R: Effects of aprotinin on anticoagulant monitoring: Implications in cardiovascular surgery. Ann Thorac Surg 55:662–666, 1993.
47. Van Oeveren W, Van Oeveren D, Wildevuur CHR: Anticoagulation policy during use of aprotinin in cardiopulmonary bypass. J Thorac Cardiovasc Surg 104:210–211, 1992.
48. Guidelines for monitoring heparin by the activated clotting time when aprotinin is used during cardiopulmonary bypass. J Thorac Cardiovasc Surg 104:211–212, 1992.
49. Desmet AAEA, Joen MCN, Van Oeveren W, et al: Increased anticoagulation during cardiopulmonary bypass by aprotinin. J Thorac Cardiovasc Surg 100:520–527, 1990.
50. Von Segesser LK, Weiss BM, Pasic M, et al: Experimental evaluation of heparin coated cardiopulmonary bypass equipment with low systemic heparinization and high dose aprotinin. Thorac Cardiovasc Surg 39:251–256, 1991.
51. Dobell ARC, Jain AK: Catastrophic hemorrhage during redo sternotomy. Ann Thorac Surg 37:273–278, 1984.
52. Bidstrup BP, Royston D, Taylor KM, Sapsford RN: Effect of aprotinin on need for blood transfusion in patients with septic endocarditis having open heart surgery. Lancet i:366–367, 1988.
53. Blakeman BP, Sullivan HJ: Surgical considerations for postoperative bleeding. In Pifarré R (ed): Anticoagulation, Hemostasis, and Blood Preservation in Cardiovascular Surgery. Philadelphia, Hanley & Belfus, 1993, pp 271–285.
54. Kirklin JK, Westaby S, Blackstone EH, et al: Complement and the damaging effects of cardiopulmonary bypass. J Thorac Cardiovasc Surg 86:845–852, 1993.
55. Elwood PC: Aspirin in the prevention of myocardial infarction: Current status. Drug 28:1, 1984.
56. Friedewal WT, Furberg CD, May GS: Aspirin and myocardial infarction. Cardiovasc Rev Rep 5:1285, 1984.
57. Chesbro JH, Clements IP, Fuster V, et al: A platelet inhibitory drug trial in coronary artery bypass operations: Benefits of perioperative dipyridamole and aspirin therapy on early postoperative vein graft patency. N Engl J Med 307:73–78, 1982.
58. Goldman S, Copeland J, Moritz T, et al: Improvement in early saphenous vein graft patency after coronary artery bypass surgery with antiplatelet therapy: Result of a Veterans Administration Cooperative Study. Circulation 77:1324–1332, 1988.
59. Michelson E, Morganroth J, Torosian M, MacVaugh H III: Relation of preoperative use of aspirin to increased mediastinal blood loss after coronary artery bypass surgery. J Thorac Cardiovasc Surg 76:694–697, 1978.
60. Ferraris VA, Ferraris SP, Lough FC, Berry WR: Preoperative aspirin ingestion increased operative blood loss after coronary artery bypass grafting. Ann Thorac Surg 45:71–74, 1988.
61. Bidstrup BP, Royston D, McGuinnes C, Sapsford RN: Aprotinin in aspirin pretreated patients. Perfusion 5(Suppl):77–91, 1990.

62. Royston D, Bidstrup BP, Taylor KM, et al: Aprotinin reduces bleeding after open heart surgery in patients taking aspirin and those with renal failure. Anesthesiology 71:A6, 1989.
63. Tabuchi N, Van Oeveren W, Eijsman L, et al: Preserved hemostasis during the combined use of aprotinin and aspirin in CABG operations. In Freidel N, Hetzer R, Royston D (eds): Blood Use in Cardiac Surgery. New York, Springer-Verlag, 1991, pp 245–251.
64. Efstratiadis T, Munsch C, Crossman D, Taylor KM: Aprotinin therapy after thrombolytic treatment. Ann Thorac Surg 52:1320–1321, 1991.
65. Alajmo F, Calamai G: High dose aprotinin in emergency coronary artery bypass following thrombolysis. Ann Thorac Surg 54:1022–1023, 1992.
66. Blauhut B, Gross C, Necek S, et al: Effect of high dose aprotinin on blood loss, platelet function, fibrinolysis complement and renal function after cardiopulmonary bypass. J Thorac Cardiovasc Surg 101:958–967, 1991.
67. Bohrer H, Fleischer F, Lang J, Vahl C: Early formation of thrombi on pulmonary artery catheters in cardiac surgical patients receiving high dose aprotinin. J Cardiothorac Anesth 4:222–225, 1990.
68. Youngberg JA: Aprotinin and thrombus formation on pulmonary artery catheters: A piece of a coagulation puzzle. J Cardiothorac Anesth 4:155–158, 1990.
69. Jegaden O, Vedrine C, Rossi R: Aprotinin does not compromise arterial graft patency in coronary bypass operations. J Thorac Cardiovasc Surg 106:180–181, 1993.
70. Bidstrup BP, Royston D, Taylor KM, Sapsford RN: Effect of aprotinin in aorta-coronary bypass graft patency. J Thorac Cardiovasc Surg 105:147–153, 1993.
71. Lemmer JH, Stanford W, Bonney SL, et al: Aprotinin for coronary bypass operations: Efficacy, safety, and influence on early saphenous vein graft patency: A multicenter, randomized, double-blind, placebo-controlled study. J Thorac Cardiovasc Surg 107:543–553, 1994.
72. Jegaden O, Vedrinne C, Rossi R: Aprotinin does not compromise arterial graft patency in coronary bypass operations. J Thorac Cardiovasc Surg 106:180–181, 1993.
73. Lynn GM, Stefanko K, Reed JF III, et al: Risk factors for stroke after coronary artery bypass. J Thorac Cardiovasc Surg 104:1518–1523, 1992.
74. Frye RL, Kronmal R, Schaff HV, et al: Stroke in coronary artery bypass graft surgery: An analysis of the CASS experience. Int J Cardiol 26:331–332, 1992.
75. Royston D: Controversies in the practical use of aprotinin. In Pifarré R (ed): Anticoagulation, Hemostasis, and Blood Preservation in Cardiovascular Surgery. Philadelphia, Hanley & Belfus, 1993.
76. Schomberger JP, Bredee J, Speekenbrink RG, et al: Autotransfusion of shed blood contributes additionally to blood saving in patients receiving aprotinin (2 million KIU). Eur J Cardiothorac Surg 7:474–477, 1993.
77. Schomberger JPAM, Everts PAM, Ercan H, et al: Low dose aprotinin in internal mammary artery bypass operations contributes to important blood saving. Ann Thorac Surg 54:1172–1176, 1992.
78. Schomberger JPAM, Zundertaajmvan, Bredee JJ, et al: Blood loss and use of blood in internal mammary artery and vein bypass grafting with and without adding a single, low dose of aprotinin (2 million units) to the pump prime. Acta Anaesthesiol Belg 43:187–196, 1992.
79. Sundt TM, Kouchoukos NT, Saffitz JE, et al: Renal dysfunction and intravascular coagulation after use of aprotinin in thoracic aortic operations employing hypothermic cardiopulmonary bypass and circulatory arrest. Ann Thorac Surg 55:1418–1424, 1993.
80. Fischer JH, Knupfer P: High dose aprotinin (Trasylol) therapy: Harmless to the kidney? Langenbecks Arch Chir 360:241–249, 1983.
81. Horl WH: Effect of aprotinin on renal function. In Dudziak R, Reuster HD, Kirchhoff PG, Schumann F, (eds): Proteolysis and Proteinase Inhibition in Cardiac and Vascular Surgery. Stuttgart, Schattauer Verlag, 1985, pp 127–135.
82. Fischer JH: Effects of Trasylol on the kidneys: Dependence on temperature and dose. In Dudziak R, Reuter HD, Kirchhoff PG, Schumann F (eds): Proteolysis and Proteinase Inhibition in Cardiac and Vascular Surgery. Stuttgart, Schattauer Verlag, 1985.
83. Bohrer H, Bach A, Fleischer F, Lang J: Adverse aerodynamic effects of high dose aprotinin in a paediatric cardiac surgical patient. Anaesthesia 45:853–854, 1990.
84. Proud G, Chamberlain J: Anaphylactic reaction to aprotinin. Lancet 2:48–49, 1976.
85. Levy AH: Unusual Reaction to Trasylol [letter]. Can Med Assoc J 111:1304, 1984.
86. McMahon MJ, Axon ATR: Anaphylactic reaction to aprotinin [letter]. BMJ 289:1696, 1984.
87. Paolo V, Piero C, Carmine S: Aprotinin in cardiac surgery. J Thorac Cardiovasc Surg 106:181, 1993.

**David Green, MD, PhD**
**Berit Edsberg, MD**

# 20

# Recombinant Aprotinin

In December 1993, the U.S. Food and Drug Administration approved Bayer/ Miles' bovine aprotinin (b-aprotinin), (Trasylol) for use in cardiovascular surgery, based on clinical trials which showed that the drug significantly limited blood loss and the need for blood replacement.[6,20,22] However, myocardial infarction, acute vein graft thrombosis, disseminated intravascular coagulation, renal dysfunction, and severe allergic reactions have been reported in patients receiving this agent.[13,21]

To avoid bovine tissue as the source of production, Novo Nordisk A/S has developed processes to produce recombinant aprotinin (r-aprotinin) by fermentation using *Saccharomyces cerevisiae* as the production organism. This chapter provides a description of this new recombinant substance and reviews preclinical and clinical studies in animals and humans.

## Description of r-Aprotinin

r-Aprotinin is a polypeptide composed of 58 amino acid residues and has a molecular weight of 6,512. The 58 amino acid residues are arranged in a single polypeptide chain which is cross-linked by three disulfide bridges and folded to form a pear-shaped molecule. The pilot purification process consists of five chromatographic steps and provides consistent yields of r-aprotinin with high-pressure liquid chromatographic (HPLC) purity higher than 95%,[26] free of non-aprotinin-related impurities and endotoxins.

r-Aprotinin has been characterized and compared to b-aprotinin Midran (Novo Nordisk A/S) by a number of methods, including amino acid compositions, amino acid sequence determination, carbohydrate analysis, and determination of structure by x-ray crystallography. From the test results, it has been concluded that r-aprotinin and b-aprotinin are structurally identical. However, bovine aprotinin contains small amounts of truncated aprotinin (1–57,1–56).[26]

The drug is supplied as an infusion in vials of 50 ml of colorless solution. The preparation contains no foreign proteins or preservatives and is for single dose use only. r-Aprotinin is a very stable molecule and may be stored at room temperature without loss of potency to expiry date. r-Aprotinin activity is expressed as kallikrein inactivator units (KIU). The concentration of r-aprotinin is 10,000 KIU/ml or ~ 1.4 mg/ml, corresponding to 500,000 KIU or ~ 70 mg r-aprotinin/vial.

## Preclinical Studies

### Animal Pharmacology

#### Cardiovascular System

Investigations carried out in rats, cats, and pigs show large interspecies variability in the effect of aprotinin (bovine and recombinant) on the cardiovascular system. In the anesthetized cat, intravenous administration of r-aprotinin, 4 mg/kg, caused a major and prolonged fall in systemic arterial blood pressure. This dose also caused strenuous respiration and paw edema.[7]

In the anesthetized rat, administration of r-aprotinin, 4 and 16 mg/kg, caused a transient dose-dependent fall of blood pressure.[8] r-Aprotinin at the high dose level (16 mg/kg) increased plasma glucose levels in the anesthetized rat 30 minutes after the start of glucose infusion. Full normalization of glucose levels was not evident 30 minutes after stopping the glucose infusion, probably due to hypotension. In the anesthetized pig, r-aprotinin, 4, 16, and 40 mg/kg, had no effect on systemic arterial blood pressure, pulmonary arterial blood pressure, or central venous blood pressure.[9]

#### Other Tests

Intravenous administration of r-aprotinin, 4 and 16 mg/kg, to hydrated conscious rats did not affect diuresis or excretion of $Na^+$, $K^+$, and $Cl^-$ from 0–3 hours after administration.[10] Furthermore, r-aprotinin did not affect sleeping time induced by hexobarbital or ethanol in mice.[11,12] In vitro studies showed that r-aprotinin did not affect smooth muscle activity in segments of guinea-pig ileum.[27]

The effect of recombinant aprotinin on tissue plasminogen activator (tPA)-induced bleeding was measured in a rat model.[14] tPA was infused at a rate of 0.3 mg/kg/min during a period of 40 minutes. A full transection of the ear tip was made 10 minutes after the onset of tPA infusion. Aprotinin was given in bolus doses of 0.05–5 mg/kg followed by infusion of 0.1–10 mg/kg during a period of 55 minutes. The aprotinin bolus was given simultaneously with initiation of tPA infusion. Saline was used as control. The study was blinded and randomized. In control rats, the bleeding time was 10 minutes (mean value). In rats given tPA and saline, the bleeding time was prolonged to > 45 minutes. Aprotinin reduced the tPA-induced bleeding to 11 minutes (mean value) only when given in the highest dose (5 and 10 mg/kg), whereas no effect was seen with 2 and 4 mg/kg or lower doses.

Acute arterial thrombus formation in 22 ePTFE (expanded polytetrafluoroethylene) grafts inserted in the common carotid arteries in sheep was studied in an experimental model.[17] Eleven animals were used; five received r-aprotinin as an intravenous infusion and six served as controls, receiving physiologic saline. The infusions were started at the beginning of graft insertion. The dose of r-aprotinin was 16 mg/kg for 20 minutes and 8 mg/kg for the rest of the experiment; 40–100 ml of heparinized saline (10 U of heparin/ml) was used for flushing of the grafts. Blood samples were obtained at the beginning and end of the experiments for later analysis of platelets, and [125]I-labeled homologous fibrinogen was infused. The uptake of platelets and fibrinogen over the proximal and distal anastomotic areas was measured simultaneously for 4 hours using a multichannel analyzer with two detectors over each graft. The uptake was compared with the baseline uptake before graft insertion.

The animals were sacrificed at the end of the experiments. The grafts were removed; the thrombus material was weighed. The uptake of platelets and fibrinogen was analyzed. Three of 10 grafts in the treatment group and 1 of 12 grafts in the control group occluded; this difference was not statistically significant. The median thrombus weight in both groups was < 0.1 gm. There was no difference between the treatment and control groups in uptake increase of platelets (8.1 vs. 7.9 proximally and distally) and fibrinogen (3.9 vs. 2.9 proximally, 3.5 vs. 3 distally), either at the proximal or at the distal anastomoses. The heparin activity in all samples except two (from two different animals) was below 0.05 aXa IU/ml plasma. The r-aprotinin concentration at the beginning of the experiments was 478 KIU ± 72 SD and at the end, 516 KIU ± 166 SD. The concentrations were more than twice the concentrations used in cardiopulmonary patients (200 KIU/ml).

It was concluded that in an experimental situation, administration of high-dose r-aprotinin does not increase the acute thrombus formation in ePTFE grafts.[17] None of the general pharmacology studies demonstrated a difference between the effects of r-aprotinin and bovine aprotinin.

## Animal Toxicology

Single-dose toxicity studies in rats[4] and mice[5] and repeated-dose toxicity studies in rats[2] and dogs[3] have shown that aprotinin causes dose-dependent nephrotoxic changes. There are no significant differences in the toxic response to r-aprotinin and b-aprotinin. The main lesion is seen in the proximal tubular cells, where the most prominent changes are eosinophilic globules (protein droplets). Necrosis and regeneration of epithelial cells of the proximal convoluted tubules are seen at the highest dose levels. These changes are due to accumulation of aprotinin in the proximal tubular cells.

The effect of r-aprotinin on renal glomeruli was investigated by inulin clearance in female Sprague-Dawley rats.[25] The Sprague-Dawley is among the most nephrotoxic-sensitive strains. The major findings following a single-dose of r-aprotinin to healthy anesthetized rats was a reversible drop in glomerular filtration rate in the highest dose group only (100 mg/kg). In most of the animals, microscopic examination of the kidney revealed reversible changes in the proximal tubules. In a single-dose administration study of rats given ≥ 33 mg/kg[4] and mice given ≥ 100 mg/kg,[5] histopathologic examination revealed nephrotoxic lesions. The severity of the lesions was dose-dependent. The reversibility of the nephrotoxic lesion in rats was examined. Full reversibility 28 days after dosage was demonstrated in 4 of 4 rats given 33 mg/kg and in 3 of 4 rats given 100 mg/kg. However, in rats given 100 or 300 mg/kg, kidney function was impaired as reflected in blood and urine parameters during the first week after treatment.

The effects on the kidney of repeated injections of r-aprotinin were investigated in four cynomolgus monkeys.[22] Two male and two female cynomolgus monkeys were given single intravenous injections of 10, 10, 30, and 90 mg/kg of r-aprotinin, respectively, at 2-week intervals. Kidney biopsies were taken before dosing and about 24 hours after the first and third doses. Eight-hour urine samples were collected daily for 9 days pretrial and up to a maximum of 10 days following each administration. Serum samples were collected at intervals throughout the study. On the day after the final dose, 1 male and 1 female were killed and autopsied. The remaining male and female were allowed a 6-week recovery period before they were killed and autopsied. No gross abnormalities were seen at autopsy. Intracytoplasmic protein droplets were found in the renal proximal tubules at a minimum level at 10 mg/kg in females and at 30 mg/kg (both sexes), and at a moderate level at 90 mg/kg. No droplets were seen following 6 weeks' recovery.

### Immunogenicity

The relative immunogenicity of organic b-aprotinin and r-aprotinin was evaluated in a study in rabbits.[1] The immunization was performed by subcutaneous injections twice a week with 1.0-ml emulsion composed of equal volumes of aprotinin (1.0 mg/ml saline) and Freund's incomplete adjuvant. Every 14 days, aprotinin antibodies were estimated in serum samples diluted 90,000 times by an enzyme-linked immunosorbent assay (ELISA) method. Both r-aprotinin and organic b-aprotinin caused immune responses of equal magnitude.

## Phase I Clinical Trials

### Pharmacokinetics in Volunteers

The primary objective of this study was to evaluate the pharmacokinetic properties (elimination half-life) of r-aprotinin at three dosage levels in volunteers. The secondary objective was to evaluate the immediate safety of three dosage levels of r-aprotinin in volunteers and to monitor volunteers for the development of antibodies to r-aprotinin and potential yeast contaminants as a result of a single injection of r-aprotinin. Thirty volunteers were entered into this randomized, double-blinded, placebo-controlled, dose-escalation study. All 30 volunteers completed the study successfully. They were randomized into three groups receiving 1, 2, or 4 mg/kg, respectively.

Plasma concentration-time curves have indicated that linear pharmacokinetics can be assumed (i.e., increase in dose level results in a corresponding increase in area under the curve [AUC]), and r-aprotinin showed a relatively dose-independent behavior. A two-compartmental method for estimation of pharmacokinetic parameters was used. The elimination half-life was found to be approximately 4 hours. A large volume of distribution (19.6 L) may have been due to the accumulation of r-aprotinin in renal proximal tubular cells. r-Aprotinin had a low clearance of 3.7 L/hr in these volunteers.

To limit the risk of allergic reactions, subjects who had never been treated previously with r-aprotinin were studied. No sensitivity tests were performed, as such tests may not always predict anaphylactic reactions. Serum samples were analyzed for antibody formation against r-aprotinin and potential yeast contaminants. Samples were taken before dosing, at 4 weeks, and at 3–4 months. Eighty-three percent of the volunteers developed antibodies to r-aprotinin. Antibody formation occurred in all three groups, with the highest frequency in the group receiving the largest dose of 4 mg/kg. The immune response had not declined to the background level by 3–4 months. None of the subjects developed antibodies to potential yeast contaminants in the product.[18]

The effect of r-aprotinin on proximal tubular cells was evaluated by examining the excretion of low-molecular-weight protein and enzymes. To ensure that the kidney function of the volunteers was normal on enrollment, an estimation of the endogenous creatinine clearance was performed prior to the study. In addition, volunteers saved three 24-hour urine collections for determination of microalbumin/protein, N-acetyl-β-D-glucosaminidase (NAG), retinol-binding protein, beta-2 microglobulin, glucose/sugar, acetone/ketones, hemoglobin/blood, direct microscopy, and specific gravity. Volunteers were enrolled in the study only if all of the above-mentioned parameters were within the normal range.

In the 4-mg/kg group, there was a significant increase in urine microalbumin, which was attributed to an increase in one volunteer, a 10-fold increase in beta-2 microglobulin, and a 2-fold increase in retinol-binding protein on the day of dosing. For all parameters, this increase was only transient and a return to baseline values occurred within 2 days.

## Pharmacokinetics in Patients Undergoing Cardiopulmonary Bypass

An open uncontrolled study was conducted in 12 patients between 50–70 years of age undergoing elective primary aortocoronary bypass operation with anticipated bridging of two or more vessels. After induction of anesthesia, a loading dose of 4 mg/kg was given over 20 minutes, followed by an infusion of 1 mg/kg/hr given continuously during surgery until closure of the sternum. To overcome the dilution effect of the prime in the oxygenator, 2 mg/kg/L was added to each liter of prime by replacement of an aliquot of the priming volume. The total dose of r-aprotinin was $10.84 \pm 0.65$ mg/kg. A pharmacokinetic model was fitted to the plasma concentration of r-aprotinin. The fitting was performed using the ADAPT II program (D.Z. D'Argenio and A. Schumitzky). The elimination half-life was found to be approximately 6.5 hours. Body clearance was found to be 3.66 L/hr. It was concluded that the elimination half-life is approximately 6.5 hours in patients and 4 hours in volunteers. This difference may be explained by the lower body temperature (hypothermia) in the patients undergoing cardiopulmonary bypass.

## Adverse Experiences in the Phase I Studies

In volunteers, a total of five adverse reactions were reported during the study by five subjects, and all resolved without the need for treatment or medication. No serious adverse reactions were observed. Three of the reported adverse reactions occurred in subjects receiving placebo. One placebo-treated subject experienced a rash surrounding the infusion site, one had a nose bleed, and a third had itching all over the body (no rash). One subject receiving r-aprotinin, 1 mg/kg, was found to be cold and sweaty for 5 minutes during the infusion, and another receiving 2 mg/kg noted a rash at the venipuncture site. Both of the latter adverse reactions were thought possibly related to the administration of r-aprotinin.

In patients undergoing cardiopulmonary bypass, one serious adverse event was reported during the study period. A patient with extensive atherosclerotic disease had an intraoperative myocardial infarction. The investigator assessed the relationship to r-aprotinin as unlikely.

## Phase II Study

To assess the efficacy and safety of r-aprotinin in patients undergoing cardiopulmonary bypass operations, an open-label, randomized, dose-escalation clinical trial was conducted.[15] A total of 84 patients were randomized: 60 had primary operations and 24 had reoperations. Patients were excluded if they had myocardial infarction within the past 7 days, an ejection fraction of less then 30%, intractable congestive heart failure, age over 70 years, or received aspirin within 72 hours of surgery. Two dose levels of r-aprotinin were studied; one was comparable to that currently recommended for bovine aprotinin and one was half that dose. The specific amounts of r-aprotinin given were 4 or 2 mg/kg as an intravenous bolus over 20 minutes after the induction of anesthesia, an intravenous infusion of 1 or 0.5 mg/kg/hr until the patient left the operating room, and 2 or 1 mg/kg added to each liter of lactated Ringer's solution for priming of the membrane oxygenator. Of the patients undergoing primary operations, 36 received r-aprotinin (18 at each dose level), and of the patients having reoperations, 12 received r-aprotinin (6 at each dose level).

As has been emphasized by Royston[19] and Taylor,[24] the activated clotting time (ACT) is unreliable as a measure of heparin effect in patients receiving aprotinin. Therefore, heparin was monitored intraoperatively by using a modified amidolytic anti-factor Xa assay.[16] This resulted in similar heparin dosing in r-aprotinin and control patients during surgery.

Perioperative blood loss was evaluated by examining the decline in hematocrit 5 days after surgery and by measuring the volume of red cells given during and after operation. The latter consisted of cell-saver red cells, red cells in reinfused chest tube drainage, and donor packed red cells. Overall red cell loss was calculated based on these measurements, which were used to compare r-aprotinin and control patients. In addition, blood urea nitrogen and creatinine were estimated, patients were clinically evaluated for the development of graft thrombosis or other coagulopathy, and studies were performed to detect antibodies to r-aprotinin and potential yeast contaminants.

r-Aprotinin and control patients did not differ in regard to age, sex, weight, number of coronary grafts, or preoperative hemoglobin concentration. However, patients undergoing primary operations treated with r-aprotinin had significantly less red cell loss in the chest drainage fluid; this was true for both primary surgery ($p < 0.001$) and reoperations ($p < 0.005$). Overall, red cell loss was significantly less for patients treated with the lower dose of r-aprotinin having reoperations and for those receiving the higher dose of r-aprotinin and having primary operations. Whereas the differences in red cell loss were most evident in patients receiving the higher doses of r-aprotinin, direct comparison of blood loss between the two dose levels was not statistically significant. Most importantly, fewer patients receiving r-aprotinin had transfusions of predonated blood (allogeneic or autologous) or chest tube blood, whether having primary operations or reoperations (Table 1).

In patients receiving the lower dose of r-aprotinin, there were no myocardial infarctions or deaths. At the higher dose, one patient had a profound bradycardia and died on the fifth postoperative day and two patients had late graft closures.

**TABLE 1.** Numbers of Patients Requiring Transfusions of Predonated Blood (Allogeneic or Autologous) or Chest Tube Drainage Blood (When Volume > 150 ml)

|  | Aprotinin | Control | p-Value |
|---|---|---|---|
| Predonated blood |  |  |  |
| Primary operation | 4/36 | 6/24 |  |
| Reoperation | 2/12 | 6/12 |  |
| Total | 6/48 | 12/36 | 0.02 |
| Chest tube blood |  |  |  |
| Primary operation | 9/36 | 15/24 |  |
| Reoperation | 3/12 | 5/12 |  |
| Total | 12/48 | 20/36 | <0.01 |

Two control patients had hypotension after bypass requiring intraaortic balloon pumps and one died. Changes in blood urea nitrogen and creatinine were small and did not differ between patients treated with the lower dose of r-aprotinin and controls; they were slightly greater in those receiving the higher dose. No participant experienced hypersensitivity reactions.

The conclusion from this phase II trial was that r-aprotinin was safe and effective in reducing blood loss during cardiopulmonary bypass surgery. Efficacy was observed with a lower dose of aprotinin than that currently recommended. To confirm these observations and provide guidelines for clinicians, a multicenter trial encompassing larger numbers of patients is clearly desirable. Such a trial will firmly establish the place of r-aprotinin in the operative management of the cardiac patient.

# References

1. Andersen L: Relative immunogenicity of organic bovine aprotinin and recombinant bovine aprotinin in rabbits. Novo Nordisk A/S Study 89038.
2. Chapman EA: Toxicity study by intravenous administration to CD rats for four weeks followed by a four week reversibility period. Life Science Research 90/NLP123/1332.
3. Chapman EA: Toxicity study by intravenous administration to beagle dogs for four weeks followed by a four week reversibility period. Life Science Research 91/NLP122/0044.
4. Christensen ND: Acute intravenous toxicity study with a 28-day observation period in Wistar rats. Novo Nordisk A/S Study 89097.
5. Christensen ND: Acute intarvenous toxicity study in NMRI mice. Novo Nordisk A/S Study 89113.
6. Cosgrove DM III, Heric B, Lytle BW, et al: Aprotinin therapy for reoperative myocardial revascularization: A placebo-controlled study. Ann Thorac Surg 54:1031–1038, 1992.
7. Dall V: The cardiovascular and respiratory effects of aprotinin (ge) in the anaesthetised cat: Comparison with aprotinin (bovine). Study No. 89020 (1989).
8. Dall V: Interaction with the glucose metabolism and cardiovascular effects of aprotinin (ge) in glucose loaded and anaesthetised rats: Comparison with aprotinin (bovine). Study No. 89022 (1989).
9. Dall V: The cardiovascular effects of aprotinin (ge) in the anaesthetised pig: Comparison with aprotinin (bovine). Study No. 89021 (1989).
10. Dall V: Effects of aprotinin (ge) on diuresis and electrolyte excretion in conscious rats: Comparison with aprotinin (bovine). Study No. 89023 (1989).
11. Dall V: Effects of aprotinin (ge) on the duration of ethanol induced sleep in mice: Comparison with aprotinin (bovine). Study No. 89024 (1989).
12. Dall V: Effects of aprotinin (ge) on the duration of hexobarbital induced sleep in mice: Comparison with aprotinin (bovine). Study No. 89025 (1989).
13. de Smet AAEA, Joen MCN, van Oeveren W, et al: Increased anticoagulation during cardiopulmonary bypass by aprotinin. J Thorac Cardiovasc Surg 100:520–527, 1990.

14. Erhardtsen E, Bregengaard C, Hedner U, et al: The effect of recombinant aprotinin on a tPA-induced bleeding in rats. Blood Coagul Fibrinolysis (in press).
15. Green D, Sanders J, Eiken M, et al: Recombinant aprotinin in coronary artery bypass graft surgery. J Thorac Cardiovasc Surg, in press (1995).
16. Kristensen HI, Nielsen GG: A fast amidolytic anti-factor Xa assay not influenced by aprotinin for monitoring of heparin during cardiopulmonary bypass operation. Thromb Haemost 69:395, 1993.
17. Lundell A, Bergqvist D, Lindblad B, et al: Intravenous administration of r-aprotinin does not increase acute thrombus formation in ePTFE arterial grafts—an experimental study in sheep [abstract]. Thromb Haemostas 69:572, 1993.
18. Lyng LH: Analysis of sera from phase I clinical trial UK/APR/006/KIN for antibodies against recombinant aprotinin and yeast contaminants (APR:Ab, YEAST:Ab).
19. Royston D: Controversies in the practical use of aprotinin. In Pifarré R (ed): Anticoagulation, Hemostasis, and Blood Preservation in Cardiovascular Surgery. Philadelphia, Hanley & Belfus, 1993, pp 147–166.
20. Royston D, Taylor KM, Bidstrup BP, Sapsford RN: Effect of aprotinin on need for blood transfusion after repeat open-heart surgery. Lancet ii:1289–1291, 1987.
21. Saffitz JE, Sundt TM, Stahl DJ, et al: Disseminated intravascular coagulopathy after administration of aprotinin in combination with hypothermic circulatory arrest. Circulation 86(Suppl 1):I-630, 1992.
22. Schonberger JPAM, Everts PAM, Ercan H, et al: Low-dose aprotinin in internal mammary artery bypass operations contributes to important blood saving. Ann Thorac Surg 54:1172–1176, 1992.
23. Scott E, McDonald P, Robb DT: r-Aprotinin renal toxicity study in cynomolgus monkeys after intravenous administration. Inveresk Research International, Project 652589.
24. Taylor KM: Effect of aprotinin on blood loss and blood use after cardiopulmonary bypass. In Pifarré R (ed): Anticoagulation, Hemostasis, and Blood Preservation in Cardiovascular Surgery. Philadelphia, Hanley & Belfus, 1993, pp 129–145.
25. Thomsen MK: The effect of recombinant aprotinin on renal function in anaesthetized rats: A dose-response study.
26. Vinter A, Bjorn SE, Soeberg H, Sorensen HH: Identification of aprotinin degradation products by the use of high-performance capillary electrophoresis, high-pressure liquid chromatography and mass spectrometry. J Chromatogr 516:175–184, 1990.
27. Weiss JU: Comparative study on aprotinin (ge) and bovine pancreatic aprotinin in the isolated guinea pig ileum. Novo Nordisk A/S Study No. 89030 (1989).

**Bradford P. Blakeman, MD**
**Henry J. Sullivan, MD**

# 21

# Aprotinin for Orthotopic Heart Transplant

Postoperative or perioperative bleeding is a common problem in heart transplant surgery. The incidence of mediastinal exploration after 209 heart transplants performed at Loyola Medical center between 1985 and 1992 was 11.9%.[1] The number of mediastinal explorations becomes particularly alarming when one considers that patients are immunocompromised and highly prone to infections. Other obvious problems associated with blood replacement and further exploration include diseases transmitted by blood transfusions, transfusion reactions, pulmonary problems due to blood products (adult respiratory distress syndrome), prolonged ventilation, greater risk for fluid overload, hemodynamic instability, increased risk that systemic temperature drugs will cause more blood loss and arrhythmias, and prolonged hospitalization. It therefore becomes imperative that physicians use any means available to decrease blood loss, including meticulous surgical technique, appropriate blood products, and recently the use of aprotinin. This chapter defines the multiple causes of bleeding during heart transplantation and reviews the limited literature as well as our own data related to the use of aprotinin in heart transplant surgery.

## Causes of Bleeding

Multiple factors account for increased bleeding problems in patients with heart transplants. Many patients have had previous surgery, such as coronary artery bypass, valve replacement, and implantation of a cardioverter, defibrillator, or possibly an assist device. The adhesions due to previous operations contribute greatly to increased bleeding.

The majority of patients with heart transplants are also in biventricular heart failure. Right-heart failure in particular leads to hepatomegaly and subsequent mild coagulopathies. The fact that many patients take Coumadin or aspirin contributes further to the coagulopathy. Most patients take Coumadin at home while on the waiting list. When a heart becomes available, patients are quickly admitted to the hospital with a prothrombin time that is elevated 1½ times above normal. Some patients also take aspirin, which affects platelet function for about 5–7 days after ingestion.[3,7,9]

The events that occur during surgery contribute further to the above causes of bleeding. Cardiopulmonary bypass (CPB) is responsible for bleeding problems. Significant alteration of platelet count and function is the primary reason for medical bleeding due to CPB.[1] The majority of platelets are not destroyed but simply inhibited for a few hours. Cardiotomy or "inside" suction also contributes to permanent platelet damage because of the interface between air and blood.[2] This destruction can be decreased by lowering the amount of suction.

Multiple coagulation factors have been studied to explain medical bleeding after all types of open-heart surgery. By the end of CPB all clotting factors have returned to normal or near-normal levels except for factor V and the platelets.[4,10,11,15] Factor V levels return to normal within 24 hours. This is the primary reason for elevation of the prothrombin time after surgery.

Another device used routinely for all open-heart surgery is the cell-saver apparatus (CSA), which contributes to bleeding by centrifuging off platelets and proteins, including proteins from the clotting cascade.[5] The CSA contributes to excessive bleeding if one or two blood volumes are filtered during the transplant, and multiple blood products may be needed to assist clotting.

In conclusion, not only do patients enter the surgical suite with increased bleeding problems due to previous heart surgery, heart failure, and anticoagulation, but the process of transplantation also contributes by altering platelet function and affecting the clotting cascade.

## Dosing Regimens for Aprotinin

Aprotinin is a serine proteinase inhibitor that has a platelet-sparing effect.[13] Although the exact mechanism is unknown, aprotinin is thought to affect the von Willebrand-platelet interaction.[13,14] The drug is given from the start of surgery; two dosing regimens have been used in our hospital.

In the high-dose regimen, 200 mg of aprotinin is placed in the prime solution of the CPB machine; an additional 200 mg is given intravenously by anesthesia; and a constant infusion of 50 mg/hr is given during CPB and stopped when the patient leaves the operating room. Heparin levels are maintained during CPB at 2mg/kg, and an activated clotting time (ACT) over 700 seconds is maintained throughout the pump run.

In the low-dose regimen, 100 mg of aprotinin is placed in the prime solution and 100 mg is given intravenously. The constant infusion is then repeated at 50 mg/hr. Heparin levels and ACTs are maintained at the previously mentioned levels.

## Available Data

Few patients undergoing orthotopic heart transplant have been exposed to aprotinin. A randomized study by Havel et al.[6] and a nonrandomized study by Royston[12] constitute the available literature. A comparative group of patients (only 5 of whom received aprotinin) from Loyola Medical Center is also discussed.

Havel et al. randomized 20 patients to receive low-dose aprotinin (560 mg) or placebo at the time of transplant.[6] Perioperative blood loss was significantly less in the aprotinin-treated group both at 24 and 48 hours. The aprotinin-treated group also received less transfused blood at 24 and 48 hours; 70% of aprotinin-treated patients vs. 30% of placebo-treated patients received no blood. All patients were diagnosed with cardiomyopathy, and none had had previous heart surgery. No significant complications due specifically to aprotinin were noted in Havel's report.

Royston used aprotinin in patients believed to be at high risk for bleeding.[12] The risk factors were reoperations through previous sternotomy, coagulopathy, and ingestion of any anticoagulant drug (i.e., aspirin or Coumadin). Of the 57 patients in the study, 23 received aprotinin in a nonrandomized manner according to the above criteria (17 of whom underwent reoperative sternotomies), and 34 received no aprotinin. The blood loss was significantly less for the aprotinin-treated group versus the untreated group at 24 and 48 hours. In addition, less blood was transfused in the aprotinin-treated group, and no platelet transfusions were necessary. It should be emphasized that this was a nonrandomized study.

Data from Loyola Medical Center also were derived from a nonrandomized group of patients undergoing orthotopic heart transplants, all of which involved reoperative sternotomies. The group consisted of 16 patients, 5 of whom were given aprotinin. The use of aprotinin was the surgeon's choice; no specific criteria were applied. Our data (Tables 1 and 2) revealed no significant improvement in blood loss at 24 or 48 hours and no significant reduction in blood product replacement. It must be emphasized that the patient population is small. No significant complications due to aprotinin were noted.

## Summary

In theory, aprotinin should minimize blood loss and decrease the need to transfuse blood and blood products. However, only 38 patients (including those in the literature and our own experience) have been treated with aprotinin at the time of orthotopic heart transplant. The studies by Havel et al. and Royston demonstrated less blood loss and product replacement. Our data are limited but demonstrated no

**TABLE 1.** Cardiac Transplant without Aprotinin*

| Patient | Diagnosis | Blood Products | CT Output 24 hr/Total | LOS (days) |
|---------|-----------|----------------|------------------------|------------|
| 1 | Ischemic disease | 6 U plts, 1 U cryo, 6 U FFP | 500/1610 | 14 |
| 2 | Ischemic disease | 6 U FFP | 305/705 | 12 |
| 3 | Ischemic disease | 2 U PRBCs, 3 U FFP | 675/1435 | 19 |
| 4 | Ischemic disease | 1 U RBCs, 8 U cryo, 2 U FFP, 12 U plts | 1010/2435 | 26 |
| 5 | Cardiomyopathy | 4 U FFP | 670/2130 | 98 |
| 6 | Ischemic disease | | 640/1590 | 16 |
| 7 | Ischemic disease | 2 U FFP | 790/1650 | 17 |
| 8 | Ischemic disease | | 990/2550 | 31 |
| 9 | Cardiomyopathy | 1 U RBCs, 4 U FFP | 605/1605 | 14 |
| 10 | Ischemic disease | 1 U RBCs, 8 U plts, 4 U FFP | 800/1610 | 16 |
| 11 | Valvular disease | 1 U RBCs, 2 U FFP, 16 U plts | 890/2270 | 20 |
| *Mean* | | 0.54 U PRBCs, 3.8 U plts, 3 U FFP, 0.8 U cryo | 715.9/1780.90 | 17.8 |

* All transplants involved reoperative sternotomies.
CT = chest tube, LOS = length of stay, PRBCs = packed red blood cells, FFP = fresh frozen plasma, plts = platelets, cryo = cryopreserved blood products.

**TABLE 2.** Cardiac Transplant with Aprotinin*

| Patient | Diagnosis | Blood Products | CT Output 24 hr/Total | LOS (days) |
|---|---|---|---|---|
| 1 | Ischemic disease | 3 U PRBCs | 840/7440 | Died |
| 2 | Ischemic disease | 3 U PRBCs | 350/935 | 14 |
| 3 | Congenital disease | 6 U plts, 4 U FFP | 1035/1620 | 18 |
| 4 | Ischemic disease | | 760/1530 | 21 |
| 5 | Ischemic disease | 4 U FFP | 665/2630 | 14 |
| *Mean* | | 1.2 U PRBCs, 1.6 U FFP, 1.2 U plts | 730/2831 | 13.4 |

*All transplants involved reoperative sternotomies.
CT = chest tube, LOS = length of stay, PRBCs = packed red blood cells, FFP = fresh frozen plasma, plts = platelets.

significant improvement with aprotinin. Obviously, more randomized studies are needed to gain meaningful data. No significant complications attributable to aprotinin were noted.

## References

1. Blakeman BP, Sullivan HS: Surgical considerations to postoperative bleeding. In Pifarré (ed): Anticoagulation, Hemostasis, and Blood Preservation in Cardiovascular Surgery. Philadelphia, Hanley & Belfus, 1993, pp 271–285.
2. Boonstra PW, Von Imhoff GW, Eysman L, et al: Reduced platelet activation and improved hemostasis after controlled cardiotomy suction during clinical membrane oxygenator perfusions. J Thorac Cardiovasc Surg 89:900–906, 1985.
3. Ferraris VA, Ferraris SP, Lough FC, Berry WR: Preoperative aspirin ingestion increases operative blood loss after coronary artery bypass grafting. Ann Thorac Surg 45:71–74, 1988.
4. Gralnick HR, Fischer RD: The hemostatic response to open heart operations. J Thorac Cardiovasc Surg 61:909–915, 1971.
5. Hall RI, Schweiger IM, Finlayson DC: The benefits of the Hemonetics cell saver apparatus during cardiac surgery. Can J Anaesth 37:618–622, 1990.
6. Havel M, Owen AN, Simon P, et al: Decreasing use of donated blood and reduction of bleeding after orthotopic heart transplantation by use of aprotinin. J Heart Lung Transplant 11:348–349, 1992.
7. Kitchen L, Erichson RB, Sideropoulos H: Effect of drug induced platelet dysfunction on surgical bleeding. Am J Surg 143:215–217, 1982.
8. Mayer ED, Welsch M, Tanzeem A, et al: Reduction of postoperative donor blood requirement by use of the cell separator. Scand J Thorac Cardiovasc Surg 19:165–171, 1985.
9. Michelson EL, Morgonroth J, Torosian M, MacVaugh H III: Relation of preoperative use of aspirin to increased mediastinal blood loss after coronary artery bypass graft surgery. J Thorac Cardiovasc Surg 76:694–697, 1978.
10. Milam JD, Austin SF, Martin RF, et al: Alteration of coagulation and selected clinical chemistry parameters in patients undergoing open heart surgery without transfusions. Am J Clin Pathol 76:155–162, 1981.
11. Morian M, Masure R, Havlet A, et al: Haemostasis disorders in open heart surgery with extracorporeal circulation: Importance of platelet function and the heparin neutralization. Vox Sang 32:41–51, 1977.
12. Royston D: Aprotinin therapy in heart and heart-lung transplantation. J Heart Lung Transplant 12:519–525, 1993.
13. Royston D, Bidstrup B: Reduction in postoperative blood loss in patients having open heart reoperations using high dose aprotinin (Trasylol). Anesthesiology 67:A23, 1987.
14. Royston D, Bidstrup BP, Taylor KM, Sapsford RN: Effect of aprotinin on need for blood transfusion after repeat open-heart surgery. Lancet ii:1289–1291, 1987.
15. Wolk LA, Wilson RF, Burdick M, et al: Changes in antithrombin, antiplasmin, and plasminogen during and after cardiopulmonary bypass. Am Surg 51:309–313, 1985.

Jack G. Copeland, MD

# 22

# The Use of Aprotinin in Assist Devices and the Total Artificial Heart

Little is known about the proper role of aprotinin in the implantation and management of circulatory support devices. We have learned much about support devices since the first use of the "permanent" total artificial heart[14] in 1982, the first successful bridge to transplant with a left ventricular assist device[32] in 1984, and the first successful bridge to transplant with a total artificial heart[8] in 1985. Aprotinin was recognized as an important pharmacologic therapy in blood conservation in cardiac surgical procedures using cardiopulmonary bypass in 1987.[35] Since the mid 1980s, extensive experience with devices[10] and with aprotinin[36,43] has accumulated. Bleeding at the time of implantation,[9,11] stimulation of coagulation and fibrinolysis,[34] and early and late thromboembolism[9,11] have been significant problems with support devices. Surgical implantation is associated with release of tissue plasminogen activator. Cardiopulmonary bypass (CPB) stimulates the intrinsic coagulation cascade, the fibrinolytic system, and results in a time-related platelet dysfunction.[1,20,21,25] Exposure of blood to the materials in blood-pumping devices and to turbulent flow patterns, particularly around prosthetic valves, constitutes a constant stimulus of factor XII, platelets, and the fibrinolytic system. Many of these problems might be solved by using aprotinin.

## Aprotinin and Cardiopulmonary Bypass

Extensive experience with aprotinin in the setting of CPB documents that total doses in the range of 5–6 million kallikrein inhibition units (KIU) significantly reduce bleeding[4,15,18] (7142.8 KIU = 1 mg of aprotinin; therefore, 5 million units = 700 mg, and 6 million units = 840 mg). Significantly reduced bleeding also has been documented for lower total doses in adults: 4.2 million KIU,[6] 2.5 million KIU,[13] and 2 million KIU.[38] Lower doses in adults did not decrease bleeding from CPB.[19] In children, and presumably in smaller adults, a dose of 60,000 KIU/kg (equal to 4.2 million KIU in a 70-kg person) decreased intra- and postoperative bleeding, whereas doses of 30,000 and 25,000 KIU/kg did not.[7,16] On the basis of these studies, our group decided to use a maximal total dose of 6 million KIU, including bolus, intravenous infusion, addition to the pump prime, and continuous infusion. For patients under 100 kg, we decided to use a dose of 60,000 KIU/kg.

Aprotinin also has been found to decrease CPB-associated bleeding in patients who receive aspirin preoperatively[30,39] as well as in patients who undergo heart and heart-lung transplantation.[22,37] Pae and associates at Hershey Medical Center[33] reported decreased bleeding at the time of insertion of ventricular assist devices. This chapter reviews their data in detail, along with data from our program and from the artificial heart program of La Pitié Hospital (Paris).

The mechanisms of action of aprotinin are of interest not only because they allow CPB to be done with less bleeding, but also because devices may have many of the same effects on the pro- and anticoagulant systems as CPB. The presence of foreign materials, turbulent flow, areas of stasis of flow, and shearing forces are common to both forms of support. The possibility of using aprotinin to control the nonphysiologic consequences of mechanical circulatory support on the pro- and anticoagulant systems throughout long periods of support is provocative. We have evidence that aprotinin inhibits activation of factor XII,[26] perhaps by inhibiting the kallikrein system. Because factor XII is stimulated by foreign surfaces, and because blood flows continuously over such surfaces during device support, one may expect that the intrinsic clotting system is continually activated. Can long-term treatment with aprotinin prevent this?

Several lines of evidence indicate that platelet function during CPB is preserved by pretreatment with aprotinin. First, reduced release of thromboxane A2 and beta thromboglobulin[31] indicates that pretreatment with aprotinin decreases platelet activation and degranulation. Yet platelets retain their function, as measured by aggregation studies demonstrating better aggregability in aprotinin-treated patients than in controls[27] after CPB, possibly because adhesive receptors (glycoprotein Ib) on the platelets are preserved by aprotinin therapy.[42] Because inhibition of platelet function is life-saving after heart valve replacement,[2] it must have the same effect in patients who receive support devices, at least those that contain valves. The role that aprotinin may play in stabilizing platelet function in patients with support devices beyond the time of implantation remains to be defined.

A major effect of aprotinin during CPB is inhibition of fibrinolysis. Activation of the fibrinolytic system, as measured by the presence of alpha-2-antiplasmin–plasmin complexes, was significantly less on CPB in aprotinin treated patients.[24,29] Szefner and colleagues[41] follow alpha-2 antiplasmin as an indicator of fibrinolytic activity in patients with support devices. When the level drops, indicating consumption by binding to plasmin, patients are treated with low-dose aprotinin to control fibrinolysis. This drop in alpha-2 antiplasmin is seen most commonly in the early stages of disseminated intravascular coagulation (DIC) associated with infection.

## Adverse Effects of Aprotinin

Adverse effects of aprotinin, such as thrombosis, renal failure, and anaphylaxis, have been reported occasionally. Obviously, the delicate condition of candidates for mechanical device support may increase their susceptibility to such effects. Perhaps coronary thrombosis as a potential complication has received the most attention. I am aware of no study that has shown a significant association between postoperative myocardial infarction and aprotinin therapy.[5,12,23] A trend toward an increase in such events, however, may be present. Extrapolation of such information to support devices is premature, but one must worry about the thrombotic effect of aprotinin therapy if low flows or areas of stasis are expected or encountered with any mechanical device.

Nearly all of the millions of units of aprotinin that are administered are rapidly taken up in the brush border of the convoluted tubule of the kidney and slowly metabolized. Thus far, no significant renal dysfunction has been reported for routine revascularization operations[12] or for cardiac transplantation.[3] In the series of Sundt et al.[40] 65% of 20 patients undergoing hypothermic arrest for thoracic or thoracoabdominal aortic operations experienced renal dysfunction; 5 patients required hemodialysis. All patients received 2 million KIU of aprotinin by intravenous infusion before bypass, 2 million KIU in the pump prime, and 500,000 KIU by intravenous infusion during the procedure. Avoidance of conventional high-dose aprotinin in the presence of low temperature and circulatory arrest seems prudent on the basis of Sundt's experience.

Antibody formation in response to aprotinin may cause anaphylaxis if immunoglobulin E (IgE) and/or IgG antibodies are present from a previous exposure. Miles reports that approximately 50% of patients have IgG antibodies to aprotinin 6 weeks after exposure. In the bridge-to-transplant scenario, significant bleeding is not uncommon when the support device is implanted or explanted at the time of cardiac transplantation. If aprotinin is used during implantation, care should be taken to exclude the possibility of hypersensitivity at the time of the transplant not only by administering the recommended test dose but also by intradermal testing.[28]

## Clinical Experience with Assist Devices and the Artificial Heart

Our experience at the University of Arizona Heart Center with aprotinin and support devices has been limited to 3 patients undergoing bridge to transplant with the CardioWest heart. The transplantations were successful, and all 3 patients are long-term survivors. The amount of bleeding and replacement therapy were compared in these 3 patients and 5 earlier patients who received a total artificial heart. We have not analyzed the data further because of the small numbers and considerable interpatient variability. The trend, however, seems clear: bleeding was less, and a smaller amount of blood and blood products was used in the 3 aprotinin-treated patients.

**TABLE 1.** Blood Loss and Replacement in Total Artificial Heart Patients

|  | Aprotinin (n = 3) | No Aprotinin (n = 5) |
|---|---|---|
| Drainage day 1 | 622 cc | 1098 cc |
| Drainage day 2 | 219 cc | 625 cc |
| Drainage day 3 | 148 cc | 574 cc |
| Units of packed red blood cells/patient | 2.67 | 9.8 |
| Units fresh frozen plasma/patient | 3.3 | 5.2 |
| Units platelets/patient | 1 | 12.8 |
| Cell saver units returned/patient | 1 | 2.4 |
| Cryoprecipitate units/patient | 3.67 | 9.8 |
| Total units blood products/patient | 11.6 | 42 |

We observed no thrombotic problems in the early postimplant period. Renal function was normal after implantation in the aprotinin group. The third patient treated with aprotinin experienced an episode of anaphylaxis at the time of transplantation. He was known to be antibody-positive for aprotinin. At the time of the transplant we were unaware of the type(s) of antibodies or titer(s), although this information had been provided by the manufacturer. In retrospect, the antibody was IgG, and the titer was in the lower one-third of positive titers at 6 weeks after administration. We administered the usual intravenous test dose (1 cc, 10,000 KIU) with no response. No scratch test or intradermal injection was performed. The patient, who had been stable for 68 days on the CardioWest heart at cardiac outputs of 6–7 L/min, was given a small transfusion from the pump just before CPB and suddenly lost venous and arterial blood pressure as well as cardiac output (decreased to 3 L/min). He had not yet been given an intravenous bolus with the anesthetic; 2 million KIU of aprotinin were added to the pump prime. Epinephrine and methylprednisolone in large amounts failed to correct the profound hypotension, and we were obliged to initiate CPB prematurely. Even so, large doses of epinephrine and norepinephrine were required to maintain adequate pressure on CPB and after the transplant in the intensive care unit. The patient survived the transplant and has done well for 5 months.

In 6 patients who were bridged to transplant with a Pierce-Donachy left ventricular assist device, Pae et al.[33] used the standard high dose of aprotinin: a loading dose of 2 million KIU, 2 million KIU in the heart-lung machine, and 500,000 KIU/hour intravenously until the patient reached intensive care. This group was compared with 6 historical controls. All 12 patients survived transplantation, but those treated with aprotinin at the time of device implantation had less bleeding and received less blood (Table 2). They observed no serious side effects from the aprotinin treatment.

The group at La Pitié has taken a different approach for the duration of its experience with total artificial heart implantation, which now includes 78 patients. A loading dose of aprotinin (125,000 KIU) is administered routinely in the postoperative phase and followed by a continuous infusion of 500 KIU/hr. Various diagnostic tests and drugs are used to balance the pro- and anticoagulant systems and to stabilize platelets.[3a] In patients with no evidence of ongoing fibrinolysis, as indicated by a decrease in alpha-2 antiplasmin, aprotinin is stopped after a few days. According to current information about the blood-saving effects of aprotinin, the La Pitié group uses neither an adequate dosage nor proper timing. A minimal dose of about 2 million KIU before bypass seems necessary to demonstrate significant blood saving. Since 1992, 78 patients have received total artificial heart implants, including 16 CardioWest devices; the mean blood loss at 24 hours after implantation was 1056 cc.[17] This appears to be quite respectable compared with our experience or that of Pae et al. Of interest also is the survival of 100% of the 9 patients who received CardioWest devices as bridges to transplantation.

**TABLE 2.**  Bleeding and Blood Replacement with Implantation of the Pierce-Donachy Left Ventricular Assist Device

|  | Aprotinin (n = 6) | No Aprotinin (n = 6) | p Value |
|---|---|---|---|
| Postop drainage | 743 ± 457 cc | 2036 ± 1184 cc | 0.047 |
| Units of blood/patient | 2.2 ± 2.2 U | 10.7 ± 7.1 U | 0.038 |

## Conclusion

High doses of aprotinin given before CPB and during the operative and early postoperative phases reduce blood loss and the need for blood and blood product replacement. Preliminary data from experiences with device implantation support this concept. Even more intriguing is the potential benefit of aprotinin in blood pumps, including the long-term mechanical circulatory support devices currently in use. Inhibition of contact activation of factor XII, stabilization of platelets and platelet function, and inhibition of fibrinolysis are three effects that may decrease complications attributed to constant exposure of circulating blood to foreign materials and to the abnormal flows and shearing forces in support devices.

In bridge to transplantation, second use of aprotinin involves some risk due to antibody formation. Testing with an intradermal injection seems prudent in this setting.

## References

1. Addonizio VP, Smith B, Guiod LR, et al: Thromboxane synthesis and platelet protein release during simulated extracorporeal circulation. Blood 54:371–376, 1979.
2. Alexander GG, Turpie MB, Gent M, et al: A comparison of aspirin with placebo in patients treated with warfarin after heart valve replacement. N Engl J Med 329:524–529, 1993.
3. Anderson JR, Mascaro JG, Reynolds L, et al: Aprotinin use does not contribute to early renal dysfunction following cardiac transplantation. J Heart Lung Transplant (in press).
3a. Bellon JL, Szefner J, Cabrol C: Coagulation et Coeur Artificiel. Paris, Masson, 1989.
4. Bidstrup BP, Royston D, Sapsford RN, Taylor KM: Reduction in blood loss and blood use after cardiopulmonary bypass with high dose aprotinin. J Thorac Cardiovasc Surg 97:364–372, 1989.
5. Bidstrup BP, Underwood SR, Sapsford RN: Effect of aprotinin on aorto-coronary bypass graft patency. J Thorac Cardiovasc Surg 105:147–153, 1993.
6. Blauhut B, Gross C, Necek S, et al: Effects of high-dose aprotinin on blood loss, platelet function, fibrinolysis, complement, and renal function after cardiopulmonary bypass. J Thorac Cardiovasc Surg 101:958–967, 1991.
7. Boldt J, Knothe C, Zickmann B, et al: Aprotinin in pediatric cardiac operations: Platelet function, blood loss, and use of homologous blood. Ann Thorac Surg 55:1460–1466, 1993.
8. Copeland JG, Levinson MM, Smith R, et al: The total artificial heart as a bridge to transplantation. JAMA 256:2991–2995, 1986.
9. Copeland JG: Bleeding and anticoagulation: Proceedings of the Circulatory Support Meeting. Ann Thorac Surg 47:88–95, 1989.
10. Copeland JG: The blood biomaterial interface in circulatory support devices: A cardiac surgeon's view. In Frazier OH, Graham T, Hill JD, et al (eds): Mechanical Circulatory Support. UK, Edward Arnold, Hodder & Stoughton Publishers, 1993.
11. Copeland JG: Anticoagulation and circulatory support devices. Ann Thorac Surg 55:213–216, 1993.
12. Cosgrove DM, Heric B, Lytle BW, et al: Aprotinin therapy for reoperative myocardial revascularization: A placebo-controlled study. Ann Thorac Surg 54:1031–1038, 1992.
13. Covino E, Pepino P, Marino L, et al: Low dose aprotinin as a blood saver in open heart surgery. Eur J Cardiothorac Surg 5:414–418, 1991.
14. DeVries W: The permanent artificial heart. JAMA 259:849–859, 1988.
15. Dietrich W, Spannagi M, Jochum M, et al: Influence of high dose aprotinin treatment on blood loss and coagulation patterns in patients undergoing myocardial revascularization. Anesthesiology 73:1119–1126, 1990.
16. Dietrich W, Mossinger H, Sannagl M, et al: Homeostatic activation during cardiopulmonary bypass with different aprotinin dosages in pediatric patients having cardiac operations. J Thorac Cardiovasc Surg 105:712–720, 1993.
17. Gandjbakhch I, Pavie A, Szefner J, Bors V, Cabrol C, Rabago G: Personal communication, 1994.
18. Harder MP, Eijsman L, Roozendaal KJ, et al: Aprotinin reduces intraoperative and postoperative blood loss in membrane oxygenator cardiopulmonary bypass. Ann Thorac Surg 51:936–941, 1991.

19. Hardy J-F, Descrochers J, Belisle S, et al: Low dose aprotinin infusion is not clinically useful to reduce bleeding and transfusion of homologous blood products in high-risk cardiac surgical patients. Can J Anaesth 40:625–631, 1993.
20. Harker LA, Malpass TW, Branson HE, et al: Mechanism of abnormal bleeding in patients undergoing cardiopulmonary bypass: Acquired transient platelet dysfunction associated with selective α-granule release. Blood 56:824–834, 1980.
21. Harker LA: Bleeding after cardiopulmonary bypass. N Engl J Med 22:1446–1447, 1986.
22. Havel M, Owen AN, Simon P, et al: Decreasing use of donated blood and reduction of bleeding after orthotopic heart transplantation by use of aprotinin. J Heart Lung Transplant 11:348–349, 1992.
23. Havel M, Grabenwoger F, Schneider J, et al: Aprotinin does not decrease early graft patency after coronary artery bypass grafting despite reducing postoperative bleeding and use of donated blood. J Thorac Cardiovasc Surg 107:807–810, 1994.
24. Kawasuji M, Ueyama K, Sakakibara N, et al: Effect of low dose aprotinin on coagulation and fibrinolysis in cardiopulmonary bypass. Ann Thorac Surg 55:1205–1209, 1993.
25. Khuri SK, Wolfe A, Josa M, et al: Hematologic changes during and after cardiopulmonary bypass and their relationship to bleeding time and nonsurgical blood loss. J Thorac Cardiovasc Surg 104:94–107, 1992.
26. Laurel M-T, Ratnoff OD, Everson B: Inhibition of the activation of Hageman factor (factor XII) by aprotinin. J Lab Clin Med 119:580–585, 1992.
27. Lavee J, Raviv Z, Samolinski A, et al: Platelet protection by low dose aprotinin in cardiopulmonary bypass: Electron microscopic study. Ann Thorac Surg 55:114–119, 1993.
28. Levy JH: Antibody formation after drug administration during cardiac surgery: Parameters for aprotinin use. J Heart Lung Transplant 12:S26–32, 1993.
29. Minami K, Notohamiprodjo G, Buschler H, et al: Alpha-2 plasmin inhibitor complex-plasmin complex and postoperative blood loss: Double-blind study with aprotinin in reoperation for myocardial revascularization. J Thorac Cardiovasc Surg 106:934–935, 1993.
30. Murkin JM, Lux J, Shannon NA, et al: Aprotinin significantly decreases bleeding and transfusion requirements in patients receiving aspirin and undergoing cardiac operations. J Thorac Cardiovasc Surg 107:554–561, 1994.
31. Nagaoka H, Innami R, Murayama F, et al: Effects of aprotinin on prostaglandin metabolism and platelet function in open heart surgery. J Cardiovasc Surg 32:31–37, 1991.
32. Oyer P, Hill D: Both investigators at different institutions were successful at bridge to transplantation with left ventricular assist devices in late 1984.
33. Pae WE, Aufiero TX, Weldner PW, et al: Aprotinin therapy for insertion of ventricular assist devices for staged cardiac transplantation. J Heart Lung Transplant (in press).
34. Ring ME, Feinberg WM, Levinson MM, et al: Platelet and fibrin metabolism in recipients of the Jarvik-7 total artificial heart. J Heart Transplant 8:225–232, 1989.
35. Royston D, Bidstrup BP, Taylor KM, Sapsford RN: Effect of aprotinin on the need for blood transfusion after repeat open heart surgery. Lancet 2:1289–1291, 1987.
36. Royston D: High dose aprotinin therapy: A review of the first five years' experience. J Cardiothorac Vasc Aug:76–100, 1992.
37. Royston D: Aprotinin therapy in heart and heart lung transplantation. J Heart Lung Transplant 12:S19–25, 1993.
38. Schonberger JPAM, Everts PAM, Ecran H, et al: Low dose aprotinin in internal mammary bypass operations contributes to important blood saving. Ann Thorac Surg 54:1172–1176, 1992.
39. Schonberger JPAM, Bredee JJ, van Oeveren W, et al: Preoperative therapy of low dose aspirin in internal mammary artery bypass operations with and without low dose aprotinin. J Thorac Cardiovasc Surg 106:262–267, 1993.
40. Sundt TM, Kouchoukos NT, Saffitz JE, et al: Renal dysfunction and intravascular coagulation with aprotinin and hypothermic circulatory arrest. Ann Thorac Surg 55:1418–1424, 1993.
41. Szefner J: Personal communication, 1994.
42. Van Oeveren W, Harder M, Roozendaal KJ, et al: Aprotinin protects platelets against the initial effect of cardiopulmonary bypass. J Thorac Cardiovasc Surg 99:788–797, 1990.
43. Westaby S: Aprotinin in perspective. Ann Thorac Surg 55:1033–1041, 1993.

**Philip Hornick, BSc (Hons), MB, BChir, FRCS**
**Kenneth M. Taylor, MD, FRCS**

# 23

# Aprotinin Used in Emergency Coronary Operations after Thrombolytic Therapy

The importance of thrombolytic therapy in the management of myocardial infarction is well established and has been verified by a number of prospective clinical trials. It has been shown to improve survival in selected patients.[13] Streptokinase should be administered within 6 hours following the onset of acute myocardial infarction,[20] and thrombolysis is achieved in about 50% of patients.[29] Thrombolytic therapy administered alone carries a high risk of reocclusion and reinfarction, but its ease and rapidity of administration makes thrombolytic therapy the first choice in the management of the vast majority of patients who do not exhibit any contraindications to its use.[17] Failure of thrombolysis in the face of prolonged ischemia, as judged by pain and electrocardiographic changes, will require mechanical means of blood flow restoration if ventricular function is to be preserved and mortality to be minimized. Depending on the distribution of the atheromatous stenoses in the diseased coronary vessels, the patient may proceed to percutaneous transluminal angioplasty (PTCA) or coronary artery bypass grafting (CABG). It has been reported that more patients require emergency coronary bypass surgery if PTCA is performed immediately following streptokinase therapy.[27] The scene is therefore set for increasing numbers of patients who will require urgent CABG following thrombolysis. Surgical revascularization following thrombolytic therapy presents particular concerns with regard to the initiation of a coagulopathy which results from the effects of the thrombolytic agent. The coagulopathy results in increased blood loss, transfusion requirements, and increased morbidity and mortality.

## The Nature of the Coagulopathy

Following administration of streptokinase, there is an increased production of plasmin due to activation of plasminogen activator. Plasmin degrades the fibrin mesh which is generated in clot formation. Plasmin will also degrade a multitude of serum proteins. There is uninhibited proteolysis of fibrinogen, fibrin, and coagulation factors (V and VII). There is also a concomitant increase in fibrin degradation products which themselves have coagulant effects.[23] The coagulopathy thus generated is generally estimated to last 12–24 hours. Streptokinase therefore is not fibrin-selective, unlike second-generation thrombolytic agents, e.g., tissue-type plasminogen activator.

## Duration and Consequences of the Coagulopathy Associated with CABG

Many studies support the safety of surgical revascularization following thrombolytic therapy from 3 days onwards.[3,7,14,16,21,25,30–32] These studies report no difference in postoperative bleeding or mortality as compared to patients who have not received thrombolysis. Data which exist for surgery performed within hours to 3 days following thrombolysis suggest that streptokinase therapy results in a postoperative coagulopathy,[4] increased blood loss,[12,24] and possibly greater morbidity and mortality.[18,24]

The effect of streptokinase therapy on immediate versus delayed coronary grafting was addressed by Lee et al.[15] Patients were compared who had CABG 12 hours after thrombolysis (early), 12 and 72 hours after thrombolysis (intermediate), and > 72 hours (late). Controls were patients who had CABG within the same time periods but who did not receive streptokinase. Patients in the early group had a higher in-hospital mortality and major noncardiac morbidity. Patients in the delayed and late groups had minimal postoperative complications and no mortality. These observations were not explained by differences in ischemic time, angioplasty failures, or patients in cardiogenic shock.

It appeared from this study that postoperative bleeding and the requirement for massive use of blood products were contributory. Patients who receive streptokinase are subject to a set of risk factors that are independent of the underlying disease process causing myocardial ischemia, e.g., allergic responses and intracranial hemorrhage. It has been estimated that in 8% of patients treated with streptokinase, gastrointestinal bleeding may develop.[9] In the clinical setting of emergency cardiac operations, which in themselves carry a high risk, excessive transfusion requirements will contribute to acid-base disturbances, dilutional coagulopathies, unstable hemodynamics, and an associated potential for subsequent pulmonary problems.[15] These problems are all in addition to the postoperative risk associated with massive postoperative hemorrhage per se.

## Therapeutic Strategies to Reduce Blood Loss Associated with Thrombolytic Therapy Preceding CABG

### Timing of the Operation

In the clinical setting of emergency myocardial revascularization, a delay of 12 hours following preoperative streptokinase therapy would minimize the coagulopathic effect. Twelve hours would appear to be the critical time period between infusion and operation.[15] That this delay will be frequently impossible in the context of an evolving infarct and/or ischemic instability is self-evident. Pharmacologic manipulation to correct the coagulopathic effect of fibrinolytic agents is the other option.

## Pharmacologic Manipulation

The use of vitamin K, fresh frozen plasma, cryoprecipitate, and platelets does not appear to hasten the resolution of the coagulopathy produced following administration of streptokinase.[6,15] A number of pharmacologic agents with the potential for reducing blood loss following open heart surgery have been investigated.

Desmopressin has been investigated, and its use is associated with a decrease in postoperative blood loss when it is administered at the end of cardiopulmonary bypass.[22] The use of prostacyclin (epoprostenol) has been shown to produce a decrease in postoperative blood loss in the first 6 hours following CABG surgery, but the total blood loss over 24 hours was not found to be different from the placebo group.[10] Heparin reversal is achieved by the administration of protamine following cardiopulmonary bypass. Protamine is also a myocardial depressant. Prostacyclin has been shown to reduce the requirement for heparin such that less protamine is required for its reversal. Prostacyclin, however, decreases arterial pressure due to its properties as a vasodilator and, as such, may compromise cerebral and myocardial perfusion.[19] The routine clinical use of prostacyclin can therefore not be recommended.

No reports exist as to the use of these agents in the clinical setting of thrombolytic-induced coagulopathy following emergency coronary surgery.

## Use of Aprotinin to Reduce Blood Loss in Emergency Coronary Operation Following Thrombolysis

Information on the use of aprotinin to reduce blood loss in emergency coronary operation following thrombolysis is at present limited to isolated reports. At the present time, no prospective randomized clinical trials exist. However, it is unlikely that any will be instigated, such is the efficacy of this therapy in the aforementioned clinical situation. Restriction of its use (for the purpose of controls) in patients requiring emergency surgical revascularization following thrombolysis in a trial setting would certainly raise ethical issues.

The role of aprotinin in reducing bleeding following streptokinase administration prior to aortic surgery was first described by Butler et al.[6] The first report of the use of aprotinin in emergency CABG following streptokinase therapy was in 1991 by Efstratiadis et al.[8] In this report, the authors described a patient who underwent emergency intracoronary thrombolysis followed by immediate CABG. Aprotinin was administered intraoperatively to control the potential bleeding problems. The total postoperative blood loss was 260 ml. A modified dosage regimen of $2 \times 10^6$ KIU intravenously was administered prior to cardiopulmonary bypass, with a further $2 \times 10^6$ KIU added to the pump prime. There was no electrocardiographic evidence of myocardial infarction, and there was no elevation of the serum creatinine kinase level in the perioperative period. The patient was discharged home on the seventh postoperative day following an uneventful recovery.

Since this report, other cases have been published in the literature. Akhtar and colleagues[1] reported 2 cases in which blood loss was reduced in patients undergoing emergency revascularization following streptokinase. In the first patient, the total blood loss was 1285 ml and for the second patient 215 ml. The dosage regimen chosen was $2 \times 10^6$ KIU of aprotinin 12 minutes before the institution of cardiopulmonary bypass, with another $1 \times 10^6$ KIU given into the bypass circuit. An aprotinin infusion of 500,000 KIU/hr was continued throughout the operation and for 4 hours postoperatively.

Three further patients have also been reported in the situation where high-dose aprotinin was used in emergency CABG after thrombolysis.[2] The dosage regimen was the same as reported by Akhtar and colleagues.[1] In all 3 patients, there was only trivial bleeding, with total postoperative drainage of 315, 550, and 555 ml, respectively. There were no postoperative complications.

The precise mechanism of action of aprotinin is still unclear. Although most of the recent studies of aprotinin have been demonstrated in cardiac surgical patients, the fact that the efficacy has been demonstrated in other forms of surgery might suggest that aprotinin acts in a nonspecific manner, rather than on any particular homeostatic disorder induced by the cardiopulmonary bypass circuit.[8] Two possible (though not necessarily conflicting) theories concerning the mechanism of action have been proposed: the first favors maintenance of platelet function by the preservation of surface receptors,[28] and the second favors an antifibrinolytic effect through its antiplasmin activity.[11,26]

Concerns as to vein graft patency and a theoretical prothrombotic effect of aprotinin are of little relevance in the situation of an unstable patient who has received thrombolytic therapy. The patient's outcome being affected not only by the underlying disease process but also by the induced coagulopathy, the administration of aprotinin is nonetheless highly unlikely to cause a prothrombotic state in this situation. The underlying coagulopathy immediately following streptokinase administration is so severe that any rebound thrombotic effect would be unlikely. Furthermore, in the situation where aprotinin is used without prior administration of a thrombolytic agent, graft patency is the same as when placebo alone is administered.[5]

## Conclusion

The use of the naturally occurring protease inhibitor aprotinin is now well established and is routinely practiced in many institutions around the world. In patients undergoing redo operations or operations for septic endocarditis, high doses of aprotinin have been shown to be effective in reducing hemorrhage and reducing blood transfusion and blood product requirements. Another indication for the use of aprotinin is in emergency cardiac operations following streptokinase treatment. Further research needs to be instigated to determine aprotinin's precise mechanism of action when thrombolytic therapy has been administered and, when it has not, to determine the optimal dose.

## References

1. Akhtar TM, Goodchild C, Boyan MKG: Reversal of streptokinase-induced bleeding with aprotinin for emergency cardiac surgery. Anaesthesia 47:226–228, 1992.
2. Alajma F, Calamai G: High-dose aprotinin in emergency coronary bypass after thrombolysis [letter]. Ann Thorac Surg 54:1018, 1992.
3. Anderson JL, Battistessa S, Clayton PD, et al: Coronary bypass surgery early after thrombolytic therapy for acute myocardial infarction. Ann Thorac Surg 41:176–183, 1986.
4. Becher H, Schroder C, Mathey D, et al: Coronary artery bypass grafting within 24 hours after intracoronary thrombolysis: Risk of bleeding [abstract]. Circulation 68(pt 2)(III):115, 1983.
5. Bidstrup BP, Underwood S, Sapsford RN: The effect of aprotinin (Trasylol) on aorto-coronary bypass graft patency. J Thorac Cardiovasc Surg 105:147–153, 1993.
6. Butler J, Davies AH, Westaby S: Streptokinase in acute aortic dissection. BMJ 300:517–519, 1990.

7. Cook LS, Lucas SK, Cheatham JE, et al: Cardiovascular parameters after acute myocardial infarction and streptokinase administration in patients receiving coronary artery bypass grafts. Am J Surg 148:860–863, 1984.
8. Efstratiadis T, Munsch C, Crossman D, Taylor KM: Aprotinin used in emergency coronary operation after streptokinase treatment. Ann Thorac Surg 52:1320–1321, 1991.
9. Ellis SG: Interventions in acute myocardial infarction. Circulation 81(suppl IV):43–50, 1990.
10. Fish KJ, Sarnquist F, Steennis C, et al: A prospective, randomized study of the effects of prostacyclin on platelet and blood loss during coronary bypass operations. J Thorac Cardiovasc Surg 91:436–442, 1986.
11. Hunt BJ, Cottam S, Segal H, et al: Inhibition of tPA-mediated fibrinolysis during orthotopic liver transplantation. Lancet 336:381, 1990.
12. Kay P, Ahmad A, Floten S, Starr A: Emergency coronary artery bypass surgery after intracoronary thrombolysis for evolving myocardial infarction. Br Heart J 53:260–264, 1985.
13. Kennedy JW, Ritchie JL, Davis KB, Fritz JK: Western Washington randomized trial of intracoronary streptokinase in acute myocardial infarction. N Engl J Med 309:1477–1482, 1983.
14. Krebber HJ, Mathey D, Kuck KJ, et al: Management of evolving myocardial infarct by intracoronary thrombolysis and subsequent aorta-coronary bypass. J Thorac Cardiovasc Surg 83:186–193, 1982.
15. Lee KF, Mandell J, Rankin JS, et al: Immediate versus delayed coronary grafting after streptokinase treatment. J Thorac Cardiovasc Surg 95:216–222, 1988.
16. Lolley DM, Fulton R, Hamman J, et al: Coronary artery surgery and direct coronary thrombolysis during acute myocardial infarction. Am Surg 49:296–300, 1983.
17. Merx W, Dorr R, Renrop P, et al: Evaluation of the effectiveness of intracoronary streptokinase infusion in acute myocardial infarction: Post-procedure management and hospital course in 204 patients. Am Heart J 102:1181–1187, 1981.
18. Phillips SJ, Kongtahworn C, Skinner JR, Zeff RH: Emergency coronary artery repercussion: A choice of therapy for evolving myocardial infarction. J Thorac Cardiovasc Surg 86:679–688, 1983.
19. Radegran K, Aren C, Teger-Nilsson AC: Prostacyclin infusion during extracorporeal circulation for coronary bypass. J Thorac Cardiovasc Surg 83:205–211, 1982.
20. Randomised trial of intravenous streptokinase, oral aspirin, both or neither among 17/187 cases of suspected acute myocardial infarction: ISIS-2. Lancet 2:349–360, 1988.
21. Richardson RL, Gooch JB, Robbins SG, et al: Coronary artery bypass grafts. Arch Surg 118:296–300, 1983.
22. Salzman EW, Weinstein M, Weintraub RM, et al: Treatment with desmopressin acetate to reduce blood loss after cardiac surgery: A double blind randomized trial. N Engl J Med 314:1402–1406, 1986.
23. Schmutzler R, Koller F: Thrombolytic therapy. In Poller F (ed): Recent Advances in Blood Coagulation. London, Churchill Livingstone, 1969.
24. Skinner JR, Phillips S, Zeff RH, Kongtahworn C: Immediate coronary bypass following failed streptokinase infusion in evolving myocardial infarction. J Thorac Cardiovasc Surg 87:567–570, 1984.
25. Sterling RP, Walker W, Weiland AP, et al: Early bypass grafting following intracoronary thrombolysis with streptokinase. J Thorac Cardiovasc Surg 87:487–492, 1984.
26. Tice DA, Worth M, Clauss RH, Reed GH: The inhibition by Trasylol of fibrinolytic activity associated with cardiovascular operations. Surg Gynecol Obstet 119:71–74, 1964.
27. Topol EJ, Califf RM, George BS, et al: A randomized trial of immediate versus delayed elective angioplasty after intravenous tissue plasminogen activator in acute myocardial infarction. N Engl J Med 317:581–588, 1987.
28. Van Oeveren W, Jansen NJG, Bidstrup BP, et al: Effects of aprotinin on hemostatic mechanisms during cardiopulmonary bypass. Ann Thorac Surg 44:640–645, 1987.
29. Verstraete M, Bernard R, Brower RW, et al: Randomised trial of intravenous recombinant tissue-type plasminogen activator versus streptokinase in acute myocardial infarction. Lancet i:842–847, 1985.
30. Walker WE, Smalling R, Fuentes F, et al: Role of coronary bypass surgery after intracoronary streptokinase infusion for myocardial infarction. Am Heart J 107:826–829, 1984.
31. Wellons HA, Schneider JA, Mikell FL, et al: Early operative intervention after thrombolytic therapy for acute myocardial infarction. J Vasc Surg 2:186–191, 1985.
32. Wilson JM, Held J, Wright CB, et al: Coronary artery bypass surgery following thrombolytic therapy for acute coronary thrombosis. Ann Thorac Surg 37:212–217, 1984.

José Mateo, MD
Joan C. Souto, MD
Isabel Zuazu-Jausoro, MD
Jordi Fontcuberta, MD
Miquel Rutllant, MD

# 24

# Laboratory Assessment of Fibrinolytic Function as Affected by Aprotinin during Cardiopulmonary Bypass

Blood loss is a common and important problem in patients undergoing cardiopulmonary bypass (CPB) surgery and carries a major risk of early and late complications. The cause of increased nonsurgical bleeding following a period of CPB is difficult to define because of the alterations of several factors which control normal hemostasis. Hemodilution reduces clotting factors and platelets. In addition, platelet function is impaired, and a defect in the formation of the platelet plug is thought to be one of the most important causes of bleeding. There is a prolongation of bleeding time during and after CPB. Blood contact with foreign surfaces causes a marked activation of coagulation and activation of the fibrinolytic system.[27] Excessive bleeding may also arise because of other causes, such as the prior use of antiaggregant drugs or deficient heparin neutralization by protamine.[1,2,4,13,17,22,23]

It has been widely demonstrated that aprotinin administration reduces blood loss and blood requirements in patients undergoing CPB surgery.[5–7,9,10,14,25,26,28–30] Aprotinin is a serine protease inhibitor that efficiently inactivates plasmin and kallikrein,[31] thereby inhibiting fibrinolysis and possibly preserving platelet glycoproteins of activated proteases,[29,30] but the exact mechanisms of its benefits remain unclear.

In CPB surgery, there is an increase in fibrinolytic activity which is initiated when sternotomy starts. This activity shows a marked rise throughout extracorporeal circulation and persists several hours after surgery.

In this chapter, the alterations of fibrinolytic parameters caused by CPB surgery and the influence of the aprotinin are reviewed. We discuss the effect of aprotinin on several tests performed to explore fibrinolysis and then analyze the available data of fibrinolytic parameters measured in different clinical trials on CPB surgery using aprotinin.

# Effects of Aprotinin on Fibrinolytic System in Vitro

Aprotinin is a small, soluble, and stable polypeptide, a member of a family of serpins (serine protease inhibitors) that is able to inhibit a wide range of proteases that have serine residues at their active site. It is a basic (pK$_a$ 10) peptide of 58 amino acid residues with a molecular weight of 6,512.

Aprotinin can inhibit trypsin, kallikrein, plasmin, and activated protein C. However, recently, it has been suggested that high concentrations of aprotinin can also inhibit factor XII activation, thrombin, and the tissue factor/factor VIIa complex.[8,26] The inhibition is provided by inactivation of the active serine of the protease by the lysine residue at position 15 of the aprotinin. When inhibition occurs, reversible stoichometric complexes between the enzyme and inhibitor are formed.

In pure chemical systems, the concentration of aprotinin required to inhibit serine proteases is substantially different. A concentration of 50 KIU/ml (1 $\mu$M) is required to inhibit plasmin, whereas to block kallikrein, 200 KIU/ml (4 $\mu$M) are necessary.[26] This may be important in vivo because aprotinin is frequently administered according to the following dosage schedule: 2,000,000 KIU prior to anesthesia, 2,000,000 added to the priming pump, and 500,000/hr until the end of the surgery. With this dosage, the estimated concentration of aprotinin is about 200 KIU/ml. Therefore, plasmin and kallikrein are both inhibited, but other serine proteases, including thrombin and tissue-type (tPA) and urokinase-type (uPA) plasminogen activators, need higher concentrations to become inhibited.

Recently, there have been ongoing studies to test lower doses of aprotinin against a standard high dose or placebo. The reduction of blood concentration of aprotinin may imply a detriment in the ability of aprotinin to inhibit plasmin or kallikrein, but the effect of this reduction remains to be established.

Aprotinin may interfere in the functional measurements of several components of the fibrinolytic system in vitro. Functional plasminogen evaluation with a chromogenic substrate assay has been shown to be interfered. The principle of this technique is to convert plasminogen into an active plasminogen–streptokinase complex by an excess of streptokinase. This complex and the plasmin formed catalyze the degradation of the substrate S-2251, resulting in a coloring reaction which can be measured photometrically. Aprotinin can block the degradation of the chromogenic substrate by the plasminogen–streptokinase complex and plasmin.[33] For this reason, functional plasminogen may be underestimated when aprotinin is present in the sample (Fig. 1), and mistaken conclusions could be reached about the effect of aprotinin on plasminogen consumption in aprotinin-treated patients.

In contrast, antiplasmin activity of plasma can be overestimated when aprotinin is present. In the absence of aprotinin, antiplasmin activity is almost exclusively due to alpha-2 antiplasmin. The method is based on a photometric reaction caused by the action of plasmin on the chromogenic substrate S-2251. Plasma is incubated with an excess of plasmin, which results in a rapid complex formation between plasmin and alpha-2 antiplasmin. The inhibited plasmin activity is proportional to the amount of antiplasmin. The remaining amount of plasmin hydrolyses the substrate S-2251. If aprotinin is present, antiplasmin activity in plasma is increased, which implies that measurements of functional alpha-2 antiplasmin are overestimated in patients receiving aprotinin (Fig. 2).

Assessment of functional plasminogen activators, such as functional tPA or uPA, may be interfered when the concentration of aprotinin is very high (400 KIU/ml).

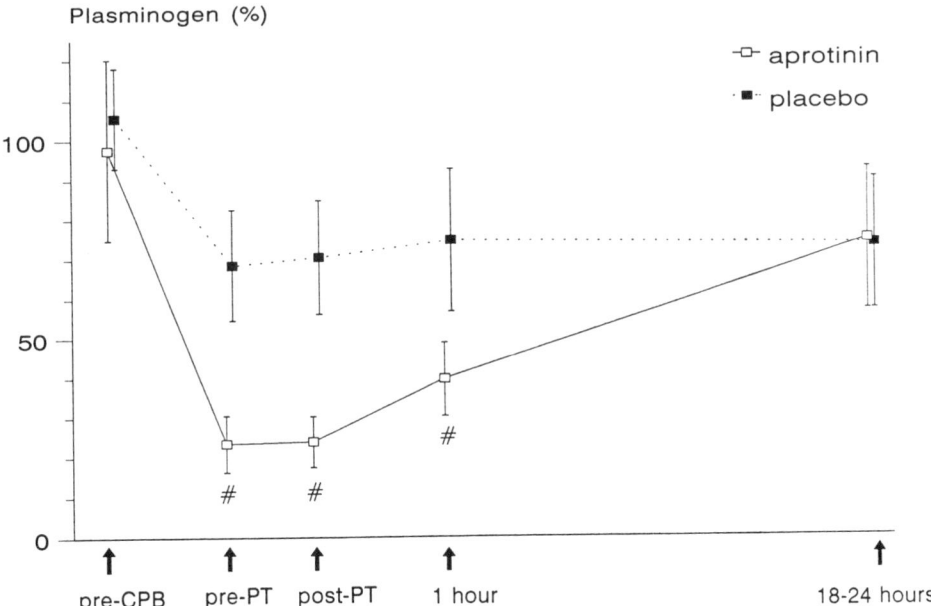

**FIGURE 1.** Plasminogen. Functional plasminogen profile throughout CPB in the placebo group shows a decrease. However, in aprotinin-treated patients, a sharp fall (# = $p < 0.05$) of plasminogen levels was seen (means ± SD). This finding can be explained because the assay was artifactually influenced by the presence of aprotinin in the sample. (PT = protamine.)

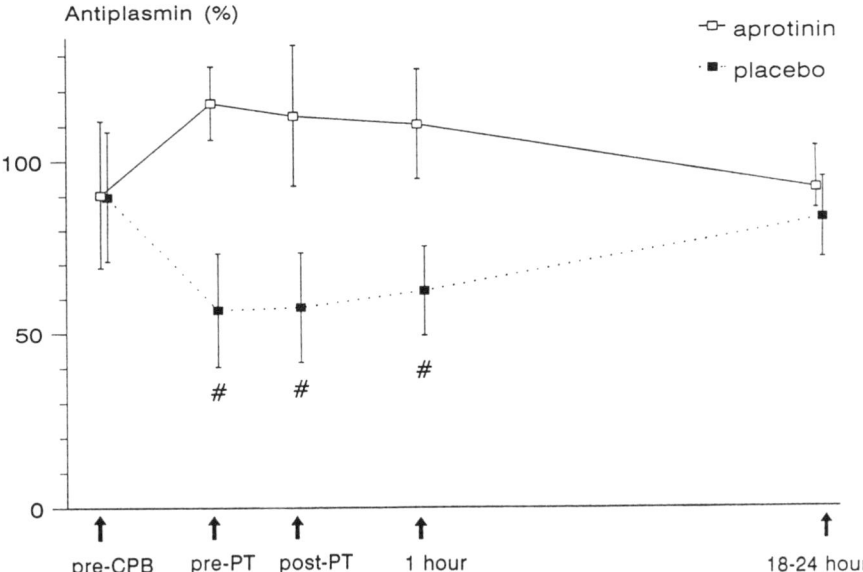

**FIGURE 2.** Alpha-2 antiplasmin. Levels of alpha-2 antiplasmin activity decreased in the placebo group. By contrast, there is an overestimate in the aprotinin-treated patients (# = $p < 0.05$), because aprotinin is able to influence this functional assay (means ± SD).

With the plasmatic concentrations that are usually reached when aprotinin is administered to patients (200 KIU/ml), the determination of both plasminogen activators seems to be reliable.[32]

In addition to plasminogen activators, the functional measurement of plasminogen activator inhibitor (PAI-1) with chromogenic substrates can be influenced only if the aprotinin concentration in plasma is higher than 400 KIU/ml.[32]

Aprotinin is also able to influence the determination of protein C. Activated protein C (APC) is an important regulator of clotting activation.[11] APC controls thrombin production by means of the inactivation of activated factors V and VIII. Moreover, APC is related to the fibrinolytic system by its ability to inhibit PAI-1. The determination of functional protein C is usually performed by clotting or photometric methods. In both cases, protein C is activated with a snake venom, and its activity is measured due to the capacity of APC to catalyze a chromogenic substrate (S-2366) or prolong the partial thromboplastin clotting time. Aprotinin is able to prevent the activation of protein C by snake venoms and can also hamper the action of APC on the chromogenic substrate. Moreover, heparin is frequently present in the sample because it is the anticoagulant used over the extracorporeal circulation and may interfere in the clotting assay. Furthermore, if heparin is present in the system, the inhibition of APC caused by aprotinin is increased. The importance of this observation in clinical situations remains to be established.[12]

The activation of fibrinolysis can be assessed by means of the determination of plasmin–alpha-2 antiplasmin complexes. When plasmin is generated, it binds to antiplasmin and results in a rapid complex formation. D-dimer can be useful also to estimate fibrinolytic activation. It is a cross-linked fibrin split product. It can be regarded as a fibrinolytic marker because it is exclusively formed by the action of plasmin over cross-linked fibrin. Both are usually measured by enzyme-linked immunosorbent assays (ELISA), which are not influenced by the presence of aprotinin.

## Effects of Aprotinin on Fibrinolysis during CPB

In most controlled assays for CPB comparing aprotinin with placebo, the results are evaluated by means of total postoperative blood loss and blood transfusion requirements. However, only in a few studies, have biological changes been investigated using plasmatic markers of coagulation and fibrinolysis activation.

In 1987, van Oeveren et al.[28] measured levels of fibrin(ogen) degradation products (FDP) in patients receiving high doses of aprotinin. They observed no increase during CPB. However, in the control group, a small but significant rise was found. They studied also tPA activity, which was found to be increased during the rewarming phase of CPB in both treated and control groups, and which developed peak values after 60 minutes of CPB.

Lu et al.[21] explored antigenic tPA and D-dimer by means of ELISA in a group of 20 patients submitted to a placebo-controlled double-blind study. An increase in plasma tPA levels was noted during the CPB. There was no statistical difference between the 10 placebo-treated patients and the 10 aprotinin-treated patients. On the contrary, the authors found a progressive increase in plasma concentration of D-dimer only in the placebo group during surgery, reflecting a substantial fibrin degradation by generated plasmin in the absence of aprotinin.

In another study,[3] levels of D-dimer and alpha-2 antiplasmin were compared in 26 patients (13 treated and 13 controls). In relation to D-dimer, the results were comparable to those mentioned above. A significant increase was observed in untreated patients. Levels of alpha-2 antiplasmin were determined with a functional assay using the chromogenic substrate S-2251. In the control group, there was a decrease from baseline, whereas in the aprotinin group levels remained essentially constant but probably levels of alpha-2 antiplasmin were overestimated. The functional plasminogen measurement was considered to be fouled by the presence of aprotinin.

In a trial performed by Havel et al.[18] a marked increase in plasma levels of thrombin–antithrombin complexes was found in all patients during extracorporeal circulation, thereby indicating an activation of coagulation. There was also a concomitant hyperfibrinolysis evaluated by measuring plasmatic cross-linked FDPs, but this was markedly less pronounced in patients receiving aprotinin.

Kawasuji et al.[20] investigated the effect of low-dose aprotinin in 27 patients undergoing CPB, and a global improvement in the hemostasis with a reduction of bleeding was observed. This improved hemostasis was attributable to the prevention of hyperfibrinolysis during CPB. They measured FDPs, functional antithrombin and functional alpha-2 antiplasmin, thrombin–antithrombin complexes and plasmin-alpha-2 antiplasmin complexes. Antithrombin levels were significantly reduced during CPB and 12 hours after operation in both groups, without differences between them. In contrast, an increase in thrombin–antithrombin complexes was seen throughout CPB. These findings denoted an activation of the coagulation system, and this activation was the same in both groups. As regards the levels of FDPs in the aprotinin group, these were significantly lower than those of the control group. The assay of alpha-2 antiplasmin was again fouled by the presence of aprotinin in the sample. However, patients from the control group showed a significant decrease during CPB. Finally, there was a marked increase in plasmin-antiplasmin complexes in the control group, whereas patients treated with aprotinin showed no significant increase.

In another study that compared patients receiving aprotinin, desmopressin, or placebo during CPB,[24] no differences in plasma levels of plaminogen, PAI-1, tPA or alpha-2 antiplasmin between groups were found. However, a significant reduction of FDPs could be demonstrated in patients receiving aprotinin.

In 1990, we carried out a double-blind randomized, prospective study comparing aprotinin and placebo in an attempt to demonstrate their effectiveness in reducing blood loss and transfusion requirements in CPB surgery.[7] We also analyzed the influence of each treatment in several hematologic and hemostatic parameters. We studied 99 patients (48 aprotinin and 51 placebo). The use of aprotinin reduced bleeding roughly by more than a half compared with placebo ($195 \pm 146$ ml/m$^2$ in the aprotinin group versus $489 \pm 361$ ml/m$^2$ in the placebo group). This reduction of hemorrhage in aprotinin-treated patients was followed by a saving of blood products: only 26% of patients receiving aprotinin needed red blood cell units, whereas 66% were transfused in the placebo group.

We measured different parameters to assess the status of coagulation and fibrinolytic activation throughout the CPB period in both groups. Blood samples were drawn as follows: (1) immediately before operation, (2) after CPB but before the administration of protamine, (3) 15 minutes after protamine, (4) 60 minutes after protamine, and (5) 18–24 hours after operation. We measured thrombin-antithrombin complexes, functional protein C (chromogenic substrate S-2366), functional plasminogen (S-2251), alpha-2 antiplasmin activity (S-2251), and plasmin-alpha-2 antiplasmin complexes, antigenic tPA, antigenic PAI-1, and split products of cross-linked fibrin (D-dimer) by means of ELISA procedures.

Activation of the coagulation system was estimated by measuring thrombin-antithrombin complex levels. A marked increase was found throughout CPB, but no differences between groups were detected. This finding could indicate that coagulation activation was similar in both groups.

Protein C, measured with a chromogenic assay (S-2366), showed a decrease during the CPB period, probably in relation to hemodilution and consumption. In the aprotinin group, protein C levels were significantly lower (Fig. 3), but the assay was probably influenced by the presence of aprotinin.

The tPA increased significantly during CPB, but no differences between groups could be found (Fig. 4). PAI-1 showed no initial changes, but levels were found higher in both groups at the fifth determination (Fig. 5), probably as a response to the endothelial release of tPA.

As discussed earlier, the evaluation of functional plasminogen and alpha-2-antiplasmin activity was not useful because both chromogenic assays were interfered with by the presence of aprotinin. In the placebo group, plasminogen and alpha-2 antiplasmin showed a decrease due to hemodilution and consumption, but the sharp fall in plasminogen and the increase in alpha-2 antiplasmin in patients treated with aprotinin may be attributed to in vitro interference with aprotinin (Figs. 1 and 2). Antigenic determinations of protein C, plasminogen, and alpha-2 antiplasmin should be recommended when aprotinin is present. Another approach could be to remove the aprotinin from the sample prior to the performance of the functional assays.[19]

Plasmin generation was evaluated by measuring plasmin–alpha-2-antiplasmin complexes. We found a significant increase in the placebo group, whereas in the

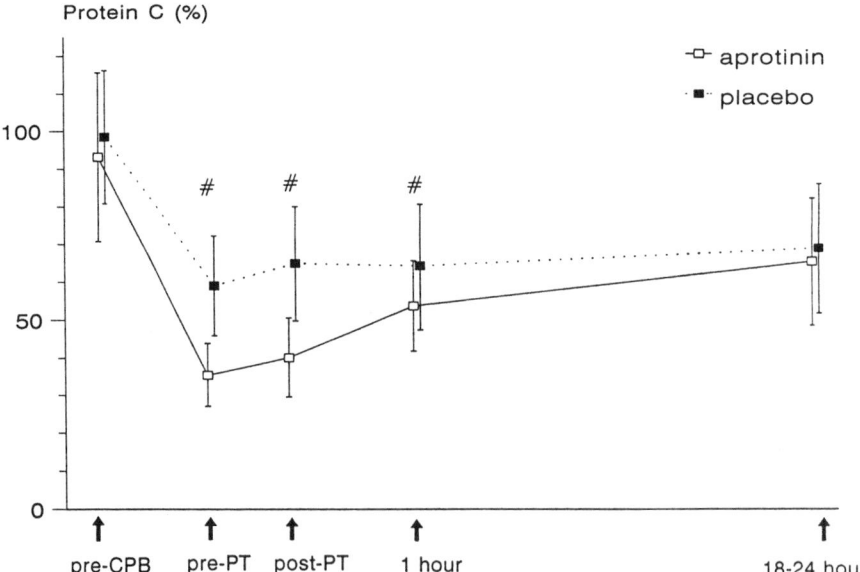

**FIGURE 3.** Protein C. Protein C levels were assessed by a chromogenic substrate assay. Different levels between both groups were found (# = $p < 0.05$), but these determinations can be artifactually influenced by aprotinin (means ± SD).

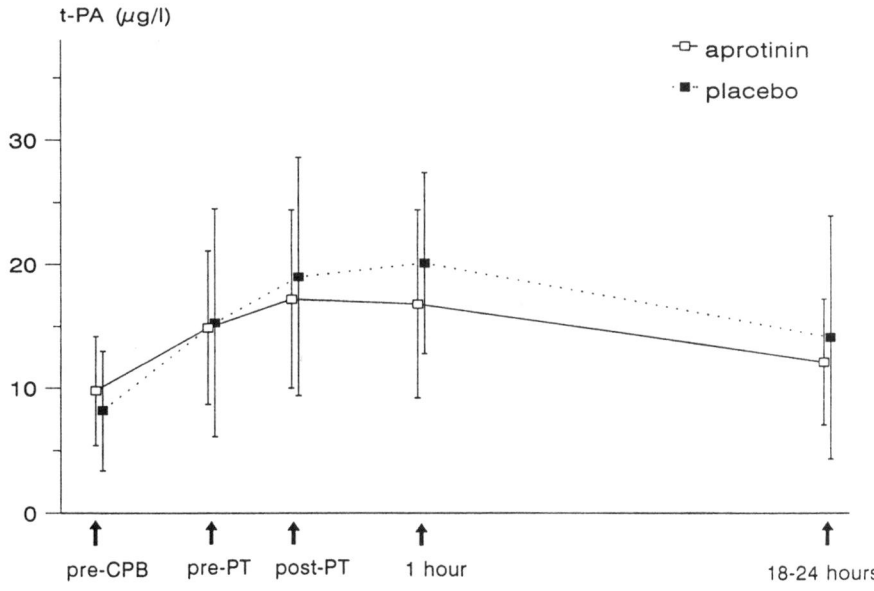

**FIGURE 4.** tPA. Antigenic tPA increased during CPB in the same way in both groups (mean ± SD).

aprotinin group, the increment was much less pronounced (Fig. 6). This could reflect the ability of aprotinin to inhibit the plasmin generated during CPB. The action of plasmin over cross-linked fibrin generates D-dimer. In our study, patients

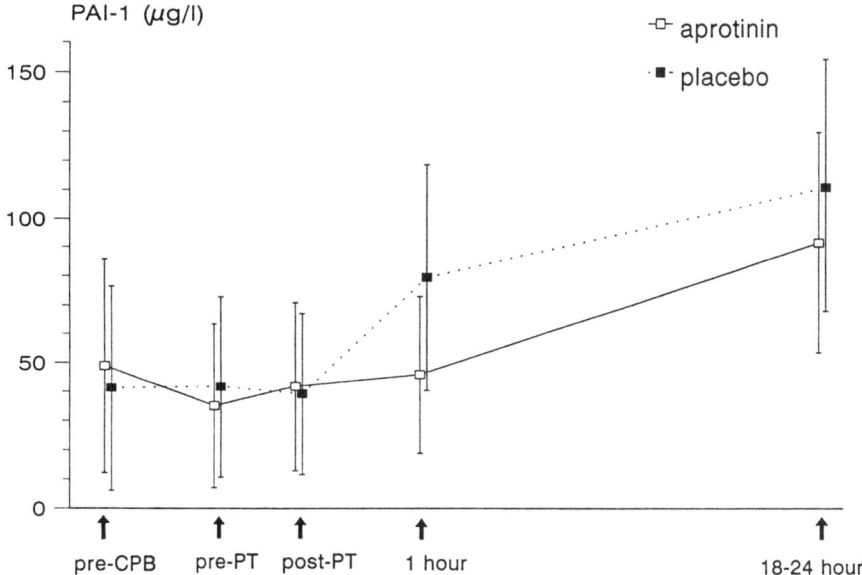

**FIGURE 5.** PAI-1. A significant increase in antigenic PAI-1 was seen at the end of CPB and in the postoperative period (18–24 hr), but no differences between groups were found (mean ± SD).

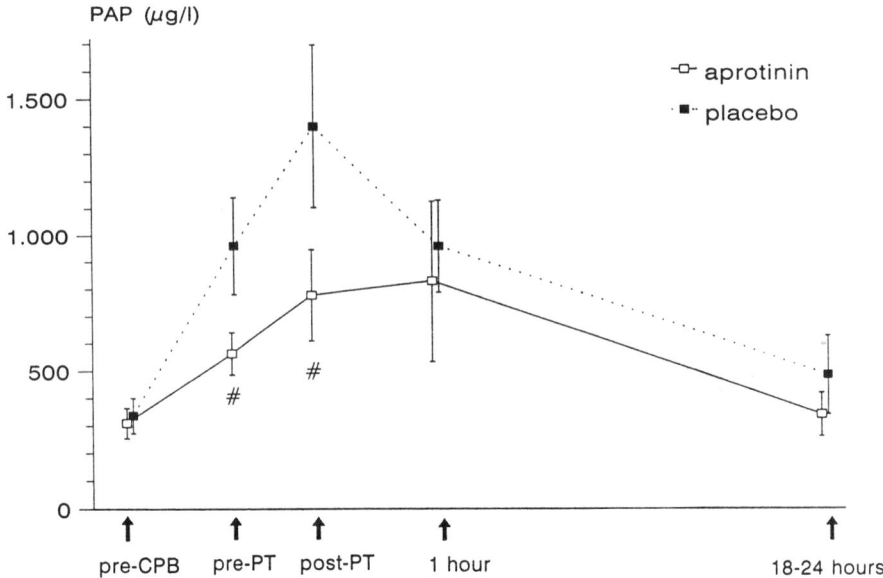

**FIGURE 6.** Plasmin–alpha-2 antiplasmin complexes (PAP). Levels of PAP complexes were raised in both groups, but the increment in the placebo group was significantly more pronounced (# = $p < 0.05$). Results are expressed as means ± SE.

who received aprotinin showed no significant increase in D-dimer levels, whereas placebo patients underwent a sharp rise (Fig. 7). Thus, patients receiving aprotinin had an efficient inhibition of fibrinolysis. CPB-associated hyperfibrinolysis has been

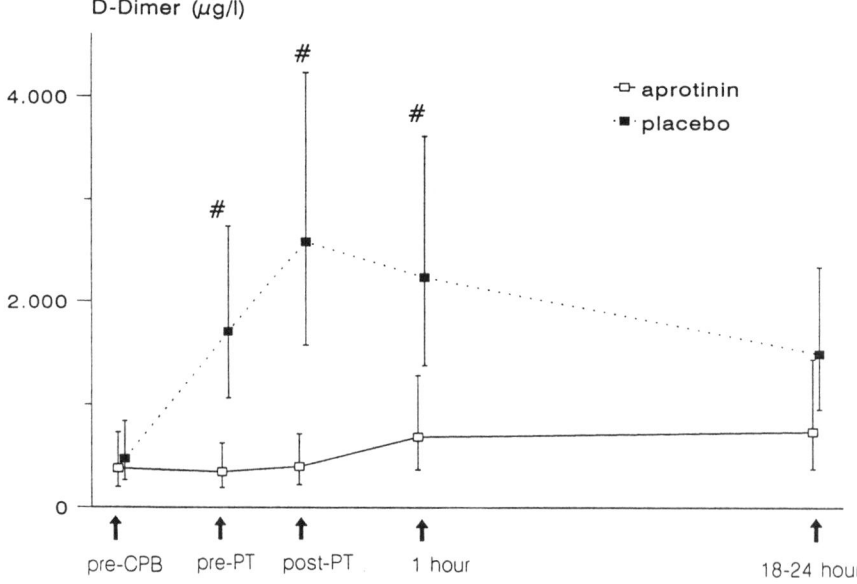

**FIGURE 7.** D-Dimer. D-Dimer markedly increased during CPB in the placebo group, but not in the aprotinin group (# = $p < 0.05$). D-Dimer levels are expressed as geometric means.

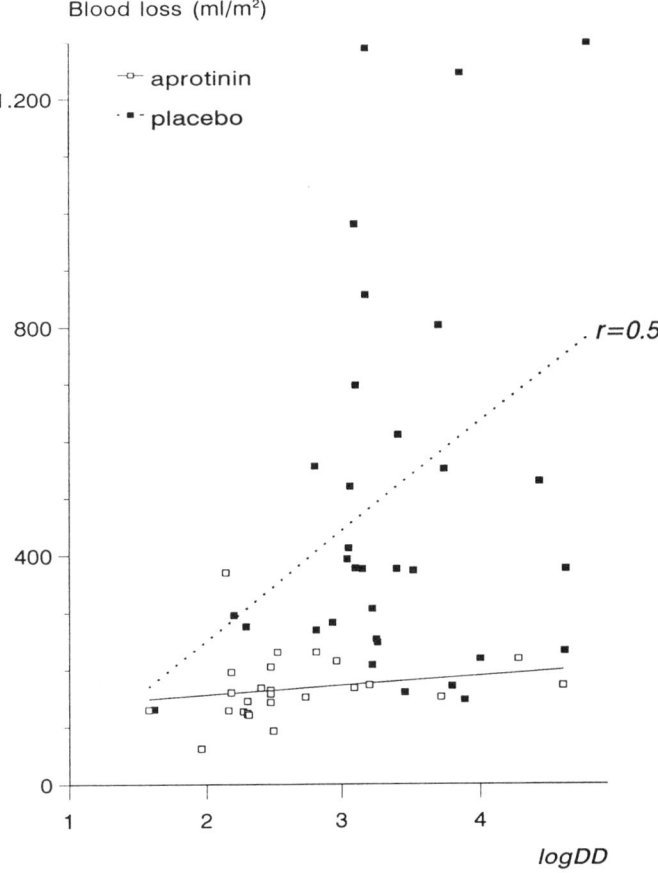

**FIGURE 8.** Blood loss. A correlation between overall blood loss (ml/m²) and D-dimer measurement after protamine neutralization was seen in the placebo group (*p* < 0.01). This correlation could not be found in the aprotinin group.

positively correlated with bleeding.[16] We found a positive correlation between overall blood loss and D-dimer in patients treated with placebo in the second (*r* = 0.5), third (*r* = 0.5), fourth (*r* = 0.5), and fifth (*r* = 0.5) determinations (all *p* < 0.01), but not in aprotinin group (Fig. 8). This finding could be of some interest in the future because this fibrinolytic marker could be used to predict bleeding tendency. In the aprotinin group, there was a poor fibrinolytic response caused by plasmin inhibition. In this group D-dimer did not significantly change during CPB, and hence no correlation with blood loss was found.

## Conclusion

The known effect of aprotinin in hemostasis is caused by its ability to inhibit plasmin and kallikrein. Kallikrein plays a role in activation of the intrinsic pathway of blood coagulation. Recently, this pathway of clotting activation has been considered to be of little importance.[15] Kallikrein also participates in the intrinsic fibrinolytic activation pathway. However, the benefit of aprotinin probably stems from its capacity to inhibit plasmin,[31] although it is still unclear whether this is its precise mode of action in the prevention of bleeding.

The available data support the idea that there is a marked activation of the fibrinolytic system throughout CPB. There is an increase in tPA and a consumption of plasminogen and its inhibitor, alpha-2 antiplasmin. Subsequently, PAI-1 increases following the tPA increment. Plasmin generation can be estimated by measuring levels of plasmin–alpha-2 antiplasmin complexes, which are increased during CPB. The marked increase in D-dimer reflects the action of plasmin over cross-linked fibrin. However, when aprotinin is administered, a similar increment of tPA and PAI-1 can be seen, but the slight increase in markers of generation and action of plasmin denotes a blockade of the fibrinolytic activation. The correlation found in our study between D-dimer and blood loss in the placebo group, but not in the aprotinin one, supports the notion that plasmin inhibition might play an important part in the ability of aprotinin to reduce bleeding in CPB surgery.

Finally, we would like to point out that because aprotinin is able to inhibit some enzymatic reactions occurring in vitro, several functional assays should be performed after the removal of aprotinin from the sample, or an antigenic procedure should be used.

## References

1. Andersen MN, Mendelow M, Alfano GA: Experimental studies of heparin-protamine activity with special reference to protamine inhibition of clotting. Surgery 46:1060–1068, 1959.
2. Bachmann F, McKenna R, Cole ER, Najafy H: The hemostatic mechanism after open heart surgery: Studies on plasma coagulation factors and fibrinolysis in 512 patients after extracorporeal circulation. J Thorac Cardiovasc Surg 70:76–85 1975.
3. Blauhut B, Gross CH, Necek S, et al: Effects of high-dose aprotinin on blood loss, platelet function, fibrinolysis, complement, and renal function after cardiopulmonary bypass. J Thorac Cardiovasc Surg 101:958–967, 1991.
4. Beurling-Harbury C, Galvan CA: Acquired decrease in platelet secretory ADP associated with increased postoperative bleeding in post-cardiopulmonary bypass patients and in patients with severe valvular heart disease. Blood 52:13–23, 1978.
5. Bidstrup BP, Royston D, Sapsford RN, Taylor KM: Effect of aprotinin on need for blood transfusion in patients with septic endocarditis having open heart surgery. Lancet 1:366–367, 1988.
6. Bidstrup BP, Royston D, Sapsford RN: Reduction in blood loss and blood use after cardiopulmonary bypass with high doses of aprotinin (Trasylol). J Thorac Cardiovasc Surg 97:364–372, 1989.
7. Casas JI, Zuazu-Jausoro I, Mateo J, et al: Aprotinin versus desmopressin for patients undergoing cardiopulmonary bypass surgery: A double-blind placebo-controlled study. (Submitted.)
8. Chabbat J, Porte P, Tellier M, Steinbuch M: Aprotinin is a competitive inhibitor of the factor VIIa–tissue factor complex. Thromb Res 71:205–215, 1993.
9. Dietrich W, Barankay A, Dilthey G, et al: Reduction of homologous blood requirement in cardiac surgery by intraoperative aprotinin application: Clinical experience in 152 cardiac surgical patients. Thorac Cardiovasc Surg 37:92–98, 1989.
10. Dietrich W, Spannagl M, Jochum M, et al: Influence of high-dose aprotinin treatment on blood loss and coagulation patterns in patients undergoing myocardial revascularization. Anesthesiology 73:1119–1126, 1990.
11. Esmon CT: The roles of protein C and thrombomodulin in the regulation of blood coagulation. J Biol Chem 264:4743–4746, 1989.
12. España F, Estellés A, Griffin JH, et al: Aprotinin (Trasylol) is a competitive inhibitor of activated protein C. Thromb Res 56:751–756, 1989.
13. Ferraris VA, Ferraris SP, Lough FC, Berry WR: Preoperative aspirin ingestion increases operative blood loss after coronary artery bypass grafting. Ann Thorac Surg 45:71–74, 1988.
14. Fraedrich G, Weber C, Bernard C, et al: Reduction of blood transfusion requirement in open-heart surgery. Lancet 37:89–91, 1989.

15. Furie B, Furie BC: Molecular and cellular biology of blood coagulation. N Engl J Med 326:800–806, 1992.
16. Gram J, Janetzko T, Jespersen J, Bruhn HD: Enhanced effective fibrinolysis following the neutralization of heparin in open heart surgery increases the risk of postsurgical bleeding. Thromb Haemost 63:241–245, 1990.
17. Harker LA, Malpass TW, Branson HE, et al: Mechanism of abnormal bleeding in patients undergoing cardiopulmonary bypass: Acquired transient platelet dysfunction associated with selective $\alpha$-granule release. Blood 56:824–834, 1980.
18. Havel M, Teufelsbauer H, Knöbl P, et al: Effect of intraoperative aprotinin administration on postoperative bleeding in patients undergoing cardiopulmonary bypass operation. J Thorac Cardiovasc Surg 101:968–972, 1991.
19. Johannessen M, Edsberg B, DeVries C, Nielsen F: A modified amidolytic assay non-affected by aprotinin for determination of $\alpha_2$-antiplasmin in plasma from patients undergoing cardiopulmonary bypass [abstract]. Thromb Haemost 69:1353, 1993.
20. Kawasuji M, Ueyama K, Sakakibara N, et al: Effect of low-dose aprotinin on coagulation and fibrinolysis in cardiopulmonary bypass. Ann Thorac Surg 55:1205–1209, 1993.
21. Lu H, Soria C, Commin PL, et al: Hemostasis in patients undergoing extracorporeal circulation: The effect of aprotinin (Trasylol). Thromb Haemost 66:633–637, 1991.
22. Mammen EF, Koets MH, Washintong BC, et al: Hemostasis changes during cardiopulmonary bypass surgery. Semin Thromb Hemost 11:291–292, 1985.
23. Musial J, Niewiarowski S, Hershock D, et al: Loss of fibrinogen receptors from the platelet surface during simulated extracorporeal circulation. J Lab Clin Med 105:514–522, 1985.
24. Rocha E, Hidalgo F, Llorens R, et al: A randomized study of aprotinin and DDAVP to reduce postoperative bleeding after cardiopulmonary bypass surgery. Circulation 90:921–927, 1994.
25. Royston D, Taylor KM, Bidstrup BP, Sapsford RN: Effect of aprotinin on need for blood transfusion after repeat open heart surgery. Lancet 2:1289–1291, 1987.
26. Royston D: High-dose aprotinin therapy: A review of the first five years' experience. J Thorac Cardiothorac Vasc Anesth 6:76–100, 1922.
27. Teufelsbauer H, Proidl S, Havel M, Vukovich TH: Early activation of hemostasis during cardiopulmonary bypass: Evidence for thrombin mediated hyperfibrinolysis. Thromb Haemost 68:250–252, 1992.
28. Van Oeveren W, Jansen NJG, Bidstrup BP, et al: Effects of aprotinin on hemostatic mechanism during cardiopulmonary bypass. Ann Thorac Surg 44:640–645, 1987.
29. Van Oeveren W, Eijsman L, Roozendaal KJ, Wildevuur CRH: Platelet preservation by aprotinin during cardiopulmonary bypass. Lancet 2:644, 1988.
30. Van Oeveren W, Harder MP, Roozendaal KJ, et al: Aprotinin protects platelets against the initial effect of cardiopulmonary bypass. J Thorac Cardiovasc Surg 99:788–797, 1990.
31. Verstrate M: Clinical application of inhibitors of fibrinolysis. Drugs 29:236–261, 1985.
32. Wendel HP, Gallimore MJ, Heller W: Aprotinin and its effects on chromogenic substrate assays for some components of the plasma defence systems [abstract]. Thromb Haemost 69:1270, 1993.
33. Wiman B: On the reaction of plasmin or plasmin-streptokinase complex with aprotinin or $\alpha_2$-antiplasmin. Thromb Res 17:143–152, 1980.

**Hanno Riess**

# 25

# The Use of Aprotinin in Liver Transplantation

Since the earliest attempts at liver transplantation in humans, survival rates and quality of life have improved dramatically. Orthotopic liver transplantation (OLT) includes excision of the diseased liver (anhepatic phase) and revascularization of an ischemic, cold-stored liver graft. This procedure has become an established therapeutic option in the treatment of fulminant hepatic failure and endstage liver disease.[43]

Soon after the start of liver transplantations about 30 years ago, increased blood loss in OLT was recognized as a significant contributory factor to postoperative morbidity and mortality. Various factors affect transfusion requirements in liver transplantation, such as severe parenchymal disease, ascites, and coagulation abnormalities.[4,40] The availability of new coagulation tests, as well as growing insight into the physiologic and pathophysiologic interactions of coagulation, fibrinolysis, platelets, leukocytes, and vessel walls, triggered new investigations of overtly disturbed hemostasis in liver transplantation. In addition, the increase in understanding of hemostasis in OLT led to clinical studies aimed at reducing bleeding complications with different kinds of drugs or blood components. Furthermore, control of bleeding and better coagulation profiles during and after liver transplantation reduced rates of surgical, immunologic, and infectious complications as well as the incidence of single or multiorgan failure.[4] As a result of such advances, along with improvements in surgical procedure, management of perioperative transfusion, and immunosuppressive regimens, the 1-year-survival rates after OLT may now be greater than 90%.

## Hemostasis in Liver Transplantation

The liver plays a pivotal role in coagulation. In addition to synthesis of clotting factors and inhibitors, the hepatic reticuloendothelial system is of major importance in the clearance and catabolism of hemostatic proteins. The pathogenesis of altered hemostasis in patients with advanced liver disease is complex and multifactorial. In

**TABLE 1.** Alterations of Hemostasis in Liver Disease

Reduced synthesis of proteases and inhibitors
Synthesis of abnormal molecules
Thrombocytopenia and platelet dysfunction
Enhanced fibrinolysis
Increased thrombin formation (low-level disseminated intravascular coagulation)
Altered cytokine network
Reduced reticuloendothelial clearance

addition to thrombocytopenia and platelet dysfunction, signs of enhanced fibrinolysis and increased disseminated intravascular coagulation (DIC) are common (Table 1). During OLT hemostasis is further disturbed by the following factors:

1. Extensive surgical trauma results from dissection of adhesions in the abdominal cavity and transsection of the many collateral vessels that were formed in response to inflammation, previous surgery, or portal hypertension during the preanhepatic phase.

2. Loss of the diseased liver, with its low-level synthetic and clearance functions during the anhepatic phase, clearly results in more severe deterioration of hemostasis compared with heterotopic liver transplantation, in which the diseased liver is left in situ.[2]

3. Reperfusion of the cold-stored graft results in complex alterations, such as reperfusion injury, systemic influx of perservation fluid and mediators released from the ischemic graft, and immediate onset of immunologic processes in the postanhepatic phase. In the operating room bleeding complications are most likely during the postanhepatic phase, presenting as diffuse oozing in a previously dry surgical field.

Hyperfibrinolysis, which is most pronounced at the end of the anhepatic phase and immediately after reperfusion, and increased thrombin formation, which begins with perfusion of the graft, characterize the deterioration of the already severely altered hemostasis in OLT (Figs. 1 and 2).[5,8,14,16,17,33-38] Both the extrinsic pathway, which is mediated by tissue-type plasminogen activator (tPA), and the intrinsic pathway, which is mediated by urokinase-type plasminogen activator (uPA), are involved in hyperfibrinolysis.[8,15,17,20,34] In the operating room hyperfibrinolysis is easily visualized by thromboelastography[24] and confirmed by increases in tPA activity, uPA activity, fibrin(ogen) degradation products, and plasmin–antiplasmin complexes as well as decreases in plasminogen.

After revascularization of the graft, systemic fibrinolysis is inhibited by steeply increasing levels of plasminogen activator inhibitor (PAI) and a DIC-like state that results in increased prothrombin activation; in addition, decreases in platelets, fibrinogen, antithrombin III, protein C, and C1 inhibitor, as well as increases in fibrin monomers, cathepsin B, and complexes of thrombin–antithrombin and elastase–proteinase inhibitor, are regularly observed.[5,14,17] Reperfusion injury, associated with mediators released from the graft and leukocyte activation, may be important in this process.[5,36,37] Release of plasminogen activators from the graft,[42] as well as nonspecific proteolysis induced by mediators released from the graft or generated in response to revascularization, such as elastase,[26,36] cathepsin B,[37] and cytokines,[10,38] may further stimulate lysis of hemostatic plugs with subsequent oozing.

Correlation between the degree of hyperfibrinolysis and blood product usage[34] suggests that antifibrinolytic therapy may decrease transfusion requirements in OLT. Indeed, epsilon aminocaproic acid (EACA), a synthetic antifibrinolytic agent, was used in the first liver transplantation done in Pittsburgh. Bleeding tendency

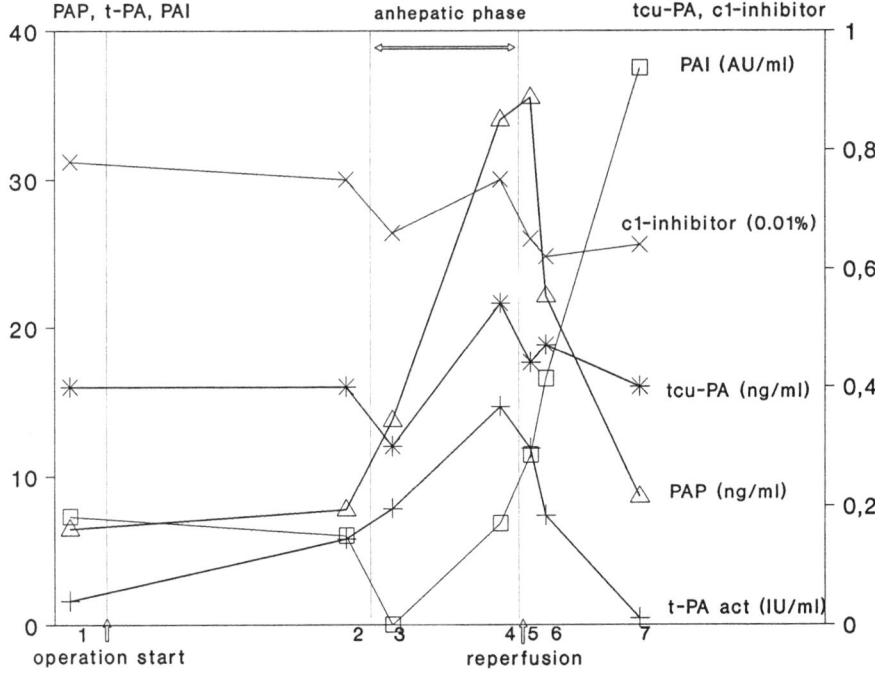

**FIGURE 1.** Plasma levels of selected parameters during OLT (n = 10). PAP = plasmin–antiplasmin complexes, PAI = plasminogen activator inhibitor, tPA = tissue-type plasminogen activator, tcu-PA = two-chain urokinase-type plasminogen activator. Time 1 = after induction of anesthesia, time 2 = 5 minutes before anhepatic phase, time 3 = 10 minutes after beginning of anhepatic phase, time 4 = 5 minutes before reperfusion, time 5 = 5 minutes after reperfusion, time 6 = 15 minutes after reperfusion, time 7 = 60 minutes after reperfusion.

was reduced, but the incidence of fatal thromboembolic complications was high. Some centers now use EACA in combination with intraoperative monitoring by thromboelastography.[23]

## Aprotinin in Orthotopic Liver Transplantation

Well-designed randomized, double-blind trials in cardiac surgery have shown that aprotinin, a potent antifibrinolytic agent, significantly reduces blood product requirements.[7,39] Because hyperfibrinolysis correlates significantly with blood loss[34] and blood loss with mortality rates during the first half year after surgery,[40] the potential role of aprotinin in liver transplantation with regard to hemostasis, transfusion requirements, and mortality warranted investigation.

### Clinical Studies

In the initial report from Neuhaus et al.[30] of its potentially beneficial effect in liver transplantation, aprotinin was given in three boluses of 0.5 million KIU each: during induction of anesthesia, immediately before the anhepatic phase, and immediately before reperfusion (Tables 2 and 3). This low-dose regimen was chosen

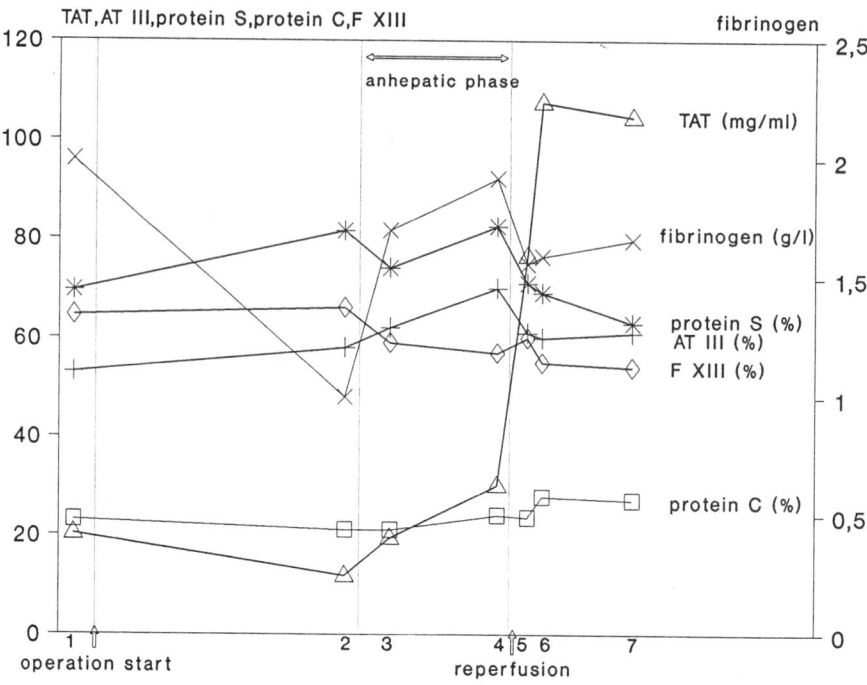

**FIGURE 2.** Plasma levels of selected parameters during OLT (n = 10). TAT = thrombin-antithrombin III complexes, AT III = antithrombin III, F XIII = coagulation factor XIII. Time 1 = after induction of anesthesia, time 2 = 5 minutes before anhepatic phase, time 3 = 10 minutes after beginning of anhepatic phase, time 4 = 5 minutes before reperfusion, time 5 = 5 minutes after reperfusion, time 6 = 15 minutes after reperfusion, time 7 = 60 minutes after reperfusion.

**TABLE 2.** Aprotinin Dose and Transfusion Requirements

| Study | Dose (million KIU) | RBC (U) | Controls | RBC (U) | n/n (p) |
|---|---|---|---|---|---|
| Neuhaus et al., 1991[3,30] | Boluses: 3 × 0.5 | 7.5 | Historic | 9.7 | 10/10 (s) |
| Grosse et al., 1991[13] | Bolus: 2.0 Inf: 0.5/hr | 8.1 | Historic | 23.3 | 40/50 (hs) |
| Mallet et al., 1991[27,28] | Bolus: 2.0 Inf: 0.5/hr 0.07/U (RBC) | 7.5 | Historic | 23.6 | 20/25 (hs) |
| Groh et al., 1992[11,12] | Bolus: 2.0 Inf: 0.5/hr | 18 | Prospectively randomized | 20 | 9/9 (ns) |
| Himmelreich et al., 1992[18] | Bolus: 0 Inf: 0.2–0.4 hr | 7 | Prospectively randomized 3 × 0.5 | 8 | 10/13 (ns) |
| Ickx et al., 1993[21] | Bolus: 0 Inf: 0.36 hr | 7 | Bolus: 0 Inf: 0.18/hr TEG monitoring | 7.4 | 5/5 (ns) |
| Suarez et al., 1993[45] | Bolus: 2.0 Inf: 0.5/hr | 7 | Nonrandomized | 11.6 | 13/15% (hs) |

Inf = infusion, RBC = red blood cells, s = significant, hs = highly significant, ns = not significant, TEG = thromboelastography.

**TABLE 3.**   Intraoperative Aprotinin Regimens in the Study by Himmelreich et al.

| Bolus (million KIU) | Time/Period | Infusion (million KIU) |
| --- | --- | --- |
| 0.5 | Induction of anesthesia | 0.2/hr |
| 0.5 | Start of anhepatic phase | 0.4/hr |
| 0.5 | Start of postanhepatic phase | 0.4/hr |

From Himmelreich G, Muser M, Neuhaus P, et al: Different aprotinin applications influencing hemostatic changes in orthotopic liver transplantation. Transplantation 53:132–136, 1992, with permission.

instead of the higher-dose continuous infusion advocated by cardiac surgeons[39] because of the fear of perioperative thromboses, since anticoagulation is not used in OLT. In addition, the large foreign surface involved in open-heart surgery results in excessive contact activation that requires higher levels of aprotinin to block activation of kallikrein.[9,46] Requirements were not expected to be as high in the venovenous bypass used in OLT. In the initial study of 10 consecutive patients with primary allografts, the clinical impression of unusually dry surgical fields after revascularization was confirmed by significant reductions in blood product requirement (see Table 2) and in operating time from revascularization to skin closure compared with 10 previous historic controls.[3,30]

The results of Neuhaus et al. were confirmed by Mallet et al.,[27,28] who used a modification of the well-established aprotinin regimen from cardiac surgery.[39] In addition to the induction bolus and continuous infusion, they added 0.7 million KIU of aprotinin to each unit of blood transfused intraoperatively. Retrospective analysis revealed significant reductions in blood product requirements, operative time, and length of stay in the intensive care unit. Two other nonrandomized studies[13,45] of the aprotinin protocol used in cardiac surgery[39] confirmed these results (see Table 2).

In contrast, the only placebo-controlled, randomized study of aprotinin in OLT with the dosing scheme of Royston et al.[39] failed to show a significant benefit for the aprotinin-treated group with regard to transfusion requirement or other clinical endpoints.[11,12] Unfortunately, 2 of 20 patients were excluded from the analysis because of massive hemorrhage and early death, resulting in a relatively small population. Furthermore, transfusion requirements in both groups were higher than in other studies in the early 1990s (see Table 2), despite the use of an intensive intraoperative monitoring system as well as intraoperative platelet transfusions and antithrombin III replacement.[12]

The total estimated dose of aprotinin used intraoperatively by the various investigators ranges from 1.5–about 5.6 million KIU,[3,11,13,21,28,45] and the range of plasma levels is even more speculative. To address the question of dosage, we performed a prospectively randomized, controlled trial[18] comparing the bolus regimen with continuous intravenous infusion (see Tables 2 and 3). With continuous infusion significantly higher concentrations of aprotinin were obtained throughout the procedure (Fig. 3). We observed a trend toward lower transfusion requirements in the infusion group; statistical significance, however, was reached only for red blood cell transfusions within the first 3 postoperative days.

## Hemostasis

Thorough investigations of hemostasis by our group and several others, using different laboratory parameters, demonstrated reductions in the increase of fibrinolysis

## INTRA-/POSTOPERATIVE APROTININ LEVELS
### Boli versus Infusion

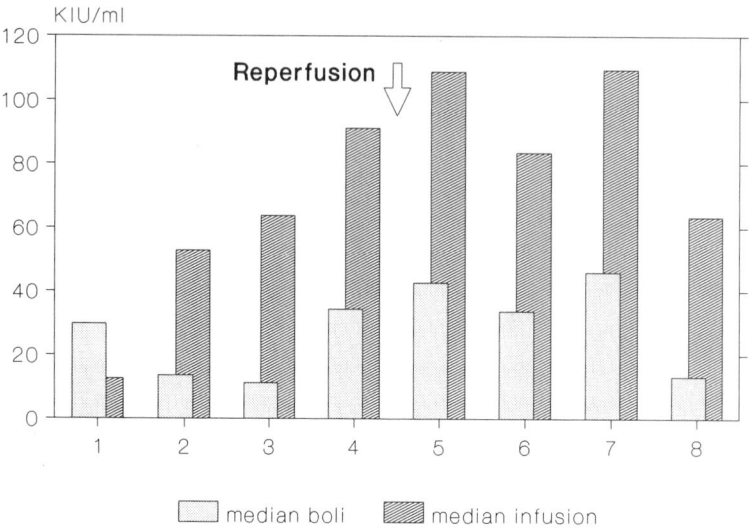

**FIGURE 3.** Plasma levels of aprotinin according to the application regimen.[18] Time 1 = after induction of anesthesia, time 2 = 5 minutes before anhepatic phase, time 3 = 10 minutes after beginning of anhepatic phase, time 4 = 5 minutes before reperfusion, time 5 = 5 minutes after reperfusion, time 6 = 15 minutes after reperfusion, time 7 = 60 minutes after reperfusion, time 8 = 12 hours after reperfusion.

in the aprotinin-treated group compared with controls. In a small randomized, controlled study, Cottam et al.[6,19] demonstrated significantly reduced levels of tPA at the end of the anhepatic phase when aprotinin was infused according to the Royston protocol. The investigators postulated that aprotinin reduces production of tPA through inhibition of kallikrein and fibrinolysis through inhibition of plasmin. Their results were confirmed by Grosse et al.[13] in a nonrandomized comparison. The antifibrinolytic efficacy of aprotinin also has been demonstrated in vitro by treating blood samples obtained during OLT with and without aprotinin before thromboelastography.[22]

According to several parameters, such as thromboelastography (Fig. 4), tPA activity, and plasmin–antiplasmin complexes, hyperfibrinolysis was better controlled with higher doses of aprotinin.[18] On the other hand, peak levels of thrombin-antithrombin complexes were higher in the infusion group, probably reflecting increased formation of thrombin when fibrinolysis is inhibited by aprotinin. Similarly, Ickx et al.[21] discuss the possibility of increased thromboembolic complications with higher doses of aprotinin. In clinical terms, however, use of our infusion protocol (see Table 2) in hundreds of patients suggests that perioperative thromboembolic complications are extremely rare.

Because oozing becomes apparent only after revascularization of the graft, is more likely in grafts with suspected severe ischemic damage, and is less severe in heterotopic liver transplantation, the donor liver may play an important role in the alteration of hemostasis. Therefore, samples of the perfusate—e.g., blood passing

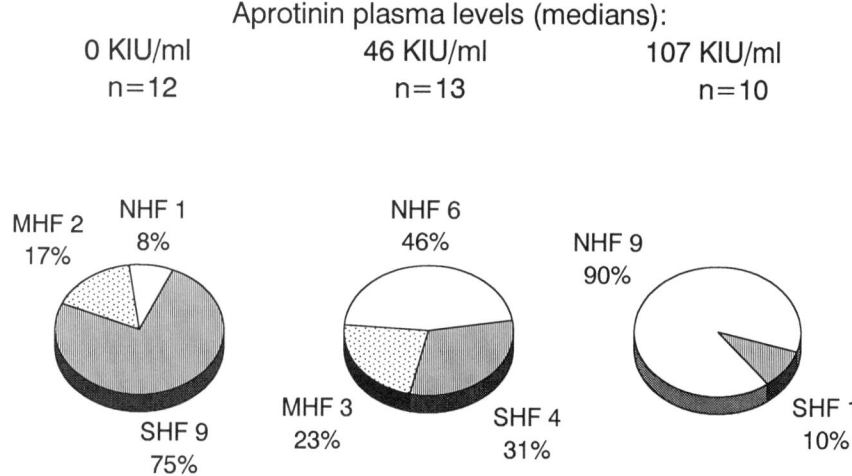

Aprotinin plasma levels (medians):

| 0 KIU/ml | 46 KIU/ml | 107 KIU/ml |
| n=12 | n=13 | n=10 |

**FIGURE 4.** Incidence of hyperfibrinolysis in thromboelastography (TEG) during OLT in relation to plasma levels of aprotinin. The incidence was estimated in two patient groups receiving different doses of aprotinin[18] and in a nonrandomized control group without aprotinin. Maximal hyperfibrinolysis detected in TEG tracings at the end of the anhepatic phase or early after reperfusion were graded according to whole-blood clot lysis time (time between end of clot formation and total spontaneous clot lysis; WBCLT). NHF = no hyperfibrinolysis (WBCLT > 120 min), MHF = mild hyperfibrinolysis (90 min < WBCLT < 120 min), SHF = severe hyperfibrinolysis (WBCLT < 90 min).

through the liver immediately after reperfusion—were collected by venting the inferior vena cava in our randomized study[18] of bolus vs. infusion aprotinin. Although the activity level of tPA antigen was lower, the activity levels of plasminogen activator inhibitor and alpha-2 antiplasmin were higher in the perfusate from patients in the infusion group (Table 4). In the infusion group, cathepsin B, released from macrophages[1] and hepatocytes, was nonsignificantly lower in the perfusate and increased significantly less in the systemic circulation.[38] Such results may reflect reduced endothelial and hepatocellular damage in the liver graft by higher levels of aprotinin during reperfusion. This view is supported by reports of the protective effects of aprotinin against myocardial and hepatocellular ischemic damage in models of warm as well as cold ischemia.[25,29,44] Similarly, continuous infusion of aprotinin in a pig model of OLT resulted in both significantly reduced hepatocellular ischemic damage and significantly prolonged survival compared with controls.[31,32]

## Conclusion

Numerous clinical investigations have shown a reduction in hyperfibrinolysis and blood product requirements, especially during the anhepatic and early postanhepatic phases of OLT, when aprotinin is administered intraoperatively.[3,6,13,18,19,27,28,30,41,45] A large multicenter trial will address questions about the role and dose of aprotinin more definitively.

On the other hand, the otherwise unusual experience of a dry operative field at the end of the surgical procedure when aprotinin is used intraoperatively—an

**TABLE 4.**   Selected Parameters (Medians and Range) Estimated in the Perfusate of the Liver Graft in OLT Using Two Different Doses of Aprotinin

| Parameter | Bolus Group (n = 13) | Infusion Group (n = 10) | p |
|---|---|---|---|
| Fibrinogen (gm/l) | 1.5 (0–2.2) | 1.5 (0–2.6) | 0.48 |
| Plasminogen (%) | 43 (3–77) | 50 (35–87) | 0.29 |
| Thrombin–antithrombin III complex (ng/ml) | 93.2 (40.5–324.2) | 73.5 (32.5–1500) | 0.29 |
| Plasmin-antiplasmin complex (ng/ml) | 61.4 (29–120) | 57.7 (34–93) | 0.49 |
| Elastase-proteinase inhibitor complex (ng/ml) | 637 (136–904) | 912 (399–1396) | 0.09 |
| Cathepsin B (U/L) | 34,710 (7,032–142,695) | 22,191 (967–524,265) | 0.40 |
| Tissue-type plasminogen activator (ng/ml) | 12.3 (7.2–26.6) | 10.1 (1.2–19.3) | 0.05 |
| Tissue-type plasminogen activator (IU/ml) | 12 (0.7–23.6) | 5 (0.7–17.7) | 0.10 |
| Antiplasmin (%) | 63 (5–95) | 93 (68–102) | 0.01 |
| Plasminogen activator inhibitor (AU/ml) | 6.4 (0–22) | 17.8 (8.8–30.4) | 0.04 |

Data from Himmelreich G, Muser M, Neuhaus P, et al: Different aprotinin applications influencing hemostatic changes in orthotopic liver transplantation. Transplantation 53:132–136, 1992, and Riess H, Jochum M, Machleidt W, et al: Role of leukocytes in hemostasis during orthotopic liver transplantation. Semin Thromb Hemost 19:197–208, 1993, with permission.

admittedly subjective impression—has led to the routine use of aprotinin in several transplantation centers. Prospective monitoring for eventual adverse effects—especially anaphylactoid reactions[47]—in more than 400 patients undergoing OLT in Berlin confirms the safety of aprotinin in this setting, even in patients with a history of aprotinin use.

# References

1. Assfalg-Machleidt I, Jochum M, Nast-Kolb D, et al: Cathepsin B: Indicator for the release of lysosomal cysteine proteinases in severe trauma and inflammation. Biol Chem Hoppeseyler 371:211–222, 1990.
2. Bakker CM, Metselaar HJ, Groenland THN, et al: Increased tissue-type plasminogen activator activity in orthotopic but not in heterotopic liver transplantation. The role of the anhepatic period. Hepatology 16:40–48, 1992.
3. Bechstein WO, Riess H, Neuhaus P, et al: The effect of aprotinin on blood product requirements during orthotopic liver transplantation. Clin Transplant 5:422–426, 1991.
4. Bontempo FA, Lewis JH, van Thiel DH, et al: The relation of preoperative coagulation findings to diagnosis, blood usage, and survival in adult liver transplantation. Transplantation 39:532–536, 1985.
5. Carrell RW, Luddington RJ, Jennings I, et al: Coagulation changes following hepatic revascularization during liver transplantation. Transplantation 48:603–607, 1989.
6. Cottam S, Hunt B, Segal H, et al: Aprotinin inhibits tissue plasminogen activator-mediated fibrinolysis during orthotopic liver transplantation. Transplant Proc 23:1933, 1991.
7. Dietrich W, Barankay A, Dilthey G, et al: Reduction in homologous blood requirement in cardiac surgery by intraoperative aprotinin application. J Thorac Cardiovasc Surg 37:92–98, 1989.
8. Dzik WH, Arkin CF, Jenkins RL, et al: Fibrinolysis during liver transplantation in humans: Role of tissue-type plasminogen activator. Blood 71:1090–1095, 1988.

9. Fritz H, Wunderer G, Jochum M: Biochemistry and applications of aprotinin, the kallikrein inhibitor from bovine organs. Arzneimittelforschung Drug Res 33:479–494, 1983.

10. Függer R, Hamilton G, Steininger R, et al: Intraoperative estimation of endotoxin, TNFa, and IL-6 in orthotopic liver transplantation and their relationship to rejection and postoperative infection. Transplantation 52:302–306, 1991.

11. Groh J, Welte M, Azad SC, et al: Does aprotinin affect blood loss in liver transplantation? Lancet 340:173, 1992.

12. Groh J, Welte M, Azad SC, et al: Does aprotinin really reduce blood loss in orthotopic liver transplantation? Semin Thromb Hemost 19:306–308, 1993.

13. Grosse H, Lobbes W, Frambach M, et al: The use of high dose aprotinin in liver transplantation. The influence of fibrinolysis and blood loss. Thromb Res 63:287–297, 1991.

14. Harper PL, Luddington RJ, Jennings I, et al: Coagulation changes following hepatic revascularization during liver transplantation. Transplantation 48:603–607, 1989.

15. Himmelreich G, Dooijewaard G, Breinl P, et al: Evolution of urokinase-type plasminogen activator (u-PA) and tissue-type plasminogen activator (t-PA) in orthotopic liver transplantation (OLT). Thromb Haemost 69:56–59, 1993.

16. Himmelreich G, Hundt K, Neuhaus P, et al: Decreased platelet aggregation after reperfusion in orthotopic liver transplantation. Transplantation 58:582–586, 1992.

17. Himmelreich G, Kierzek B, Neuhaus P, et al: Coagulation changes and the influence of the early perfusate in the course of orthotopic liver transplantation (OLT) when aprotinin is used intraoperatively. Blood Coagul Fibrinol 2:51–59, 1991.

18. Himmelreich G, Muser M, Neuhaus P, et al: Different aprotinin applications influencing hemostatic changes in orthotopic liver transplantation. Transplantation 53:132–136, 1992.

19. Hunt BJ, Cottam S, Segal H, et al: Inhibition by aprotinin by tPA—mediated fibrinolysis during orthotopic liver transplantation. Lancet 336:381, 1990.

20. Ichinose A, Fujikawa K, Suyama T: The activation of pro-urokinase by plasma kallikrein and its inactivation by thrombin. J Biol Chem 261:3486–3489, 1989.

21. Ickx B, Pradier O, Degroote F, et al: Effect of two different dosages of aprotinin on perioperative blood loss during liver transplantation. Semin Thromb Hemost 19:300–301, 1993.

22. Kang Y, de Wolf AM, Aggarwal S, et al: In vitro study of the effects of aprotinin on coagulation during orthotopic liver transplantation. Transplant Proc 23:1934–1935, 1991.

23. Kang YG, Lewis JH, Navalgung A, et al: Epsilon-aminocaproic acid for treatment of fibrinolysis during liver transplantation. Anesthesiology 66:766–773, 1987.

24. Kang YG, Martin DJ, Marques J, et al: Intraoperative changes in blood coagulation and thrombelastographic monitoring in liver transplantation. Anaesth Analg 64:888–896, 1985.

25. Lie TS, Seger R, Hong GS, et al: Protective effect of aprotinin in ischemic hepatocellular damage. Transplantation 48:396–399, 1989.

26. Machovic R, Owen WG: The elastase-mediated pathway of fibrinolysis. Blood Coagul Fibrinol 1:79–90, 1990.

27. Mallet SV, Rolles K, Cox D, et al: Intraoperative use of aprotinin (Trasylol) in orthotopic liver transplantation. Transplant Proc 23:1931–1932, 1991.

28. Mallet SV, Cox D, Burroughs A, et al: Aprotinin and reduction of blood loss and transfusion requirements in orthotopic liver transplantation. Lancet 336:886–887, 1990.

29. Morgan GR, Harvey PRC, Strasberg SM: Aprotinin for the pretreatment of liver allograft donors. Transplantation 49:1203, 1990.

30. Neuhaus P, Bechstein WO, Lefèbre B, et al: Effect of aprotinin in intraoperative bleeding and fibrinolysis in liver transplantation. Lancet 2:924–925, 1989.

31. Oldhafer KJ, Hauss J, Spiegel HU, et al: Tisue $P_{O_2}$ and reperfusion injury in the transplanted liver after application of aprotinin. Transplant Proc 25:2555–2555, 1993.

32. Oldhafer KJ, Schüttler W, Wiehe B, et al: Treatment of preservation/reperfusion liver injury by the protease inhibitor aprotinin after cold ischemic storage. Transplant Proc 23:2380–2381, 1991.

33. Palareti G, Legnani C, Mazziotti A, et al: The "lytic state" during orthotopic liver transplantation: Plasminogen activators and other protease activities. Semin Thromb Hemost 19:290–291, 1993.

34. Porte RJ, Bontempo FA, Knot EAR, et al: Systemic effects of tissue plasminogen activator-associated fibrinolysis and its relation to thrombin generation in orthotopic liver transplantation. Transplantation 47:978–984, 1989.

35. Porte RJ, Knot EAR, Bontempo FA: Hemostasis in liver transplantation. Gastroenterology 97:488–501, 1989.

36. Riess H, Jochum M, Machleidt W, et al: Possible role of extracellularly released phagocyte proteinases in the coagulation disorder during liver transplantation. Transplantation 52:482–490, 1991.
37. Riess H, Jochum M, Machleidt W, et al: Possible role of the phagocytic proteinases cathepsin B and elastase in orthotopic liver transplantation. Transplant Proc 23:1947–1949, 1991.
38. Riess H, Jochum M, Machleidt W, et al: Role of leukocytes in hemostasis during orthotopic liver transplantation. Semin Thromb Hemost 19:197–208, 1993.
39. Royston D, Bidstrup BP, Taylor KM: Effect of aprotinin on need for blood transfusion after repeat open-heart surgery. Lancet ii:1289–1291, 1987.
40. Shaw BW Jr, Wood RP, Gordon RD, et al: Influence of selected patient variables and operative blood loss on six month survival following liver transplantation. Semin Liver Dis 5:385–393, 1985.
41. Smith O, Hazlehurst G, Brozovic B, et al: Impact of aprotinin on blood transfusion requirements in liver transplantation. Trans Med 3:97–102, 1993.
42. Smokovitis A: Normal liver actually possesses a high vascular plasminogen activator activity. Experientia 35:776–777, 1979.
43. Starzl TE, Iwatsuki S, Thiel DH, et al: Evolution of liver transplantation. Hepatology 2:614–636, 1982.
44. Suamori M, Amano J, Kameda T, et al: Additive protection of aprotinin, proteinase inhibitor of cold cardioplegia from ischemic myocardium. Jpn Circ J 44:771–778, 1980.
45. Suarez M, Sangro B, Herrero J, et al: Effectiveness of aprotinin in orthotopic liver transplantation. Semin Thromb Hemost 19:292–296, 1993.
46. Verstraete M: Clinical applications of inhibitors of fibrinolysis. Drugs 29:236–261, 1985.
47. Wüthrich B, Schmid P, Schmid ER, et al: IgE-mediated anaphylactic reaction to aprotinin during anaesthesia. Lancet 340:173–174, 1992.

**Marc Janssens**
**Maurice Lamy**

# 26

# The Use of Aprotinin in Orthopedic Surgery

Blood loss during orthopedic surgery frequently necessitates transfusion. A recent multicenter study of hip surgery[46] showed that blood loss averaged 3–4 units and that the mean transfusion requirement was 2–3 units of packed red cells per patient. Some centers have reported losses as high as 2 L.[24,52] Under these conditions, all available techniques of blood savings must be used to avoid excessive transfusion. Currently used strategies include techniques which involve preferential use of the patient's blood (autologous transfusion) and/or techniques aimed at reducing the blood loss itself. Autologous blood can be obtained before surgery using predonation, at the start of surgery using normovolemic hemodilution, or during the operation using salvage of shed blood. Anesthetic techniques, such as controlled hypotension or locoregional anesthesia (epidural, three-in-one block), diminish blood loss and thus transfusion requirements.

Another possibility to reduce bleeding involves use of pharmacologic substances to improve hemostasis. Aprotinin has been shown to reduce blood loss in cardiac surgery,[1,6,7,13,20,40,41] liver transplantation,[31] and abdominal aortic surgery,[45] all surgical procedures that may result in severe bleeding. Although the full range of aprotinin's effects has yet to be elucidated, several mechanisms have been proposed.[14] First, high-dose aprotinin inhibits fibrinolytic activity both by direct inhibition of plasmin[49] and by inhibition of the kinin-kallikrein system.[13] Decreased production of bradykinin reduces the release of tissue plasminogen activator, resulting in decreased production of plasmin.[22] Second, high dose aprotinin may partially inhibit the intrinsic coagulation pathway while leaving the extrinsic pathway intact.[10,11,13,18] Finally, a protective effect of aprotinin on glycoprotein Ib receptors, responsible for platelet adhesion, and on glycoprotein IIb-IIIa receptors, responsible for platelet aggregation, has also been suggested.[7,40,47,48,51]

During cardiac surgery, extracorporeal circulation modifies platelet receptors[30,50] and activates several biochemical systems involved in coagulation,[29] potentially leading to bleeding. Patients scheduled for liver transplantation may suffer severe preoperative hemostatic disorders. In orthopedic surgery, bleeding seems to be more dependent upon surgical approach and skill than on surgically induced biochemical coagulation abnormalities. This explains why recent studies have been performed to confirm the efficacy of aprotinin in this type of surgery.

Until now, aprotinin has only been used for hip surgery. Its efficacy, both in terms of reduction of intra- and postoperative blood loss as well as on reduction of transfusion requirements has been evaluated by several authors.[19,24,52] The appearance of side effects, especially thromboembolic phenomena, has been carefully sought.[19,24] The effect of aprotinin on renal function, as well as the appearance of allergic manifestations, has also been studied. An attempt at elucidating the mechanism of action of aprotinin in orthopedic surgery has also been carried out.[24]

## Blood Loss Reduction

The first report of a reduction of blood loss by aprotinin in hip surgery was made by Wollinsky et al. in 1991.[52] Forty patients undergoing total hip replacement were studied. Twenty patients received a bolus of 4 mg/kg aprotinin ($\pm$ 1.5 $\times$ 10$^6$ kallikrein inactivator units [KIU]) prior to incision, followed by a continuous infusion of 1 mg/kg/hr ($\pm$ 5 $\times$ 10$^5$ KIU/hr). This study showed a significant reduction in postoperative bleeding in the patients treated with aprotinin ($p < 0.01$), especially during the first 6 hours after surgery. There was a trend to lower intraoperative losses, but this did not reach statistical significance. Globally, the aprotinin group lost 1578 ml versus 1952 ml in the controls. Salvage of shed blood allowed recovery of 750 ml and 1100 ml in the aprotinin and control groups, respectively ($p < 0.01$). Loss of hemoglobin to drainage was also less in the treated group ($p < 0.01$).

In a randomized, double-blind study, Haas et al.[19] also showed that aprotinin (1.5 $\times$ 10$^6$ KIU at the start of surgery) reduced postoperative blood loss from 800 ml in the controls to 580 ml in the treated patients ($p < 0.05$). Postoperative hematomas were also less frequent in the aprotinin group (15% versus 28%).

Recently, 40 patients scheduled for primary elective total hip replacement were randomly allocated to receive, in a double-blind fashion, either preservative-free aprotinin given as a bolus injection of 2 $\times$ 10$^6$ KIU over 30 minutes followed by an infusion of 5 $\times$ 10$^5$ KIU/hr until the end of surgery, or the same volume of normal saline according to the same protocol.[24] Surgical technique, which consisted in a posterolateral approach with osteotomy of the greater trochanter, was standardized and performed in all patients by the same surgeon. When non-cemented prostheses were placed, cancellous screws were used to secure the acetabular component. Cemented prostheses were equally distributed between the two groups (7 in the aprotinin group, 10 in the placebo group). All operations were carried out using a standardized general anesthesia technique. Except for predonation in 17 patients in the placebo group and 14 patients in the aprotinin group, no special blood-saving techniques (such as intra- or postoperative shed-blood recovery or intentional preoperative normovolemic hemodilution) were used. The anesthesiologist estimated intraoperative blood loss by measuring the volume in the suction bottles and counting sponges ($\pm$ 5 ml/sponge). At the end of the surgery, the surgeon evaluated bleeding on a four-point rating scale as slight, moderate, heavy, or very heavy. Postoperative blood loss also was measured from the surgical drains over the first 5 hours, from the 5th to the 24th hour, and on the 2nd postoperative day. After the first 5 hours, the hematocrit of the drainage fluid was measured.

**TABLE 1.** Perioperative Blood Loss in ml

| | Intraoperative | | | Postoperative (Drains) | | | | Total |
|---|---|---|---|---|---|---|---|---|
| | Suction | Sponges | Total | 0–5 hr | 5–24 hr | 24–48 hr | Total | |
| Aprotinin group (n = 20) | 588 ± 273 | 205 ± 77 | 793 ± 332 | 181 ± 83 | 261 ± 163 | 211 ± 171 | 653 ± 306 | 1446 ± 514 |
| Placebo group (n = 20) | 833 ± 422 | 280 ± 100 | 1113 ± 494 | 427 ± 220 | 219 ± 92 | 184 ± 78 | 830 ± 334 | 1943 ± 700 |
| p value | <0.05 | <0.05 | <0.05 | <0.001 | NS | NS | NS | <0.05 |

Values are mean ± SD. NS = not significant.

In this study, total blood loss (peri- and postoperative) was reduced by 26% in the aprotinin group ($p < 0.05$) (Table 1). This reduction in bleeding occurred both during ($p < 0.05$) and in the first 5 hours after surgery ($p < 0.001$). Subsequent losses were comparable in the two groups. No significant difference in total bleeding was noted between cemented and noncemented prostheses in both groups (Table 2). However, in the placebo group, early postoperative blood loss (during the first 5 hours postoperatively) was significantly greater in the case of cement-free prostheses as compared with cemented prostheses ($p < 0.05$). In the aprotinin group, blood loss associated with noncemented prostheses was significantly greater as compared with cemented prostheses during the postoperative period between the 5th and the 24th hour ($p < 0.05$). Multiple regression statistical analysis demonstrated that, intraoperatively, only treatment with aprotinin significantly influenced bleeding. Postoperatively, treatment and the type of prostheses were significant determinants of blood loss. Whereas the effect of treatment is predominant during the first 5 hours postoperatively, thereafter the benefit of cemented prostheses in terms of reduction of bleeding becomes more apparent. In this study, aprotinin infusion was interrupted at the end of the surgical procedure. Considering that the plasma half-life of aprotinin is approximately 150 min, it is reasonable to expect aprotinin's pharmacologic effect to last for 4–8 hours after the interruption of the aprotinin infusion. The reduction in blood loss between aprotinin and placebo groups was clinically evident: The bleeding intensity score given by the surgeon was significantly lower for the operations performed with aprotinin ($p < 0.01$) (Table 3).

**TABLE 2.** Cemented versus Noncemented Blood Loss in ml

| | Intra-operative | Postoperative (Drains) | | | Total |
|---|---|---|---|---|---|
| | | 0–5 hr | 5–24 hr | 24–48 hr | |
| Aprotinin group | | | | | |
| Cemented (n = 7) | 662 ± 214 | 199 ± 74 | 147 ± 94* | 251 ± 223 | 1259 ± 493 |
| Noncemented (n = 13) | 863 ± 369 | 172 ± 89 | 322 ± 161* | 190 ± 142 | 1547 ± 516 |
| Placebo group | | | | | |
| Cemented (n = 10) | 1002 ± 434 | 329 ± 139* | 204 ± 69 | 165 ± 85 | 1700 ± 573 |
| Noncemented (n = 10) | 1223 ± 548 | 525 ± 247* | 235 ± 113 | 202 ± 69 | 2185 ± 759 |

*$p < 0.05$ between cemented and noncemented prosthesis. Values are mean ± SD.

**TABLE 3.** Bleeding Intensity Scores

|  | Slight | Moderate | Heavy | Very Heavy |
|---|---|---|---|---|
| Aprotinin group | 9 | 6 | 5 | 0 |
| Placebo group | 1 | 4 | 10 | 5 |

Difference between aprotinin and placebo groups, $p < 0.01$ (chi-squared analysis).

In addition, as in Wollinsky's study, the hematocrit of the drainage fluid was significantly lower ($p < 0.05$) in the aprotinin group ($18 \pm 7\%$) than in the placebo group ($23 \pm 6\%$). No statistical differences between the blood hematocrit of the two groups were observed except on postoperative day 1, when the hematocrit of the placebo group was lower ($p < 0.01$) (Fig. 1).

Thus, these studies show that in patients undergoing total hip replacement, a high-dose regimen of aprotinin decreases external blood loss. The reduction in blood loss seen with aprotinin is probably underestimated. Indeed, Wollinsky et al.[52] and Janssens et al.[24] noted a lower hematocrit in the drainage fluid from the aprotinin group. Consistent with this, the surgeon routinely reported less oozing in the surgical field in the treated group. Moreover, postoperative bleeding was assessed only by measuring drainage fluid. All blood lost is not, however, recovered in the surgical drains. As was seen with external blood loss, the occult undrained blood loss, which was not objectively evaluated in these two studies, may well have been reduced in the aprotinin group. Haas et al.[19] noted a lower incidence of wound hematoma in the group receiving aprotinin. Moreover, in Janssens' study, the hematocrit of the placebo group, which was similar to that of the aprotinin group 5 hours after surgery, was significantly lower than that of the aprotinin group on postoperative day 1, despite similar external blood loss (Table 1 and Fig. 1) and transfusion protocols.

## Transfusion Requirements

In Wollinsky et al.'s study,[52] full use of autologous transfusion, including preoperative plasmapheresis, normovolemic hemodilution, and shed-blood recovery, was sufficient

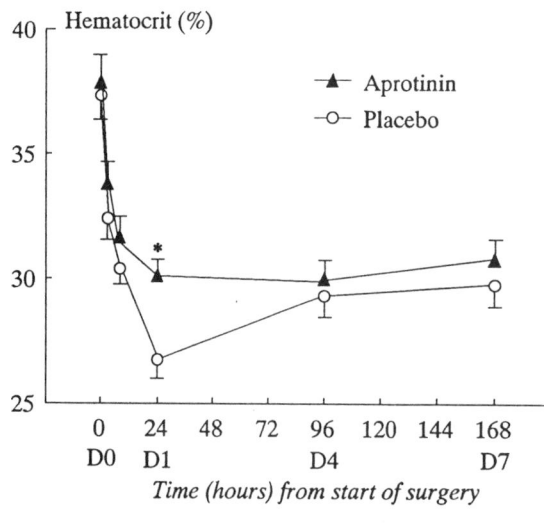

**FIGURE 1.** Time course of hematocrit in aprotinin versus placebo groups (mean ± SEM). D0 = day of surgery; D1, D4, D7 = postoperative days 1, 4, and 7. The asterisk (*) indicates $p < 0.01$ as compared with placebo.

for all patients, and no homologous blood was used in either group. Nevertheless, significantly less blood was recovered by the blood recuperation system ($p < 0.01$) in the treated group. Haas et al.[19] transfused significantly fewer patients in the aprotinin group compared with controls (12% versus 21%; $p < 0.01$).

Janssens et al.[24] used a standardized transfusion protocol in all patients. Hematocrit was monitored both during and after surgery. Autologous, if available, or homologous packed red blood cells were transfused to maintain a hematocrit of 30%. No fresh frozen plasma or other blood components were transfused. Aprotinin treatment resulted in a significant reduction in blood transfusion, which for the aprotinin group was $1.8 \pm 1.2$ U/patient and for the placebo group $3.4 \pm 1.3$ U/patient ($p < 0.001$) (Table 4). This reduction was noted not only perioperatively (from the day of surgery to postoperative day 1) ($p < 0.05$), but also during the postoperative period (day 1–7) ($p < 0.05$). Significantly fewer patients in the treated group required more than 3 units of red blood cells: two in the aprotinin group versus nine in the placebo group ($p < 0.05$). Three patients from the placebo group did not donate blood preoperatively; all required homologous blood transfusion. Four patients from this group who had predonated only 2 units of autologous blood received homologous blood. On the other hand, in the aprotinin group, two of six patients who had no autologous blood available did not require blood transfusion, whereas the single unit of autologous blood predonated by two patients was sufficient to avoid homologous transfusion. Four patients in this group did not require any transfusion.

Any technique or treatment that allows a reduction in the number of units of packed red cells transfused is a potentially useful adjunct to other strategies for reducing transfusion-related risks. Janssens et al.'s study indicates that aprotinin treatment alone, without normovolemic hemodilution or blood recovery, is not sufficient to avoid transfusion in most patients undergoing total hip replacement using Moore's posterolateral approach. However, 90% of patients in the aprotinin group received fewer than 4 units of packed red blood cells. Therefore, the association of treatment with aprotinin and of predonation of 3 units of packed red blood cells, a goal achievable by most patients, should allow 90% of patients to undergo such surgery without homologous blood transfusion. As in Wollinsky et al.'s study, combination of aprotinin with other blood conservation and/or anesthetic techniques (controlled hypotension or regional anesthesia) may further reduce or eliminate the need for homologous blood transfusion. When perioperative blood loss associated with other surgical techniques is low, the potential benefits of aprotinin are probably smaller. It seems reasonable that aprotinin should be considered as a supplementary weapon in the armamentarium of blood-sparing

**TABLE 4.** Units of Packed Red Cells Transfused

|  | Perioperative (Day 0–Day 1) | Postoperative (Day 1–Day 7) | Total |
|---|---|---|---|
| Aprotinin group |  |  |  |
| Mean ± SD | $1.1 \pm 0.97$ | $0.7 \pm 0.98$ | $1.8 \pm 1.24$ |
| Median (range) | 1 (0–3) | 0 (0–3) | 2 (0–4) |
| Placebo group |  |  |  |
| Mean ± SD | $1.95 \pm 1.28$ | $1.45 \pm 1.10$ | $3.4 \pm 1.31$ |
| Median (range) | 2 (0–5) | 1 (0–4) | 3 (1–6) |
| $p$ Value | $< 0.05$ | $< 0.05$ | $< 0.001$ |

techniques, to be used when anticipated blood loss is high and conventional techniques are impossible or insufficient.

## Possible Adverse Effects

### Thromboembolic Phenomena

The issue that has been raised many times, especially by surgeons, is whether a drug can prevent bleeding without an increased risk of thromboembolic phenomena. Böhrer et al. reported early formation of thrombi on pulmonary artery catheters when aprotinin was used in cardiac surgery.[8] Anecdotal reports of graft occlusion or perioperative myocardial infarction in patients who have received high-dose aprotinin can be found in the literature.[9] The risk of graft occlusion after coronary artery bypass, however, does not seem to be increased by aprotinin.[5] In European studies,[38] the incidence of complications related to the cardiovascular system was no different if high-dose aprotinin was used when compared to controls. Moreover, aprotinin therapy in cardiac surgery seems to reduce postoperative neurologic sequelae related to thrombotic episodes.[12] Nevertheless, this potential problem cannot be neglected in orthopedic surgery, which is associated with a high incidence of deep venous thrombosis (DVT).[32]

Using classical prophylaxis with 5000 IU of heparin twice daily, with the first injection 2 hours prior to onset of surgery, Haas et al.[19] did not observe significant differences in the incidence of DVT (as diagnosed by the radiofibrinogen uptake test) between aprotinin-treated patients and controls.

In Janssens et al.'s study,[24] DVT prophylaxis was optimized. Prophylaxis was based on the use of low-molecular-weight heparin: 40 IU/kg were injected subcutaneously 12 hours before surgery, 12 hours after surgery, and once per day thereafter. Because thromboembolic risk increases in total hip replacement patients from the third or fourth postoperative day, with a parallel decrease in hemorrhagic risk,[42] this dose was increased to 60 IU/kg on the fourth postoperative day. Passive normovolemic hemodilution (hematocrit 30%) was maintained in all patients. As a complement to DVT prophylaxis, 500 ml of 6% hydroxyethyl starch (200,000 d) was infused during surgery, 500 ml in the postanesthetic care unit, and 500 ml over postoperative day 1. Antistasis stockings were applied preoperatively to the nonoperative leg and as soon as possible to the other leg. Mobilization was routinely started on the first postoperative day. All patients were examined daily for signs of DVT in the lower limbs. Any clinical sign (swelling or increase in the diameter of the calf, pain on palpation, or localized redness) prompted immediate venography.

To characterize the potential hemostatic effect of aprotinin and its effect on thromboembolic phenomena, three possible mechanisms of action were explored. First, the effect on fibrinolysis was assessed by measuring the appearance of D-dimers in patients' blood. Second, prothrombin time and activated partial thromboplastin time (aPTT) were measured to assess the extrinsic and intrinsic coagulation pathways, respectively, whereas activation of the coagulation system was estimated by assay of thrombin–antithrombin complexes and fibrinopeptide A. Finally, platelet function was explored: platelet counts and plasma levels of beta-thromboglobulin, which reflects in vivo platelet activation, were measured; adenosine diphosphate and collagen-induced aggregation were used to assess in vitro aggregability. Bleeding

**TABLE 5.** Number of Patients with D-Dimers Greater Than Normal ($\geq 0.5$ $\mu$g/ml)

| | Preoperative | PACU | | Postoperative Day | | |
|---|---|---|---|---|---|---|
| | | *Arrival* | *Discharge* | *1* | *4* | *7* |
| Aprotinin group (n = 20) | 1 | 1 | 1 | 1 | 2 | 4 |
| Placebo group (n = 20) | 1 | 7 | 8 | 1 | 0 | 1 |

Nonsignificant statistical differences. PACU = postanesthesia care unit.

time by the Ivy method was measured on the day before surgery, immediately after surgery, and on postoperative day 7.

The incidence of clinical DVT was not increased by aprotinin treatment. Instead, a trend toward reduction of DVT was observed ($p = 0.10$). In the aprotinin group, only one patient had clinical signs of DVT, which was ruled out by venography. On the other hand, in the placebo group, four clinically suspected cases of DVT (20%) (one in the deep femoral vein and three below the poplital fossa) were confirmed with venography. No clinically evident pulmonary emboli were diagnosed in this study. The incidence of DVT is consistent with data in the literature.[21] DVT, confirmed by bilateral phlebography on the 10th postoperative day after total hip replacement, was reported in 12.9% of patients given the same prophylactic regimen (3.6% proximal and 9.3% distal).[43]

Postoperatively, fewer patients in the aprotinin group had increases in D-dimers, but this was not statistically significant (Table 5). Whereas the extrinsic coagulation pathway (prothrombin time) was not affected by treatment and did not change during the perioperative period, the intrinsic pathway (aPTT) was significantly inhibited by aprotinin during the early postoperative period ($p < 0.001$) (Fig. 2). Similar activation of the coagulation system was observed in both groups. Plasma levels of thrombin-antithrombin complexes and fibrinopeptide A increased after surgery and returned to normal by 1 week after surgery (Fig. 3). The platelet count and bleeding time, similar in both groups, did not change significantly. No evidence of platelet activation was found: beta-thromboglobulin remained normal throughout the study. No significant changes in in vitro platelet aggregability were observed in either group.

**FIGURE 2.** Time course of activated partial thromboplastin time (aPTT) during and after total hip replacement in aprotinin versus placebo groups (mean ± SEM). The asterisk (*) indicates $p < 0.001$ as compared with placebo. S = surgery.

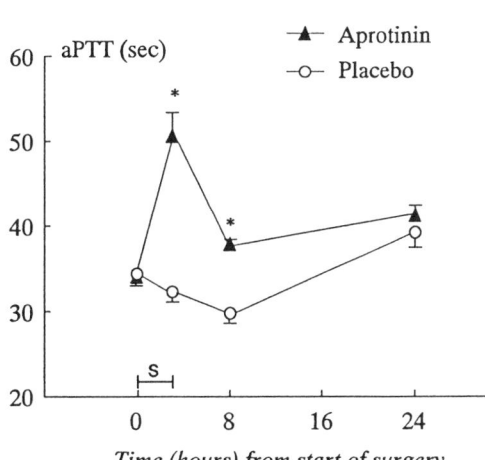

*Time (hours) from start of surgery*

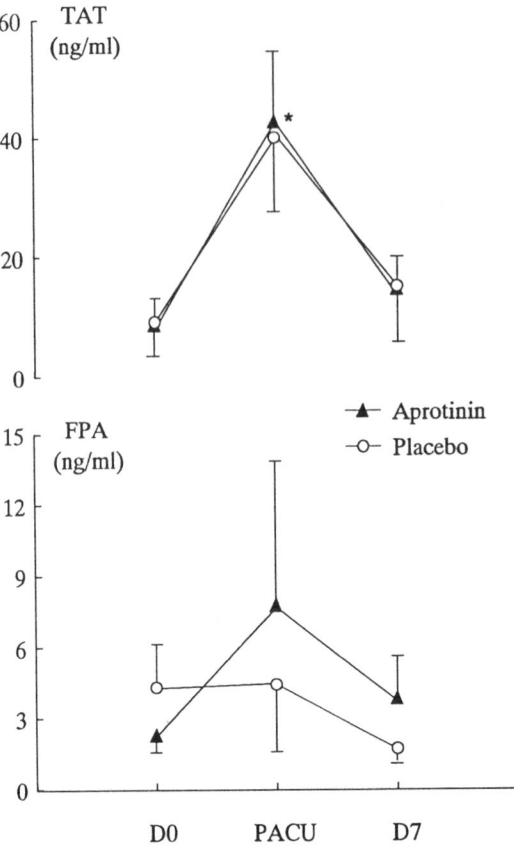

**FIGURE 3.** Time course of thrombin–antithrombin complexes (TAT) and fibrinopeptide A (FPA) in aprotinin versus placebo groups (mean ± SEM). The asterisk (*) indicates *p* < 0.05 compared with D0 (day of surgery) and D7 (postoperative day 7). PACU = postanesthesia care unit.

The increase of thrombin-antithrombin complexes and, to a lesser extent, of fibrinopeptide A reflected in vivo formation of thrombin and fibrin, respectively. Despite this activation of coagulation, Janssens et al. observed a significant prolongation of the aPTT in the aprotinin group, suggesting an anticoagulant effect of aprotinin. The antifibrinolytic effect of aprotinin, which is a serine proteinase inhibitor, has been correlated with an anticoagulant effect, originating at the activation phase of the contact system[2,3,13] and at the initial phase of the intrinsic pathway.[37] The apparent discrepancy between an anticoagulant effect of aprotinin and the observed activation of coagulation might be due to the removal of platelets from blood before the aPTT test. In vivo, the anticoagulant property of aprotinin might be masked by the procoagulant activity of platelets and other blood cells, as well as by the release of tissue thromboplastin from the surgical field. This hypothesis, which needs further investigation, may explain why aprotinin can reduce bleeding despite moderate anticoagulant activity.

In orthopedic surgery, most thromboses form during surgery itself.[32] During hip surgery, both patient position and surgical manipulation can cause endothelial microlesions and liberation of tissue thromboplastin. Inhibition of the intrinsic clotting process, confirmed by increased aPTT, will reduce the likelihood of thrombus formation initiated by contact of blood with negatively charged surfaces, such as collagen and similar subendothelial matrix substances. Consistent with this, aprotinin partially inhibits the thromboembolic phenomena induced by intravenous injection of thromboplastin in the dog.[33,34] It reduces the effects of disseminated intravascular coagulation induced by injection of sodium polyanethol sulfonate (Liquoïd), leading to decreased tissue damage and improved survival.[28] Finally, postoperative platelet hyperaggregability also contributes to DVT in orthopedic surgery.[35] Some evidence suggests that administration of aprotinin leads to inhibition of platelet adhesion to glass beads.[25] Because of its antiplatelet action, aprotinin has already been used as prophylaxis to prevent DVT in patients having hip surgery.[26] Janssens et al.[24] were, however, unable to show any difference in platelet number or in vitro aggregability between the two groups.

In fact, the small number of patients in Janssens' study does not allow firm conclusions to be drawn about the lower incidence of DVT in the aprotinin group. A possible additive effect of a putative anticoagulant property of aprotinin to the antithrombotic effect of low-molecular-weight heparin cannot be excluded and deserves further investigation.

## Effect on Renal Function

Aprotinin is eliminated by binding to the brush border of renal tubular epithelial cells.[17] Use of high doses could theoretically lead to alterations in renal function. In cardiac surgery, it has been shown that urine output and fractional excretion of sodium were increased in aprotinin-treated patients.[7,15] This effect was transient and returned to normal in the early postoperative period. No effects on creatinine clearance or plasma creatinine concentration were observed. In orthopedic surgery, Janssens et al.[24] measured serum concentrations of urea and creatinine during the perioperative period to assess renal function. These values remained normal in all patients throughout the study, suggesting that high-dose aprotinin has no effect on renal function when used in orthopedic surgery. All patients had normal renal function before surgery; further studies are necessary to determine the effects of aprotinin in the presence of preoperative renal failure.

## Allergic Phenomena

Because aprotinin is a polypeptide derived from bovine organs, there is a theoretical possibility of immunologic reaction after its administration in humans. The risk of anaphylactic reactions following previous exposure to aprotinin is estimated to be approximately 1%.[16] Janssens et al. noted neither allergic reactions nor hypotension during the loading dose of aprotinin.[24] However, the current incidence of anaphylactic reactions should be assessed and reconsidered because of the routine use of high-dose aprotinin in cardiac surgery and liver transplantation in many institutions. Furthermore, a proportion of patients who have had initial cardiac surgery with aprotinin will need to undergo a second cardiac surgical procedure. Reoperations are potentially more hemorrhagic than primary surgery and may perhaps require a second administration of aprotinin. The benefits of aprotinin must therefore be balanced against the risks when the indications for its use are discussed.

It is interesting to note that the hypotensive reaction occurring after insertion of acrylic cement into the femoral medullary cavity may be prevented by the use of aprotinin.[4] By its inhibitory effects on the kallikrein-kinin system, aprotinin may reduce the production of bradykinin, a powerful vasodilatator, thus blunting the systemic cardiovascular effects of acrylic cement. This beneficial effect of aprotinin was not confirmed in Janssens' study, where no hypotensive reaction was found during implantation of cement in any group.

## Mechanism of Action

Aprotinin's mechanism of action remains incompletely understood. It is likely that several mechanisms are involved (Fig. 4). Depending on the dose used and the type of surgery, certain of these mechanisms predominate in determining the drug's efficacy. Aprotinin is a relatively nonspecific serine protease inhibitor. It is capable of inhibiting various proteases involved in the coagulation, fibrinolytic, and inflammatory cascades. Based on theoretical calculations and certain clinical studies, the plasma concentration of aprotinin necessary to inhibit individual enzymes has been estimated.[36] Thus, 25 KIU/ml are necessary to inhibit trypsin, 50 KIU/ml for plasmin, 125 KIU/ml for tissue kallikrein, 200 KIU/ml for plasmatic kallikrein, and > 600 KIU/ml for thrombin. These concentrations may vary as a

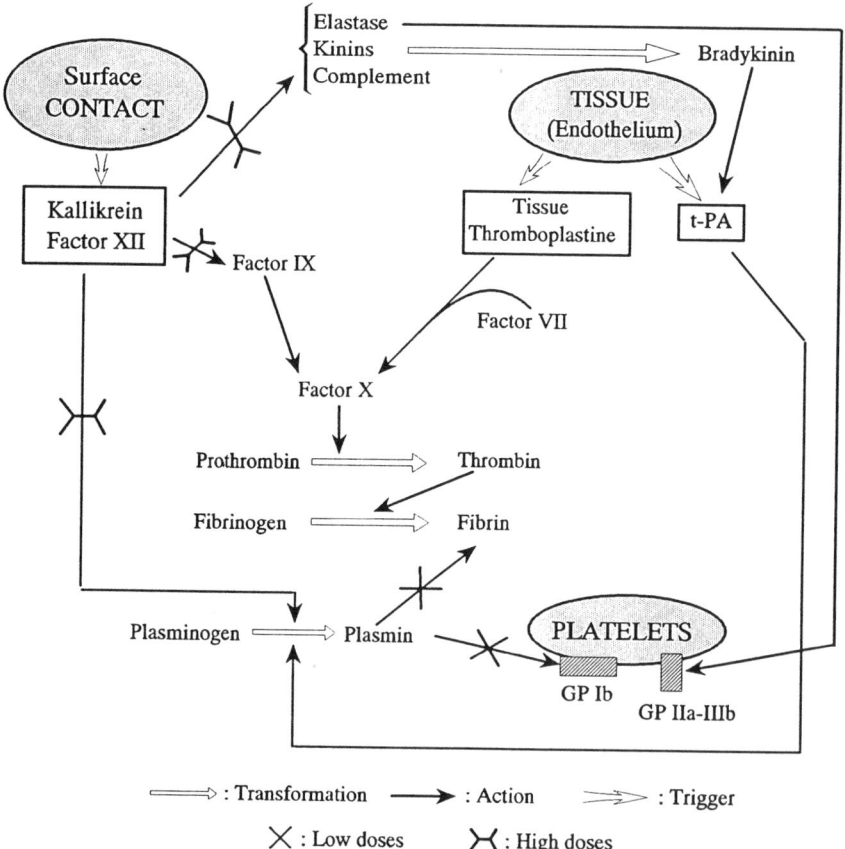

**FIGURE 4.** Aprotinin's proposed mechanism of action. Low-doses = plasmin inhibition; high-doses = kallikrein inhibition; tPA = tissue plasminogen activator.

function of the activation state of the various enzymes and the local concentrations of substrate.

Depending on the dose administered, the mechanism of action seems to vary.[23] At low doses, with plasma levels sufficient to inhibit plasmin, the principal effect is likely produced by stopping fibrinolysis. In procedures in which liberation of plasminogen activator is a primary cause of abnormal bleeding (prostate surgery, ear nose and throat surgery, liver transplantation), the hemostatic effect of aprotinin is probably related to inhibition of fibrinolytic activity. While certain studies have shown moderate activation of fibrinolysis during cardiac surgery,[44] the major hemostatic defect is related to altered platelet function.[27] Inhibition of plasmin with low-dose aprotinin could, as suggested by van Oeveren,[47,48] allow sparing of platelet glycoprotein Ib receptors, responsible in part for platelet adhesion.

The use of high doses of aprotinin further reduces blood loss in cardiac surgery. With sufficiently high blood levels, inhibition of kallikrein leads to blockade of the contact system (factor XII, kallikrein), with consequent inhibition of the intrinsic coagulation pathway. This occurs while the extrinsic system remains largely intact. Inhibition of the intrinsic pathway has been demonstrated in both cardiac[10,18] and orthopedic surgery.[24] This anticoagulant effect of aprotinin could play a role in prevention of DVT and/or in the maintenance of coronary vein graft permeability.[39] Inhibition of the contact system also leads to reduction of intrinsic fibrinolysis; formation of plasmin by factor XII is reduced. This effect is additive with the direct inhibition of plasmin already seen at low doses of aprotinin. Although not statistically significant, the reduced levels of D-dimers seen in treated orthopedic patients (Table 5) would seem to indicate that at least some of the reduction in bleeding is due to the antifibrinolytic effects of aprotinin. The trend would possibly have reached significance had a large number of patients been studied. Finally, inhibition of kallikrein reduces the organism's response to surgical aggression.[29,39] Activation of the complement cascade may be reduced, kinin formation inhibited,[22] and lesser stimulation of polymorphonuclear neutrophils may be seen. Royston showed reduced release of granulocyte elastase when high-dose aprotinin was administered.[40] He speculated that elastase acts on platelets to expose glycoprotein IIb-IIIa receptors, which are partially responsible for aggregation. The beneficial effect of aprotinin on platelet function may be related to inhibition of this phenomenon, although this remains speculative.

During cardiac surgery, extracorporeal circulation activates several biochemical systems involved in coagulation and is associated with alterations of platelet receptors.[27] These modifications result in significant changes in coagulation tests and platelet function, which may facilitate detection of an effect of aprotinin on these systems. The differences in the perturbations of coagulation occurring during cardiac surgery and total hip replacement surgery might explain why Janssens et al. were unable to relate aprotinin's mechanisms of action in orthopedic surgery to those reported after cardiac surgery. In this study, low-dose aprotinin would have been sufficient to produce an antifibrinolytic effect via inhibition of plasmin. Use of sufficiently high doses to block the kallikrein-kinin system increased the antifibrinolytic activity and added a moderate anticoagulant effect. If the effect of high-dose aprotinin on the incidence of DVT is confirmed, it would seem prudent to use such dosing regimens to reduce bleeding without increasing the risk of thromboembolic phenomena. Further studies, however, are necessary to confirm this hypothesis.

## Conclusion

Aprotinin has been shown to reduce blood loss in cardiac surgery and liver transplantation. In orthopedic surgery, which also may be associated with substantial bleeding requiring blood transfusion, the use of aprotinin deserves to be carefully evaluated. Until now, it has been used only during total hip replacement, where high-dose aprotinin reduces both bleeding and the amount of blood transfused. No adverse effects due to the agent were seen; renal function was not altered by the treatment, and the incidence of clinically suspected DVT was not increased in the treated group. The prolongation of the aPTT test, which reflects inhibition of the intrinsic coagulation pathway, was associated with a trend to decreased incidence of DVT in the treated group, suggesting a possible protective effect of aprotinin on thrombotic phenomena. However, further studies are necessary to confirm this hypothesis and to elucidate the mechanism of aprotinin's hemostatic activity in orthopedic surgery. The risk of anaphylactic reactions following administration of aprotinin cannot be neglected. This is why routine use of aprotinin is not recommended in orthopedic surgery. However, it may be useful in procedures where heavy blood loss is expected, e.g., spinal surgery or reoperative hip surgery. In these cases, the benefits of this molecule must be balanced against the risk of sensitization. In fact, aprotinin should be considered as a supplementary weapon in the armamentarium of blood-sparing techniques and used when conventional techniques are impossible or insufficient.

## References

1. Alajmo F, Calamai G, Perna AM, et al: High-dose aprotinin: Hemostatic effects in open heart operations. Ann Thorac Surg 48:536–539, 1989.
2. Amris CJ: Inhibition of fibrinolytic and thromboplastic activity by Trasylol. Scand J Haematol 3:19–32, 1966.
3. Amris CJ, Hilden M: Inhibition of thromboplastic activity by Trasylol. Scand J Haematol 4:3–10, 1967.
4. Arac SS, Ercan ZS, Türker RK: Prevention by aprotinin of the hypotension due to acrylic cement implantation into the bone. Curr Ther Res 28:554–557, 1980.
5. Bidstrup BP: Aorto-coronary bypass graft patency after high dose aprotinin [abstract]. Presented at the 72th meeting of the American Association for Thoracic Surgery, Los Angeles, 40:142–143, 1992.
6. Bidstrup BP, Royston D, McGuinness C, Sapsford RN: Aprotinin reduces bleeding in patients taking aspirin at the time of open heart surgery [abstract]. Circulation 80:158, 1989.
7. Bidstrup BP, Royston D, Sapsford RN, Taylor KM: Reduction in blood loss and blood use after cardiopulmonary bypass with high dose aprotinin (Trasylol). J Thorac Cardiovasc Surg 97:364–372, 1989.
8. Böhrer H, Fleischer F, Lang J, Vahl CH: Early formation of thrombi on pulmonary artery catheters in cardiac surgical patients receiving high-dose aprotinin. J Cardiothorac Anesth 4:222–225, 1990.
9. Cosgrove DM, Heric B, Lytle BW, et al: Aprotinin therapy for reoperative myocardial revascularization: A placebo-controlled study. Ann Thorac Surg 54:1031–1038, 1992.
10. De Smet AA, Joen MCN, van Oeveren W, et al: Increased anticoagulation during cardiopulmonary bypass by aprotinin. J Thorac Cardiovasc Surg 100:520–527, 1990.
11. Dietrich W, Barankay A, Dilthey G, et al: Reduction of homologous blood requirement in cardiac surgery by intraoperative aprotinin application: Clinical experience in 152 cardiac surgical patients. Thorac Cardiovasc Surg 37:92–98, 1989.
12. Dietrich W, Barankay A, Niekau E: High-dose aprotinin in cardiac surgery: Old drug–new aspects of homologous blood requirement. In Birnbaum DE, Hoffmeister HE (eds): Blood Saving in Open Heart Surgery. New York, Schattauer, 1990, pp 76–82.

13. Dietrich W, Spannagl M, Jochum M, et al: Influence of high-dose aprotinin treatment on blood loss and coagulation patterns in patients undergoing myocardial revascularization. Anesthesiology 73:1119–1126, 1990.
14. Emerson TE: Pharmacology of aprotinin and efficacy during cardiopulmonary bypass. Cardiovasc Drug Rev 7:127–140, 1989.
15. Fraedrich G, Neukamm K, Schneider T: Safety and risk/benefit assessment of aprotinin in primary CABG. In Freidel N, Hetzer R, Royston D (eds): Blood Use in Cardiac Surgery. New York, Springer-Verlag, 1991, pp 221–231.
16. Freeman JG, Turner GA, Venables CW: Serial use of aprotinin and incidence of allergic reactions. Curr Med Res Opin 8:559–561, 1983.
17. Fritz H, Wunderer G: Biochemistry and applications of aprotinin, the kallikrein inhibitor from bovine organs. Arzneimittelforschung Drug Res 33:479–494, 1983.
18. Fuhrer G, Gallimore MJ, Heller W, Hoffmeister HE: Studies on components of the plasma kallikrein-kinin system in patients undergoing cardiopulmonary bypass. Adv Exp Med Biol 198:385–391, 1986.
19. Haas S, Fritsche HM, Ritter H, et al: Is the risk of postoperative thrombosis increased after perioperative therapy with the plasmin inhibitor aprotinin? In Betzler M, Quintmeier A, Raute M (eds): Chirurgisches Forum 1991 für experimentelle und klinische Forschung. Munchen, Springer-Verlag, 1991, pp 371–374. (In German, English abstract.)
20. Havel M, Teufelsbauer H, Knöbl P, et al: Effect of intraoperative aprotinin administration on postoperative bleeding in patients undergoing cardiopulmonary bypass operation. J Thorac Cardiovasc Surg 101:968–972, 1991.
21. Hirsh J: Prevention of venous thrombosis in patients undergoing major orthopaedic surgical procedures. Acta Chir Scand 556:30–35, 1990.
22. Hunt BJ, Cottam S, Segal H, et al: Inhibition by aprotinin of tPA-mediated fibrinolysis during orthotopic liver transplantation. Lancet 336:381, 1990.
23. Hunt BJ, Yacoub M: Aprotinin and cardiac surgery. BMJ 303:660–661, 1991.
24. Janssens M, Joris J, David JL, et al: High-dose aprotinin reduces blood loss in patients undergoing total hip replacement surgery. Anesthesiology 80:23–29, 1994.
25. Ketterl R, Haas S, Heiss A, et al: Zur Wirkung des natürlichen Proteinaseninhibitors Aprotinin auf die Plätchenfunktion beim alloarthroplastischen Hüftgelenkersatz. Med Welt 33:480–486, 1982.
26. Ketterl R, Haas S, Lechner F, et al: Wirkung von Aprotinin auf die Thrombozytenfunktion während Hüft-totalendoprothesenoperationen. Med Welt 31:1239–1243, 1980.
27. Mammen EF, Koets MH, Washington BC, et al: Hemostasis changes during cardiopulmonary bypass surgery. Semin Thromb Hemost 11:281–292, 1985.
28. Müller-Berghaus G, Maul FD, Lasch HG: Prevention of the Liquoid-induced consumption coagulopathy by the protease inhibitor aprotinin. Thromb Diathes Haemorrh 27:396–406, 1972.
29. Murphy WG, Davies MJ, Eduardo A: The haemostatic response to surgery and trauma. Br J Anaesth 70:205–213, 1993.
30. Musial J, Niewiarowski S, Hershock D, et al: Loss of fibrinogen receptors from the platelet surface during simulated extracorporeal circulation. J Lab Clin Med 105:514–522, 1985.
31. Neuhaus P, Bechstein WO, Lefebre B, et al: Effect of aprotinin on intraoperative bleeding and fibrinolysis in liver transplantation. Lancet ii:924–925, 1989.
32. Nicolaides AN: Benefits of prophylaxis in general surgery. Acta Chir Scand 556:25–29, 1990.
33. Nordström S: Inhibition of thromboplastin-induced intravascular coagulation by heparin and Trasylol. Acta Physiol Scand 79:390–404, 1970.
34. Nordström S: Effect of Trasylol on thromboplastin-induced arterial hypotension. Acta Physiol Scand 79:469–474, 1970.
35. Paramo JA, Rocha E: Deep vein thrombosis and related platelet changes after total hip replacement. Haemostasis 15:389–394, 1985.
36. Philipp E: Calculations and hypothetical considerations on the inhibition of plasmin and plasma kallikrein by Trasylol. Prog Chem Fibrinol Thromb 3:291–295, 1978.
37. Prentice CR, MacNicol GP, Douglas AS: Studies on the anticoagulant action of aprotinin (Trasylol). Thromb Diathes Haemorrh 24:265–272, 1970.
38. Royston D: Aprotinin in open heart surgery: Background and results in patients having aorto-coronary bypass grafts. Perfusion 5:63–72, 1990.
39. Royston D: High-dose aprotinin therapy: A review of the first five years' experience. J Cardiothorac Vasc Anesth 6:76–100, 1992.
40. Royston D, Bidstrup BP, Taylor KM, Sapsford RN: Effect of aprotinin on need for blood transfusion after repeat open-heart surgery. Lancet ii:1289–1291, 1987.

41. Royston D, Bidstrup BP, Taylor KM, Sapsford RN: Aprotinin decreases the need for postoperative blood transfusions in patients having open heart surgery. Bibl Cardiol 43:73–82, 1988.

42. Schöndof TH, Hey D: Modified (low dose) heparin prophylaxis to reduce thrombosis after hip joint operations. Thromb Res 12:153–163, 1978.

43. Simon P, Kindermans A, Kempf JF, Postel M: Efficacité et tolérance d'une héparine de bas poids moléculaire dans la prévention des thromboses veineuses profondes lors des arthroplasties totales de hanche réglées: Essai prospectif, multicentrique. J Chir 127:252–257, 1990.

44. Tanaka K, Takao M, Yada I, et al: Alterations in coagulation and fibrinolysis associated with cardiopulmonary bypass during open heart surgery. J Cardiothorac Anesth 3:181–188, 1989.

45. Thompson JF, Roath OS, Francis JL, et al: Aprotinin in peripheral vascular surgery [letter]. Lancet 335:911, 1990.

46. Toy PTCY, Kaplan EB, McVay PA, et al: Blood loss and replacement in total hip arthroplasty: A multicenter study. Transfusion 32:63–67, 1992.

47. Van Oeveren W, Eijsman L, Roozendaal KJ, Wildevuur CRH: Platelet preservation by aprotinin during cardiopulmonary bypass [letter]. Lancet ii:644, 1988.

48. Van Oeveren W, Harder MP, Roozendaal KJ, Wildevuur CRH: Aprotinin protects platelets against the initial effect of cardiopulmonary bypass. J Thorac Cardiovasc Surg 99:788–797, 1990.

49. Van Oeveren W, Jansen NJG, Bidstrup BP, et al: Effects of aprotinin on haemostatic mechanisms during cardiopulmonary bypass. Ann Thorac Surg 44:640–645, 1987.

50. Wenger RK, Lukasiewicz H, Mikuta BS, et al: Loss of platelet fibrinogen receptors during clinical cardiopulmonary bypass. J Thorac Cardiovasc Surg 97:235–239, 1989.

51. Wildevuur CRH, Eijsman L, Roozendaal KJ, et al: Platelet preservation during cardiopulmonary bypass with aprotinin. Eur J Cardiothorac Surg 3:533–538, 1989.

52. Wollinsky KH, Mehrkens HH, Freytag T, et al: Vermindert Aprotinin den intraoperativen Blutverlust? Anästhesiol Intensivmed Notfallmed Schmerzther 26:208–210, 1991. (In German, English abstract.)

**John M. Murkin, MD, FRCPC**

# 27

# Blood Conservation and Thromboembolic Disease after Aprotinin Use for Complex Total Hip Arthroplasty

Patients undergoing hip arthroplasty tend to be older; frequently suffer from hypertension, heart disease, or diabetes as well as degenerative joint disease; and often take multiple medications, including aspirin. All of these factors influence perioperative morbidity. Complex hip arthroplasty, which includes such procedures as revision total hip arthroplasty (rTHA) or bilateral primary total hip arthroplasty (bTHA), further increases intraoperative and postoperative complications. The most frequent complications are increased blood loss and transfusion requirements, whereas the most common life-threatening complications are thromboembolism, myocardial infarction, and congestive heart failure. The average mortality rate in total hip arthroplasty is about 1.2%.[20]

## Blood Loss in Hip Arthroplasty

### Blood Loss and Transfusion

Total hip arthroplasties that involve loss of less than 500 ml of blood require no specific replacement therapy, either intraoperatively or postoperatively.[20] Most series reported in the literature, however, demonstrate much higher rates of blood loss. Blood loss is increased when considerable soft tissue must be released, as in rTHA; when components and cement must be removed; and when the patient has undergone more extensive prior surgery, such as Girdlestone arthroplasty.[20]

In a series of patients undergoing rTHA, an average of 2.4 units of homologous blood was transfused in those managed without intraoperative autologous transfusion.[15] In another assessment of intraoperative autologous transfusion in patients undergoing rTHA, patients in the control group lost a total of 2245 ml of blood and received a total of 1160 ml of homologous blood.[54] A series of 34 patients who underwent primary THA received an average of 2.7 units of homologous blood and lost an average of 1300 ml of blood.[48] In 100 patients undergoing primary or revision THA, Woolson et al. reported that total blood loss was approximately 1800 ml and patients required an average blood replacement of 1500 ml.[56]

## Fibrinolysis

Tissue injury incites processes involved with thrombus formation as well as induces release of substances involved with limiting clot formation. Tissue plasminogen activator (tPA), protein C, prostacyclin (PG12), and antithrombin III (ATIII), which are released from endothelial surfaces, activate various enzymes circulating in zymogen form and thus initiate diverse aspects of the clotting/fibrinolytic cascades.

Plasmin, the potent enzyme responsible for dissolution of fibrin clot, acts to limit extent of thrombus formation and to allow recannalization of thrombosed vessels. Free plasmin is quickly degraded by circulating alpha-antiplasmin and cleared from the circulation. Plasminogen, the precursor zymogen form of plasmin, is formed in the liver and circulates freely in plasma. It becomes incorporated into fibrin clot through lysine-binding sites that adhere to specific lysine residues of fibrin. Enzymatic cleavage by the serine proteases tPA or kallikrein and, to a lesser extent, factor XIIa, converts plasminogen to plasmin within platelet-fibrin clot, exposing the serine-histidine enzymatic site.[52] Plasmin incorporated within fibrin clot dissolves fibrin polymer, producing x, y, and E fragments and D-dimer. These fibrin degradation products (FDPs) in turn slow coagulation by inhibiting factor IX and fibrin cross-linkage.

As a nonspecific inhibitor of serine protease, aprotinin binds to various proteolytic enzymes in a dose-dependent manner. The lysine-analogue antifibrinolytics, epsilon-aminocaproic acid and tranexamic acid, inhibit plasminogen and plasmin activity by blocking the lysine-binding sites. In contrast, aprotinin inhibits plasmin activity by binding directly to the active serine enzymatic site.[52] In patients undergoing orthotopic liver transplantation, aprotinin has been shown to inhibit release of tPA. This may represent another important mechanism whereby aprotinin exerts its hemostatic effects.[21]

## Aprotinin Pharmacology

Aprotinin, a serine protease inhibitor isolated commercially from bovine lung, has been known since the 1930s.[28,29] It was first reported in clinical use in 1953 for the treatment of acute pancreatitis and later for shock syndromes and hyperfibrinolytic hemorrhage.[52] In 1987 Royston and colleagues reported that high doses of aprotinin were found to reduce blood loss and blood replacement associated with open heart surgery.[41] This finding was confirmed in later studies both in patients undergoing routine cardiac surgery and in patients at risk of high blood loss (e.g., reoperation or septic endocarditis).[5]

The measure of aprotinin activity is the kallikrein inactivator unit (KIU), i.e., the amount of aprotinin that decreases the activity of 2 biologic kallikrein units by 50%.[12] Aprotinin is a strongly basic molecule with a pKa of 10.5 and a molecular weight of 6512; it contains 58 amino acid residues and is remarkably stable in solution against denaturation by high temperature, acids, alkalis, and proteolytic degradation.[12] Equivalency of concentration and activity of aprotinin is expressed by 100,000 KIU/L = 14 mg = 2.15 $\mu$mol/L = 50 KIU/ml.[52] Animal studies demonstrate an extremely low toxicity (median lethal dose in mice = $2.5 \times 10^6$ KIU/kg), but rapid intravenous injection of large doses may cause anaphylaxis due to release of histamine in response to high basicity.[12] After an intravenous bolus, plasma levels of aprotinin decline rapidly due to redistribution into extracellular fluid and subsequent accumulation in the brush border epithelial cells of the proximal renal tubules. It is metabolized almost entirely into small peptides by lysozomal activity of the kidney: thus biologically active aprotinin is not excreted in the urine.[12,52] Inhibition of renal tissue and urinary kallikreins has been postulated as the cause of the reduction in glomerular filtration rate that has been reported periodically after aprotinin administration.[52]

The reactive site on the aprotinin molecule has been characterised as Lys-15-Ala-16. Various proteolytic enzymes that have serine residues at their functional sites (serine proteases) are inhibited in a dose-dependent manner by formation of competitive aprotinin-protease complexes; reaction of lysine with the serine residues blocks the active proteolytic site. Binding affinity for various proteases differs: the extremely low dissociation constant (Ki) for trypsin (Ki = 0.00006 nmol/L) indicates highly stable binding, whereas plasmin (Ki = 1.0 nmol/L), kallikrein (Ki = 30 nmol/L), and leukocyte elastase (Ki = 3.5 $\mu$mol/L), are inhibited only at progressively higher concentrations of aprotinin.[12,52] In clinical practice, the usual plasma concentration of aprotinin after a loading dose of 2 million KIU plus infusion of 0.5 million KIU/hr ranges from 100–200 KIU/ml[37] or approximately 2.1–4.3 $\mu$mol/L. A wide variety of proteolytic enzymes, including those involved in the inflammatory response, are thus inhibited to variable degrees by plasma concentrations of aprotinin achieved with the usual clinical dosages. The half-life of elimination for aprotinin is biphasic: in the initial rapid phase the half-life is 0.7 hr, whereas in the slower phase the half-life is 7 hr.[12]

## Aprotinin and Hemostasis

Aprotinin has been shown to decrease blood loss in patients undergoing a variety of cardiac surgical procedures.[5,11,41] Aprotinin also benefits patients undergoing noncardiac procedures such as liver transplantation[31,38] and major vascular reconstruction.[49] In addition, several recent studies have demonstrated decreased blood loss and transfusion requirements in aprotinin-treated patients undergoing primary hip arthroplasty. Woolinsky et al. administered an average of 2.5 million KIU of aprotinin to 20 patients undergoing THA under regional anesthesia; another 20 patients in the same group served as controls.[55] The authors demonstrated a significant reduction in total blood loss of approximately 20% in aprotinin-treated patients. Janssens et al. demonstrated a reduction in blood loss of approximately 26% and in transfusion requirements of 47% in a group of 20 patients undergoing primary THA after treatment with an average of 3.5 million KIU aprotinin in comparison with a saline-treated control group.[23] Haas et al. administered 1.5 million KIU aprotinin or saline to 120 patients undergoing THA and also demonstrated a 30% reduction in postoperative blood loss and significantly lower transfusion requirements in the aprotinin-treated group.[17]

In a recent study of cardiac surgical patients who received aspirin within 48 hrs of surgery, aprotinin was shown to reduce total blood loss by over 50% in comparison with placebo.[36] In addition, transfusion of packed red blood cells (PRBCs) was reduced by 60%. Intraoperative transfusions of PRBCs, fresh frozen plasma (FFP), or platelets were significantly reduced in the aprotinin-treated group.

This effect persisted for the duration of hospitalization; overall transfusion of any type-specific blood products (PRBC, FFP, or platelets) was significantly decreased from 88% in the placebo group to 59% in the aprotinin-treated group. Hemoglobin concentration was similar in the two groups at 24 hours and at 7 days; thus treatment with aprotinin did not substitute anemia for transfusion. The demonstrated efficacy of aprotinin administration in the presence of aspirin therapy may be of especial relevance to patients undergoing THA, a variable number of whom take aspirin as a component of their antiarthiritic regimen.

The mechanisms whereby aprotinin decreases blood loss are unclear but may involve enhanced antifibrinolytic activity. Various studies demonstrate suppression of the rise in FDPs, preservation of alpha-2-antiplasmin activity, and decreased plasmin activity during CPB.[17,19,51] Preservation of platelet membrane-binding receptors also has been demonstrated.[50] In addition, aprotinin has a weak anticoagulant effect,[40] probably through inhibition of intrinsic pathway clotting factors[53] and reversible inhibition of platelet activation.[18] Aprotinin has undergone preliminary assessment for thromboembolic prophylaxis in patients undergoing prosthetic hip replacement surgery.[27]

## Thromboembolic Disease in Hip Arthroplasty

The classic triad described by Virchow identifies three primary factors in the development of thromboembolic disease: stasis, tissue injury, and hypercoagulability. In the context of total hip arthroplasty, elements of all three factors are operative and give rise to a disproportionate risk of venous thromboembolism. Consideration must be given to the possibility that hemostatic agents administered to decrease blood loss may exacerbate thrombotic complications, particularly in such a high-risk population.

Venous thromboembolic syndrome includes deep venous thrombosis (DVT) and its associated complications, pulmonary embolism (PE) and chronic deep venous insufficiency. Usually DVT is further characterized as proximal (popliteal vein or above) or distal (calf veins); clinically significant PE is believed to arise primarily from proximal DVT.[25,42] Thrombi of iliac, femoral, and popliteal veins carry a 50% risk of PE vs. a 1–2% risk with calf-vein thrombi.[35] The most common serious complication of total hip arthroplasty is venous thromboembolism, which is reported to occur in over 50% of untreated patients.[16] It accounts for the majority of postoperative mortality and is the most common cause of death within 3 months of surgery.[24] PE occurs in up to 20% of patients who receive no antithrombotic prophylaxis after THA; the mortality rate of PE is as high as 6% in contrast to 0.1–0.8% in general surgery patients.[16]

### Thrombus Formation

To clarify the relationship between THA and DVT and the implications of aprotinin administration to patients undergoing THA, relevant aspects of the blood coagulation system are reviewed briefly.

Both activation of the coagulation system, involving clotting factors and platelets, and inhibition of the fibrinolytic system are involved in thrombus formation. Maintaining the fluidity of blood within the vascular tree, while retaining the ability to form a localized coagulum for defence against blood loss, requires a dynamic interplay between the circulating proenzymes responsible for coagulation and those responsible for clot lysis as well as the structural and biochemical involvement of both platelets and vasculature. Increasing evidence suggests that perioperative factors, particularly during lower limb surgery, can upset the dynamic balance of the coagulation system, giving rise to a prothrombotic state.

## Vascular Responsiveness and Endothelial Injury

Vasoconstriction after injury is an intrinsic reaction of small blood vessels, particularly arterioles and precapillary sphincters. Arteries, arterioles, and venules contain longitudinal smooth muscle fibers that constrict with severance. Constriction causes retraction into soft tissue, thus facilitating extravascular tamponade and also producing intense vasospasm. This phenomenon does not appear to be mediated via autonomic nerves; instead, it is an intrinsic response of the vasculature, augmented by release of thromboxane A2 (TXA2) from activated platelets, which in turn are stimulated by release of tissue thromboplastins (TTP) from injured vessels.

Under certain conditions this mechanical function of the vasculature may be lost. During surgery, particularly arthroplastic surgery, alterations of the vascular tonus and associated endothelial disruptions have been demonstrated. Intraoperative dilation in veins distant to the operative site has been demonstrated in dogs. Venodilation was associated with mild focal endothelial damage in dogs undergoing abdominal operations and with much more serious endothelial damage in dogs undergoing THA.[43,46] The venodilation was believed to reflect the release of humoral substances due to surgically induced muscle trauma. The attendant endothelial damage is of particular concern, because it may give rise to thrombus formation. Similar intraoperative venodilatation and implied endothelial damage have been demonstrated in patients undergoing THA and correlated with development of DVT.[47] In addition, several prospective trials that assessed the efficacy of heparin combined with dihydroergotamine, a relatively specific venoconstrictor, have demonstrated significant reductions in both DVT and PE with intraoperative venoconstrictor therapy.[16]

In addition, intraoperative phlebography has been used to demonstrate severe distortion of the femoral vein during surgical manipulation of the operative leg.[45] This distortion likely results in direct endothelial damage and initiation of thrombus formation and may account for the preponderance of DVT at the level of the greater trochanter in the femoral vein of the operative leg, where maximal intraoperative trauma to the femoral vein occurs.[2] The incidence of DVT may be significantly influenced by surgical technique. With the posterior approach, in which retraction of femoral vessels is unnecessary, DVT is found in 9% of patients, whereas the modified Charnley technique with external rotation of the leg, which requires medial retraction of vessels, may give rise to a 40% incidence of proximal DVT.[13]

Vascular injury leads to exposure of subendothelial collagen, which initiates platelet adhesion. Von Willebrand factor (vWF) is released from endothelial cells and is essential for platelet adhesion, acting as an adhesive protein by binding with glycoprotein (GP) Ib receptors on both collagen fibers and platelets. Fibronectin, another ubiquitous adhesive protein that is found in plasma and subendothelial tissue matrix, also is synthesized by endothelial cells and platelets. It appears to be involved in platelet aggregation by binding to GP IIb/IIIa receptors and by enhancing vWF binding to GP Ib. Evidence suggests that aprotinin protects platelet GP receptors against plasmin-mediated damage; this may be an important mechanism of the hemostatic action of aprotinin.[50]

Hemostatic substances synthesized and released by endothelial cells include the high-molecular-weight subunit of factor VIII (vWF, which is considered to be an acute-phase reactant), platelet activation factor (PAF), and TTP. In particular, TTP is responsible for initiating the extrinsic limb of the coagulation cascade, whereas PAF activates platelets and stimulates release of TXA2, thus massively amplifying platelet aggregation and release and initiating the sequence that leads to formation of a platelet thrombus.

Prostacyclin (PGI2), a potent vasodilator released from endothelial cells, also decreases platelet adhesion to reduce stasis and prevent clot propagation. Synthesis and release of PGI2 from the endothelium may be induced by histamine, thrombin, bradykinin, and serotonin. PGI2 binds to specific membrane receptors to stimulate production of cyclic adenosine monophosphate (cAMP) and is both a potent vasodilator and an inhibitor of platelet biosynthesis and adhesion to vessel walls.

## Coagulation Cascade

The clotting cascade refers to a self-amplifying series of enzymatic cascades, with conversion of each of the various clotting factors to its active, serine protease enzymatic form, which in turn activates the next factor in the clotting sequence. Factors within the intrinsic limb of the cascade, particularly factors XIIa and IXa, are partially inhibited by aprotinin in clinically relevant concentrations, tending to decrease contact-activated coagulation (Figs. 1 and 2). With exposure of blood to a negatively charged surface, as occurs with endothelial disruption, factor XII and high-molecular-weight kinogen (HMWK) attach directly to the negatively charged surface at which factor XII undergoes activation to factor XIIa. Prekallikrein and factor XI are bound to HMWK and in the presence of factor XIIa are converted to factor XIa and kallikrein. This conversion incites a positive-feedback amplification loop that leads to rapid generation of excessive factor XIa, which in turn activates

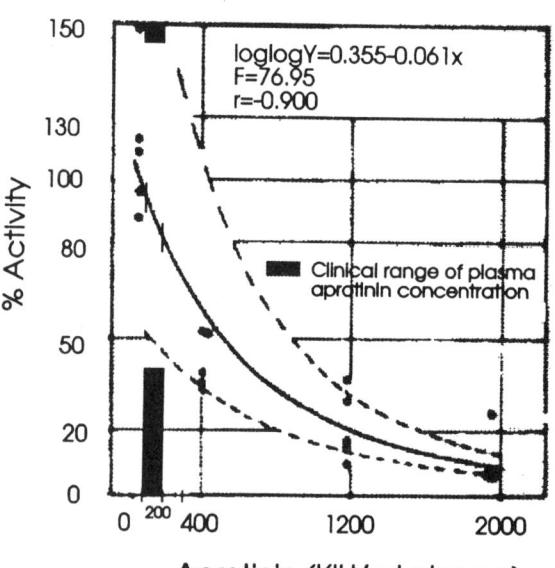

**FIGURE 1.** Percent inhibition of factor XIIa activity by increasing concentration of aprotinin. The usual plasma concentrations of aprotinin achieved in adults with a loading dose of 2 million KIU and infusion of 0.5 million KIU/hr is shown. (Redrawn from Harke H, Gennrich T: Aprotinin-ACD-Blood: I. Experimental studies on the effect of aprotinin on the plasmatic and thrombocytic coagulation. Anaesthetist 29:266–276, 1980, with permission.)

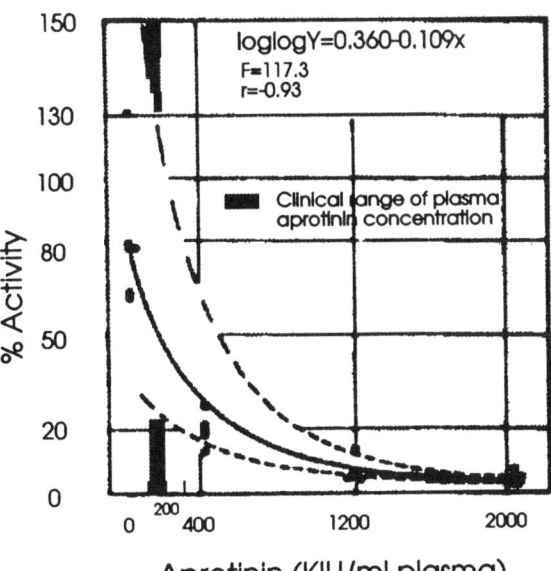

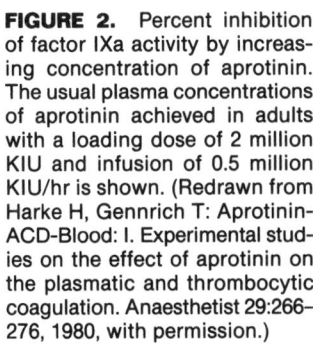

**FIGURE 2.** Percent inhibition of factor IXa activity by increasing concentration of aprotinin. The usual plasma concentrations of aprotinin achieved in adults with a loading dose of 2 million KIU and infusion of 0.5 million KIU/hr is shown. (Redrawn from Harke H, Gennrich T: Aprotinin-ACD-Blood: I. Experimental studies on the effect of aprotinin on the plasmatic and thrombocytic coagulation. Anaesthetist 29:266–276, 1980, with permission.)

**Aprotinin (KIU/ml plasma)**

factor IX to factor IXa—the initial steps of the intrinsic cascade (Fig. 3). Alternatively, tissue injury exposes tissue factor, which binds factor VII and acts as a weak protease to convert factor X to factor Xa. This sequence accelerates activation of factor VIIa and production of factor Xa, a self-amplifying process.[1,6]

## CLASSICAL COAGULATION CASCADE

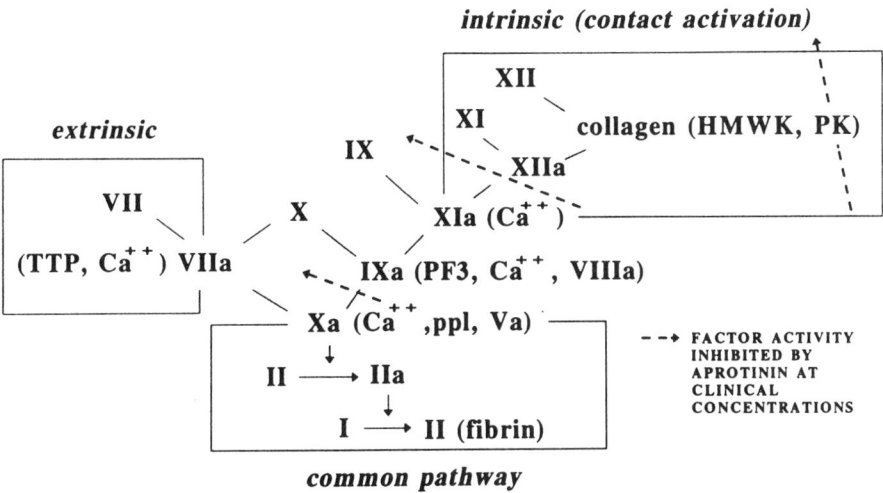

**FIGURE 3.** Coagulation cascade comprised of both contact activated pathway and extrinsic pathway. Role of clinical concentrations of aprotinin in inhibiting activation through the contact pathway by inhibiting activity of both XIIa and IXa, as well as inhibiting kallikrein activity, is shown. PK = prekallikrein, HMWK = high-molecular-weight kininogen.

Endothelial cells bind factors IXa and X. With secretion of PAF, factor IXa forms a calcium-linked complex with factor VIII on the platelet surface that activates factor X. Combining with the phospholipid platelet factor 3 (PF3) and factor V via a calcium bridge on platelet surface, this reaction complex cleaves prothrombin to thrombin (II). Thrombin is a tremendously potent activator and amplifier of coagulation and cleaves fibrinogen to fibrin, which forms cross-linkages to stabilize platelet thrombus.[1,6] Harke and Gennrich investigated the effects of aprotinin on hemostatic mechanisms and documented inhibition of both coagulation factors and platelet activity.[19] At clinically relevant plasma concentrations, aprotinin has been shown in vitro to decrease factor XIIa activity by 20% and factor IXa activity by greater than 50% (see Figs. 1 and 2). In addition, aprotinin was shown to prolong partial thromboplastin time (PTT) in a dose-related fashion in vitro (Fig. 4). Similarly, in a recent study by Murkin et al. of patients undergoing complex THA, intraoperative activated partial thromboplastin time (aPTT)—a measure of contact activation reflecting activity of the intrinsic pathway of the coagulation cascade—was higher in the aprotinin-treated group than in a placebo-treated group, whereas prothrombin time was unaffected. (Fig. 5).[37] Because micronized silicate was used as the activator in the aPTT studies, the results were not due to in vitro celite-aprotinin interaction, which has been reported as the cause of a prolonged activated clotting time (ACT),[53] but rather most likely reflected inhibition of coagulation factor activity by aprotinin (see Fig. 3).

## Platelet Activity

With a half-life of 10–14 days, platelets perform both a mechanical and a biochemical role in hemostasis. When exposed to damaged endothelial surfaces, platelets

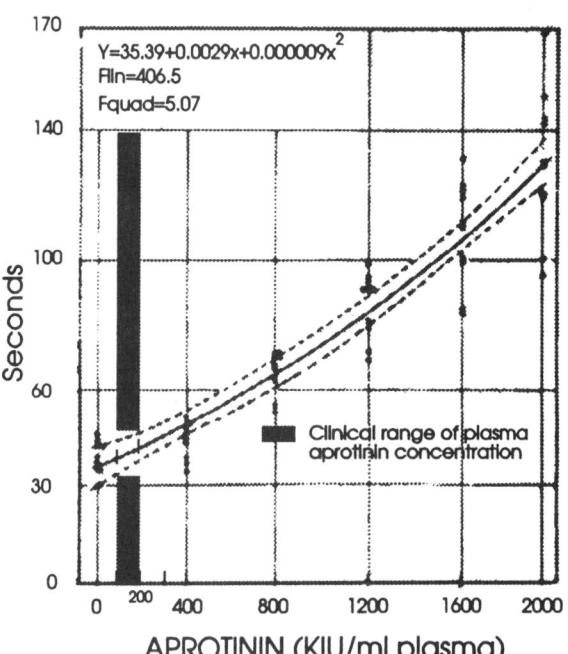

$$Y=35.39+0.0029x+0.000009x^2$$
Flin=406.5
Fquad=5.07

Clinical range of plasma aprotinin concentration

**FIGURE 4.** Prolongation of partial thromboplastin time (PTT) by increasing concentration of aprotinin, reflecting suppression of contact activation. (Redrawn from Harke H, Gennrich T: Aprotinin-ACD-Blood: I. Experimental studies on the effect of aprotinin on the plasmatic and thrombocytic coagulation. Anaesthetist 29: 266–276, 1980, with permission.)

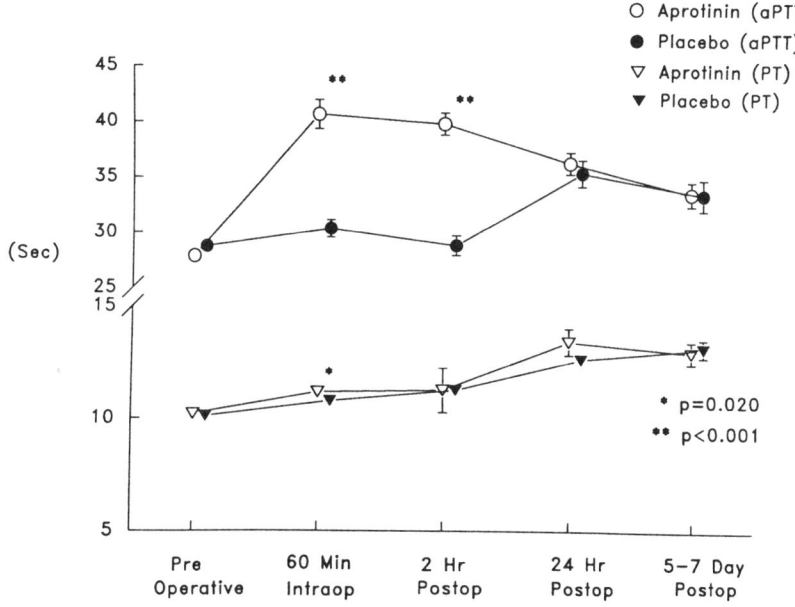

**FIGURE 5.** Perioperative activated partial thromboplastin time (aPTT) and prothrombin time (PT) in patients undergoing bilateral or revision total hip arthroplasty treated with aprotinin (n = 29) or placebo (n = 24). At both 60 min and 2 hr postoperatively aPTT was higher in aprotinin-treated patients, as was PT at 60 min. This finding likely reflects partial inhibition of the intrinsic coagulation pathway by aprotinin.( Data = mean ± SEM.)

adhere to exposed collagen via GP 1b receptors; become activated, producing a burst of metabolic activity with release of adenosine diphosphate (ADP) and the potent platelet agonist TXA2; and undergo a spherical shape change. This process results in exposure of a lipoprotein surface that incorporates PF3—a cofactor for activation of the intrinsic system and production of TXA2, one of the most powerful vasoconstrictive substances and a potent mediator of platelet aggregation and release. Platelet GP IIb/IIIa receptors are exposed through a membrane conformational change that is augmented by TXA2 and that facilitates fibrin cross-linking between platelets and resultant platelet aggregation. Platelet aggregation initiates degranulation with release of ADP and TXA2 and results in a self-amplifying cycle of platelet aggregation.

Aspirin inhibits the synthesis of prostacyclin (PGI2) and TXA2, both of which depend on cyclooxygenase activity. Irreversible acetylation of cyclooxygenase in nucleus-free platelets after even low dosages of aspirin (e.g., 80–100 mg) results in dysfunction of the platelet for its lifespan. Synthesis of PGI2, however, may be restored after cessation of aspirin therapy via synthesis of functional cyclooxygenase by the nucleated endothelial cells.[14,26] Because aspirin therapy is a component of the antiarthritic regimen of a variable number of patients undergoing THA, the attendant platelet dysfunction may be a factor in increasing blood loss.

Postoperative thrombocytosis and increases in platelet adhesiveness have been documented within the first postoperative day in surgical patients.[3] One mechanism by which aprotinin may act to decrease the incidence of DVT is inhibition of surgically induced platelet activation. In orthopedic patients, both collagen-induced platelet aggregability and glass-bead platelet retention, measures of surgically induced platelet activation, were shown to be significantly decreased by aprotinin.[27] Some evidence suggests that this reversible inhibition of platelet adhesion and aggregation may represent a membrane-stabilizing effect due to binding of aprotinin to membrane-bound enzyme systems.[19] Van Oeveren and colleagues have shown that aprotinin preserves platelet membrane receptors GP Ib and GP IIb/IIIa,[50] and others have shown that nonspecific platelet activation during CPB, evidenced as increases in plasma concentration of thromboxane $B_2$ (stable metabolite of TXA2), is significantly inhibited by aprotinin.[7] In addition, a study using scanning electron microscope techniques demonstrated significantly better preservation of platelet aggregation after CPB in an aprotinin-treated group in comparison with a control group.[30] Alternatively, this finding may reflect an indirect effect. Both leukocyte tumor necrosis factor (TNF) and platelet activating factor (PAF) increase with surgical trauma and interact synergistically to cause platelet activation, which may result in thrombus formation. Aprotinin has been shown to suppress both leukocyte TNF and PAF.[22]

## Regional Anesthesia and Deep Venous Thrombosis

Several studies have demonstrated that regional anesthesia, using either the spinal or epidural technique, significantly reduces the incidence of thromboembolic disease in patients undergoing THA. Modig and colleagues conducted several prospective randomized studies that assessed risk of DVT in this population.[32,33] A series of 60 patients undergoing THA were randomized to receive either general anesthesia (GA) and postoperative parenteral analgesics or epidural anesthesia and postoperative epidural analgesia for 24 hours.[32] The incidence of DVT in popliteal and femoral veins was significantly decreased from 67% to 13%, whereas pulmonary emboli were decreased from 33% to 10% in the GA group vs. the epidural group, respectively. No antithrombotic drug prophylaxis was used in either group. The beneficial effects of epidural anesthesia were ascribed to enhanced venous blood flow or "hyperkinetic lower limb circulation," which decreased venous stasis.[34] Davis et al. demonstrated similar results in a series of 129 patients undergoing a total of 140 THAs and randomized to either spinal or GA.[10] Again, routine pharmacological antithrombotic prophylaxis was not used, and the rate of DVT was significantly lower in the spinal group than in patients receiving GA (13% vs. 27%, respectively). In a review of 441 patients undergoing primary THA with a posterior approach, all of whom received epidural anesthesia and 650 mg aspirin daily as thromboprophylaxis, the overall rate of detected DVT was 15%; DVTs occurred significantly more often in longer procedures (> 70 min, 20.3% vs. < 70 min 9.5%).[44]

These studies are consistent with the theory that venous stasis due to intra-operative obstruction of the femoral vein and the added risks from endothelial damage are significant factors in the formation of venous thrombosis.[4,45] In this context, prolonged surgery promotes stasis and vessel trauma, wheras regional anesthesia enhances vessel flow. Similar effects have been ascribed to aprotinin, which has been reported to increase the speed of venous blood flow postoperatively by producing arterial dilatation and venous constriction.[39] Such effects help to mitigate the tendency for venous stasis and thrombus formation.

## Aprotinin and Venous Thrombosis

The estimated incidence of DVT in patients undergoing THA who receive oral anticoagulant prophylaxis is 19%[8] (Table 1). In two recent studies of patients undergoing THA and receiving Coumadin as antithrombotic prophylaxis, the incidence of DVT in the control groups ranged from 12% to 20% and thus is consistent with the expected incidence reported in the literature. In a total of 49 patients treated with aprotinin, however, no DVT was detected.[23,37] In the study by Janssens et al.,[23] DVT was documented in 4 of 20 placebo-treated patients but in none of 20 aprotinin-treated patients. In a study of complex THA, Murkin et al. reported that 3 of 24 patients receiving placebo developed postoperative DVT. Of these, 2 patients were diagnosed with acute proximal femoral vein thrombosis.[37] In both patients DVT occurred in the operative limb, and one of them suffered a concomitant postoperative cerebrovascular accident (CVA), documented on brain imaging as consistent with multiple emboli. After postsurgical convalescence of 6–18 days, both patients were discharged to other hospitals for continuing therapy. A third patient in the placebo-treated group was diagnosed by ultrasound as having a probable postoperative DVT in the popliteal vein. Evidence of definite DVT was detectable on repeat Doppler study 3 weeks postoperatively. No DVT was detected in 29 aprotinin-treated patients.

When assessed independently, the above studies show no significant difference in the incidence of DVT between aprotinin-treated patients and controls, despite a strong trend to decreased incidence with aprotinin treatment. When taken together, they are important indicators of the safety of aprotinin in patients undergoing THA, who are at greatly increased risk of venous thromboembolic disease. The studies demonstrate at the very least that aprotinin does not increase the risk of venous thrombosis but rather shows a trend to decreased risk.

Various enzyme systems exhibit differing sensitivities to inhibition by aprotinin, and effects on intrinsic coagulation and platelet activity are dose-related.[19] Evidence suggests that the plasma concentration of aprotinin necessary to decrease blood loss is lower than the concentration that may be antithrombotic. In a prospective study

**TABLE 1.** Thromboembolic Prophylaxis after Elective Hip Replacement*

| Regimen | No. of Trials | No. of Patients | No. of Patients with DVT | Incidence (%) | 95% Confidence Limits |
|---|---|---|---|---|---|
| Untreated controls | 10 | 459 | 232 | 51 | 46–56 |
| Low-dose heparin | 6 | 257 | 88 | 34 | 29–40 |
| Adjusted-dose heparin | 2 | 78 | 9 | 12 | 5–21 |
| Low-dose heparin/DHE | 3 | 223 | 83 | 37 | 31–43 |
| Low-molecular-weight heparins | 6 | 581 | 93 | 16 | 13–19 |
| Oral anticoagulants | 3 | 162 | 30 | 19 | 13–26 |
| Dextran 70 | 5 | 229 | 68 | 30 | 24–36 |
| Aspirin | 6 | 418 | 189 | 45 | 40–50 |
| Leg compression | 2 | 109 | 26 | 24 | 16–33 |
| Elastic stockings | 2 | 137 | 52 | 38 | 30–47 |

* Pooled data from trials using routine phlebography to assess the risk of deep venous thrombosis. DVT = deep venous thrombosis, DHE = dihydroergotamine. (From Gallus A, Salzman EU, Hirsch J: Prevention of venous thromboembolism. In Colman RW, Hirsch J, Marder VJ, Salzman Ew (eds): Hemostasis and Thrombosis: Basic Principles and Clinical Practice, 3rd ed. Philadelphia, J.B. Lippincott, 1994, pp 1331–1345, with permission.)

of 120 orthopedic patients randomized to receive either 1.5 million KIU of aprotinin or placebo, blood loss and transfusion requirements were significantly lower in the aprotinin-treated patients.[17] Radiofibrinogen uptake showed no differences between groups, however, in incidence of venous thrombosis therefore, it appears likely that plasma concentrations of aprotinin achieved with higher dosages are necessary to exert any potential antithrombotic effect.

## Aprotinin in Complex Total Hip Arthroplasty[37]

### Rationale

Given the potential benefit ascribed to aprotinin administration in a variety of patients undergoing cardiac and noncardiac surgery, and the lack of increased risk of thrombotic complications, Murkin et al.[37] investigated another population of patients at increased risk of blood loss: those undergoing complex total hip arthroplasty.

### Protocol

The study enrolled 53 consecutive patients undergoing rTHA or bTHA. Patients were assigned to receive either aprotinin or an equivalent volume of saline placebo, administered from uniformly blinded bottles. Before induction of anesthesia a test dose of 5 ml of the study drug was administered over 5 minutes followed by a continuous infusion for the duration of surgery and for 1 hour postoperatively. Patients weighing between 60 and 80 kg and randomized to receive aprotinin received a loading dose of 2 million KIU (200 ml) over 15 minutes followed by an infusion of 0.5 million KIU (50 ml)/hour, whereas patients weighing less than 60 kg or more than 80 kg received a loading dose of 2.8 ml/kg (10,000 KIU/ml) dose and an infusion of 0.7 ml/kg/hr. Placebo-treated patients received an equivalent volume of 0.9% saline.

To assess equivalency of surgical procedures in both groups, all operative procedures were reviewed retrospectively by an independent, blinded observer and categorized as routine if the following criteria were met: (1) first revision; (2) use of a standard long-stem femoral component revision prosthesis (i.e., a calcar replacement-type prosthesis was not used); (3) no requirement of structural bone grafting; and (4) no operative complications. Procedures not meeting all of these criteria were categorized as complex.

To assess risk of development of DVT, both preoperatively and within 5–7 days postoperatively, patients underwent bilateral compression color Doppler ultrasound of the lower limbs.[56] Patients with clinical symptoms of DVT underwent venography and were anticoagulated as required. Twenty-five patients in the aprotinin group and 22 in the placebo group were treated with Coumadin prophylaxis (10 mg orally on the night before surgery and maintenance doses of 5–7.5 mg orally for the duration of hospitalization), whereas the remainder received heparin (5,000 U subcutaneously) within 24 hours before surgery and until discharge. Patients were routinely discharged from the postoperative recovery area to the orthopedics ward within 2–4 hours postoperatively. All patients received postoperative physiotherapy and leg compression exercises and were mobilized as early as possible. At 6-week follow-up, patients were examined and questioned specifically about symptoms or signs suggestive of DVT. Clinically significant DVT included all proximal DVT diagnosed until the 6-week follow-up.

To avoid possible confounding factors associated with regional anesthesia, all patients underwent general anaesthesia using $N_2O/O_2$ and isoflurane, with supplemental opioids as clinically indicated. Monitoring was routine, and arterial blood pressure was maintained within clinically acceptable limits. Hypotensive anesthesia was not specifically used.

An independent, blinded observer assessed intraoperative blood loss by measurement of suction losses and weight of sponges; postoperative blood loss was measured from volumetric wound drains. Transfusion criteria for PRBCs were defined prospectively. The amount of transfused blood products was recorded and totalled for the duration of hospitalization. The effect of aprotinin treatment on perioperative red cell mass was assessed by measurement of hemoglobin and hematocrit as well as platelet count and white blood cell (WBC) fractionation for neutrophils, lymphocytes, and monocytes. Renal function was assessed by measuring urea, creatinine, sodium, potassium, chloride, and bicarbonate, whereas fibrinogen, bilirubin, alkaline phosphatase, and aspartate aminotransferase (AST) were measured to screen for any influence on hepatic function. The effect of aprotinin on contact activation and the extrinsic coagulation cascade was determined by serial measurements of prothrombin time and activated partial thromboplastin time. For all of the above measures, venous blood was obtained preoperatively, 60 minutes after incision, within 2 hours postoperatively and at 24 hours and 5–7 days postoperatively. To assess the efficacy of the dosing schedule, plasma concentration of aprotinin was measured using the 60-minute postincision sample.

## Results

All patients survived the procedure, and surgery was deemed successful in all members of both placebo and aprotinin-treated groups. Twenty-nine patients received aprotinin, whereas 24 received placebo treatment. Demographics and operating-room characteristics are reported in Table 2. There were no differences between the two groups in age, gender, duration of operation, time till ambulation, or duration of hospitalization. In the placebo group 12 operations were categorized as complex, whereas 16 were characterized as complex in the aprotinin-treated group.

Aprotinin-treated patients experienced significantly less postoperative blood loss and total blood loss (Table 3). Of patients who were transfused, aprotinin-treated

**TABLE 2.** Demographics and Perioperative Results (Mean ± SEM)

|  | Aprotinin | Control |
|---|---|---|
| N (patients) | 29 | 24 |
| Age (yrs) | 66.9 ± 2.8 | 65.5 ± 3.4 |
| Gender (M/F) | 9/20 | 11/13 |
| Weight (kg) | 72 ± 3 | 78 ± 3 |
| (range) | (38–99.5) | (45–118) |
| Diabetes mellitus | 6 (20.7%) | 0 |
| Preoperative hypertension | 2 | 1 |
| Aspirin use | 7/29 | 4/24 |
| Duration of surgery (min) | 180 ± 7.5 | 194 ± 11.0 |
| Hospitalization (days) | 13.1 ± 1.7 | 11.4 ± 1.3 |

From Murkin JM, Shannon NA, Bourne RB, et al: Aprotinin significantly decreases blood loss in patients undergoing bilateral or revision total hip joint replacement. Anesth Analg 1994 (in press), with permission.

**TABLE 3.**   Blood Loss (Mean ± SEM)

|  | Aprotinin (n = 29) | Control (n = 24) | p-Value |
|---|---|---|---|
| Intraoperative (ml) | 996 ± 81 | 1318 ± 145 | 0.060 |
| Postoperative (ml) | 502 ± 62 | 778 ± 118 | 0.046 |
| Total (ml) | 1498 ± 110 | 2096 ± 223 | 0.022 |

From Murkin JM, Shannon NA, Bourne RB, et al: Aprotinin significantly decreases blood loss in patients undergoing bilateral or revision total hip joint replacement. Anesth Analg 1994 (in press), with permission.

patients required significantly less PRBCs (Table 4). No patient in either group received transfusion compontent therapy other than PRBCs, such as platelets or fresh frozen plasma. Preoperative and intraoperative hemoglobin (Hb) concentration was similar in the two groups. At 24 hours and 5–7 days postoperatively, however, hemoglobin concentration was significantly higher in aprotinin-treated patients . In addition, at 60 minutes intraoperatively both aPTT and PT and at 2 hours postoperatively aPTT were higher in the aprotinin-treated group (see Fig. 5). In both treatment groups, WBC count, platelet count, and fibrinogen concentrations were similar. Also, there were no clinically important differences between biochemical indices of renal or hepatic function between groups.

Average plasma concentration of aprotinin (131.7 ± 4.7 KIU/ml) did not vary between patients receiving fixed-dose aprotinin (n = 10; 131.9 ± 5.4 KIU/ml) and patients receiving a weight-based dosage (n = 19; 131.5 ± 6.6 KIU/ml). In addition, there appeared to be no relationship between either blood loss or transfusion requirements and plasma concentration of aprotinin, which ranged from 105 KIU/ml to 160 KIU/ml in patients receiving a fixed dose, and from 74 KIU/ml to 206 KIU/ml in patients receiving a weight-based dosage.

The similarity between plasma concentration with either fixed-dose or weight-based regimens implies that in adult patients the relatively simpler fixed-dose regimen can be used effectively without sacrificing effective plasma concentrations. Furthermore, the plasma concentration of 132 KIU/ml is well above the 50 KIU/ml required to inhibit plasmin activity completely but appears to be less than the 200 KIU/ml required for kallikrein inhibition in vitro.[12] This finding may indicate that aprotinin achieves hemostasis primarily through inhibition of plasmin rather than through inhibition of kallikrein-mediated release of bradykinin/tissue plasminogen activator (tPA).[54] Thus, similar efficacy may be achieved by targeting plasmin inhibition with a plasma concentration of 50 KIU/ml. Whether such a lower dosage would also exhibit a salutary effect on venous thrombosis is less certain.[17]

**TABLE 4.**   Transfusions in Patients Receiving Blood Products (Mean ± SEM)

|  | Aprotinin (n = 29) | Control (n = 24) | Confidence Interval of Difference |
|---|---|---|---|
| Patients transfused | 18 (62.1%) | 17 (70.8%) |  |
| Transfusion of red blood cells (units) | 2.0 ± 0.2 | 2.9 ± 0.4 | −1.69, −0.07 |

From Murkin JM, Shannon NA, Bourne RB, et al: Aprotinin significantly decreases blood loss in patients undergoing bilateral or revision total hip joint replacement. Anesth Analg 1994 (in press), with permission.

## Summary

In the randomized, double-blind clinical trial undertaken by Murkin and colleagues, aprotinin resulted in significantly less blood loss and lower transfusion requirements in patients undergoing bTHA or rTHA surgery. Aprotinin-treated patients also had higher postoperative levels of Hb at 24 hours and at 5–7 days, a finding consistent with the previously observed hemostatic effects of aprotinin. Thus the lower transfusion requirement in aprotinin-treated patients did not result in anemia but rather in conservation of red cell mass. The lower blood loss and transfusion requirements are consistent with results reported in patients undergoing primary hip replacement surgery.[17,23,55] Patients undergoing bTHA or rTHA, as in our study population, are at increased risk for excessive blood loss as a result of the increased complexity and duration of the surgery.[21,56]

The results of all studies to date indicate that the efficacy of aprotinin, as measured by a decrease in blood loss and lower transfusion requirements, is not contingent on the complexity of the procedure and remains high for both primary and revision hip arthroplasty. In addition, aprotinin therapy can be undertaken without risk of increased thrombotic complications, even in high-risk patients, when combined with a routine of pharmacologic antithrombotic prophylaxis.

## References

1. Babior BM, Stossel TP: The clotting cascade and its regulation: Congenital and acquired clotting factor disorders. In Barry BK (ed): Hematology: A Pathophysiological Approach, 2nd ed. New York, Churchill Livingstone, 1990, pp 181–248.
2. Bell WR, Tomasulo PA, Alving BM: Prospective study in 52 patients. Ann Intern Med 85:155, 1976.
3. Bennett PN: Postoperative change in platelet adhesiveness. J Clin Pathol 20:708–709, 1967.
4. Bibbs M, Pho R: Femoral, vein occlusion during total hip arthroplasty. Clin Orthop 255:168–172, 1990.
5. Bidstrup BP, Harrison J, Royston D, et al: Aprotinin therapy in cardiac operations: A report on use in 41 cardiac centres in the United Kingdom. Ann Thorac Surg 55:971–976, 1993.
6. Bithell TC: The physiology of primary hemostasis. In Wintrobe MM (ed): Clinical Hematology. Philadelphia, Lee & Febiger, 1993, pp 540–613.
7. Blauhut LB, Gross C, Necek S, et al: Effects of high-dose aprotinin on blood loss, platelet function, fibrinolysis, complement, and renal function after cardiopulmonary bypass. J Thorac Cardiovasc Surg 101:958–967, 1991.
8. Clagett GP, Anderson FA, Levine MN, et al: Prevention of venous thromboembolism. Chest 102:391S–407S, 1992.
9. Cronan JJ: Ultrasound evaluation of deep venous thrombosis. Semin Roentgen 27:39–52, 1992.
10. Davis FM, Laurenson VG, Gillespie WJ, et al: Deep vein thrombosis after total hip replacement. J Bone Joint Surg 71B:181–185, 1989.
11. Dietrich W, Barankay A, Dilthey G, et al: Reduction of homologous blood requirements in cardiac surgery by intraoperative aprotinin application: Clinical experience in 152 cardiac surgical patients. J Thorac Cardiovasc Surg 37:92–98, 1989.
12. Fritz H, Wunderer G: Biochemistry and applications of aprotinin, the kallikrein inhibitor from bovine organs. Drug Res 33:479–494, 1983.
13. Gallus A, Raman K, Darby T: Venous thrombosis after elective hip replacement—the influence of preventive intermittent calf compression and of surgical technique. Br J Surg 70:17, 1983.
14. George J, Shattil SJ: The importance of acquired abnormalities of platelet function. N Engl J Med 324:27–29, 1991.
15. Goulet JA, Bray TJ, Timmerman LA, et al: Intraoperative autologous transfusion in orthopaedic patients. J Bone Joint Surg 71B:3–7, 1989.
16. Haake DA, Berkman SA: Venous thromboembolic disease after hip surgery. Risk factors, prophylaxis and diagnosis. In Urist MR (ed): Clinical Orthopaedics and Related Research. Philadelphia, J.B. Lippincott, 1989, pp 212–231.

17. Haas S, Fritsche HM, Ritter H, et al: Fuhrt eine perioperative Gabe des plasmainhibitors Aprotinin zu einer Steigerung des postoperativen Thromboserisikos? In Hartel W, Bager HG, Ungeheuer E (eds): Chirurgisches Forum '91, Berlin, Springer-Verlag, 1991, pp 371–374.

18. Haas S, Ketterl R, Stemberger A, et al: The effect of aprotinin on platelet function, blood coagulation and blood lactate level in total hip replacement—a double-blind clinical trial. Adv Exp Med Biol 167:287–297, 1984.

19. Harke H, Gennrich T: Aprotinin-ACD-Blood:I. Experimental studies on the effect of aprotinin on the plasmatic and thrombocytic coagulation. Anaesthetist 29:266–276, 1980.

20. Harkess JW: Arthroplasty of hip. In Crenshaw AH (ed): Campbell's Operative Orthopaedics, vol. 1. St. Louis, Mosby, 1992, pp 441–626.

21. Hunt BJ, Cottam S, Segal H, et al: Inhibition by aprotinin of tPA-mediated fibrinolysis during orthotopic liver transplantation [letter]. Lancet 336:381, 1990.

22. Hunyadi J, Szabo Kenderessy A, Duda E, et al: Platelet-activating factor antagonists (BN 52021 and BN 50730) inhibit tumor necrosis factor-alfa-mediated cytotoxicity on murine L929 tumor cells. Mol Immunol 30:517–579, 1993.

23. Janssens M, Joris J, David JL, et al: High-dose aprotinin reduces blood loss in patietns undergoing total hip replacement surgery. Anesthesiology 80:23–29, 1994.

24. Johnson R, Green JR, Charnley J: Pulmonary embolism and its prophylaxis following the Charnley total hip replacement. Clin Orthop 127:123–132, 1977.

25. Kavanagh BF, Heit JA: Thromboembolic disease and its prophylaxis. In Morrey BF (ed): Joint Replacement Arthroplasty. New York, Churchill Livingstone, 1992, pp 881–890.

26. Kessler CM: The pharmacology of aspirin, heparin, coumarin, and thrombolytic agents. Chest 99:97S–101S, 1991.

27. Ketterl R, Haas S, Lechner F, Blumel G: Wirkung von Aprotinin auf die Thrombozytenfunktion wahrend Huft-Totalendoprothesenoperation. Med Welt 31:1239–1243, 1980.

28. Kraut E, Frey EK, Werle E: Uber die Inaktivierung des Kallikreins. Hoppe-Seyler Z Physiol Chem 192:1–21, 1930.

29. Kunitz M, Northrop JH: Isolation from beef pancreas of crystalline trypsinogen, trypsin, atrypsin inhibitor and an inhibitor trypsin compound. J Gen Physiol 19:991–1007, 1936.

30. Lavee J, Savion N, Smolinsky A, et al: Platelet protection by aprotinin in cardiopulmonary bypass: Electron microscopic study. Ann Thorac Surg 53:477–481, 1992.

31. Mallett SV, Cox D, Burroughs AK, Rolles K: Aprotinin and reduction of blood loss and transfusion requirements in orthotopic liver transplantation [letter]. Lancet 2:886–887, 1990.

32. Modig J, Borg T, Karlstrom G, et al: Thromboembolism after total hip replacement: Role of epidural and general anesthesia. Anesth Analg 62:174–180, 1983.

33. Modig J, Hjelmstedt A, Sahlstedt B, et al: Comparative influences of epidural and general anaesthesia on deep venous thrombosis and pulmonary embolism after total hip replacement. Acta Chir Scand 147:125–130, 1981.

34. Modig J, Malmberg P, Karlstrom G: Effect of epidural versus general anaesthesia on calf blood flow. Acta Anaesthesiol Scand 24:305–309, 1980.

35. Moser KM, LeMoine JR: Is embolic risk conditioned by location of deep vein thrombosis? Ann Intern Med 94:439, 1981.

36. Murkin JM, Lux JA, Shannon NA, et al: Aprotinin significantly decreases bleeding and transfusion requirements in patients receiving aspirin and undergoing cardiac operations. J Thorac Cardiovasc Surg 107:554–561, 1994.

37. Murkin JM, Shannon NA, Bourne RB, et al: Aprotinin significantly decreases blood loss in patients undergoing bilateral or revision total hip joint replacement. Anesth Analg (in press).

38. Neuhaus P, Bechstein WO, Lefebre O, et al: Effect of aprotinin on intraoperative bleeding and fibrinolysis in liver transplantation. Lancet 2:924–925, 1989.

39. Pauschinger P, Matis P, Rieckert H: Circulatory changes in the area of the lower extremities secondary to inactivity and the influence exerted on them by Trasylol. In Haberland GL, Matis P (eds): New Aspects of Trasylol Therapy, vol. 3. Stuttgart, Schattauer Verlag, 1970, pp 83–90.

40. Quereshi A, Lamont J, Burke P, et al: Aprotinin: The ideal anticoagulant? Eur J Vasc Surg 6:317–320, 1992.

41. Royston D, Bidstrup BP, Taylor KM, Sapsford RN: Effect of aprotinin on the need for blood transfusion after repeat open heart surgery. Lancet 2:1289–1291, 1987.

42. Salzman EW, Rosenberg RD, Smith MH, et al: Effects of heparin and heparin fractions on platelet aggregation. J Clin Invest 65:64, 1980.

43. Schaub RG, Lynch PR, Stewart GJ: The response of canine veins to three types of abdominal surgery: A scanning and transmission electron microscopic study. Surgery 83:411–424, 1978.
44. Sharrock NE, Ranawat CS, Urquhart B, Peterson M: Factors influencing deep vein thrombosis following total hip arthroplasty under epidural anesthesia. Anesth Analg 76:765–771, 1993.
45. Stamatakis JD, Kakkar VV, Sagar S, et al: Femoral vein thrombosis and total hip replacement. BMJ 2:223–225, 1977.
46. Stewart GJ, Alburger PD, Stone EA, et al: Total hip replacement induces injury to remote veins in a canine mode. J Bone Joint Surg 65:97–102, 1983.
47. Stewart GJ, Ziskin MC, Alburger PD: Correlation of venous dilation during hip arthroplasty and subsequent development of deep vein thrombosis (DVT): Clinical study using intraoperative ultrasound (US) monitoring. Thromb Haemost 4:247–250, 1985.
48. Thomson JD, Callaghan JJ, Savory CC, et al: Prior deposition of autologous blood in elective orthopaedic surgery. J Bone Joint Surg 69A:320-324, 1987.
49. Thomson JF, Roath OS, Francis FL, et al: Aprotinin in vascular surgery. Lancet 336:911, 1990.
50. van Oeveren W, Harder MP, Roozendaal KJ, et al: Aprotinin protects platelets against the initial effect of cardiopulmonary bypass. J Thorac Cardiovasc Surg 99:788–797, 1990.
51. van Oeveren W, Jansen NJ, Bidstrup BP, et al: Effects of aprotinin on hemostatic mechanisms during cardiopulmonary bypass. Ann Thorac Surg 44:640–645, 1987.
52. Verstaete M: Clinical application of inhibitors of fibrinolysis. Drugs 29:236–261, 1985.
53. Wang J-S, Lin C-Y, Hung W-T, Karp RB: Monitoring of heparin-induced anticoagulation with kaolin-activated clotting time in cardiac surgical patients treated with aprotinin. Anesthesiology 77:1080–1084, 1992.
54. Wilson WJ: Intraoperative autologous transfusion in revision total hip arthroplasty. J Bone Joint Surg 71B:8–14, 1989.
55. Wollinsky KH, Mehrkens HH, Freytag T, et al: Vermindert Aprotinin den intraoperativen Blutverlust? Anasthesiol Intensivmed Notfallmed Schmerzther 26:208–210, 1991.
56. Woolson ST, Marsh JS, Tanner JB: Transfusion of previously deposited autologous blood for patients undergoing hip-replacement surgery. J Bone Joint Surg 69:325-328, 1987.

# Index

Page numbers in **boldface type** indicate complete chapters.

**390**